MW00447145

BASIC AND CLINICAL ANATOMY OF THE

SPINE, SPINAL CORD,
AND ANS

Basic and Clinical Anatomy of the Spine, Spinal Cord, and ANS

Gregory D. Cramer, D.C., Ph.D.

Associate Professor and Chairperson
Department of Anatomy
The National College of Chiropractic

Susan A. Darby, Ph.D.

Associate Professor
Department of Anatomy
The National College of Chiropractic

Illustrator

Sally A. Cummings, M.A., M.S.

Photographer

Ron Mensching

with 293 illustrations

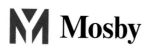 Mosby

St. Louis Baltimore Boston Carlsbad Chicago Naples New York Philadelphia Portland
London Madrid Mexico City Singapore Sydney Tokyo Toronto Wiesbaden

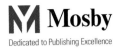

Mosby
Dedicated to Publishing Excellence

**A Times Mirror
Company**

Executive Editor: Martha Sasser
Associate Developmental Editor: Kellie F. White
Project Manager: Patricia Tannian
Production Editor: Melissa Mraz
Senior Book Designer: Gail Morey Hudson
Cover Designer: Teresa Breckwoldt
Manufacturing Supervisor: Tim Stringham

Copyright ©1995 by Mosby–Year Book, Inc.

All rights reserved. No part of this publication may be reproduced,
stored in a retrieval system, or transmitted, in any form or by any
means, electronic, mechanical, photocopying, recording, or otherwise,
without prior written permission from the publisher.

Permission to photocopy or reproduce solely for internal or personal
use is permitted for libraries or other users registered with the Copyright
Clearance Center, provided that the base fee of $4.00 per chapter plus $.10
per page is paid directly to the Copyright Clearance Center, 27 Congress
Street, Salem, MA 01970. This consent does not extend to other kinds
of copying, such as copying for general distribution, for advertising or
promotional purposes, for creating new collected works, or for resale.

Printed in the United States of America
Composition by Graphic World, Inc.
Printing/binding by Von Hoffmann Press, Inc.

Mosby-Year Book, Inc.
11830 Westline Industrial Drive
St. Louis, Missouri 63146

Library of Congress Cataloging in Publication Data

Cramer, Gregory D.
   Basic and clinical anatomy of the spine, spinal cord, and ANS /
Gregory D. Cramer, Susan A. Darby; illustrator, Sally A. Cummings;
photographer, Ron Mensching.
      p.   cm.
   Includes bibliographical references and index.
   ISBN 0-8016-6467-5
    1. Spinal cord—Anatomy.   2. Spine—Anatomy.   3. Autonomic nervous
system—Anatomy.   I. Darby, Susan A.   II. Title.
    [DNLM: 1. Spinal Cord—anatomy & histology.   2. Autonomic Nervous
System—anatomy & histology.   WL 400 C889b 1995]
QM465.C73   1995
611′.82—dc20
DNLM/DLC
for Library of Congress   94-30169
                                             CIP

95 96 97 98 99 / 9 8 7 6 5 4 3 2 1

Contributors

WILLIAM E. BACHOP, Ph.D.

Professor
Department of Anatomy
The National College of Chiropractic

BARCLAY W. BAKKUM, D.C., Ph.D.

Assistant Professor
Department of Anatomy
The National College of Chiropractic

DARRYL L. DALEY, Ph.D.

Assistant Professor
Division of Natural Science and Mathematics
Snow College

CHAE-SONG RO, M.D., Ph.D.

Associate Professor
Department of Anatomy
The National College of Chiropractic

PETER C. STATHOPOULOS, M.Ed., M.S., D.C.

Professor
Department of Anatomy
The National College of Chiropractic

To

Chris and David
Dave, Katherine, and Jason

Thank you for your invaluable support, patience, and encouragement
throughout the writing of this text.

Forewords

Drs. Cramer and Darby, with the able assistance of colleagues in Anatomy and Physiology at the National College of Chiropractic, have created a remarkable resource for both clinicians and students.

Basic and Clinical Anatomy of the Spine, Spinal Cord, and ANS is designed to facilitate a learner's understanding of important anatomic concepts and their relationship to clinical practice. The most important aspects of this book include comprehensive coverage of spinal anatomy and related neuroanatomy with clear explanations of structural relationships; the extensive use of illustrations and photographs to enhance anatomic detail; and numerous well-referenced clinical pearls that relate anatomy to clinical care.

Anatomy faculty and students will find that this book goes beyond a mere description of the structure of the spine and nervous system. It sets out to explain how a structure developed, to uncover patterns of distribution, and to foster an appreciation of the morphologic basis of variation. Anatomic facts are presented within the context of their mutual relationships and clinical relevance.

This inevitably leads to comprehension of the underlying principles involved and facilitates anatomic reasoning and easier acquisition of additional morphologic facts and concepts.

For the clinician, this book provides essential background knowledge for the safe and appropriate care of patients with neuromusculoskeletal disorders of the spine. Valuable chapters have been included on the surface anatomy of the back, muscles that influence the spine, pain of spinal origin, and the microscopic anatomy of the zygapophyseal joints and intervertebral discs. Special emphasis is placed on structures that may be affected by manual spinal techniques. Each chapter is extensively referenced. I highly recommend this invaluable resource to all students and practitioners who regularly care for patients with spinal disorders.

Alan H. Adams, D.C.

Vice President for Professional Affairs
Los Angeles College of Chiropractic
Whittier, California

Medical textbooks are usually targeted at the interests and needs of undergraduate medical students. While on one hand this helps provide a common language among health care providers, it frequently does not do justice to several special areas of concern to those students and practitioners interested in neuromusculoskeletal function. Nowhere is that deficiency more apparent than in the anatomy of the spine and of the autonomic nervous system, two areas that are of particular relevance to clinical practice. This has placed a burden on those involved in the teaching of anatomy, as well as on those desiring to extend their knowledge beyond the rather terse descriptions of these topics available in most anatomy texts.

Therefore I received with enthusiasm the news that Drs. Cramer and Darby were embarking on a project to create a text that would remediate many of the deficiencies in existing anatomic textbooks. Some of my excitement came from the fact that I have known these authors for many years and have recognized their commitment to undergraduate and graduate education. My optimism was based on the knowledge that their teaching methods and style of exposition had been "field tested" on literally thousands of students over more than a decade. I am pleased to say that the product does not disappoint. The authors present difficult concepts clearly and concisely. The selection of material is appropriate for both the undergraduate student and for anyone in the field wishing to solidify their foundations or "brush up" for examinations.

In recognition of the highly visual nature of anatomy, the text is supplemented with detailed illustrations, many in full color. In addition, many high-quality photographs taken of careful cadaver dissections reinforce further important concepts in the anatomy of spinal regions. I believe that this is particularly helpful to the student of anatomy who is asked to dissect the spinal region aided only by atlases, which do not do justice to the region. Finally, I am very pleased by the addition of radiographs, computed tomograms, and magnetic resonance images. With the proliferation of diagnostic imaging technology in clinical practice comes a special importance in presenting radiographic anatomy in a manner that supports further study of radiographic pathology. In short, I believe that this text fills an important deficiency in modern medical anatomy textbooks and will be a valuable addition to any library.

Rand S. Swenson, D.C., M.D., Ph.D.

Department of Anatomy and Section of Neurology
Dartmouth Medical School and Dartmouth-Hitchcock Medical Center
Editor, *Journal of the Neuromusculoskeletal System*

Preface

Current anatomy texts that describe the spine, spinal cord, and autonomic nervous system frequently discuss this material in a rather general way. Often the pages devoted to these topics are scattered throughout the text, deemphasized, or relegated to later chapters. At the other end of the spectrum, several highly specialized texts on spinal anatomy describe a single region of the spine. In some instances even subregions of the vertebral column, such as the intervertebral discs or intervertebral foramina, become the sole topic of the text. These general and specialized texts both serve important purposes. However, we felt that a need existed for a cohesive, well-illustrated text covering spinal anatomy, which included the neuroanatomy of the spinal cord and the autonomic nervous system as well.

The purpose of this book is threefold:

◆ To provide an accurate and complete text for students studying the spine, spinal cord, and autonomic nervous system.
◆ To serve as a reliable reference to spinal anatomy and related neuroanatomy for clinicians and researchers.
◆ To help bridge the gap between the basic science of anatomy and the applied anatomy of clinical practice.

To accomplish the first purpose the anatomy of the spine, spinal cord, and autonomic nervous system is organized with both the student and the clinician in mind. The first chapter on surface anatomy provides both the neophyte and the seasoned clinician with a valuable resource—a comprehensive view of surface landmarks and the vertebral levels of clinically relevant structures. General concepts also are emphasized throughout the book through many illustrations and photographs to help the reader establish a three-dimensional image of the spine, spinal cord, and autonomic nervous system.

The second purpose of the text was accomplished with a thorough search of the current literature in spinal anatomy, with the results of many of these clinically relevant studies included in the text. Even though the science of anatomy is very old, a surprisingly large number of studies related to spinal anatomy continue to appear in the scientific literature. The past 15 years have also seen an explosion of new neuroanatomic information.

Including the results of recent investigative studies also provided a means by which the third objective of this book was attained. This objective was to serve as a bridge between the basic science of anatomy and the applied anatomy of clinical practice. Throughout the text the results of clinically relevant research have been presented with a red rule running beside, thus providing a rapid reference to this clinically applicable information. In addition, a chapter on pain generators and pain pathways of the back has been included (Chapter 11). This chapter focuses on those structures that can be a source of back pain and details the manner by which the resulting nociceptive stimuli are transmitted and perceived by the patient.

Numerous magnetic resonance imaging scans have been included throughout this text. The purpose of these scans is not only to demonstrate clinically relevant anatomy, but also to aid the unfamiliar reader beginning the exciting process of learning cross-sectional spinal anatomy, which is often clearly demonstrated on these scans.

This book is designed to serve the needs and interests of many groups. The basic anatomy and concepts should be an aid to the beginning student of spinal anatomy whether they be allopathic, osteopathic, chiropractic, or physical therapy students. The text should also provide a ready source for those in clinical practice desiring a rapid reference on a specific topic related to the spine, since the book is arranged topically and exhaustively indexed. Finally, the inclusion of the results of recent research studies, as well as discussions on clinically related topics, will hopefully spark interest and highlight the importance of the spine for the new students, as well as the experienced individual.

Gregory D. Cramer
Susan A. Darby

Introduction

This book has been organized with two groups of readers in mind: those studying the spine for the first time, and those clinicians and researchers who have previously studied the spine in detail. Therefore we have accepted the daunting task of designing a book to act as a source of reference and as a book that is "readable." To this end an outline has been included at the beginning of each chapter. This format should help the reader organize his or her thoughts before beginning the chapter and also provide a quick reference to the material of interest. A complete subject index is also included at the end of the text for rapid referencing. In addition, items of particular clinical relevance and the results of clinically relevant research appear with a red rule beside the material throughout the book.

This highlighting procedure is meant to aid students and clinicians alike in focusing on areas that are thought to be of particular current importance in the detection of pathologic conditions or in the treatment of disorders of the spine, spinal cord, and the autonomic nervous system. Discussions of the clinical relevance of anatomic structures are included to relate anatomy to clinical practice as efficiently as possible.

Chapter 1 discusses surface anatomy. It contains information not only useful to the student who has yet to palpate his or her first patient, but also to the clinician who examines patients on a daily basis. Chapters 2 and 3 relate the general characteristics of the spine and spinal cord, using a basic approach. These chapters are directed primarily to the beginning student. A quick review of these chapters, with attention focused on the sections highlighted by a red rule, should also be of benefit to the more advanced student. Chapter 2 includes a section on advanced diagnostic imaging. This section is provided for the individual who does not routinely view computed tomography and magnetic resonance imaging scans. A brief description of the strengths and weaknesses of both imaging modalities and a concise overview of other less frequently used advanced imaging procedures are included. Chapters 3 and 4 relate soft tissues to the "bones" by describing the spinal cord and its meningeal coverings, and the muscles that surround and influence the spine. This material is followed by a detailed study of the regional anatomy of the spine in Chapters 5 through 8. These chapters also include information concerning the ligamentous tissues of the spine. A more thorough presentation of the anatomy of the spinal cord and autonomic nervous system is found in Chapters 9 and 10, and the development and histologic makeup of the spine and spinal cord are found in Chapters 11 and 12.

Please note that the first four chapters provide the groundwork for later chapters that are more detailed and contain additional information with specific clinical relevance. Therefore certain material is occasionally discussed more than once. For example, Chapters 2 and 3 are concerned with general characteristics of the spine and spinal cord with a discussion of the various components of a typical vertebra, the vertebral canal, and the spinal cord within the canal. These structures are discussed again regionally (Chapters 5 through 8) to a much greater depth to explore their relative importance and clinical significance in each region of the spine and to appreciate the neuroanatomic connections within the spinal cord (Chapter 9).

Chapter 11 is devoted to pain producers (those structures that receive nociceptive innervation), the neuroanatomic pathways for nociception from spinal structures, and the spinal and supraspinal modulation of these impulses. This chapter is designed for readers who have already completed study in spinal anatomy and neuroanatomy. Chapter 12 discusses the development of the spine and is designed for use by students studying spinal anatomy and for clinicians who wish to refresh their knowledge of the development of the spine and spinal cord. Chapter 13 describes the microscopic anatomy of the zygapophyseal joints and the intervertebral discs. Since much of the current research on the spine is focused at the tissue, cellular, and subcellular levels, both students and clinicians should find this chapter useful at some point in their careers. Because of the rather specialized nature of the last three topics, they have been positioned at the end of the book.

CLARIFICATION OF ABBREVIATIONS AND TERMS

Vertebral levels are frequently abbreviated throughout this text. The initials C, T, and L are used to abbreviate cervical, thoracic, and lumbar, respectively. Vertebral levels can then be easily identified by placing the appropriate number after the abbreviated region. For example, "T7" is frequently used rather than "the seventh thoracic vertebra."

In addition, some potentially confusing terminology should be clarified. Throughout this text the term **kyphosis** is used when referring to a spinal curve that is concave anteriorly, and the term **lordosis** is used for a curve that is concave posteriorly. The term **hyperlordosis** refers to an accentuation of a lordosis beyond what is usually accepted as normal, and the term **hyperkyphosis** is used for an accentuation of a kyphosis beyond the range of normal. This is in contrast with the terminology of some texts that refer to normal spinal curves as being "concave anteriorly" or "concave posteriorly" and reserve the terms "kyphosis" and "lordosis" for curves that are deeper than normal. Although both sets of terminology are correct, the prior one was chosen for this text because we felt that this terminology would lend the most clarity to subsequent discussions.

Finally, we hope that you, the reader, believe as we do that the long-standing interest of clinicians in the anatomic sciences is not an accident. Greater awareness of structure leads to a keener perception of function, and an increased understanding of pathologic conditions is the natural consequence. This results in a better comprehension of current therapeutic approaches and the development of new treatment procedures based upon a scientific foundation. Therefore astute clinicians keep an eye toward developments in the structural sciences, being aware that their concepts of human mechanisms may be influenced by new discoveries in these disciplines. Whenever new knowledge of the causes underlying dysfunction is developed, new therapeutic approaches are sure to follow, and clinicians who have kept abreast of these recent discoveries will find themselves as leaders in their field.

Acknowledgments

This project would not have been possible had it not been for the support of the members of the administration, faculty, students, and staff of The National College of Chiropractic, who allowed us the time and facilities necessary to review the literature, to write several drafts of text, and to work on the development of supporting figures. We greatly appreciate their support of, and in some instances commitment to, this work.

In addition, many people have helped with the production of this book. We would like to take this opportunity to thank those who helped with proofreading portions of various drafts of this work and whose suggestions were extremely helpful in the development of the final manuscript. These people include Carol Muehleman, Ph.D.; Joe Cantu, D.C.; Richard Dorsett; Kris Gongaware; James McKay; Ken Nolson; and John DeMatte.

We would also like to thank Patrick W. Frank for his beautiful dissections of the muscles of the back, which appear in Chapter 4. The work of Victoria Hyzny in the dissection of the neck and her assistance with the dissection of the autonomic nervous system is greatly appreciated. Photographs of these dissections appear in Chapters 5 and 10. We also thank Sheila Meadows for organizational help with photographs and illustrations, and we are also grateful for the computer graphics added by Dino Juarez to several of the magnetic resonance imaging scans found in Chapters 11 and 13. Mr. Juarez also produced many of the illustrations in Chapter 10. We are extremely grateful for all of his contributions.

The magnetic resonance imaging scans, computed tomograms, and x-ray films were graciously provided by William V. Glenn, M.D., who is in the private practice of radiology in Carson, California, and Dennis Skogsbergh, D.C., DABCO, DACBR, Chairman of the Department of Diagnostic Imaging at The National College of Chiropractic. We would like to thank them for providing these important images.

We are particularly indebted to Michael L. Kiely, Ph.D., for his review of the entire manuscript. His comments were always useful and were presented with the delicate precision of a master teacher.

We would also like to gratefully acknowledge our parents, Dr. and Mrs. David Cramer and Mr. and Mrs. George Anderson, whose encouragement and early instruction gave us a strong desire to learn more and to help others.

The outstanding teaching of Drs. Joseph Janse, Delmas Allen, Liberato DiDio, William Potvin, and Frank Saul will never be forgotten. Their example provided much of the motivation for beginning, and completing, this endeavor.

Thank you all very much.

G.C.
S.D.

Contents

BASIC AND CLINICAL ANATOMY OF THE

SPINE, SPINAL CORD, AND ANS

PART I

CHARACTERISTICS OF THE SPINE AND SPINAL CORD

CHAPTER 1

Surface Anatomy of the Back and Vertebral Levels of Clinically Important Structures

Barclay W. Bakkum

Surface anatomy is defined as the configuration of the surface of the body, especially in relation to deeper parts. A thorough knowledge of surface anatomy is necessary for the proper performance of a physical examination. Information gathered by the eyes (inspection) and fingers (palpation) is often critical in the assessment of a patient. An understanding of the topography of the human body also allows the health care provider to locate the position of deep structures that may need further evaluation.

The locations of structures in reference to the surface of the body are always approximations. Individual variations are common and are influenced by such factors as age, sex, posture, weight, and body type. Respiratory movements also can have marked effects on the locations of structures, especially those of the thorax. Determining the position of the contents of the abdomen can be particularly challenging, and the precise location of abdominal viscera can be established only by verification with appropriate diagnostic imaging procedures.

In keeping with the scope of this text, the surface anatomy included in this chapter is limited to the back. Spinous processes and posterior bony landmarks are used as points of reference in the first part of the chapter. One reason for the use of these as landmarks is to help clinicians with examination and treatment of the back and spine when the patient is in the prone position. In addition, the vertebral levels of structures of the anterior neck and trunk, which are either visible by means of advanced imaging procedures (magnetic resonance imaging or computed tomography) or palpable during physical examination, are included. Knowledge of the normal relationships between the viscera and the spine is becoming increasingly important in clinical practice, as clinicians are asked with greater frequency to interpret or review studies employing these advanced imaging procedures. On a more practical level, knowledge of these relationships helps the clinician quickly become oriented with the vertebral level of diagnostic images taken in the horizontal plane.

Because other texts discuss the location of organs with regard to abdominal regions or quadrants, that method of locating organs is not covered here.

THE BACK

The back, or dorsum, is the posterior part of the trunk and includes skin, muscles, vertebral column, spinal cord, and various nerves and blood vessels (Gardner, Gray, & O'Rahilly, 1975). The 24 movable vertebrae consist of, from superior to inferior, 7 cervical (C), 12 thoracic (or dorsal) (T), and 5 lumbar (L). Inferior to the lumbar vertebrae, five sacral vertebrae (S) fuse in the adult to form the sacrum. The lowermost three to five vertebrae fuse late in adult life to form the coccyx (Co).

Intervertebral discs are located between the anterior portions of the movable vertebrae and between L5 and the sacrum. There is no disc located between the

3

occiput and C1 (atlas), or between C1 and C2 (axis). The discs are named for the vertebra located immediately above the disc, that is, the T6 disc is located between the T6 and T7 vertebrae.

Seven processes arise from the posterior portion of the typical vertebra. Several atypical vertebrae have variations in their anatomy and are discussed in Chapters 5, 6, and 7. The spinous process is a midline structure that is directed posteriorly and to a variable degree inferiorly. The transverse processes are a pair of lateral projections. The other four processes are articular, and each vertebra has a superior pair and an inferior pair. These processes are discussed in greater detail in Chapter 2.

The remainder of this chapter discusses visual landmarks of the back; palpatory landmarks of the back; spinal cord levels versus vertebral levels; and vertebral levels of structures in the anterior neck and trunk. This information enables the clinician to gain a thorough understanding of surface anatomy and serves as a reference for future patient assessment, both in the physical examination and through diagnostic imaging procedures, including x-ray examination, computed tomography, and magnetic resonance imaging.

Visual Landmarks of the Back

In the midline of the back is a longitudinal groove known as the median furrow (Fig. 1-1). Superiorly it begins at the external occipital protuberance (EOP) (see the following discussion) and continues inferiorly as the gluteal (anal, natal, or cluneal) cleft to the level of the S3 spinous tubercle, the remnants of the spinous process of S3. It is very shallow in the lower cervical region and deepest in the lumbar region. The median furrow widens inferiorly to form an isosceles triangle with a line connecting the posterior superior iliac spines (PSISs) forming the base above, and the gluteal cleft forming the apex of the triangle below. The PSISs are often visible as a pair of dimples located 3 cm lateral to the midline at the level of the S2 spinous tubercle. The gluteal fold is a horizontal skin fold extending laterally from the midline and corresponds with the inferior border of the gluteus maximus muscle. This fold marks the lower extent of the buttock.

Several muscles are commonly visible in the back region. The trapezius is a large, flat, triangular muscle that originates in the midline from the EOP to the spinous process of T12 and inserts laterally onto the spine of the scapula. Its upper fibers form the "top of the shoulder," where the neck laterally blends into the thorax. The latissimus dorsi, extending from the region of the iliac crest to the posterior border of the axilla, forms the lateral border of the lower thoracic portion of the back. This muscle is especially noticeable when the upper extremity is adducted against resistance. Between the trapezius medially and the latissimus dorsi laterally, the inferior angle of the scapula may be seen at about the level of the T7 spinous process. The erector spinae muscles form two large longitudinal masses in the lumbar region that extend about a handbreadth (10 cm) laterally from the midline. These muscle masses are responsible for the deepening of the median furrow in this region.

Besides these muscles, several bony landmarks are usually visible in the region of the back. The spinous process of C7 (the vertebra prominens) is usually visible in the lower cervical region. The spinous process of T1 is often also visible and is actually the most prominent spinous in 30% to 40% of the population. When the patient's head is flexed, the spinous processes of C7 and T1, and often C6, are usually easily seen.

In the adult the vertebral column has several normal curves that are visible. In the cervical and lumbar regions the spine is anteriorly convex (lordotic), and in the thoracic and sacral areas it is posteriorly convex (kyphotic). Normally there is no lateral deviation of the spinal column, but when present this curvature is known as scoliosis. These curves are covered in more detail in Chapter 2.

Palpatory Landmarks of the Back

The following structures are not usually visible, but can be located upon palpation. Some of the structures in this discussion of palpable landmarks cannot normally be felt, but their relation to landmarks that can be localized is given.

Cervical Region. In the center of the occipital squama is the external occipital protuberance (inion) (EOP) (Fig. 1-2). Extending laterally from the EOP is the superior nuchal line. The transverse process of the atlas may be found directly below and slightly anterior to the mastoid process of the temporal bone. Because of the relatively fragile styloid process of the temporal bone that lies just in front, and the great auricular nerve that ascends in the fascia superficial to the C1 transverse process, care must be taken when palpating this structure.

The spinous process of the axis is the first readily palpable bony structure in the posterior midline below the EOP (Fig. 1-2), although according to Oliver and Middleditch (1991) the posterior tubercle of C1 may be palpable in some people between the EOP and the spinous process of C2. In the midline below the spinous process of the axis, the second prominent palpable structure is the spinous process of C7 or the vertebra prominens. In 60% to 70% of the population the vertebra prominens is the most prominent spinous process, whereas in the other 30% to 40% the spinous process of T1 is more evident. The other cervical spinous processes

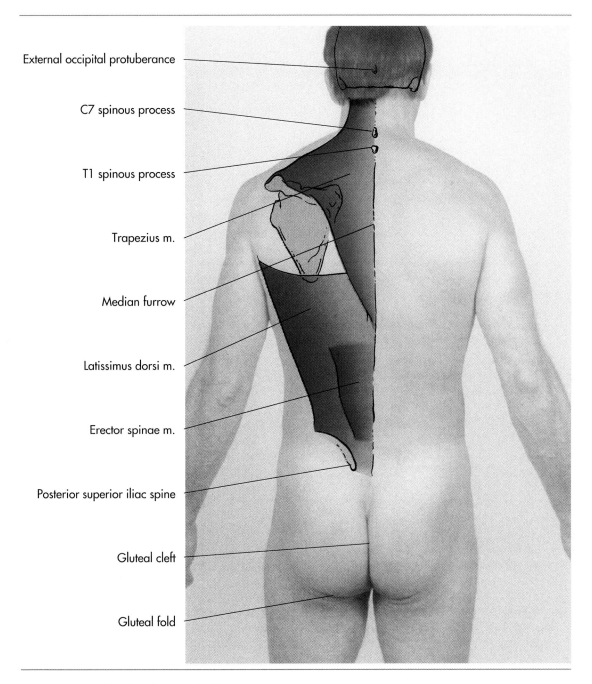

External occipital protuberance

C7 spinous process

T1 spinous process

Trapezius m.

Median furrow

Latissimus dorsi m.

Erector spinae m.

Posterior superior iliac spine

Gluteal cleft

Gluteal fold

FIG. 1-1   Visual landmarks of the back.

are variably more difficult to palpate. The spinous process of C3 is the smallest and can be found at the same horizontal plane as the greater cornua of the hyoid bone. The spinous process of C6 is the last freely movable spinous process with flexion and extension of the neck. It is usually readily palpable with full flexion of the neck.

The facet joints between the articular processes of the cervical vertebrae (collectively known as the articular pillars) can be found 1.5 cm lateral of the midline in the posterior neck. With the exception of C1, the tips of transverse processes of the cervical vertebrae are not individually palpable, but the posterior tubercles of these processes form a bony resistance that may be palpated along a line from the tip of the mastoid process to the root of the neck, approximately a thumb breadth (2.5 cm) lateral of the midline. The anterior aspects of the transverse processes of the cervical vertebrae may be found in the groove between the larynx and sternocleidomastoid muscle (SCM). It may be necessary to slightly retract the SCM laterally in order to palpate these structures. The anterior tubercles of the transverse processes of C6 are especially large and are known as the carotid tubercles (Fig. 1-2). These may be palpated at

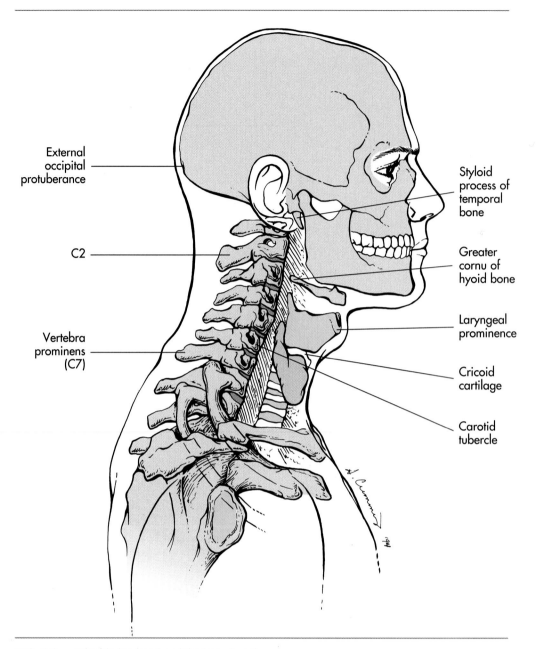

External occipital protuberance

C2

Vertebra prominens (C7)

Styloid process of temporal bone

Greater cornu of hyoid bone

Laryngeal prominence

Cricoid cartilage

Carotid tubercle

FIG. 1-2 Palpable landmarks of the lateral neck.

the level of the cricoid cartilage. Care must be taken when locating the carotid tubercles (and the other cervical transverse processes), since they are in the proximity of the common carotid arteries, and they should always be palpated unilaterally.

Anteriorly, the superior border of the thyroid cartilage, forming the laryngeal prominence (Adam's apple) in the midline, may be used to find the horizontal plane of the C4 disc. The body of C6 is located at the same horizontal level as the cricoid cartilage and the first tracheal ring.

Thoracic Region. The spinous process of T1 is the third prominent bony structure in the midline below the

EOP, the spinous processes of C2 and C7 being the first and second, respectively (Fig. 1-3). The spinous process of T3 is located at the same horizontal plane as the root of the spine of the scapula. The spinous process of T4 is located at the extreme of the convexity of the thoracic kyphosis and therefore is usually the most prominent spinous process below the root of the neck.

When patients are standing or sitting with their upper extremities resting along the sides of their trunk, the inferior scapular angle usually is at the horizontal level of the spinous process of T7. This changes when the patient is lying prone with his or her upper extremities resting toward the floor in a flexed position (the most common posture of the patient when this region of the

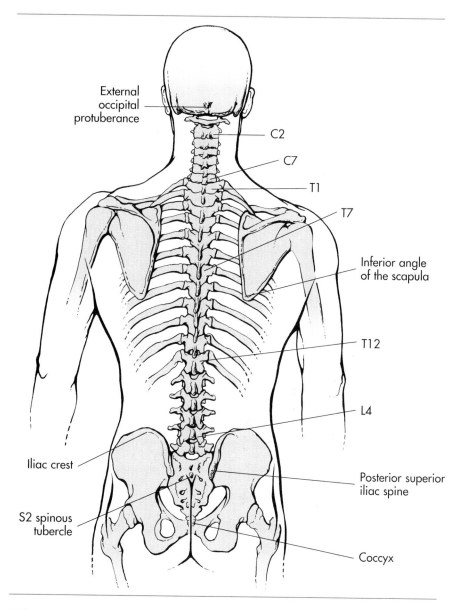

FIG. 1-3   Palpable landmarks of the back.

back is palpated). In this position the scapulae are rotated so that the T6 spinous process is more commonly found at the level of the inferior scapular angle.

The spinous processes of T9 and T10 are often palpably closer together than other thoracic spinous processes, but this is not a consistent finding. Located approximately halfway between the level of the inferior angle of the scapula and the superior margin of the iliac crests is the spinous process of T12.

Since the spinous processes of the thoracic vertebrae project in an inferior direction to different degrees, the remainder of the vertebrae are located variably superior to the spinous process of the same vertebral segment (Keogh & Ebbs, 1984). The tips of the transverse processes of T1-4 and T10-12 are located one spinous interspace superior to the tip of the spinous process of the same segment. The tips of the transverse processes of

T5-9 are located two spinous interspaces superior to the tips of their respective spinous processes since these spinous processes project inferiorly to a greater degree. For example, the tips of the transverse processes of T3 are located in the same horizontal plane as the inferior tip of the spinous process of T2, whereas the tips of the transverse processes of T8 are at the same horizontal plane as the inferior tip of the spinous process of T6. The transverse processes of the thoracic vertebrae progressively get shorter from superior to inferior, so that the tips of the transverse processes of T1 are located 3 cm lateral to the midline, although those of T12 are 2 cm. The transverse processes of T12 are sometimes very small and not readily palpable. The angles of the ribs may be palpated 4 cm lateral to the midline at the horizontal levels of their respective transverse processes.

Lumbosacral Region. The posterior aspect of the spinous processes of the lumbar vertebrae differ from the thoracic vertebrae in that they present a flat surface. The spinous processes of L4 and L5 are shorter than the other lumbar spinous processes and are difficult to palpate, especially that of L5. The spinous process of L4 is the last spinous process with palpable movement of the spine with flexion and extension of the trunk. It is usually in a horizontal plane with the superior margin of the iliac crests, although in approximately 20% of the population the iliac crests are even with the spinous process of L5 (Oliver & Middleditch, 1991).

The tips of the transverse processes of the lumbar vertebrae are located approximately 5 cm lateral to the midline and are not usually palpable. The mamillary processes are small tubercles on the posterior-superior aspect of the superior articular processes of the lumbar vertebra. They are located about a finger breadth (2 cm) lateral to the midline at the level of the spinous process of the vertebra above and are not readily palpable.

The second spinous tubercle, the remnants of the spinous process of S2, is located at the extreme of the convexity of the sacral kyphosis and is the most prominent spinous tubercle on the sacrum. It is also on the same horizontal plane as the posterior superior iliac spines. The third spinous tubercle is located at the upper end of the gluteal cleft. The lowest palpable depression in the midline of the posterior aspect of the sacrum is the sacral hiatus. There are four pairs of posterior sacral foramina located 2.5 cm lateral to the midline and 2.5 cm apart, but these are not usually palpable. The tip of the coccyx is the last palpable bony structure of the spine and can be found in the gluteal cleft approximately 1 cm posterior to the anus.

SPINAL CORD LEVELS VERSUS VERTEBRAL LEVELS

The spinal cord is the extension of the central nervous system outside the cranium (Fig. 1-4). It is encased by the vertebral column and begins, on a gross anatomical level, at the foramen magnum, located halfway between the inion and the spinous process of C2. In the third fetal month the spinal cord extends the entire length of the embryo, and the spinal nerves exit the intervertebral foramina (IVFs) at their level of origin (Langman, 1975). With increasing development, however, the vertebral column and the dura mater lengthen more rapidly than does the neural tube, and the terminal end of the spinal cord gradually assumes a relatively higher level. At the time of birth the tip of the spinal cord, or conus medullaris, lies at the level of the L3 vertebral body. In the adult the conus medullaris is usually found at the L1-2 level (L1 body–26%, L1 disc–36%, L2 body–20%), but

may be found as high as the T12 disc (12%) or as low as the L2 disc (6%) (Fitzgerald, 1985).

As a result of this unequal growth, the portion of the spinal cord from which the respective pairs of spinal nerve roots begin, known as the spinal cord level, is more superior than the level of the IVF from which the corresponding spinal nerve exits. Therefore the spinal nerve roots run obliquely inferior inside the vertebral (spinal) canal from their spinal cord level to their corresponding IVF. This obliquity is not equal throughout the length of the vertebral column. At the most superior levels of the vertebral column, the spinal nerve roots are nearly horizontal, and at more inferior levels they are progressively more oblique. In the lumbosacral region of the vertebral canal, the spinal nerve roots are nearly vertical and form a bundle known as the cauda equina.

A convenient method of locating various structures of the neck and trunk is to relate them to which vertebra, or portion of a vertebra, that lies at the same horizontal level as that structure. This plane is known as the vertebral level of a structure. Unless otherwise noted, the vertebral body serves as the source of reference for the vertebral level. Table 1-1 lists the vertebral levels of many of the clinically important visceral structures in the anterior neck and trunk. When locating structures within the vertebral canal, it is important to distinguish spinal cord levels from vertebral levels. The cervical spinal cord levels lie at even intervals between the foramen magnum and the spinous process of C6 (Keogh & Ebbs, 1984). The upper six thoracic spinal cord levels are between the spinous processes of C6 and T4, and the lower six thoracic spinal cord levels are between the spinous processes of T4 and T9. The lumbar, sacral, and coccygeal spinal cord levels are located between the spinous processes of T10 and L1, where the spinal cord ends as the conus medullaris.

The diameter of the spinal cord increases in two regions. These spinal cord enlargements are formed by the increased numbers of nerve cells required to innervate the limbs. The cervical enlargement includes the C4-T1 spinal cord levels and is at the level of the vertebral bodies of C4-7, or the spinous processes of C3-6 (Keogh & Ebbs, 1984). The lumbar enlargement is composed of the L2-S3 spinal cord levels and is found at the level of the T10-L1 vertebral bodies or the spinous processes of T9-12.

VERTEBRAL LEVELS OF STRUCTURES IN THE ANTERIOR NECK AND TRUNK

This section describes the vertebral levels of most of the clinically important structures found in the anterior neck and trunk. A knowledge of the surface locations for the deep structures of the anterior neck and trunk is essential for relating those structures to the whole person,

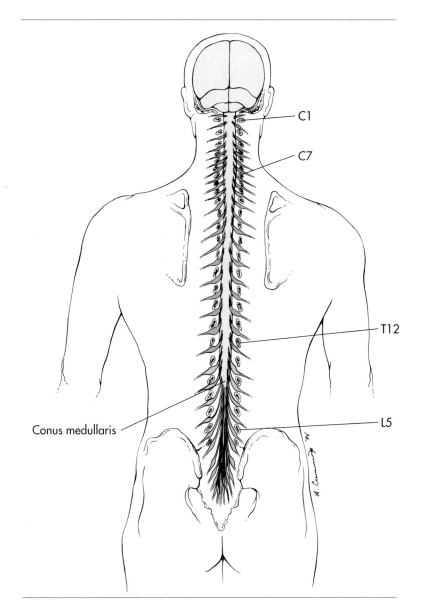

C1

C7

T12

L5

Conus medullaris

FIG. 1-4   Relationship between vertebral levels and spinal cord levels.

especially during the physical examination. This information is summarized in Table 1-1.

Visual Landmarks

In the anterior neck region the most obvious visible structure is the laryngeal prominence (Fig. 1-5). It can be seen in the midline at the level of the C4 disc and is larger in adult males versus females. Moving inferiorly, the jugular notch of the sternum, or suprasternal notch, is at the superior margin of the manubrium and corresponds with the horizontal plane of the T2 disc or T1-2 interspinous space. The sternal angle (of Louis) at the inferior margin of the manubrium is at the level of the T4 disc. Near the inferior end of the sternum the xiphisternal junction is found. It corresponds not only with the

body of T9 but also with the inferior margin of the pectoralis major muscle and the fifth costal cartilages. These relationships are quite variable depending on body type. Laterally, the lowest portion of the costal margin is made up of the tenth costal cartilages. The horizontal plane at this level is termed the subcostal plane and goes through the body of L3 (Moore, 1992).

The transpyloric plane is the horizontal plane at the halfway point between the upper border of the symphysis pubis and the suprasternal notch. It corresponds with the L1 disc and is usually one handbreadth (10 cm) inferior to the xiphisternal junction. The vertebral level of the umbilicus is typically at the level of L3, but this is quite variable depending upon body type and weight. The pubic crest is identified with the level of the superior margin of the pubic symphysis. It extends 2.5 cm

Table 1-1 Vertebral Levels of Clinically Important Structures

Vertebral level	Structure	Vertebral level	Structure
C1	Transition of medulla into spinal cord		aspects of lungs
	Hard palate		Superior extent of left hemidiaphragm
	Anterior portion of soft palate		Superior pole of spleen
C2	Inferior border of free edge of soft palate		Left extent of inferior border of liver
	Nasopharynx and oropharynx join	T10	Apex of heart
C2 disc	Superior cervical ganglion		Anteroinferior ends of oblique fissures
C3	Epiglottis		of lungs
	Oropharynx becomes laryngopharynx		Esophageal hiatus (diaphragm)
C3 disc	Common carotid arteries split into internal	T11	Lowest extent of lungs (inferolateral angles of
	and external carotid arteries		posterior aspects of lungs)
	Carotid sinus		Inferior extent of esophagus
C3 spinous	Greater cornua of hyoid bone		Cardiac orifice of stomach
C4 disc	Laryngeal prominence		Left suprarenal gland
C5	Vocal folds	T12	Aortic hiatus (diaphragm)
	Erb's point		Costodiaphragmatic recesses
	Superior margin of lobes of thyroid gland		Inferior pole of spleen
C6	Middle cervical ganglion		Tail of pancreas
	Cricoid cartilage		Orifice of gallbladder
	First tracheal ring		Superior poles of kidneys (right slightly
	Transition of larynx to trachea		lower than left)
	Transition of laryngopharynx to esophagus		Right suprarenal gland
C7	Inferior cervical ganglion	L1	Pyloric orifice of stomach
T1	Stellate ganglion		Superior horizontal (first) part of duodenum
	Inferior margin of thyroid gland		Left colic (splenic) flexure
	Subclavian and internal jugular veins	L1 disc	Transpyloric plane
	unite to form the brachiocephalic		Conus medullaris
	veins		Hila of kidneys (right slightly below and
	Apices of lungs		left slightly above)
T2	Brachiocephalic veins unite to form	L2	Duodenal-jejunal junction
	superior vena cava		Right colic (hepatic) flexure
T2 disc	Suprasternal notch		Head of pancreas
T4	Aortic arch	L3	Subcostal plane (lowest portion of costal
T4 disc	Sternal angle (of Louis)		margin made up from the tenth costal carti-
T5	Pulmonary trunk divides into right and		lage)
	left pulmonary arteries		Umbilicus (inconsistent)
	Pulmonary artery and primary bronchus		Inferior horizontal (third) part of duodenum
	enter right lung		Right extent of lower border of liver
	Trachea divides into primary bronchi		Inferior poles of kidneys (right slightly lower
	Posterosuperior ends of oblique		than left)
	fissures of lungs	L4	Beginning of sigmoid colon
T6	Base of heart	L4 disc	Aorta divides into common iliac arteries
	Pulmonary artery and primary bronchus	L5	Common iliac veins unite to form inferior
	enter left lung		vena cava
	Pulmonary veins exit right lung		Ileocecal junction
	Superior vena cava enters right atrium		Vermiform appendix arises from cecum
T7	Pulmonary veins exit left lung	L5 disc	Anterior superior iliac spine
	Inferior vena cava enters right atrium		Superolateral end of inguinal ligament
	Horizontal fissure of right lung	S3	Beginning of rectum
T8	Caval hiatus (diaphragm)	Lower sacrum	Superior extent of uterus
	Superior extent of right hemidiaphragm	Coccyx	Pubic crest
	Superior border of liver		Ganglion impar
T9	Xiphisternal junction		Superior margin of pubic symphysis
	Fifth costal cartilage		Inferomedial end of inguinal ligament
	Inferior border of pectoralis major muscle		Bladder (empty)
	Inferomedial angles of posterior		

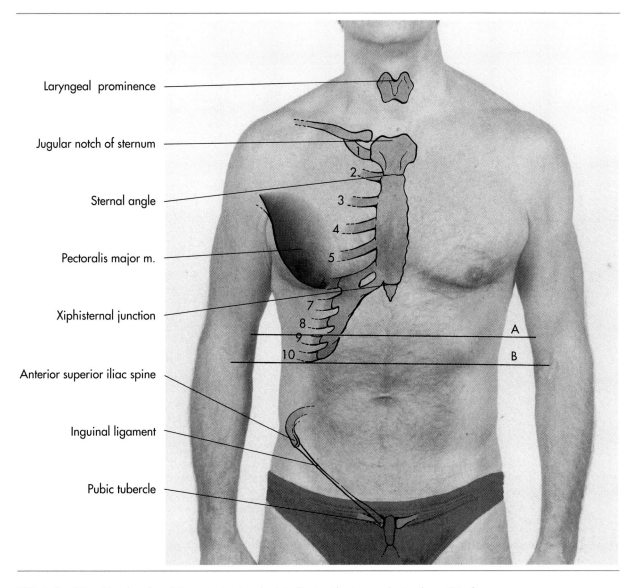

Laryngeal prominence

Jugular notch of sternum

Sternal angle

Pectoralis major m.

Xiphisternal junction

Anterior superior iliac spine

Inguinal ligament

Pubic tubercle

FIG. 1-5   Visual landmarks of the anterior trunk. *A* indicates the transpyloric plane. *B* indicates the subcostal plane. Note that the ribs have been numbered.

lateral to the midline and has a prominence on its lateral aspect known as the pubic tubercle. Typically the pubic crest is in the same plane as the coccyx, but again weight and body type can alter the tilt of the pelvis and therefore this relationship. The inguinal ligament extends from the anterior superior iliac spine at the level of the L5 disc to the pubic tubercle and demarcates the beginning of the thigh region.

Deeper Structures

Neural Structures. At the level of the atlas, the gross anatomical transition of the medulla oblongata into the spinal cord occurs as it exits the cranium via the foramen magnum. The conus medullaris, the inferior tip of the spinal cord, is usually found at the L1-2 level (see previous discussion).

The sympathetic trunks (Fig. 1-6) extend along the entire anterolateral aspect of the spinal column. In the cervical region the trunks are approximately 2.5 cm lateral to the midline. They are somewhat more laterally located in the thoracic and lumbar regions. Along the anterior surface of the sacrum the trunks begin to converge until they meet as the ganglion impar on the anterior surface of the coccyx. Sympathetic ganglia are located at fairly regular intervals along these trunks. Typically there are three ganglia in the cervical region (Fig. 1-6). The superior cervical ganglion can be found at the C2-3 interspace. The middle and inferior cervical ganglia typically are found at the C6 and C7 levels,

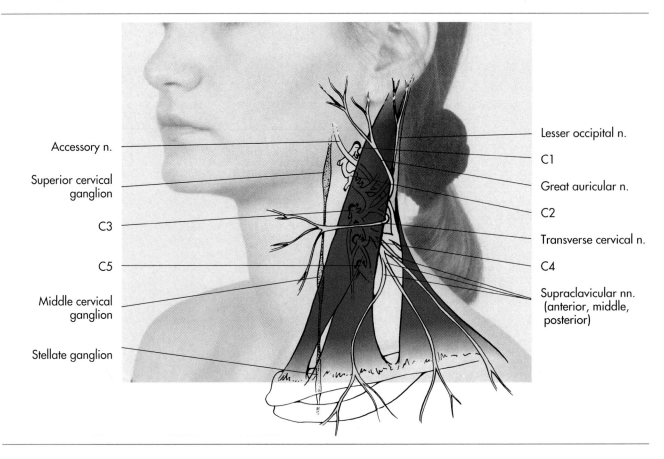

Accessory n.

Superior cervical
ganglion

C3

C5

Middle cervical
ganglion

Stellate ganglion

Lesser occipital n.

C1

Great auricular n.

C2

Transverse cervical n.

C4

Supraclavicular nn.
(anterior, middle,
posterior)

FIG. 1-6   Erb's point and the cervical sympathetic trunk. Note Erb's point is located midway
along the posterior border of the sternocleidomastoid muscle. Also note the sympathetic trunk
connecting the cervical sympathetic ganglia.

respectively. Sometimes the inferior cervical ganglion
and the first thoracic ganglion unite to form the stellate
(or cervicothoracic) ganglion, which is found at the T1
level. The sympathetic trunks are described in more detail in Chapter 10.

Several peripheral nerves become superficial about
midway along the posterior border of the sternocleidomastoid muscle (SCM) (Fig. 1-6). This area is sometimes
called Erb's point and is approximately at the C5 level.
These nerves include the transverse cervical nerve,
which supplies the skin of the throat region; the lesser
occipital nerve, which supplies the skin in the area of
the mastoid process; and the great auricular nerve,
which innervates the skin in the vicinity of the ear. In
addition, the supraclavicular nerves arise by a common
trunk that emerges from Erb's point. This trunk divides
into three branches alternately referred to as anterior,
middle, and posterior *or* medial, intermediate, and lateral, which go to the skin of the upper chest region.
Finally, the accessory nerve (cranial nerve XI), after
sending motor branches into the deep surface of the
SCM, becomes superficial in this region. It then courses
in a posterolateral direction to reach the deep surface of

the trapezius muscle, which it also supplies with motor
innervation.

The roots of the brachial plexus, which arise from the
ventral rami of the C5-T1 spinal nerves, are located just
posterior to the lower one third of the SCM (Keogh &
Ebbs, 1984). The upper (lateral) margin of the plexus
runs along a line from the junction of the middle and
lower thirds of the SCM to the tip of the coracoid
process of the scapula. The lower (or medial) border of
the plexus extends from the junction of the posterior
border of the SCM with the clavicle to one finger
breadth (2 cm) inferior and medial to the tip of the coracoid process of the scapula.

Vascular Structures.   The shape of the heart may be
thought of as an isosceles triangle with a superior base
and an inferior apex directed to the left of the midline
(Fig. 1-7). The base of the heart can usually be found at
the level of T6. The horizontal position of the apex of
the heart is usually said to be at the level of T10, but this
is variable depending upon the patient's body type. It
may be found as high as T9 (Moore, 1992) or as low as
T11 (Gardner et al., 1975).

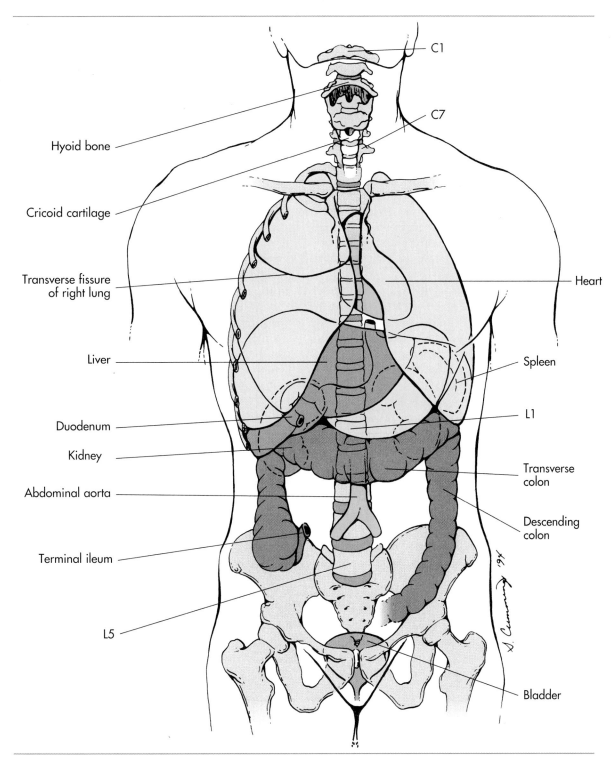

FIG. 1-7 Vertebral levels of deeper structures of the anterior neck and trunk.

The ascending aorta emerges from the left ventricle of the heart approximately in the midline and runs superiorly. It then turns to the left and forms the aortic arch that can be found at the level of the T4 body. The thoracic portion of the descending aorta begins in the plane of the T4 disc and runs inferi-orly slightly left of the midline along the anterior surface of the thoracic vertebrae. It becomes the abdominal aorta as it passes through the aortic hiatus of the diaphragm in the midline at the level of T12 (Moore, 1992). The abdominal aorta descends along the anterior surface of the lumbar vertebrae and divides into the common iliac arteries just anterior to the L4 disc, slightly left of the midline.

The aortic arch has three branches. The first is the brachiocephalic trunk. This trunk gives rise to the right common carotid and right subclavian arteries. The left common carotid artery is the second branch of the aortic arch, and the left subclavian artery is the third branch of the aortic arch. The subclavian arteries supply blood to the upper extremities, and the common carotid arteries supply the head and neck region. The common carotid arteries ascend on either side of the anterolateral neck to the level of the C3 disc where they each split into an internal and external carotid artery. This is the region of the important carotid sinus, which monitors the blood pressure of the body. Therefore care must be taken when palpating these structures, and they should always be palpated only unilaterally.

The pulmonary trunk arises from the right ventricle of the heart and divides into the right and left pulmonary arteries in a plane with T5. The pulmonary arteries enter (and the pulmonary veins exit) their respective lungs via a hilum. The pulmonary artery enters the right lung opposite T5 and enters the left lung at the level of T6 (Williams et al., 1989). The pulmonary veins exit the lungs about one vertebral level lower than the arteries enter. There is some variation of these levels with body type, and both of the pulmonary arteries may enter their respective lungs as low as T7 (Gardner et al., 1975).

The internal jugular and subclavian veins of each side of the body unite several centimeters lateral to the midline at the level of T1 to form the brachiocephalic veins. The brachiocephalic veins then unite to form the superior vena cava slightly right of the midline at the T2 level (Williams et al., 1989). The superior vena cava runs inferiorly and ends in the upper portion of the right atrium of the heart at approximately the level of T6.

The common iliac veins unite to form the inferior vena cava at the level of the L5 body, a little to the right of the midline. The inferior vena cava then ascends in front of the vertebral column, on the right side of the abdominal aorta. Passing through the caval hiatus of the diaphragm in the horizontal plane of the body of T8 (Moore, 1992), the inferior vena cava enters the lower portion of the right atrium just above that level at T7.

Visceral Structures. The respiratory system begins with the nasal cavity, which is separated from the oral cavity by the hard palate. The hard palate lies in the same horizontal plane as the atlas. The nasal cavity becomes continuous with the nasopharynx in the region of the soft palate also at the level of C1. The nasopharynx joins the oropharynx at the inferior border of the posterior margin of the soft palate just anterior to the C2 body, and for several centimeters the alimentary and respiratory systems share a common passageway. At the superior border of the epiglottis, the oropharynx becomes the laryngopharynx. In this region the alimentary and respiratory tracts again become separate. Anteriorly the respiratory tract continues as the larynx. Its lumen is protected during deglutition by the epiglottis, which may be found at the C3 level. The adjacent hyoid bone provides attachment sites for several muscles involved in deglutition and vocalization, and its greater cornua can be found at the C3 spinous process level. The most anterior projection of the thyroid cartilage, the laryngeal prominence, is at the level of the C4 disc, and the vocal folds, or cords, are slightly lower in the C5 plane. The cricoid cartilage, the lowest portion of the larynx, joins the first tracheal ring, the highest portion of the trachea, at the level of C6. The lobes of the thyroid gland are located anterior and lateral to the larynx and trachea and extend from the C5 to T1 levels. The trachea descends in the midline anterior to the esophagus to the level of the upper border of the T5 body where it divides into the primary bronchi (Williams et al., 1989). The primary bronchi enter the lungs via their respective hila at approximately the same levels as the pulmonary arteries, which are T5 on the right and T6 on the left.

The apex of each lung extends superiorly to the level of the T1 body (Fig. 1-7). On their posterior aspects, the inferomedial angles of both lungs are approximately at T9 and the inferolateral angles, the lowest portion of the lungs, extend inferiorly to T11. The anterior inferior border of each lung is approximately one vertebral level higher than the posterior border. With full inspiration these levels may descend nearly two vertebral segments (Williams et al., 1989).

The left lung is divided into upper and lower lobes by an oblique fissure. This fissure extends from the T5 level posterosuperiorly to T10 anteroinferiorly. The right lung not only has an oblique fissure very similar to that of the left lung, but also has a horizontal fissure at the level of T7. The right lung is therefore divided into three lobes: upper, middle, and lower.

The diaphragm extends several vertebral levels superiorly in its center and is shaped like a dome. Therefore the diaphragm makes an impression on the inferior surface of each of the lungs. The right half of the diaphragm, often termed the right hemidiaphragm, reaches the T8 level and is about 1 cm higher than the level of the left hemidiaphragm because of the underlying liver (Moore, 1992). With full inspiration, these levels may descend as much as two vertebral levels (Williams et al., 1989). Normally, the pleural cavity extends slightly lower than the inferolateral angles of the lungs and forms the costodiaphragmatic recesses at the level of T12. Because of the domelike shape of the diaphragm, these recesses represent the lowest points of the thoracic cavity and are potential sites of fluid accumulation in the chest.

The alimentary canal begins as the oral cavity, which becomes the oropharynx in the region of the soft palate at the C1 level. The oropharynx, after being joined by the nasopharynx at the inferior border of the free edge of the soft palate just in front of the C2 body, turns into the laryngopharynx at the superior border of the epiglottis at the level of C3. The laryngopharynx continues inferiorly on the posterior aspect of the larynx and changes into the esophagus at the level of C6. The esophagus runs inferiorly in the chest on the anterior aspect of the vertebral column slightly anterior and to the right of the descending thoracic aorta. Passing through the diaphragm via the esophageal hiatus at the T10 level, the esophagus enters the abdomen (Williams et al., 1989) and ends at the cardiac orifice of the stomach slightly left of the midline at T11.

The stomach is the most dilated portion of the alimentary canal. Curving inferiorly and to the right, the stomach becomes continuous with the small intestine at the pyloric orifice at the level of L1. The duodenum, the first part of the small intestine, is shaped like a U lying on its side and has four parts. The first, or superior horizontal, part continues from the pyloric orifice horizontally to the right at the level of L1. The second (descending) part proceeds inferiorly to the horizontal plane of L3 where it turns to the left to become the third, or inferior horizontal, part. The third part continues to the left, crosses the midline, and bends slightly superiorly to give rise to the fourth (ascending) part that runs obliquely superior and ends as the duodenal-jejunal junction at the level of L2.

The rest of the small intestine continues as a series of loops and ends by connecting with the large intestine at the junction of the cecum and the ascending portion of the colon in the right lower quadrant of the abdomen at the L5 level. The proximal two fifths and the distal three fifths of the small intestine distal to the duodenum are called the jejunum and ileum, respectively.

The large intestine, or colon, begins as the cecum, which is a cul-de-sac located in the right iliac fossa (Fig. 1-7). The ileum connects with the upper portion of the cecum at the L5 level. The vermiform appendix usually arises from the cecum approximately one finger breadth (2 cm) inferior to the ileocecal junction. The large intestine continues in a superior direction above the ileocecal junction as the ascending colon. At the level of L2 the ascending colon makes a sharp turn to the left and continues as the transverse colon. This sharp turn is termed the right colic flexure, or hepatic flexure, since it is just below the liver. The transverse colon continues horizontally and slightly superiorly across the midline to the left side of the abdomen where it turns sharply inferior. This left colic flexure occurs at the L1 level, which is slightly more superior than the right colic flexure. The left colic flexure, located just below the spleen, sometimes is

termed the splenic flexure. The large intestine then continues inferiorly on the left side of the abdominal cavity as the descending colon. At the L4 level, the large intestine becomes somewhat tortuous and is called the sigmoid colon. The sigmoid colon then continues into the true pelvis and becomes the rectum in the midline at the S3 level.

The head of the pancreas can be found within the curve of the duodenum. It is usually described as being located at the level of L2 (Williams et al., 1989). The neck and body of the pancreas extend superiorly and obliquely to the left. The body of the pancreas ends as the tail of the pancreas, which can be found at the lower pole of the spleen in the left upper quadrant at T12. The superior pole of the spleen is adjacent to the left hemidiaphragm at about the level of T9.

The liver, the largest gland of the body, is found mostly in the upper right quadrant of the abdomen, but its left lobe does extend somewhat across the midline. Superiorly, the liver is in relation to the diaphragm and fills the domelike hollow of the right hemidiaphragm. The superior border of the liver therefore extends up to the T8 level. The inferior border runs diagonally from the right side of the abdomen at the level of L3 to the left hemidiaphragm at the T9 horizontal plane (Williams et al., 1989). The gallbladder rests in a fossa in the inferior border of the right lobe of the liver. The orifice of the gallbladder is usually found at the T12 level.

The urinary system begins with the kidneys. The superior poles of the kidneys lie at the level of T12 and their inferior poles at L3. The right kidney is slightly lower than the left kidney, probably because of its relationship with the liver (Williams et al., 1989). The suprarenal, or adrenal, glands are located on the anterosuperior borders of the kidneys. As with the kidneys, the left suprarenal gland is located somewhat more superior than the right. These endocrine glands can be found at the T11 and T12 levels, respectively. The hilum of the left kidney is just above the level of the L1 disc (transpyloric plane), and that of the right kidney just below it. A ureter arises from the hilum of each kidney, and both run to the bladder in an inferior and slightly medial direction. The bladder is a midline structure in the true pelvis posterior to the pubic symphysis at the coccygeal level. When distended the bladder may expand upward and forward into the abdominal cavity.

In the female the uterus lies posterior to the bladder and anterior to the rectum. Superiorly, the uterus extends above the superior border of the bladder to the lower sacral levels, and because of its anteverted and anteflexed position, the superior portion of the uterus usually lies on the posterior portion of the superior surface of the empty bladder. The ovaries are situated one on either side of the uterus near the lateral wall of the true pelvis. The position of the ovaries is variable, since they are displaced during the woman's first pregnancy and probably never return to their original position (Williams et al., 1989).

We hope that you will refer to this chapter often as you continue through the rest of this text. Knowledge of the structures of the body that are visible and palpable through the skin and an awareness of the surface locations of deeper structures are important tools in the proper examination and evaluation of patients. Therefore this chapter is designed not only as a beginning reference point for the rest of the text, but also as a quick reference for the health care provider.

REFERENCES

Basmajian, J.V. (1983). *Surface anatomy: An instruction manual.* Baltimore: Williams & Wilkins.

Fitzgerald, M.J.T. (1985). *Neuroanatomy basic & applied.* London: Bailliere Tindall.

Gardner, E., Gray, D.J., & O'Rahilly, R. (1975). *Anatomy.* Philadelphia: WB Saunders.

Keogh, B., & Ebbs, S. (1984). *Normal surface anatomy.* London: William Heinemann Medical Books.

Langman, J. (1975). *Medical embryology.* Baltimore: Williams & Wilkins.

Lumley, J.T. (1990). *Surface anatomy: The basis of clinical examination.* Edinburgh: Churchill Livingstone.

Moore, K.L. (1992). *Clinically oriented anatomy.* Baltimore: Williams & Wilkins.

Oliver, J., & Middleditch, A. (1991). *Functional anatomy of the spine.* Oxford: Butterworth-Heinemann.

Williams, P.L. et al., (Eds.). (1989). *Gray's anatomy* (ed 37). Edinburgh: Churchill Livingstone.

CHAPTER 2

General Characteristics of the Spine

Gregory D. Cramer

The purpose of this chapter is to discuss the basic and clinical anatomy of the spine as a whole, that is, to introduce many of the features that are common to the major regions of the spine (cervical, thoracic, and lumbar). Some of the topics listed are discussed in more detail in later chapters.

FUNCTION AND DEVELOPMENT OF THE SPINE

The anatomy of the human spine can best be understood if the functions are considered first. The spine has three primary functions: support of the body, protection of the spinal cord and spinal nerve roots, and movement of the trunk. These varied functions are carried out by a series of movable bones, called vertebrae, and the soft tissues that surround these bones. A brief explanation of the development of the vertebrae and the related soft tissues is given to highlight the detailed anatomy of these structures. A more thorough discussion of spinal development is presented in Chapter 12.

Development of the Spine

Following the early development of the neural groove into the neural tube and neural crest (see Fig. 12-5), paraxial mesoderm condenses to form somites (see Figs. 12-5 and 12-10 A). The somites, in turn, develop into dermatomes, myotomes, and sclerotomes. Dermatomes develop into the dermis and the subcutaneous tissue, whereas myotomes develop into the axial musculature. The sclerotomes migrate centrally to surround the neural tube and notochord (see Fig. 12-10 B). The sclerotomal cells then form the vertebral column and associated ligaments.

While the paraxial mesoderm is developing into somites, the more inferior portion of the neural tube differentiates into the ependymal, mantle, and marginal layers of the future spinal cord. The ependymal layer surrounds the future central canal region of the spinal cord. The mantle layer develops into the cells of the nervous system (neurons and glia), and the outer marginal layer of the tube consists of the axons of tract cells. The neural crest develops into the sensory neurons of the peripheral nervous system and the postganglionic neurons of the autonomic nervous system.

Chondrification Centers and Primary Ossification Centers. Cells of sclerotomal origin condense to form vertebral chondrification centers (three pairs). This results in the development of a cartilage model of each vertebra (see Fig. 12-11). Each vertebra then develops three primary centers of ossification (see Fig. 12-11). One primary center is located in the anterior part of the future vertebra. This region is known as the centrum and helps to form the future vertebral body. The remaining two primary ossification centers are located on each side of the portion of the vertebra that surrounds the developing neural tube. This region is known as the posterior arch or neural arch. The two ossification centers at the neural arch normally unite posteriorly to form the spinous process. Failure to fuse at these centers results in a condition known as spina bifida. This condition is discussed in more detail in Chapter 12.

Anteriorly, the left and right sides of the neural arch normally fuse to the vertebral body. Known as the neurocentral synchondrosis, this region is actually located within the area that becomes the posterior aspect of the vertebral body. The fusion that occurs unites the primary ossification centers of the neural arch with the centrum, consequently forming a vertebral body from both the centrum and a small part of the neural arch. Because of this the vertebral arch is somewhat smaller than its developmental predecessor, the neural arch, and the vertebral body is somewhat larger than its predecessor, the centrum.

The precise time of fusion between the neural arch and centrum at the neurocentral synchondrosis remains a topic of current investigation. Some authors state that closure occurs as early as 3 to 6 years of age, and other investigators state that the neurocentral cartilage remains until as late as 16 years of age (Vital et al., 1989). Part of the function of the neurocentral cartilage is to ensure growth of the posterior arch of the vertebrae. Early fusion of the neurocentral synchondrosis has been implicated in the development of scoliosis (Vital et al., 1989). Scoliosis is discussed in more detail in Chapter 6. Occasionally the vertebral body develops from two primary centers of ossification, left and right. If one of these centers fails to develop, only one half of the vertebral body remains. This is known as a cuneiform vertebra, or a hemivertebra, and can result in lateral curvature of the spine. Frequently a hemivertebra at one level is compensated for by the same condition at another level on the opposite side.

During development the vertebral bodies may appear to be wedge shaped—narrower anteriorly than posteriorly. This can give the appearance of a compression fracture (Fesmire & Luten, 1989). Wedging that occurs in several consecutive vertebrae is seen as an indication of a normal variant. However, if it occurs at only one level, and the vertebrae above and below are more rectangular in appearance, a compression fracture of the wedge-shaped vertebra must be ruled out.

Secondary Ossification Centers. Between the ages of 10 and 13, five secondary centers of ossification appear in the vertebral column (Fig. 12-11). One secondary center of ossification is located on each of the vertebral end plates. These centers are known as the annular epiphyses or ring epiphyses (Williams et al., 1989). A secondary center of ossification is also found on each of the transverse processes, and another is located on the single spinous process. The centers on the transverse processes and spinous process enable the rapid growth of these processes that occurs during the adolescent years.

The two centers of ossification associated with the upper and lower surfaces of the vertebral bodies (annular epiphyses) do not help with the longitudinal growth of the vertebral bodies and for this reason are frequently termed ring apophyses (Bogduk & Twomey, 1991; Theil, Clements, & Cassidy, 1992). These centers incorporate the outer layers of the anulus fibrosus (Fardon, 1988), which explains the bony attachment of the outer layers of the anulus, whereas the more central layers are attached to the cartilage of the vertebral end plates (Bogduk & Twomey, 1991).

All of the secondary ossification centers listed previously fuse with the remainder of the vertebrae between the ages of 14 and 25 (Bogduk & Twomey, 1991; Williams et al., 1989), and no further growth can occur after their fusion. Before they have fused, these centers can be mistaken as sites of fracture.

Fully Developed Vertebral Column. The first accurate description of the number of movable vertebrae in the fully developed spine was that of Galen between 100 and 200 AD (Shapiro, 1990). However, perhaps because of the many anatomic errors made by Galen in other areas, controversy ensued over the precise number of vertebrae until the publication of Vesalius' *De Humani Corporis Fabrica* in 1543 (Shapiro, 1990). This publication showed that the vertebral column develops into 24 vertebrae (Fig. 2-1), which are divided into 7 cervical, 12 thoracic, and 5 lumber vertebrae (expressed as C1-7, T1-12, and L1-5). The L5 vertebra rests upon the bony sacrum (made of five fused segments). The coccyx

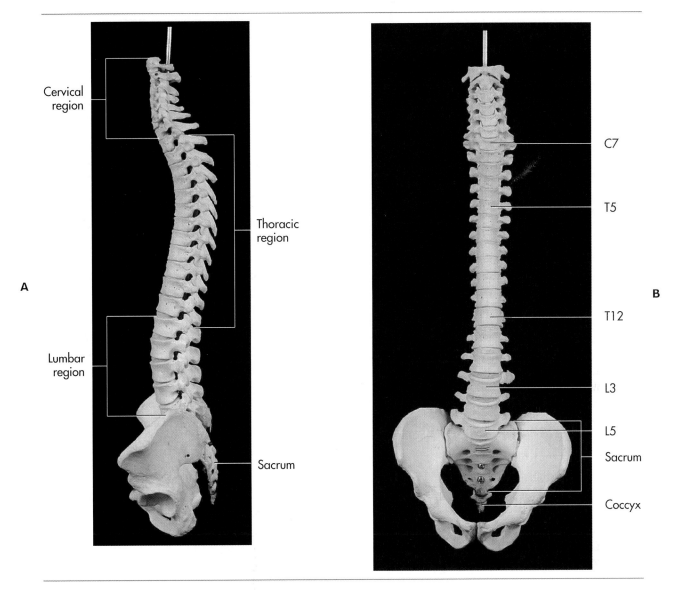

FIG. 2-1 Three views of the vertebral column. **A,** Lateral view showing the cervical, thoracic, lumbar, and sacral regions. Also notice the cervical and lumbar lordoses and the thoracic and sacral kyphoses. **B,** Anterior view. *Continued.*

(three to five fused segments) is suspended from the sacrum. All of these bones join to form the vertebral column.

CURVES OF THE SPINE

The spine develops four anterior to posterior curves, two kyphoses and two lordoses (see Introduction of text for further clarification of the terms lordosis and kyphosis). Kyphoses are curves that are concave anteriorly, and lordoses are curves that are concave posteriorly. The two primary curves are the kyphoses. These include the thoracic and pelvic curvatures (Fig. 2-1). They are referred to as primary curves because they are seen from

the earliest stages of fetal development. The thoracic curve extends from T2 to T12 and is created by the larger superior to inferior dimensions of the posterior portion of the thoracic vertebrae (see Chapter 6). The pelvic curve extends from the lumbosacral articulation throughout the sacrum to the tip of the coccyx. The concavity of the pelvic curve faces anteriorly and inferiorly.

The two secondary curves are the cervical lordosis and lumbar lordosis (Fig. 2-1). These curves are known as secondary or compensatory curves because even though they can be detected during fetal development, they do not become apparent until the postnatal period. The cervical lordosis begins late in intrauterine life but becomes apparent when an infant begins to lift his or

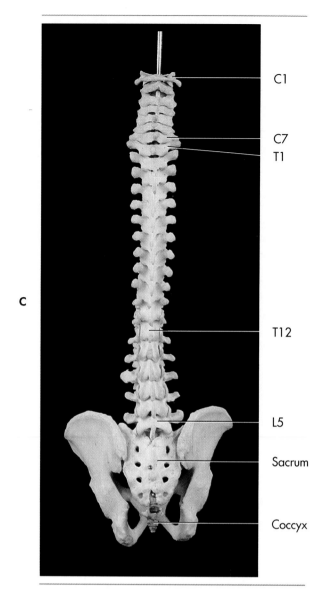

FIG. 2-1, cont'd. **C,** Posterior view of the vertebral column.

lumbosacral articulation and is more pronounced in females than in males. The region between L3 and the lumbosacral angle is more prominently lordotic than the region from T12 to L2. Following infancy, the lumbar lordosis is maintained by the shape of the intervertebral discs and the shape of the vertebral bodies. Each of these structures is taller anteriorly than posteriorly in the lumbar region of the spine.

A slight lateral curve is normally found in the upper thoracic region. The convexity of the curve is on the left in left-handed people and on the right in those who are right handed. Such deviations are probably the result of asymmetric muscle use and tone.

The kyphoses and lordoses of the spine, along with the intervertebral discs, help to absorb the loads applied to the spine. These loads include the weight of the trunk, along with loads applied through the lower extremities during walking, running, and jumping. In addition, loads are applied by carrying objects with the upper extremities, the pull of spinal muscles, and the wide variety of movements that normally occur in the spine. The spinal curves, acting with the intervertebral discs, dissipate the increased loads that would occur if the spine were shaped like a straight column. Yet even with these safeguards, the vertebrae can be fractured as a result of falling and landing on the feet or buttocks, objects falling onto the head, or diving and landing on the head. Such injuries usually compress the vertebral bodies. Cervical compression usually occurs between C4 to C6 (Foreman & Croft, 1988). When the force comes from below, T9 through L2 are the most commonly affected through compression. Flexion injuries can also result in a compression fracture of vertebral bodies. Again, C4 through C6 are the most commonly affected in the cervical region, whereas T5 and T6 and the upper lumbar vertebrae are usually affected in the thoracic and lumbar regions (White & Panjabi, 1990).

ANATOMY OF A TYPICAL VERTEBRA

A typical vertebra can be divided into two basic regions, a vertebral body and a vertebral arch (also referred to as the posterior arch or dorsal arch). The bone in both regions is composed of an outer layer of compact bone and a core of trabecular bone (Fig. 2-2). The shell of compact bone is thin on the discal surfaces of the vertebral body and is thicker in the vertebral arch and its processes. The outer compact bone is covered by a thin layer of periosteum that is innervated by nerve endings, which transmit both nociception and proprioception (Edgar & Ghadially, 1976). The outer compact bone also contains many small foramina to allow passage for numerous nutrient arteries and also for veins. The trabecular interior of a vertebra contains red marrow and one or two large canals for the basivertebral vein(s).

her head from the prone position (approximately 3 to 4 months after birth). This forces the cervical spine into a lordotic curve. The cervical lordosis is further accentuated when the small child begins to sit upright and stabilizes his or her head, while looking around in the seated position. This occurs at approximately 9 months of age. Further details of the cervical curvature are given in Chapter 5.

The action of the erector spinae muscles (Chapter 4), pulling the lumbar spine erect in order to achieve the position necessary for walking, creates the posterior concavity known as the lumbar lordosis (Fig. 2-1). The lumbar lordosis therefore develops approximately 10 to 18 months after birth as the infant begins to walk upright. The lumbar lordosis extends from T12 to the

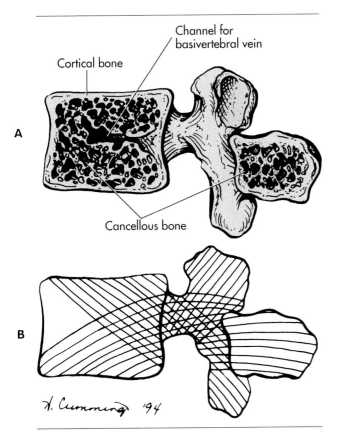

Cortical bone

Channel for
basivertebral vein

Cancellous bone

A

B

A. Cummings '94

FIG. 2-2 Midsagittal view of a vertebra. **A,** The central cancellous, or trabecular bone of the vertebral body and spinous process. Also, notice the more peripheral cortical bone. **B,** The pattern of trabeculation, which develops along the lines of greatest stress.

The density of bone in the vertebrae varies from individual to individual but seems to increase significantly in most people during puberty (Gilsanz, 1988), reaching a peak during the midtwenties, when closure of the growth plates of the secondary centers of ossification occurs (Gilsanz et al., 1988). A decrease in bone density to below normal limits is known as osteoporosis. Osteoporosis is of particular clinical relevance in the spine because of the weight-bearing function of this region, and a decrease in bone density increases the likelihood of vertebral fracture (Mosekilde & Mosekilde, 1990). Osteoporosis has been associated with aging (Mosekilde & Mosekilde, 1990) and particularly with menopause (Ribot et al., 1988). Ribot and colleagues (1988) found that spinal bone density in French women remained stable in the young adult years and in women over 70 years of age. An average rate of apparent bone loss of approximately 1% per year was found between the years of 45 and 65. This represented approximately 75% of the total bone loss occurring within the individuals of their sample population (510 women). Ribot and colleagues (1988) also found that the bone mineral

density in their population of French women appeared to be between 5% and 10% lower than reported values in the United States. Mosekilde and Mosekilde (1990), studying the L2 and L3 vertebrae, found relatively few sex-related differences in vertebral body density. However, Mosekilde (1989) did find a sex-related difference in vertebral trabecular architecture with age. Consistent with the findings of Ribot et al. (1988), Mosekilde (1989) discovered that in both sexes bone density diminished by 35% to 40% from 20 to 80 years of age. She also found that the trabecular center (cancellous bone) of the vertebral body lost more bone mass than the outer cortical rim.

The regions of the vertebral body and the vertebral arch are discussed separately in the following sections of this chapter. Elaboration on each component of the vertebra, with special emphasis placed on the characteristics unique to each region of the spine, is included in the chapters on the cervical, thoracic, and lumbar regions of the spine (Chapters 5 through 7). The ligaments of the spine are discussed from superior to inferior with the region in which they first occur (e.g., ligamentum nuchae and anterior longitudinal ligament with the cervical spine; supraspinous ligament with the thoracic spine). Thereafter, the ligaments are mentioned only when they have unique characteristics in a specific region. The intervertebral disc is covered later in this chapter.

Vertebral Body

The vertebral body (Fig. 2-3) is the large anterior portion of a vertebra that acts to support the weight of the human frame. The vertebral bodies are connected to one another by fibrocartilaginous intervertebral discs. The vertebral bodies, combined with their intervening discs, create a flexible column or pillar that supports the weight of the trunk and head. The vertebral bodies also must be able to withstand additional forces from contraction of the axial and proximal limb muscles. The bodies are cylindric in shape and have unique characteristics in each named region of the spine. The transverse diameter of the vertebral bodies increases from C2 to L3. This is probably due to the fact that each successive vertebral body is required to carry a slightly greater load. There is variation in the width of the last two lumbar vertebrae, but the width steadily diminishes from the first sacral segment to the apex (inferior tip) of the coccyx.

Moskilde and Moskilde (1990) found the cross-sectional area of vertebral bodies to be larger in men than in women. They also found that the cross-sectional area of the vertebral bodies increased with age in men, but no similar finding was discovered in women.

The superior and inferior surfaces of vertebral bodies range from flat, but not parallel (Williams et al., 1989), to

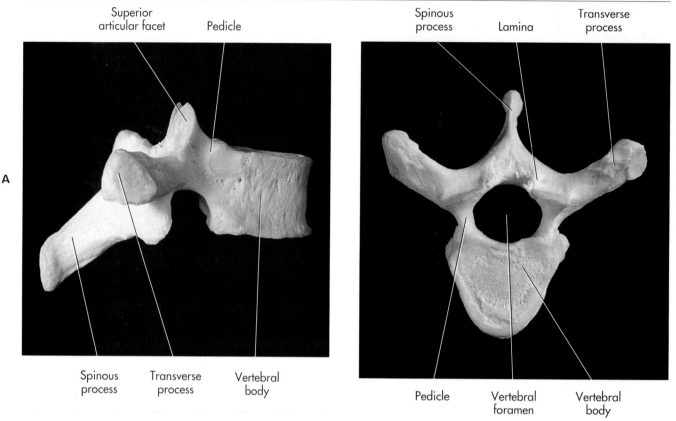

FIG. 2-3 Typical vertebra. **A,** Lateral view. **B,** Superior view.

interlocking (see Cervical region, Chapter 5). A raised, smooth region around the edge of the vertebral body is formed by the annular epiphysis. Inside the annular epiphysis, the vertebral body is rough.

Most vertebral bodies are concave posteriorly (in the transverse plane) where they help to form the vertebral foramina. Small foramina for arteries and veins appear on the front and sides of the vertebral bodies. Posteriorly there are small arterial foramina and one or two large, centrally placed foramina for the exiting basivertebral vein(s) (Williams et al., 1989).

Vertebral Arch

The vertebral (posterior) arch has several unique structures (Fig. 2-3). These include the pedicles, laminae, superior articular, inferior articular, transverse, and spinous processes. Each of these subdivisions of the vertebral arch is discussed separately in the following sections.

   Pedicles. The pedicles (Fig. 2-3) create the narrow anterior portion of the vertebral arch. They are short, thick, and rounded and attach to the posterior and lateral aspects of the vertebral body. They also are placed

superior to the midpoint of a vertebral body. Because the pedicles are smaller than the vertebral bodies, a groove, or vertebral notch, is formed above and below the pedicles. These are known as the superior and inferior vertebral notches, respectively. The superior vertebral notch is more shallow and smaller than the inferior vertebral notch.

The percentage of compact bone surrounding the inner cancellous bone of the pedicles varies from one region of the spine to another and seems to depend on the amount of motion that occurs at the given region (Pal et al., 1988). More compact, stronger bone is found in regions with more motion. Therefore the pedicles of the middle cervical and upper lumbar regions contain more compact bone than the relatively immobile thoracic region. The thoracic pedicles are made primarily of cancellous bone (Pal et al., 1988).

   Laminae. The laminae (singular, *lamina*) are continuous with the pedicles. They are flattened from anterior to posterior and form the broad posterior portion of vertebral arch (Fig. 2-3). They curve posteromedially to unite with the spinous process, completing the vertebral foramen.

Spinous
process   Lamina

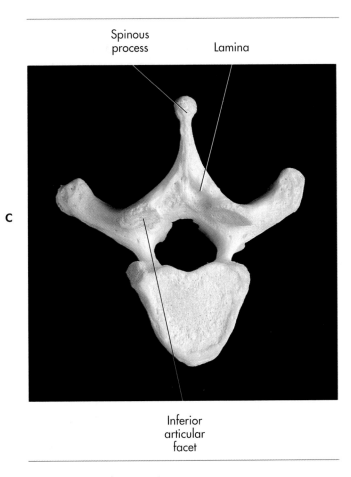

C

Inferior
articular
facet

FIG. 2-3, cont'd.   C, Inferior view.

Spinous Process. The spinous process (spine) of each vertebra (Fig. 2-3) projects posteriorly and often inferiorly from the laminae. The size, shape, and direction of this process vary greatly from one region of the vertebral column to the next (see individual regions). A spinous process may also normally deviate to the left or right of the midline, and this can be a source of confusion in clinical practice.

Therefore a deviated spinous process seen on x-ray film or palpated during a physical examination frequently is not associated with a fracture of the spinous process or a malposition of the entire vertebra.

The spinous processes throughout the spine function as a series of levers both for muscles of posture and for muscles of active movement (Williams et al., 1989). Most of the muscles that attach to the spinous processes act to extend the vertebral column. Some muscles attaching to the spinous processes also rotate the vertebrae to which they attach.

Lateral to the spinous processes are the vertebral grooves. These grooves are formed by laminae in the cervical and lumbar regions. They are much broader in the thoracic region and are formed by both the laminae and transverse processes. The left and right vertebral

grooves serve as gutters. These gutters are filled with the deep back muscles that course the entire length of the spine.

The spinous processes of a specific vertebra frequently can be identified by its relationship to other palpable landmarks of the back. Chapter 1 provides a rather detailed account of the relationship between the spinous processes and other anatomic structures.

Vertebral Foramen and the Vertebral Canal. The vertebral foramen is the opening within each vertebra that is bounded by the structures discussed thus far. Therefore the vertebral body, the left and right pedicles, the left and right laminae, and the spinous process form the borders of the vertebral foramen in a typical vertebra (Fig. 2-3). The size and shape of the vertebral foramina vary from one region of the spine to the next, and even from one vertebra to the next. The vertebral canal is the composite of all of the vertebral foramina. This region houses the spinal cord, nerve roots, meninges, and many vessels. The vertebral canal is discussed in more detail later in this chapter.

Transverse Processes. The transverse processes project laterally from the junction of the pedicle and the lamina (pediculolaminar junction) (Fig. 2-3). Like the spinous processes, their exact direction varies considerably from one region of the spine to the next. The transverse processes of typical cervical vertebrae project obliquely anteriorly between the sagittal and coronal planes and are located anterior to the articular processes and lateral to the pedicles. The left and right cervical transverse processes are separated from those of the vertebrae above and below by successive intervertebral foramina. The thoracic transverse processes are quite different and project obliquely posteriorly and are located behind the articular processes, pedicles, and the intervertebral foramina (see Fig. 6-1). They also articulate with the ribs. The lumbar transverse processes (see Fig. 7-1) lie in front of the lumbar articular processes and posterior to the pedicles and the intervertebral foramina.

The transverse processes serve as muscle attachment sites and are used as lever arms by spinal muscles. The muscles that attach to the transverse processes maintain posture and induce rotation and lateral flexion of single vertebrae and the spine as a whole.

Each transverse process is composed of the "true" transverse process (diapophysis) and a costal element. Each costal element (pleurapophysis) develops as part of the neural arch. The costal elements of the thoracic region develop into ribs. Elsewhere the costal elements are incorporated with the diapophysis and help to form the transverse process of the fully developed vertebra. The cervical costal elements are composed primarily of the anterior tubercle but also include the intertubercular lamella and a part of the posterior tubercle. The lumbar costal elements are the anterior aspects of the transverse processes, and the left and right sacral alae represent the costal processes of the sacrum. The cervical and lumbar costal processes may occasionally develop into ribs. This occurs most frequently in the lower cervical and upper lumbar regions. These extra ribs may be a cause of discomfort in some individuals. This is particularly true of cervical ribs (see Chapter 5).

Superior Articular Processes. Like the transverse processes, the superior articular processes (zygapophyses) and facets also arise from the pediculolaminar junction (Fig. 2-3). The superior articular processes project superiorly, and the articular surface (facet) faces posteriorly, although the precise direction varies from posteromedial in the cervical and lumbar regions to posterolateral in the thoracic region. The superior and inferior articular facets are discussed in more detail under Zygapophyseal Joints later in this chapter.

Inferior Articular Processes. The inferior articular processes (zygapophyses) and facets project inferiorly from the pediculolaminar junction, and the articular surface (facet) faces anteriorly (Fig. 2-3). Again, the precise direction in which they face varies from anterolateral (cervical region) to anteromedial (thoracic and lumbar regions).

Adjoining zygapophyses form zygapophyseal joints (Z joints), which are small and allow for limited movement. Mobility at the Z joints varies considerably between vertebral levels. The Z joints also help to form the posterior border of the intervertebral foramen. The anatomy of the Z joint is discussed later in this chapter.

Functional Components of a Typical Vertebra

Each region of a typical vertebra is related to one or more of the functions of the vertebral column mentioned at the beginning of this chapter (support, protection of the spinal cord and spinal nerve roots, and movement). In general, the vertebral bodies help with support, whereas the pedicles and laminae protect the spinal cord. The superior and inferior articular processes help determine spinal movement by the facing of their facets. The transverse and spinous processes aid movement by acting as lever arms upon which the muscles of the spine act.

The posterior arches also act to support and transfer weight (Pal et al., 1988), and the articular processes of the cervical region form two distinct pillars (left and right) that bear weight. In addition, the laminae of C2, C7, and the upper thoracic region (T1 and T2) are much thicker than those of their neighbors. These

specific laminae also help to support weight. Therefore a laminectomy at these levels results in marked cervical instability (Pal et al., 1988), whereas a laminectomy from C3 to C6 is relatively safe.

The pedicles also act to transfer weight from the posterior arch to the vertebral body, and vice versa, in the cervical region (Pal et al., 1988), but only from the posterior arch to the vertebral bodies in the thoracic region. The role of the pedicles in the transfer of loads is yet to be completely determined in the upper lumbar region, but the trabecular pattern of the L4 and L5 pedicles seems to indicate that the majority of load may be transferred from the vertebral bodies to the region of the posterior arch. This is discussed in further detail in Chapter 7, which is devoted to the lumbar spine.

ZYGAPOPHYSEAL JOINTS

The articulating surface of each superior and inferior articular process (zygapophysis) is covered with a 1 to 2 mm thick layer of hyaline cartilage. The hyaline-lined portion of a superior and inferior articular process is known as the articular facet. The junction between the superior and inferior articular facets on one side of two adjacent vertebrae is known as a zygapophyseal joint. Therefore a left and right Z joint are between each pair of vertebrae. Fig. 2-4, *A*, shows the Z joints of the cervical, thoracic, and lumbar regions. These joints are also referred to as facet joints or interlaminar joints (Giles, 1992). The Z joints (Fig. 2-4, *B*) are classified as synovial (diarthrodial), planar joints. They are rather small joints, and although they allow motion to occur, they are perhaps more important in their ability to determine the direction and limitations of movement that can occur between vertebrae. The Z joint is of added interest to those who treat spinal conditions because, as is the case in any joint, loss of motion or aberrant motion may be a primary source of pain (Paris, 1983).

Each Z joint is surrounded posterolaterally by a capsule. The capsule consists of an outer layer of dense fibroelastic connective tissue, a vascular central layer made up of areolar tissue and loose connective tissue, and an inner layer consisting of a synovial membrane (Giles & Taylor, 1987). Fig. 2-4, *B*, shows the previously listed regions of the capsule. The anterior and medial aspects of the Z joint are covered by the ligamentum flavum. The synovial membrane lines the articular capsule, the ligamentum flavum (Xu et al., 1991), and the synovial joint folds (see the following), but not the hyaline articular cartilage that covers the joint surfaces of the articular processes (Giles, 1992).

The Z joint capsules throughout the vertebral column are thin and loose and are attached to the margins of the opposed superior and inferior articular facets of the adjacent vertebrae (Williams et al., 1989). Superior and inferior external protrusions of the joint capsules,

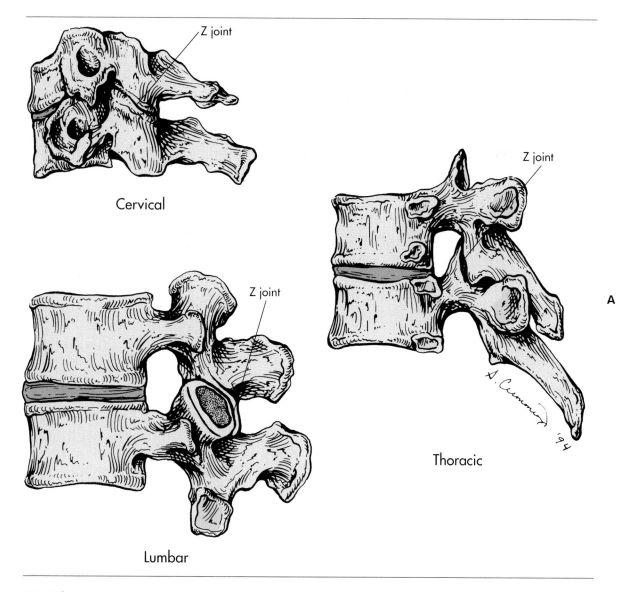

FIG. 2-4   **A,** Typical Z joints of each vertebral region.

Continued.

known as recesses, bulge out from the joint and are filled with adipose tissue. The inferior recess is larger than the superior recess (Jeffries, 1988). The capsules are longer and looser in the cervical region than in the lumbar and thoracic regions.

Innervation of the Zygapophyseal Joints

The Z joint capsule receives a rich supply of sensory innervation (Fig. 2-5). The sensory supply is derived from the medial branch of the posterior primary division (dorsal ramus) at the level of the joint, and each joint also receives a branch from the medial branch of the posterior primary division of the level above and the level below (Jeffries, 1988). This multilevel innervation is probably one reason why pain from a Z joint frequently has a very broad referral pattern (Jeffries, 1988). Chapter 11 deals with the phenomenon of referred pain in more detail.

In addition, Wyke (1985) states that there are three types of sensory receptors in the joint capsule of the Z joints. These are as follows*:

◆ Type I—very sensitive static and dynamic mechanoreceptors that fire continually, even to some extent when the joint is not moving
◆ Type II—less sensitive mechanoreceptors that fire only during movement
◆ Type IV—slow conducting nociceptive mechanoreceptors

Wyke (1985) asserts that type I and II receptors have a pain suppressive effect (a Melzack and Wall gate control type of mechanism). He also states that there is a reflexogenic effect created by type I and II fibers that causes a normalization of muscle activity on both sides

---

*Type III receptors are nociceptive fibers found in joints of the extremities, and Wyke (1985) did not find these in the Z joints.

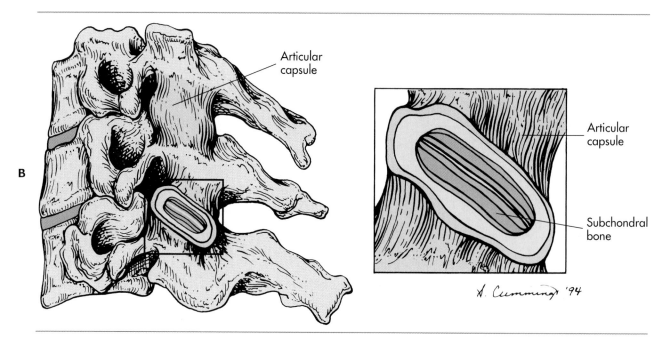

FIG. 2-4, cont'd.   B, Typical Z joint. The layers of the Z joint as seen in parasagittal section *(inset)* are color coded as follows: *light blue,* joint space; *violet,* articular cartilage; *brown,* subchondral bone; *orange,* synovial lining of articular capsule; *peach,* vascularized, middle layer of the articular capsule; *turquoise,* fibrous, outer layer of the articular capsule.

of the spinal column when stimulated. This reflexogenic effect is thought to occur at the level of the site of stimulation, as well as the levels above and below. Of possible interest is the fact that Isherwood and Antoun (1980) found similar nerve endings within the interspinous and supraspinous ligaments and the ligamentum flavum. These ligaments are discussed in Chapters 5 and 6 on the cervical and thoracic regions.

Zygapophyseal Joint Synovial Folds

Z joint synovial folds are synovium-lined extensions of the capsule that protrude into the joint space to cover part of the hyaline cartilage. The synovial folds vary in size and shape in the different regions of the spine. Fig. 2-6 shows a photomicrograph by Singer, Giles, and Day (1990) demonstrating a large Z joint synovial fold.

Kos in 1969 described the typical intraarticular fold (meniscus) (Fig. 2-7) as being attached to the capsule by loose connective tissue. Distal to the attachment was synovial tissue and blood vessels, followed by dense connective tissue (Bogduk & Engel, 1984).

Engle and Bogduk in 1982 reported on a study of 82 lumbar Z joints. They found at least one intraarticular fold within each joint. The intraarticular structures were categorized into three types. The first was described as a connective tissue rim found running along the most peripheral edge of the entire joint. This con-

nective tissue rim was lined by a synovial membrane. The second type of meniscus was described as an adipose tissue pad, and the third type was identified as a distinct, well-defined, fibroadipose meniscoid. This latter type of meniscus was usually found entering the joint from either the superior or inferior pole or both poles of the joint.

Giles and Taylor (1987) studied 30 Z joints, all of which were found to have menisci. The menisci were renamed zygapophyseal joint synovial folds because of their histologic make-up. Free nerve endings were found within the folds, and the nerve endings met the criteria necessary for classification as pain receptors (nociceptors). That is, they were distant from blood vessels and were of proper diameter (6 to 12 microns). Therefore the synovial folds (menisci) themselves were found to be pain sensitive. This meant that if the Z joint synovial fold became compressed by, or trapped between, the articular facets making up the Z joint, back pain could result (Fig. 2-7).

Zygapophyseal Joints as a Source of Back Pain

Various Clinical Approaches to Pain Management. The Z joints have been shown to be a source of back pain (Mooney & Robertson, 1976; Lippitt, 1984; Jeffries, 1988), and several therapeutic approaches have been designed to treat pain originating from the Z joints.

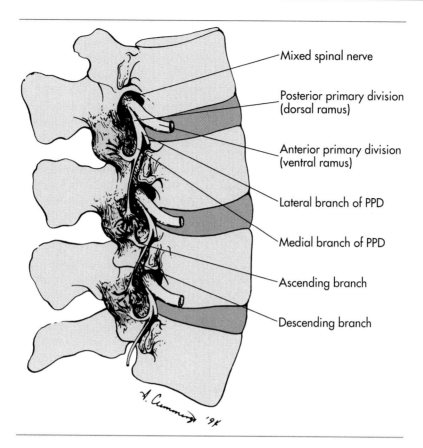

- Mixed spinal nerve
- Posterior primary division (dorsal ramus)
- Anterior primary division (ventral ramus)
- Lateral branch of PPD
- Medial branch of PPD
- Ascending branch
- Descending branch

FIG. 2-5 Innervation of the Z joints. Each mixed spinal nerve divides into a medial and lateral branch. The medial branch has an ascending division, which supplies the Z joint at the same level, and a descending division, which supplies the Z joint immediately below.

Physical therapy in the form of ice, moist heat, or exercise is frequently used. Acupuncture has also been used. Injection of the Z joints with local anesthetic or corticosteroids is carried out with some frequency, and denervation of the Z joints has been performed by a number of clinicians and researchers (Shealy, 1975). Surgical transection of the posterior primary divisions innervating these joints was the first method used to denervate the joint. This technique has been replaced by radiofrequency neurotomy (Shealy, 1975). Others are not yet convinced that this is the method of choice for treating pain arising from these structures (Lippitt, 1984). Spinal adjusting (manipulation) to introduce movement into a Z joint suspected of being hypomobile has also been frequently used to treat pain of Z joint origin. Mooney and Robertson (1976) stated that spinal manipulation may produce therapeutic benefit by relieving the Z joint articular capsule or its synovial lining from chronic reaction to trauma. Such chronic reaction to trauma resulting in Z joint pain would include the catching of a synovial fold between the joint capsule and an articular process and also the entrapment of zygapophyseal joint menisci (synovial folds) deep within the Z joint (Fig. 2-7).

Entrapped Z joint menisci may be a direct source of pain since they are supplied by pain-sensitive nerve endings (Giles & Taylor, 1987). A spinal adjustment (manipulation) may have the effect of slightly separating (gapping) the opposed articular surfaces of the Z joint. This separation may relieve direct pressure on the meniscus, and also provide traction to the Z joint articular capsule that, by its attachment to the Z joint meniscus, could pull the meniscus peripherally, away from the region of previous entrapment (Kos & Wolf, 1972). Bogduk and Engel (1984) felt that entrapment of a Z joint meniscus would tear it away from its capsular attachment. If this were the case, the nerve endings leading to the synovial fold would probably be torn as well. This could result in transient pain. Bogduk and Engel (1984) also stated that a meniscus that had torn away from its capsular attachment could conceivably result in a loose body being found in the Z joint, similar to those that are sometimes found in the knee. This, they felt, may be amenable to spinal manipulation. However, the frequency with which this scenario actually occurs in clinical practice was questioned (Bogduk & Engel, 1984). Further research is needed to clarify the frequency with which

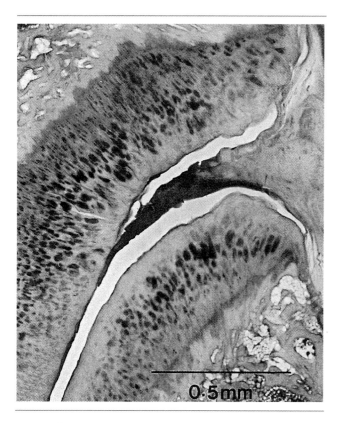

FIG. 2-6 A fibrous synovial fold is shown protruding between the articular surfaces of a Z joint. (From Singer, K., Giles, D., & Day R. [1990] Intra-articular synovial folds of thoracolumbar junction zygapophyseal joints. *Anat Rec, 226,* 147-152.)

Z joint menisci (synovial folds) actually tear away from their capsular attachments to become loose bodies. Additional study is also needed to determine whether menisci can become entrapped while remaining attached to the capsule and their nerve supply.

Mooney and Robertson (1976) used facet joint injections of local anesthetic and corticosteroids to treat pain arising from the Z joint. They felt such injections helped to relieve intraarticular adhesions that had been seen to develop during the degenerative phase of progressive back pain. Perhaps the removal of this type of adhesion could be another positive effect of Z joint manipulation.

MOVEMENT OF THE SPINE

Movement between two typical adjacent vertebrae is slight, but when the movement between many segments is combined, the result is a great deal of movement. The movements that can occur in the spine include flexion, extension, lateral flexion (side bending), rotation, and circumduction (Fig. 2-8). Circumduction is a combination of flexion, lateral bending, rotation, and extension.

The intervertebral discs help to limit the amount of movement that can occur between individual vertebrae. Therefore the thicker intervertebral discs of the cervical and lumbar regions allow for more movement to occur in these regions. In addition, the shape and orientation of the articular facets determine the movements that can occur between two adjacent segments and also limit the amount of movement that can occur between segments.

The specific ranges of motion of the spine are discussed with each vertebral region (Chapters 5 through 7). However, this section discusses the factors limiting spinal motion and the phenomenon of coupled motion.

Structures that Limit Spinal Movement

Spinal motion is limited by a series of bony stops and ligamentous brakes (Louis, 1985). Table 2-1 shows some of the structures limiting spinal motion.

Other factors associated with each type of spinal motion include the following:

- Flexion—the anterior longitudinal ligament is relaxed, and the anterior aspects of the discs are compressed. The intervals between laminae are widened; the inferior articular processes glide upward on the superior articular processes of the subjacent vertebrae. The lumbar and cervical regions allow for more flexion than the thoracic region (Williams et al., 1989).
- Extension—motion is more restricted in the thoracic region because of thinner discs and the effects of the thoracic skeleton and musculature.
- Lateral flexion—sides of the intervertebral discs are compressed. Lateral flexion is greatest in the cervical region, followed by the lumbar region, and finally the thoracic region (White & Panjabi, 1990).

Rotation with Lateral Flexion

As a result of the facing of the superior and inferior articular facets, lateral flexion of the cervical and lumbar regions is accompanied by axial rotation (Fig. 2-9). This is known as coupled motion. However, the direction of the rotation is opposite in these two regions, and more rotation occurs with lateral flexion in the cervical region than in the lumbar region (Moroney et al., 1988). Lateral flexion of the cervical spine is accompanied by rotation of the vertebral bodies into the concavity of the arch formed by the lateral flexion (vertebral body rotation to the same side as lateral flexion). For example, right lateral flexion of the cervical region is accompanied by right rotation of the vertebral bodies (Fig. 2-9). Since the spinous processes move in the direction opposite that of the vertebral bodies during rotation, right lateral flexion of the cervical region is accompanied by left rotation of the spinous processes.

Lateral flexion of the lumbar spine, on the other hand, is accompanied by rotation of the vertebral bodies

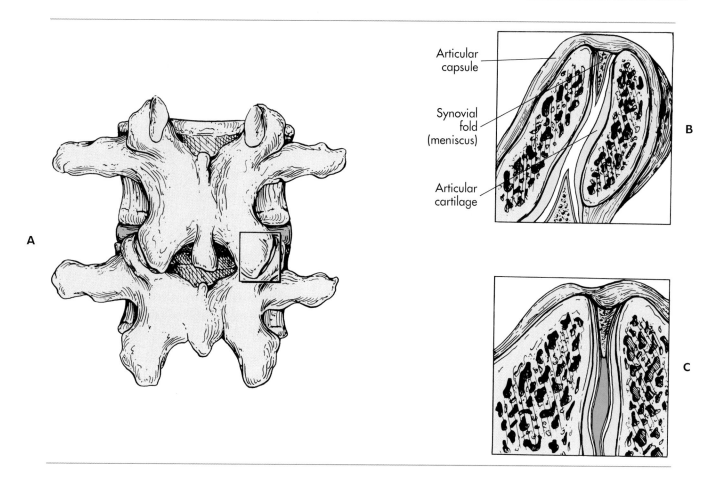

FIG. 2-7 Z joint synovial folds. **A,** Posterior view of the lumbar Z joint. **B,** A coronal section similar to that demonstrated in A. This coronal section shows the Z joint synovial folds. Notice the synovial lining of these folds, the articular cartilage, and the joint space. The synovial fold is attached to the articular capsule. **C,** An entrapped synovial fold. The distal portion of the fold is fibrous, and the proximal portion contains vessels and adipose tissue. Giles and Taylor (1987) have also found sensory nerve endings within the Z joint synovial folds.

toward the convexity of the arch formed by lateral flexion (vertebral body rotation away from the side of lateral flexion). For example, left lateral flexion of the lumbar region is accompanied by right rotation of the vertebral bodies and left rotation of the spinous processes (Fig. 2-9).

The upper four thoracic vertebrae move in a fashion similar to that of the cervical vertebrae during lateral flexion (i.e., vertebral body rotation into the side of concavity), whereas the lower four thoracic vertebrae mimic the motion of lumbar vertebrae (i.e., vertebral body rotation toward the side of convexity). The middle four thoracic vertebrae have little coupled motion (White & Panjabi, 1990).

INTERBODY JOINT AND INTERVERTEBRAL DISC

The intervertebral discs (IVDs) are structures of extreme clinical importance. IVD disease can be not only a pri-

mary source of back pain, but also can result in compression of exiting dorsal roots and spinal nerves, which can result in radicular symptoms. A thorough knowledge of the IVD is essential for those who treat disorders of the spine. This section discusses those aspects of the IVD common to all regions of the spine. Future chapters discuss those characteristics of the IVD unique to the cervical, thoracic, and lumbar regions.

The IVDs develop from the notochord and from somitic mesenchyme (sclerotome). The somitic mesenchyme surrounds the notochordal cells and differentiates into the 12 to 20 relatively thin layers that make up the anulus fibrosus. The notochordal tissue becomes the centrally located nucleus pulposus. Notochordal cells are replaced in the neighboring vertebral body by osteoblasts and in the cartilage end plate primarily by chondroblasts. However, remnants of notochordal cells in the cartilage end plate (see the following discussion) can cause it to weaken. This can lead to herniation of the nucleus pulposus into the cartilage end plate and

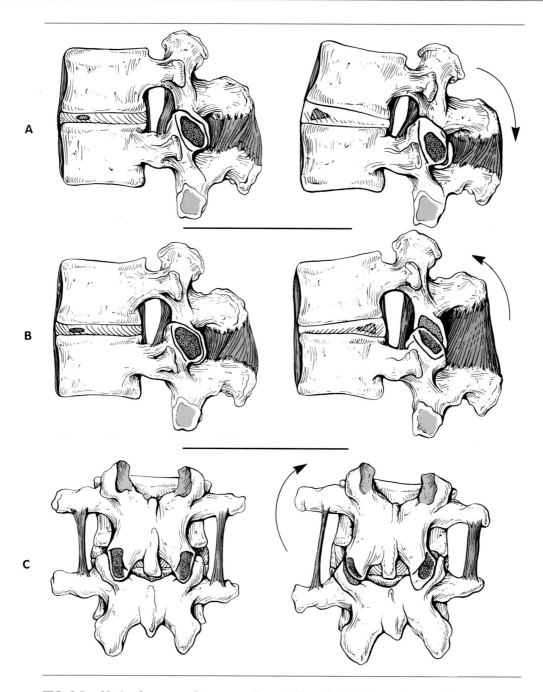

FIG. 2-8 Motion between adjacent vertebrae. **A** through **C**, *Left*, Vertebrae in their neutral position. **A**, *Right*, Vertebrae in extension. The anterior longitudinal ligament is becoming taut. **B**, *Right*, Vertebrae in flexion. Notice that the interspinous and supraspinous ligaments, as well as the ligamentum flavum, are being stretched. **C**, *Right*, Vertebrae in lateral flexion. The left intertransverse ligament is becoming taut, and the right superior articular process is making contact with the right lamina.

vertebral body later in life. This type of herniation is known as a Schmorl's node and can result in more rapid degeneration of the IVD.

During the fetal stage and shortly after birth, the IVDs have a rich vascular supply. However, the blood vessels narrow and diminish in number until the second decade

of life, when the IVD is almost completely avascular (Taylor, 1990).

Each IVD is located between adjacent vertebral bodies from C2 to the interbody joint between L5 and the first sacral segment (Fig. 2-1). The joint formed by two adjacent vertebral bodies and the interposed IVD is classified

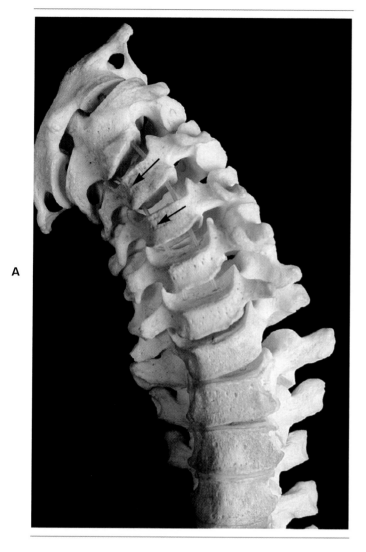

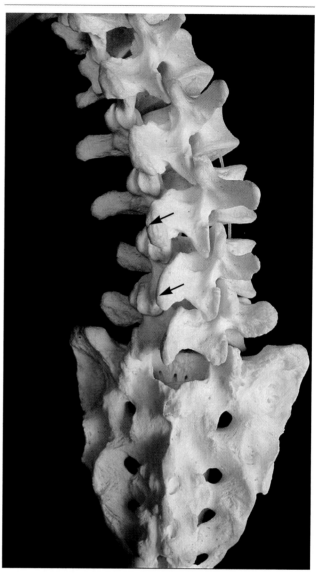

FIG. 2-9 Coupled motion. **A,** Lateral flexion of the cervical region results in concomitant axial rotation of the vertebrae. The cervical vertebral bodies rotate toward the side of lateral flexion. **B,** Lateral flexion of the lumbar region results in axial rotation to the opposite side. The lumbar vertebral bodies in this case rotate away from the side of lateral flexion, and the spinous processes rotate into the side of lateral flexion.

as a symphysis (Williams et al., 1989). No disc is located between the occiput and the atlas and the atlas and the axis, but a small disc exists between the sacrum and the coccyx. Therefore 24 IVDs are located in the spine: 6 cervical, 12 thoracic, 5 lumbar (including the L5-S1 disc), and 1 between the sacrum and coccyx. Occasionally a small disc remains between the first and second coccygeal segments, and additional discs are sometimes found between the fused sacral segments (these can frequently be seen well on magnetic resonance imaging scans). The IVDs make up approximately one fourth of the height of the vertebral column (Coventry, 1969). Because of the strong and intimate connections with the

vertebral bodies of two adjacent vertebrae, the IVD and the adjacent vertebrae constitute the most fundamental components of the vertebral unit, or motor segment. The function of the disc is to maintain the changeable space between two adjacent vertebral bodies. The disc aids with flexibility of the spine and at the same time acts as a shock absorber, helping to properly assimilate compressive loads. The mechanical efficiency of the healthy disc appears to improve with use. Therefore pathologic changes within the disc have a strong impact on spinal biomechanics (Humzah & Soames, 1988).

The discs are usually named by using the two vertebrae that surround the disc, for example the C4-C5 disc

Table 2-1 Factors Limiting Spinal Motion

Motion	Structures limiting motion
Flexion	Posterior longitudinal ligament
	Ligamenta flava
	Interspinous ligament
	Supraspinous ligament
	Posterior fibers of the intervertebral disc
	Articular capsules
	Tension of back extensor muscles
	Anterior surface of inferior articular facet against posterior surface of superior articular facet
Extension	Anterior longitudinal ligament
	Anterior aspect of intervertebral disc
	Approximation of spinous processes, articular processes, and laminae
Lateral flexion	Contralateral side of intervertebral disc and intertransverse ligament
	Approximation of articular processes
	Approximation of uncinate processes (cervical region)
	Approximation of costovertebral joints (thoracic region)
	Antagonist muscles
Rotation	Tightening of lamellar fibers of anulus fibrosus
	Orientation and architecture of articular processes

Data from Williams et al. (1989). *Gray's Anatomy* (37th ed). Edinburgh: Churchill Livingstone.

or the T7-T8 disc. A disc also may be named by referring to the vertebra directly above the disc. For example, the C6 disc is the IVD directly below C6. This can be more easily remembered if the vertebra is pictured as "sitting" on its disc (W. Hogan, personal communication, November 15, 1991).

The shape of an IVD is determined by the shape of the two vertebral bodies to which it is attached. The thickness of the IVDs varies from one part of the spine to the next. The discs are thickest in the lumbar region and thinnest in the upper thoracic region (Williams et al., 1989). The cervical discs are about two fifths as tall as the vertebral bodies, the thoracic discs about one fifth as tall as their vertebral bodies, and the lumbar discs about one third the height of lumbar vertebral bodies. The discs of the cervical and lumbar regions are thicker anteriorly than posteriorly, helping to create the lordoses found in these regions (Williams et al., 1989). The thoracic discs have a consistent thickness from anterior to posterior.

The discs are connected to the anterior and posterior longitudinal ligaments. The attachment to the posterior longitudinal ligament is firm throughout the spine. The anterior longitudinal ligament generally has a strong attachment to the periosteum of the vertebral bodies, particularly at the most superior and inferior aspects of the anterior vertebral bodies, but this ligament has a rather loose attachment to the anterior aspect of the intervertebral disc (Humzah & Soames, 1988). However, Panjabi, Oxland, & Parks (1991) have found a strong discal attachment to the anterior longitudinal ligament in the cervical region. The thoracic discs are also connected to the intraarticular ligaments, which connect the thoracic IVDs to the crests of the heads of the second through the ninth ribs.

Composition of the Intervertebral Disc

Like cartilage elsewhere in the body, the disc is made up of water, cells (primarily chondrocytelike cells and fibroblasts), proteoglycan aggregates, and type I and type II collagen fibers (see Chapter 13). The proteoglycan aggregates are composed of many proteoglycan monomers attached to a hyaluronic acid core. However, the proteoglycans of the IVD are of a smaller size and a different composition than the proteoglycans of cartilage found in other regions of the body (articular cartilage, nasal cartilage, and cartilage of growth plates) (Buckwalter et al., 1989). The cartilaginous IVD is a dynamic structure that has been shown to be able to repair itself and is capable of considerable regeneration (Humzah & Soames, 1988; Mendel et al., 1992; Nitobe et al., 1988).

The IVD is composed of three regions (Fig. 2-10) known as the anulus fibrosus, the nucleus pulposus, and the vertebral (cartilage) end plate (Humzah & Soames, 1988). Together the regions make up the anterior interbody joint or intervertebral symphysis. Each region consists of different proportions of the primary materials that make up the disc (water, cells, proteoglycan, and collagen). Table 2-2 compares some of the characteristics of the anulus fibrosus with those of the nucleus pulposus.

Although each region of the disc has a distinct composition, the transition between the anulus fibrosus and the nucleus pulposus is rather indistinct. The main difference between the two regions is their fibrous structure (Humzah & Soames, 1988). Type I collagen (typical in tendons) predominates in the anulus fibrosus, and type II collagen (typical for articular cartilage) predominates in the nucleus pulposus. The histologic and biochemical make-up of the IVD is currently an active field of research and has a great deal of potential clinical relevance. Chapter 13 discusses the histologic characteristics of the IVD in more detail. The gross morphologic characteristics of the three regions of the disc are discussed in the following sections.

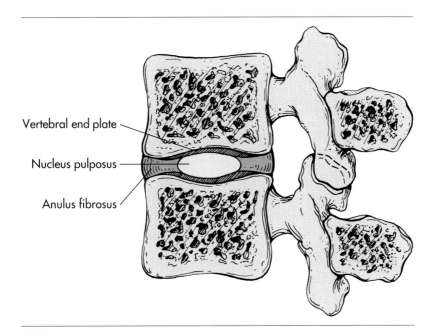

FIG. 2-10 Midsagittal section of two adjacent lumbar vertebrae and the intervertebral disc separating the two vertebral bodies. Notice the components of the intervertebral disc: anulus fibrosus, nucleus pulposus, and vertebral end plate.

Anulus Fibrosus

The anulus fibrosus is made up of several fibrocartilaginous lamellae, or rings, that are convex externally (Figs. 2-10 and 2-11). The lamellae are formed by closely arranged collagen fibers and a smaller percentage (10% of the dry weight) of elastic fibers (Bogduk & Twomey, 1991). The majority of fibers of each lamella run parallel with one another at approximately a 65° angle from the vertical plane. The fibers of adjacent lamellae overlie each other, forming a 130° angle between the fibers of adjacent lamellae. However, the direction of the lamella varies considerably from individual to individual and from one vertebra to the next (Humzah & Soames, 1988). The most superficial lamellae of the anulus fibrosus attach via Sharpey's fibers (see Chapter 13 and Fig. 13-10) directly to the vertebral bodies in the region of the ring epiphysis. They anchor themselves to the zone of compact bone that forms the outside of the vertebral rim, as well as the adjacent vertebral body and the periosteum that covers it (Humzah & Soames, 1988). The inner lamellae of the anulus fibrosus attach to the cartilaginous vertebral end plate.

The anulus fibrosus has been found to be the primary load-bearing structure of the disc. It can perform this function even when the nucleus has been experimentally removed (Humzah & Soames, 1988). The anterior aspect of the disc is stronger than the rest, whereas the posterolateral aspect of each disc is the weakest region. Therefore the posterolateral aspect of the IVD is the region most prone to protrusion and herniation.

The most superficial lamellae of the anulus are innervated by general somatic afferent nerves and general visceral afferent nerves (which run with sympathetic efferent fibers). Specifically, the recurrent meningeal nerve innervates the posterior aspect of the anulus and separate nerves arising from the ventral ramus, and the sympathetic chain innervate the lateral and anterior aspects of the anulus.

CLINICAL IMPLICATIONS

Weinstein, Claverie, and Gibson (1988) investigated the pain associated with discography. Discography is the injection of radiopaque dye into a disc and the subsequent visualization of the disc on x-ray film. They found neuropeptides, which are frequently identified as neurotransmitters associated with inflammation (substance P, calcitonin gene related peptide, and vasoactive intestinal peptide), in the remaining lamellae of the anulus fibrosus and in the dorsal root ganglia of dogs that had undergone surgical removal of an intervertebral disc (discectomy). They state that the dorsal root ganglion may be a mediator of the sensory environment of the motor unit and that discs with anular disruption may be sensitized to further irritation. Therefore fibers whose cell bodies

Table 2-2 Composition of Anulus Fibrosus and Nucleus Pulposus

Region*	% Water	Collagen type†	Disc weight (%) Collagen‡	Disc weight (%) Proteoglycan§
Anulus fibrosus	60-70	I	50-60	20/50-60
Nucleus pulposus	70-90	II	15-20	65/25

*Values are for the lumbar spine (Bogduk & Twomey, 1991).
†I, II, III, IV.
‡Percentage of dry weight of disc made up of collagen.
§Percentage of dry weight of disc made up of proteoglycan/percentage of proteoglycan found in aggregated form.

reside in the dorsal root ganglion may release the neurotransmitters listed previously into the region of the anulus fibrosus, making the anulus more sensitive to injury. This may mean that a torn or otherwise diseased disc could be more sensitive to further irritation and therefore more capable of nociceptive (pain) stimulation than the discs of adjacent vertebrae. This may help to explain the heightened sensitivity of patients with disc disorders. Weinstein (1988) used his findings to help explain why the chemical irritants found in the radiopaque dye (Renografin) injected into a disc during discography (Fig. 2-12) reproduce the patient's symptoms. However, the procedure is not generally associated with pain when the dye is injected into a neighboring healthy disc of the same individual.

The lamellae of the anulus fibrosus are subject to tearing. These tears occur in two directions, circumferentially and radially. Many investigators believe that circumferential tears are the most common. This type of tear represents a separation of adjacent lamellae of the anulus. The separation may cause the lamellae involved to tear away from their vertebral attachments. The second type of tear is radial in direction. These tears run from the deep lamellae of the anulus to the superficial layers. Most authors (Ito et al., 1991) believe these types of tears follow circumferential tears in chronology and that the circumferential tears make it easier for radial tears to occur. This is because the radial tears are able to connect the circumferential ones. When the connection occurs, the nucleus pulposus may be allowed to bulge or even extrude into the vertebral canal. This is known as intervertebral disc protrusion (bulging) or herniation (extrusion).

However, Lipson (1988) recently challenged the long-held assumption that disc herniations were the result of the nucleus pulposus' entering the vertebral canal through a tear in the anulus fibrosus. He showed that the material seen in IVD herniations did not consist of nucleus pulposus. He found the free edge of the herniated material to be very cellular in nature and very similar in

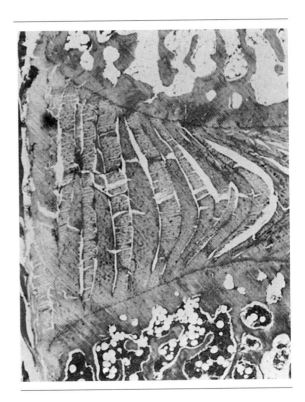

FIG. 2-11 Low power photomicrograph demonstrating the lamellar arrangement of the anulus fibrosus. (Courtesy of Vernon-Roberts, from Jayson M. [1992] *The lumbar spine and back pain* (4th ed.) New York: Churchill Livingstone.)

light microscopic appearance to anulus fibrosus. However, the material was found to be younger than the surrounding anulus. After augmenting his work with biochemical studies, Lipson (1988) concluded that the material herniated in disc prolapse was actually metaplastic fibrocartilage (cartilage cells growing at a more rapid rate than surrounding cells) from the anulus fibrosus. He concluded that a herniated disc is a slowly progressing disease. He explained that the process may begin with a mechanical insult to the disc, resulting in a shift of the metabolic pathways within the cells of the anulus fibrosus. The metabolic shift would result in metaplastic change and growth of anular cells until protrusion occurred. This theory of disc protrusion is quite different from the currently held belief that disc herniation is the result of the nucleus pulposus' pushing through tears in the outer anulus fibrosus. Future study is required to either confirm or challenge Lipson's theory. Perhaps such metaplastic change occurs in a subpopulation of individuals with disorders of the IVD.

Nucleus Pulposus

The nucleus pulposus is a rounded region located within the center of the IVD (Fig. 2-10). The nucleus pulposus is thickest in the lumbar region, followed in thickness by

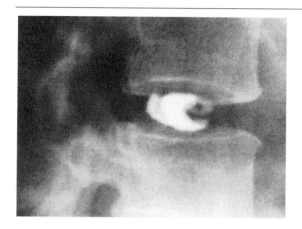
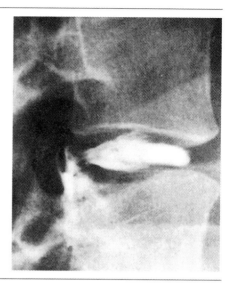

FIG. 2-12 Normal discogram *(left)* and discogram demonstrating extrusion of nuclear material through the lamellae of the anulus fibrosus *(right)*. (Courtesy of Park, from Jayson M. [1980] *The lumbar spine and back pain* (2nd ed.) Baltimore: Urban & Schwarzenburg and Pitman Publishing.)

the cervical region; it is the thinnest in the thoracic region. It is most centrally placed within the horizontal plane in the cervical region and is more posteriorly placed in the lumbar region (Humzah & Soames, 1988).

The nucleus pulposus develops from the embryologic notochord. It is gelatinous and relatively large just after birth, and several multinucleated notochordal cells can be found within its substance (Williams et al., 1989). The remnants of the notochord can be recognized in magnetic resonance imaging (MRI) scans as an irregular dark band, usually confined to the nucleus pulposus (Breger et al., 1988). The notochordal tissue has been found to be more apparent in fetal spines than in the spines of infants (Ho et al., 1988). The notochordal cells decrease in number over time and are almost completely replaced by fibrocartilage by approximately the eleventh year of life (Williams et al., 1989). As the notochordal cells are replaced, the outer aspect of the nucleus pulposus blends with the inner layer of the anulus fibrosus, making it difficult to determine the border between the two regions. Notochordal cells may remain anywhere throughout the spine. These remnants are known as notochordal "rests" and may develop into neoplasms known as chordomas. Chordomas most commonly occur at the base of the skull and in the lumbosacral region (Humzah & Soames, 1988).

The disc is an avascular structure, except for the most peripheral region of the anulus fibrosus, and the nucleus pulposus is responsible for absorbing the majority of the fluid received by the disc. The process by which a disc absorbs fluid from the vertebral bodies above and below has been termed imbibition. The disc loses water when a load is applied but retains sodium and potassium. This increase in electrolyte concentration creates an osmotic gradient that results in rapid rehydration when the loading of the disc is stopped (Kraemer et al., 1985). The disc apparently benefits from both activity during the day (Holm & Nachemson, 1983) and the rest it receives during the hours of sleep. As a result the disc is thicker (from superior to inferior) after rest than after a typical day of sitting, standing, and walking. However, too much rest may not be beneficial. A decrease in the amount of fluid (hydration) of the IVDs has been noted on MRIs after 5 weeks of bed rest (LeBlanc et al., 1988). The disc reaches its peak hydration at about the age of 30, and the process of degeneration begins shortly thereafter (Coventry, 1969). As the disc ages, it becomes less gelatinous in consistency, and its ability to absorb fluid diminishes. The changes in composition and structure that are common to all sources of cartilage with aging occur earlier and to a greater extent in the IVD (Bayliss et al., 1988). Breakdown of the proteoglycan aggregates and monomers (see Fig. 13-6) is thought to contribute to this process of degeneration. The breakdown of proteoglycan results in a decreased ability of the disc to absorb fluid, which leads to a decrease in the ability of the disc to resist loads placed on it. The degeneration associated with the decrease in ability to absorb fluid (water) has been identified through use of computed tomography (CT) (Bahk & Lee, 1988) and MRI and has been correlated with histologic structure and fluid content. As the disc degenerates, it narrows in the superior to inferior dimensions and the adjacent vertebral bodies may become sclerotic (thickened and opaque on x-ray film).

Much of the disc thinning seen with age may also be the result of the disc sinking into the adjacent vertebral bodies over the course of many years (Humzah & Soames, 1988).

Pathologic conditions of the IVD are frequently seen in clinical practice. As mentioned previously, the nucleus pulposus may cause bulging of the outer anular fibers or may protrude (herniate) through the anulus. This was first described by Mixter and Barr (1934). Bulging or herniation of the disc may be a primary source of pain, or pain may result because of pressure on the exiting nerve roots within the medial aspect of the intervertebral foramen. Such bulging is usually associated with heavy lifting or trauma, although such a history may be absent in as many as 28% of patients with confirmed disc protrusion (Martin, 1978). Some investigators believe proteoglycan leaking out of a tear in the anulus may also cause pain by creating a chemical irritation of the exiting nerve roots. The pain that results from pressure on or irritation of a nerve root radiates in a dermatomal pattern (see Chapter 11). Such pain is termed radicular pain because of its origin from the dorsal root (radix) or dorsal root ganglion. Treatment for herniation of the nucleus ranges from excision of the disc (discectomy), to chemical degradation of the disc (chymopapain chemonucleolysis) (Alcalay et al., 1988; Dabezies et al., 1988), to conservative methods (Sanders & Stein, 1988).

Vertebral End Plate

These cartilaginous plates limit all but the most peripheral rim of the disc superiorly and inferiorly. They are attached both to the disc and to the adjacent vertebral body (Fig. 2-12). Although a few authors consider the vertebral end plate to be a part of the vertebral body, most authorities consider it to be an integral portion of the disc (Bogduk, 1991; Coventry, 1969). The end plates are approximately 1 mm thick peripherally and 3 mm thick centrally. They are composed of both hyaline cartilage and fibrocartilage. The hyaline cartilage is located against the vertebral body, and the fibrocartilage is found adjacent to the remainder of the IVD. The end plates help to prevent the vertebral bodies from undergoing pressure atrophy and, at the same time, contain the anulus fibrosus and nucleus pulposus within their normal anatomic borders.

The vertebral end plates are very important for proper nutrition of the disc (Humzah & Soames, 1988). The end plates are very porous and allow fluid to enter and leave the anulus fibrosus and nucleus pulposus by osmotic action (Humzah & Soames, 1988). Very early in postnatal life, small vascular channels enter the vertebral side of the vertebral end plate and a few channels enter the outermost lamella of the anulus fibrosus. These channels disappear with age and are almost completely gone by the age of 30, leaving the IVD to obtain its nutrition by means of imbibition through the vertebral end plate.

The nucleus pulposus may rupture through the vertebral end plate, causing a lesion known as Schmorl's node. These nodes cause the vertebrae surrounding the lesion to move closer together. This movement is thought to increase pressure on the posterior and anterior joints between the vertebrae, increasing the degenerative process of the anterior interbody joint (the remainder of the IVD). In addition, the disc thinning or narrowing that results from these end plate herniations causes more force to be borne by the Z joints and may result in more rapid degeneration of these structures as well.

The vertebral end plates begin to calcify and thin with advancing years. This leaves them more brittle. The central region of the end plate in some vertebrae of certain individuals may be completely lost in the later years of life.

Innervation of the Intervertebral Discs

The outer third of the anulus fibrosus of the IVDs has been found to receive both sensory and vasomotor innervation (Bogduk, Tynan, & Wilson, 1981). The sensory fibers are probably both nociceptive (pain sensitive) and proprioceptive in nature, and the vasomotor fibers are associated with the small vessels located along the superficial aspect of the anulus fibrosus. The posterior aspect of the disc receives its innervation from the recurrent meningeal nerve (sinuvertebral nerve). The posterolateral aspect of the anulus receives both direct branches from the anterior primary division and also branches from the gray communicating rami of the sympathetic chain. The lateral and anterior aspects of the disc receive their innervation primarily from branches of the gray communicating rami and also branches from the sympathetic chain.

The fact that the disc has direct nociceptive innervation is clinically relevant. The IVD itself is most likely able to generate pain. Therefore disorders affecting the IVDs alone (e.g., internal disc disruption, tears of the outer third of the anulus fibrosus, and possibly even marked disc degeneration) can be the sole cause of back pain. The disc can also generate pain by compressing (entraping) an exiting dorsal root. As mentioned previously, leakage of nerve irritating (histamine-like) molecules from disrupted IVDs also has been found to be a cause of irritation to the exiting dorsal root. These latter conditions cause a sharp, stabbing pain that radiates along a dermatomal pattern. This type of pain is known as radicular pain because it results from irritation of a nerve root (radix). Chapter 11 covers the differentiation of radicular pain from somatic referred pain. The unique characteristics of the innervation to the IVDs of the specific spinal regions are covered in Chapters 5 through 7.

RELATIONSHIP OF THE SPINAL NERVES TO THE INTERVERTEBRAL DISC

The first seven spinal nerves exit through the intervertebral foramen (IVF) located above the vertebra of the same number (example, C5 nerve exits the C4-C5 IVF). This relationship changes at the eighth cervical nerve. Because there are eight cervical spinal nerves and only seven cervical vertebrae, the eighth cervical nerve exits the IVF between C7 and T1 (i.e., inferior to C7). All spinal nerves located below the C8 cervical nerve exit inferior to the vertebra of the same number (i.e., the T5 nerve exits below T5, through the T5-T6 IVF). Figure 3-6 shows this relationship.

The previous information is of clinical importance. Because of the relationships just discussed, a disc herniation occurring at the level of the C3-C4 disc usually affects the exiting C4 nerve. However, a disc protrusion of the T3-T4 IVD normally affects the T3 spinal nerve. The anatomic relationships of a disc protrusion in the lumbar spine are unique. As expected the exiting spinal nerve passes through the IVF located below the vertebra of the same number (L3 nerve through the L3-L4 IVF). However, the spinal cord ends at the L1-L2 disc (see Chapter 3), and below this the lumbar and sacral roots descend inferiorly, forming the cauda equina. To exit an IVF, the sharply descending nerve roots must make a rather dramatic turn laterally, and as each nerve root exits, it "hugs" the pedicle of the most superior vertebra of the IVF (Fig. 2-13). Because they leave at such an angle, the nerve roots are kept out of the way of the IVD at the same level. Even though they are positioned away from the disc at their level of exit, they do pass across the IVD above their level of exit. This is approximately where they enter the dural root sleeve, and this is also where the nerve roots may be compressed by disc protrusions. The other nerve roots of the cauda equina are not as vulnerable at this location because only the nerve beginning to exit the vertebral canal has entered its dural root sleeve. Once in the sleeve, the exiting nerve roots are contained and more or less held in place as they descend to exit the IVF. This more firmly positions the exiting roots against the disc above the level of exit (Fig. 2-13). The other nerve roots of the cauda equina, within the subarachnoid space of the lumbar cistern, "float" away from a protruding disc. The result is that a lumbar disc protrusion normally affects the nerve roots exiting the

subjacent IVF (for example, a L3 disc protrusion affects the L4 nerve roots).

SYNDESMOSES OF THE SPINE

In addition to the Z joints and the interbody symphysis, the spine also contains a number of joints classified as syndesmoses. Recall that a syndesmosis is a joint consisting of two bones connected by a ligament. The spine is unique in that it has several examples of such joints. The spinal syndesmoses include the following:
- Axial-occipital syndesmosis (between odontoid and clivus, ligaments include cruciform, apical-odontoid, and alar)
- Ligamentum nuchae (syndesmosis between occiput and C1-C7)
- Laminar syndesmosis (ligamentum flavum)
- Intertransverse syndesmosis (intertransverse ligament)
- Supraspinous syndesmosis (supraspinous ligament)
- Interspinous syndesmosis (interspinous ligament)

These joints are innervated by the posterior primary division (dorsal ramus) exiting between the two vertebrae connected by the ligaments. Afferent nerves running with sympathetic nerves also innervate these joints. The ligaments forming these joints are discussed in Chapters 5 through 7.

VERTEBRAL CANAL

The chapter has thus far been devoted to a discussion of the relatively solid elements of the spine (e.g., bones, ligaments, and joints). The remainder of the chapter is devoted to the "holes" (Latin = *foramen,* singular; *foramina,* plural) of the spine, what runs through them, and the clinical significance of these openings.

A vertebral foramen (Fig. 2-3) is the opening within a vertebra through which the spinal cord or cauda equina runs. The vertebral foramen can be best defined by listing its boundaries. The boundaries of a typical vertebral foramen include the following:
- Vertebral body
- Left and right pedicles
- Left and right laminae
- Spinous process

The boundaries of a vertebral foramen are shown in Fig. 2-3. Two congenital anomalies can affect the vertebral foramen. The first is failure of the posterior elements of a vertebra to fuse during development. This is known as spina bifida (see Chapter 12). Another congenital anomaly of the vertebral foramen is the development of a fibrous or bony bridge between the vertebral body and the spinous process. Such a bridge may divide the spinal cord midsagitally at that level. This condition,

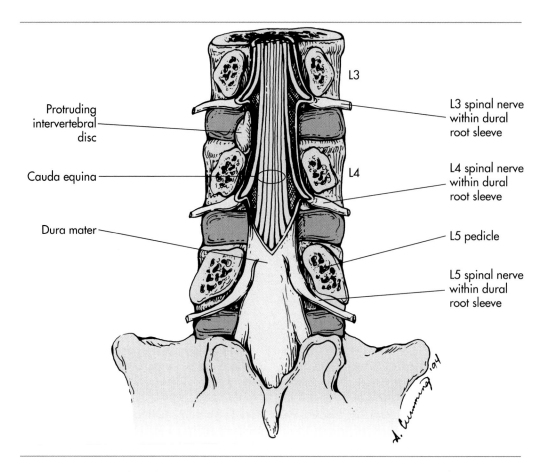

Protruding intervertebral disc

Cauda equina

Dura mater

L3

L4

L3 spinal nerve within dural root sleeve

L4 spinal nerve within dural root sleeve

L5 pedicle

L5 spinal nerve within dural root sleeve

FIG. 2-13 Relationship of exiting nerve roots to the intervertebral discs. Notice the L4 nerve roots are vulnerable to a protrusion of the L3 disc.

known as diastematomyelia, may go unnoticed throughout life or may become symptomatic later in life or following trauma.

The collection of all of the vertebral foramina is known as the vertebral (spinal) canal. Therefore the IVDs and the posteriorly located ligamenta flava (*ligamentum flavum*, singular) also participate in the formation of the vertebral canal. The ligamenta flava are discussed in detail in Chapter 5.

The vertebral canal is fairly large in the upper cervical region but narrows from C3 to C6. In fact the spinal cord fills 75% of the vertebral canal at the C6 level. Therefore the lower cervical cord is particularly vulnerable to a wide variety of pathologic entities that can compromise the cord within the vertebral canal. These include IVD protrusion, hypertrophy of the ligamentum flavum, space-occupying lesions, and arteriovenous malformations.

The vertebral canal follows the normal contour of the curves of the spine. It is relatively large and triangular in the cervical (see Fig. 5-1) and lumbar regions (see Fig. 7-1), where there is a great deal of spinal movement. The vertebral canal in the thoracic region is smaller and almost circular in configuration (see Fig. 6-1). This may be due to the fact that the thoracic spine undergoes less movement than the other regions of the spine. Also, the vertebral canal in the thoracic region does not need to be as large as in the cervical region. This is because the thoracic spinal cord is narrower than the cervical cord, which contains the cervical enlargement.

The size of the vertebral canal has been assessed by several investigators, most of whom were interested in the condition of spinal (vertebral) canal stenosis. This condition is defined as a narrowing of either the anteroposterior or the transverse diameter of the vertebral canal. Some investigators have shown a change in vertebral dimensions and canal size with normal aging (Leiviska, 1985). However, spinal canal stenosis seems to have a strong developmental component and may be due, in part, to prenatal and perinatal growth disruption (Clarke et al., 1985). Vertebral canal growth is approximately 90% complete by late infancy. Since canal diameters do not undergo "catch-up growth" (Clarke et al., 1985) factors affecting canal size must occur before infancy. A significant relationship has been found between a decrease in anteroposterior vertebral foramen size and spinal cord constriction. As little as 2 mm in anteroposterior diameter separates persons with or without low back pain, and Clarke and colleagues (1985) suggest that as many as 53% of low back pain patients may have anteroposterior spinal stenosis. Clarke and colleagues (1985) believe that spinal stenosis and sciatica may have a developmental basis and that perhaps there is a higher association between canal size and low back pain than was previously realized (Clarke et al., 1985). They believe that attention to prenatal and neonatal nutrition may play an important role in preventing back pain from this origin. In addition, they state that maternal smoking and other environmental factors have been shown to significantly reduce head circumference. They hypothesize that the same phenomenon may occur with the vertebral canal (Clarke et al., 1985). If this is shown to be the case, reduction in maternal smoking may prevent future of back pain in the offspring. The effect of smoking on back pain in adults is still a subject of much debate, and many prominent surgeons strongly suggest that a person stop smoking before undergoing a surgical procedure on the spine (Herkowitz et al., 1992).

External Vertebral Venous Plexus

Before investigating the contents of the vertebral canal it is necessary to discuss a plexus of veins that surrounds the outside of the vertebrae and the vertebral canal. This network of veins surrounding the external aspect of the vertebral column is known as the external vertebral venous plexus. The external vertebral venous plexus is associated with both the posterior and anterior elements of the vertebral column and can be divided into an anterior external vertebral venous plexus surrounding the vertebral bodies and a posterior external vertebral venous plexus associated with the neural arches of adjacent vertebrae. These plexuses communicate with segmental veins throughout the spine (deep cervical veins, intercostal veins, lumbar veins, and ascending lumbar veins) and also with the internal vertebral venous plexus, which lies within the vertebral canal. The external and internal vertebral plexuses communicate through the IVFs and also directly through the vertebral bodies. The veins, which run through the IVFs to connect the two plexuses, surround the exiting spinal nerve and form a vascular cuff around the nerve (Humzah & Soames, 1988).

Epidural Space

The region immediately beneath the bony and ligamentous elements forming the vertebral canal is known as the epidural space (see dura mater in Fig. 2-13). The epidural space is sometimes entered at the L3-L4 interspinous space for the purpose of administering anesthetics. The depth to the epidural space at this level is 4.77 ± 0.55 cm in males and 4.25 ± 0.55 cm in females.

The range of depth is 3.0 to 7.0 cm (1.2 to 2.8 inches), and there is a positive correlation between both body weight and body height with the depth to the epidural space (Chen et al., 1989).

The epidural space contains a venous plexus embedded in a thin layer of adipose tissue. The adipose tissue is known as the epidural adipose tissue, or epidural fat, and the venous plexus is known as the internal vertebral venous plexus.

Internal Vertebral Venous Plexus

The internal vertebral venous plexus is located beneath the bony elements of the vertebral foramina (laminae, spinous processes, pedicles, and vertebral body). As previously mentioned, it is embedded in a layer of loose areolar tissue known as the epidural (extradural) adipose tissue. The internal vertebral venous plexus is a clinically important plexus, and perhaps for this reason it has been given many names. It is known as the internal vertebral venous plexus, the epidural venous plexus, the extradural venous plexus, and also as Batson's channels.

The internal vertebral venous plexus consists of many interconnected longitudinal channels. Several run along the posterior aspect of the vertebral canal, and several run along the anterior aspect of the canal. The anterior channels drain the vertebral bodies via large basivertebral veins. The basivertebral veins pierce the center of each vertebral body and communicate posteriorly with the internal plexus and anteriorly with the external vertebral venous plexus. The posterior communication of the basivertebral veins with the anterior internal vertebral venous plexus occurs by means of small veins that run from the basivertebral veins and around the posterior longitudinal ligament to reach the anterior internal vertebral venous plexus.

The veins of the internal vertebral venous plexus contain no valves; therefore the direction of drainage is posture and respiration dependent. Inferiorly this plexus is continuous with the prostatic venous plexus of the male, and superiorly (in both sexes), it is continuous with the occipital dura mater venous sinus of the posterior cranial fossa. Therefore prostatic carcinoma may metastasize via this route to all regions of the spine and to the meninges and the brain.

The walls of the veins of the internal vertebral venous plexus are very thin and may collapse from the pressure of an IVD protrusion. This fact has been used in a procedure known as epidural venography (Fig. 2-14) to aid in the diagnosis of IVD disease. In epidural venography, radiopaque dye is injected into the epidural veins and x-ray films are taken. This allows the veins filled with dye to be visualized (Jayson, 1980). Pressure from a disc protrusion prevents the veins from filling and is seen as an area devoid of dye on the x-ray film.

Spinal epidural hematoma is a condition in which bleeding occurs into the space surrounding the dura mater. It is usually the result of a ruptured epidural vein and is rather rare, with only 250 cases reported in the literature. Of these approximately 50% are spontaneous and of unknown cause. The causes of the remainder of the cases include trauma, anticoagulant therapy, and arteriovenous malformation. Spinal epidural hematoma may simulate IVD protrusion but can usually be identified through MRI (Mirkovic & Melany, 1992). Treatment is usually removal of pressure (decompression) by the removal of a lamina (laminectomy), although several cases with spontaneous recovery have been reported (Sei et al., 1991).

Meningeal and Neural Elements Within the Vertebral Canal

The meningeal and neural elements of the vertebral canal are thoroughly discussed in Chapter 3. This section focuses on the neural elements that enter and leave the vertebral canal.

Beneath the epidural venous plexus and epidural adipose tissue lie the meninges, which surround the spinal cord (Fig. 2-15). These layers of tissue are known as the dura mater, arachnoid mater, and pia mater.

The spinal cord lies under the arachnoid and pia mater (Fig. 2-15). Beneath the transparent pia mater, dorsal and ventral rootlets can be seen attaching to the spinal cord. These rootlets divide the spinal cord into spinal cord segments (see Chapter 3). A spinal cord segment is the region of the spinal cord delineated by those exiting dorsal and ventral rootlets that eventually unite to form a single mixed spinal nerve. Spinal cord segments can be easily identified on a gross specimen of the spinal cord(see Figure 3-8, *C*). The rootlets combine to form dorsal roots (from dorsal rootlets) and ventral roots (from ventral rootlets). The dorsal and ventral roots then unite to form a mixed spinal nerve. The rootlets are "exceedingly delicate and vulnerable and when implicated in fibrous adhesions from whatever cause, undergo irreversible changes" (Domisse & Louw, 1990).

Formation of the Mixed Spinal Nerve and Anterior and Posterior Primary Divisions. The dorsal and ventral roots unite within the IVF to form the mixed spinal nerve (Fig. 2-16; also see Chapter 3). As the mixed spinal nerve exits the IVF, it divides into two parts: a posterior primary division (dorsal ramus) and an anterior primary division (ventral ramus) (Fig. 2-15). The posterior primary division further divides into a medial branch, which supplies the Z joints and transversospinalis group of deep back muscles, and a lateral branch, which supplies the sacrospinalis group of deep

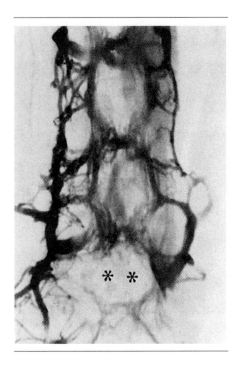

FIG. 2-14 Epidural venogram. Radiopaque dye was injected into the epidural venous plexus, x-ray films were taken, and extraneous tissue was removed using digital subtraction techniques. *Asterisks,* An intervertebral disc protrusion; notice that the dye has not filled the veins in this region (Courtesy of Park, from Jayson M. [1980] *The lumbar spine and back pain* [2nd ed.] Baltimore: Urban & Schwarzenberg and Pitman.)

back muscles (see Chapter 4). The anterior primary division may unite with other anterior primary divisions to form one of the plexuses of the body. Anterior primary divisions also innervate the body wall; the intercostal nerves serve as a prime example of this function. The plexuses of the anterior primary divisions and the specific innervation of spinal structures by the posterior primary divisions are discussed in the chapters covering the specific regions of the spine (see Chapters 5 through 8). The plexuses are discussed in the chapter dealing with the spinal region from which they arise.

Arterial Supply to the Spine

The external aspect of the vertebral column receives its arterial supply from branches of deep arteries "in the neighborhood." The cervical region is supplied by the left and right deep cervical arteries (from the costocervical trunks) and also the right and left ascending cervical arteries (from the right and left inferior thyroid arteries). The thoracic region of the spine is supplied by intercostal arteries, and the lumbar region is supplied by lumbar segmental arteries.

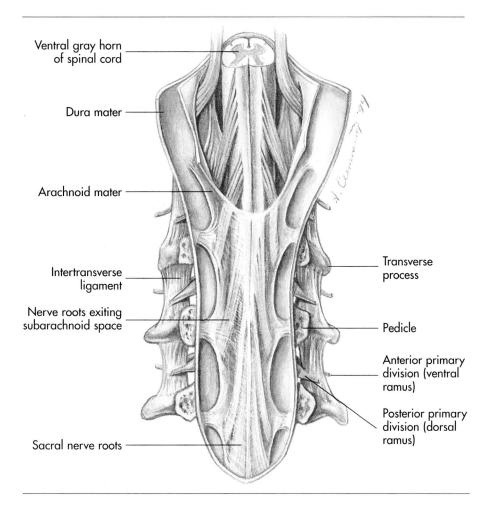

Ventral gray horn
of spinal cord

Dura mater

Arachnoid mater

Intertransverse
ligament

Nerve roots exiting
subarachnoid space

Sacral nerve roots

Transverse
process

Pedicle

Anterior primary
division (ventral
ramus)

Posterior primary
division (dorsal
ramus)

FIG. 2-15 The vertebral canal with the posterior vertebral arches removed. Notice the dura mater, arachnoid, and neural elements within the canal.

The internal aspect of the vertebral canal receives its arterial supply from segmental arteries that send spinal branches into the IVFs. The segmental arteries are branches of the vertebral artery in the cervical region, the intercostal arteries in the thoracic region, and the lumbar arteries in the lumbar region.

On entering the IVF, each spinal branch of a segmental artery further divides into three branches. One branch courses posteriorly to supply the posterior arch structures of the neighboring vertebrae. Another branch courses anteriorly to supply the posterior longitudinal ligament, the posterior aspect of the vertebral body, and the surrounding tissues. The third branch of each segmental artery, known as the neural branch, runs to the mixed spinal nerve. Unique characteristics of the blood supply to each region of the spine are discussed in further detail in the chapters on specific regions of the spine (Chapters 5 through 8). The spinal cord, the vasculature of the cord, and its meningeal coverings are discussed in detail in Chapter 3.

INTERVERTEBRAL FORAMEN

The second major opening, or foramen, of the spine is the intervertebral foramen. The IVF is an area of great biomechanical, functional, and clinical significance (Williams et al., 1989). Much of its importance stems from the fact that the IVF provides an osteoligamentous boundary between the central nervous system and the peripheral nervous system. This foramen is unlike any other in the body in that the spinal nerve and vessels running through it are passing through an opening formed by two movable bones (vertebrae) and two joints (anterior interbody joint and the Z joint) (Amonoo-Kuofi et al., 1988). Because of this the IVFs change size during movement. They become larger in spinal flexion and smaller in extension (Amonoo-Kuofi et al., 1988; Awalt et al., 1989; Mayoux-Benhamou et al., 1989). Compression of the exiting spinal nerves or other foraminal contents has been reported to be an important cause of back pain and pain radiating into the extremities (Amonoo-Kuofi et al., 1988). Hasue et al. (1983) found evidence that osseous tissue can constrict neurovascular tissue in the nerve root tunnel (IVF). Therefore knowledge of the specific anatomy of this clinically important area is important in the differential diagnosis of back and extremity pain and can help with the proper management of individuals with compromise of this region.

A pair (left and right) of IVFs are located between all of the adjacent vertebrae from C2 to the sacrum. The sacrum also has a series of paired dorsal and ventral foramina (Chapter 8). There are no IVFs between C1 and C2. Where present, the IVFs lie posterior to the vertebral bodies and between the superior and inferior vertebral notches of adjacent vertebrae. Therefore the pedicles of adjacent vertebrae form the roof and floor of this region. The width of the pedicles in the horizontal plane gives depth to these openings, actually making them neural canals (Czervionke et al., 1988) rather than foramina, but the name intervertebral foramina remains.

Six structures form the boundaries of the IVF (Fig. 2-16, *A* and *B*). Beginning from the most superior border (roof) and continuing anteriorly in a circular fashion, the boundaries include the following:

- The pedicle of the vertebra above (more specifically, its periosteum)
- The vertebral body of the vertebra above (again, its periosteum)
- The IVD (posterolateral aspect of the anulus fibrosus)
- The vertebral body of the vertebra below, and in the cervical region, the uncinate process (periosteum)
- The pedicle of the vertebra below forms the floor of the IVF (periosteum). A small part of the sacral base (between the superior articular process and the body of the S1 segment) forms the floor of the L5-S1 IVF.
- The Z joint forms the "posterior wall." Recall that the Z joint is made up of *(a)* the inferior articular process (and facet) of the vertebra above, *(b)* the superior articular process (and facet) of the vertebra below, and *(c)* the anterior articular capsule, which is composed of the ligamentum flavum (Giles, 1992; Xu et al., 1991).

The IVFs are smallest in the cervical region, and generally there is a gradual increase in IVF dimensions to the L4 vertebra. The left and right IVFs between L5 and S1 are unique in size and shape (see the following discussion). The unique characteristics of the cervical, thoracic, and lumbar IVFs are covered in the chapters on regional anatomy of the spine (Chapters 5 through 7).

As mentioned previously the IVFs are actually canals. These canals vary in width from approximately 5 mm

(Hewitt, 1970) in the cervical region to 18 mm (Pfaundler, 1989) at the L5-S1 level.

Many structures traverse the IVF (Fig. 2-16). They include the following:

- The mixed spinal nerve (union of dorsal and ventral roots)
- The dural root sleeve
- Lymphatic channel(s)
- The spinal branch of a segmental artery. This artery divides into three branches: one to the posterior aspect of the vertebral body, one to the posterior arch, and one to the mixed spinal nerve (neural branch)
- Communicating (intervertebral) veins between the internal and external vertebral venous plexuses
- Two to four recurrent meningeal (sinuvertebral) nerves

Adipose tissue surrounds all of the listed structures.

The dorsal and ventral roots unite to form the mixed spinal nerve in the region of the IVF, and the mixed spinal nerve is surrounded by the dural root sleeve. The dural root sleeve is attached to the borders of the IVF by a series of fibrous bands. The dural root sleeve becomes continuous with the epineurium of the mixed spinal nerve at the lateral border of the IVF (Fig. 2-16). The arachnoid blends with the perineurium proximal to the dorsal root ganglion and at an equivalent region of the ventral root (Hewitt, 1970). Occasionally the arachnoid extends more distally, and in such cases the subarachnoid space extends to the lateral third of the IVF.

Each recurrent meningeal nerve (sinuvertebral nerve of Von Luschka) originates from the most proximal portion of the ventral ramus. It receives a branch from the nearest gray communicating ramus of the sympathetic chain before traversing the IVF. This nerve provides sensory innervation (including nociception) to the posterior aspect of the anulus fibrosus, the posterior longitudinal ligament, anterior epidural veins, periosteum of the posterior aspect of the vertebral bodies, and the anterior aspect of the spinal dura mater. Usually several recurrent meningeal nerves enter the same IVF. These nerves are discussed in more detail in Chapters 5 and 11.

Since the beginning of the twentieth century, the IVF has been a region that has received much attention from those engaged in the treatment of the spine. The effects of spinal adjusting on the nerve roots and spinal nerves is an area of acute interest and much debate. Lumbar IVFs have received much scrutiny because of their extreme clinical importance in lumbar IVD protrusion and lumbar intervertebral foraminal (canal) stenosis. In the words of Lancourt, Glenn, & Wiltse (1979), "The importance of the nerve root entrapment in the nerve root canals cannot be overemphasized." The arteries, veins, lymphatics, and particularly the neural

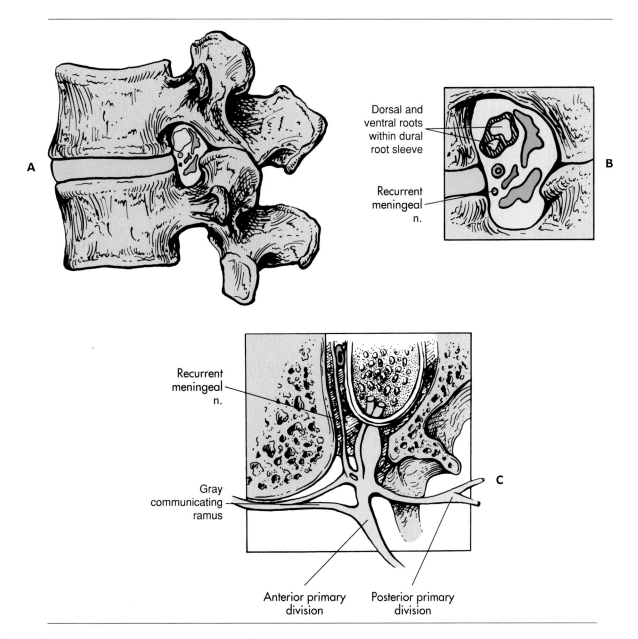

Dorsal and
ventral roots
within dural
root sleeve

Recurrent
meningeal
n.

Recurrent
meningeal
n.

Gray
communicating
ramus

Anterior primary
division

Posterior primary
division

FIG. 2-16   Lumbar intervertebral foramen. In addition to the structures labeled, notice the intervertebral veins *(blue)*, the spinal branch (ramus) of a lumbar segmental artery *(red)*, and a lymphatic channel *(green)*. **C,** Horizontal section through the intervertebral foramen. Notice the recurrent meningeal nerve originates from the most proximal portion of the anterior primary division and receives a branch from the gray communicating ramus. It then passes medially to enter the intervertebral foramen.

elements may be adversely affected by pathologic conditions of one or more of the following structures (Williams et al., 1989):

- ◆ Fibrocartilage of the anulus fibrosus
- ◆ Nucleus pulposus (especially in earlier decades)
- ◆ Red bone marrow of the vertebral bodies
- ◆ Compact bone of the pedicles
- ◆ Z joints
    Capsules
    Synovial membranes
    Articular cartilage

Fibroadipose meniscoids
Fat pads
Connective tissue rim (fibrous labra)
- ◆ Costocorporeal joints (in the thoracic region)

Even though there have been a few well-documented studies of the IVF, very little is known about the normal size of this region in the living. For the first time the imaging modalities of CT and MRI allow for accurate evaluation of the IVF in the living. Previous studies have shown both methods to be reliable in measuring the IVF in the sagittal plane (Cramer et al., 1992a).

Fig. 2-17 shows three parameters measured from MRI scans of the lumbar IVFs of normal human subjects. Table 2-3 shows the average values obtained from the left lumbar IVFs of 37 subjects (17 females and 20 males), and Table 2-4 gives the same values for the right side. Figs. 2-18 and 2-19 show the values displayed graphically. Notice that the values are very much the same from left to right. In fact the relationship between left and right IVFs at the same level is statistically significant (Cramer et al., 1992b). The greatest superior to inferior dimension of the IVF is at L2. IVF dimension then diminishes until L5, where it is the smallest. The anteroposterior dimensions are smaller than the vertical dimensions and remain quite constant throughout the lumbar region, with the more superior of the two anteroposterior measurements shown in Fig. 2-17 being larger. Therefore the IVFs from L1 to L4 are similar in shape. They are shaped like an inverted pear. The L5 IVF is distinct in shape. It is more oval than the others, with the superior to inferior dimension being greater than the anteroposterior dimension.

The databases, such as those shown in the previously mentioned tables, and figures are compiled to benefit biomechanic and clinical researchers. The normative data may be used as a source of comparison when studying the IVF in healthy and diseased states. Perhaps more importantly these databases may aid clinicians in determining the relative patency of the lumbar IVFs in their patients with suspected intervertebral foraminal stenosis (narrowing). Such stenosis can occur as the result of disc degeneration (Crock, 1976), ligamentum flavum hypertrophy, or Z joint arthrosis (increased bone formation because of increased weight bearing or torsional stress). Of further interest to clinicians is the fact that the dimensions of the IVF have been found to be significantly related to anteroposterior vertebral canal diameters. However, transverse diameters of the vertebral canals and vertebral body heights do not correlate with IVF dimensions (Clarke et al., 1985). Clarke and colleagues (1985) suggest that spinal stenosis and sciatica may both have a developmental basis, and perhaps a higher association exists between canal size and low back pain than was previously realized (Clarke et al., 1985). They speculate that prenatal and neonatal growth disruption may be a primary cause of abnormally small vertebral canal and IVF size. This is certainly an important area for future investigation.

Accessory Ligaments of the Intervertebral Foramen

In 1969 Golub and Siverman first used the term *transforaminal ligament* (TFL) when describing a ligamentous band that crosses the IVF at any level of the spine. These ligaments vary considerably in size, shape, and

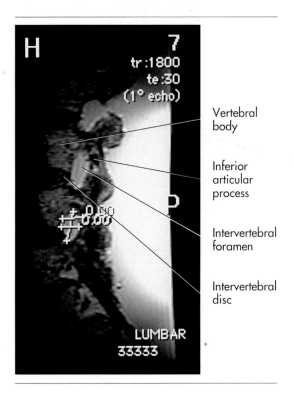

FIG. 2-17 Three measurements made of the lumbar intervertebral foramina. These measurements were made on the parasagittal MRI scans of 37 individuals to generate the data used to create Table 2-3 and 2-4. The measurements of this figure read "0.00" because the scale was set to zero before this photograph was taken. This was done to avoid a distracting overlap of numbers on the screen. Normally each measurement would be made separately and the intervertebral foramen would be cleared of lines following each measurement.

Table 2-3 Dimensions of Left Lumbar IVFs*

IVF	Superior to inferior dimension	SAP	IAP
LL1	19.50 (1.75)	9.05 (1.25)	7.96 (1.45)
LL2	21.12 (1.51)	10.09 (1.80)	7.83 (1.58)
LL3	20.53 (1.75)	10.78 (2.70)	8.07 (1.79)
LL4	19.30 (1.85)	10.47 (1.99)	7.43 (1.82)
LL5	16.40 (2.20)	10.93 (1.92)	9.30 (2.11)

(From Cramer et al. [1992b]. *Proc 1992 Internatl Conf Spin Manipulation*, 1, 3-5.) *SAP*, Superior, anteroposterior measurement taken at the level of the Z joint. *IAP*, Inferior, anteroposterior measurement taken at the level of the inferior vertebral end plate.
*The average size of the left L1-L5 IVFs for three measured parameters (Fig. 2-17). Values given in millimeters with standard deviations in parentheses. Values calculated from 37 human subjects: 17 females and 20 males.

location from one IVF to another. The authors found that the spinal arteries and veins ran above this structure and the anterior primary division ran underneath it. Fig. 2-20 shows a TFL at the L5-S1 level of a cadaveric spine.

Table 2-4 Dimensions of Right Lumbar IVFs*

IVF	Superior to inferior dimension	SAP	IAP
RL1	—	9.28 (1.51)	8.18 (1.51)
RL2	21.44 (2.11)	10.30 (1.94)	8.08 (1.73)
RL3	20.70 (1.75)	10.75 (1.92)	8.23 (1.56)
RL4	19.07 (2.01)	10.73 (2.06)	7.79 (1.86)
RL5	16.72 (2.01)	9.98 (1.67)	8.24 (1.87)

(From Cramer et al. [1992b]. *Proc 1992 Internatl Conf Spin Manipulation*, 1, 3-5.) *SAP*, Superior, anteroposterior measurement taken at the level of the Z joint. *IAP*, Inferior, anteroposterior measurement taken at the level of the inferior vertebral end plate.
*The average size of the right L1-L5 IVFs for three measured parameters (Fig. 2-17). Values given in millimeters with standard deviations in parentheses. Values calculated from 37 human subjects: 17 females and 20 males.

Fig. 2-21 shows two MRIs of the same cadaveric spine. The TFL is shown on the MRI of Fig. 2-21, *B*.

Bachop and Janse (1983) reported that the higher the ligament is placed, the less space remains for the spinal vessels, which could conceivably lead to ischemia or venous congestion. They also postulated that lower placement of the ligament would increase the possibility of sensory and motor deficits.

Bachop and Hilgendorf (1981) studied 15 spines and from these dissected the lumbar IVFs (a total of 150 IVFs). From these dissections they found the following:

- 26 (17.3%) of IVFs had TFLs
- 13 (50%) of TFLs were at L5-S1
- 11 (73.3%) of the 15 spines had 1 or 2 TFLs at L5-S1
- 2 (13.3%) of the 15 spines had TFLs at L5-S1 on both the left and right sides

The term *corporotransverse ligament* is used when referring to a TFL that runs between the vertebral body and the transverse process at the L5-S1 junction (Bachop and Janse, 1983). Bachop and Hilgendorf (1981) found that the corporotransverse ligaments were of two basic types: broad and flat, and rodlike. The rodlike ligaments were usually tougher (firmer) than the flat type. Golub and Silverman (1969) reported that the rodlike ligaments could calcify and be seen on x-ray film. Bachop and Ro (1984) found the gray sympathetic ramus running through the opening above the corporotransverse ligament.

Bachop and Janse (1983) felt that the corporotransverse ligament could have a constricting effect on the anterior primary division (ventral ramus). That is, in patients with sciatica, as the leg is raised, the anterior primary division could be stretched across the ligament, possibly mimicking the thigh and leg pain of a disc protrusion.

Breig and Troup (1979) and Rydevik and colleagues (1984) have reported on increased sensitivity of in-

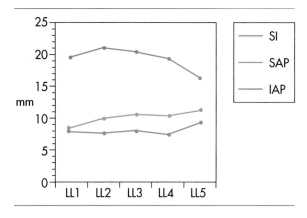

FIG. 2-18 Dimensions of the left lumbar intervertebal foramina of 37 normal human subjects. Notice the two anteroposterior measurements (SAP and IAP) remain almost the same throughout the lumbar region. The superior to inferior dimension (S-I) is the greatest at L2 and then becomes progressively smaller.

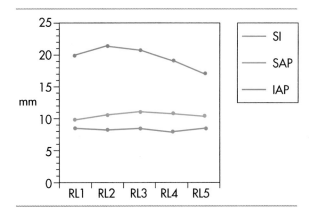

FIG. 2-19 Dimensions of the right lumbar intervertebral foramina IVFs of the same 37 subjects studied in Fig. 2-18. Notice that the values are similar to those of the left intervertebral foramina charted in Fig. 2-18.

flamed nerve roots. Factors such as facet arthrosis, disc protrusion, and ligamentum flavum hypertrophy could conceivably increase intraforaminal pressure. The presence of a corporotransverse ligament could further increase this pressure and possibly cause a subclinical problem to become clinical. Other ligaments that might impinge on nerves and blood vessels have been described by Bogduk (1981) and Nathan, Weizenbluth, & Halperin (1982).

Amonoo-Kuofi has recently discussed accessory ligaments of the IVF (1988). He found them consistently throughout the lumbar region and mapped out the relationship of the spinal nerve, segmental veins and arteries, and the recurrent meningeal nerve through the openings between the ligaments. He concluded that the

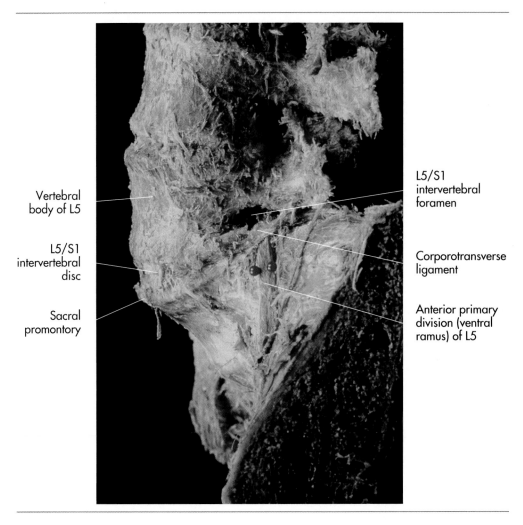

Vertebral body of L5

L5/S1 intervertebral disc

Sacral promontory

L5/S1 intervertebral foramen

Corporotransverse ligament

Anterior primary division (ventral ramus) of L5

FIG. 2-20   Lateral view of a cadaveric lumbar spine. The red pins pass beneath a corporotransverse ligament that spans the left L5-S1 intervertebral foramen. Notice the anterior primary division (ventral ramus) passing beneath this ligament (between the red pins).

accessory ligaments tend to hold the previously mentioned structures in their proper place.

Nowicki and Haughton (1992a) also recently studied these structures. Their findings differed somewhat from Amonoo-Kuofi's in that the total number of ligaments found at each IVF was fewer and the various types of ligaments were found with less frequency. However, Nowicki and Haughton (1992a) did find certain ligaments with great frequency, and they were able to identify several of them on MRI scans (Nowicki & Haughton, 1992b). Bakkum and Mestan (1994) found that of 49 lower thoracic and lumbar IVFs examined on four cadaveric spines, 71.4% had TFLs present in the lateral aspect (exit zone) of the IVF. They also found that when TFLs were present, the superior to inferior dimension of the compartment transmitting the anterior primary division of the spinal nerve was significantly decreased as compared with the osseous IVF (the mean decrease in size was 31.5%). Bakkum and Meastan concluded that

there is often less space at the exit zone of the IVF for the emerging anterior primary division than is traditionally thought. Further they felt that the decreased space may, at times, contribute to the incidence of neurologic symptoms in the region, especially following trauma or secondary to degenerative arthritic changes in the region of the IVF.

ADVANCED DIAGNOSTIC IMAGING

One of the most important clinical applications of the anatomy of the spine and spinal cord is in the field of advanced diagnostic imaging. The imaging modalities of CT and MRI frequently allow for extremely clear visualization of the normal and pathologic anatomy of spinal structures. Examples of these images are included in future chapters to demonstrate various anatomic structures and also to show how some of the structures discussed in the text appear on these images. A general

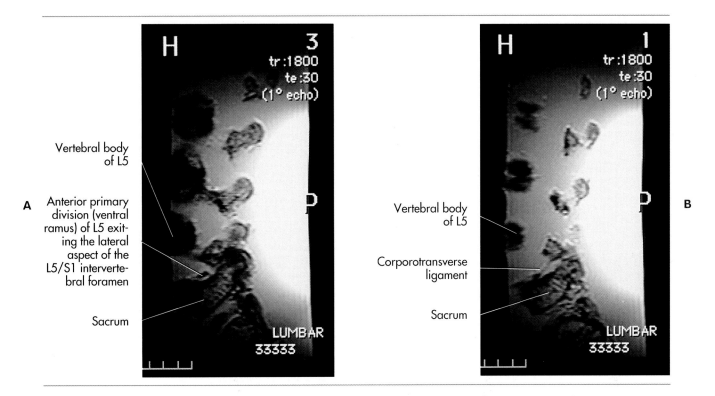

FIG. 2-21 Parasagittal MRI scans of the same cadaveric spine shown in Fig. 2-20. **A,** The anterior primary division (ventral ramus). **B,** Corporotransverse ligament.

understanding of the advantages and disadvantages of the most commonly used advanced imaging techniques helps the reader gain more information from these images. Therefore the first purpose of this section, which is written for those who do not come in contact with these films on a daily basis, is to review the general application and uses of advanced diagnostic imaging procedures. The second purpose is to discuss which atomic structures and spinal disorders can best be imaged with a specific type of modality. Areas of relevant research also are discussed when the results affect currently used imaging procedures. The final purpose is to provide a review of the literature for the student, clinician, and researcher whose major field is not related to diagnostic imaging. Because most of the principles discussed in this section are applicable to all spinal regions, diagnostic imaging included in this chapter is related to general characteristics of the spine rather than to specific spinal regions, which are discussed later in the text.

Since the advanced imaging modalities most commonly used are MRI and CT, the majority of this review deals with these two imaging modalities. Other methods, including myelography, discography, angiography, ultrasonography, three-dimensional computed tomography, radionuclide imaging, and digital imaging, also are discussed.

Magnetic Resonance Imaging

MRI is the newest of the advanced imaging techniques and has rapidly gained worldwide acceptance as a very important component of spinal imaging. MRI shows soft tissue especially well. MRI represents a quantum leap in the evaluation of patients with disc disease (Woodruff, 1988), has been found to be more sensitive than contrast-enhanced CT in demonstrating disc degeneration (Schnebel et al., 1989), and is currently the imaging modality of choice in the evaluation of lumbar disc herniation (Forristall, Marsh, & Pay, 1988; Jackson et al., 1989). MRI can also detect disruption of the posterior longitudinal ligament secondary to herniated nucleus pulposus. MRI allows for visualization of the discs, cerebrospinal fluid, cord, and the perimeter of the spinal canal in several planes without the use of intravenous contrast and is therefore currently the method of choice for detecting disorders of the spinal canal and spinal cord (Woodruff, 1988). Spinal cord tumors, syringomyelia, extramedullary tumors (e.g., meningiomas), metastatic disease to the vertebrae, and dysraphism (spina bifida) are all evaluated exceptionally well with this technology (Alexander, 1988; Woodruff, 1988). MRI has also been found to be effective in the evaluation of failed back surgery syndrome by differentiating fibrotic scar formation secondary to spinal surgery from disc herniation (Frocrain et al., 1989; Kricun et al., 1990) and is becoming the most important modality for all imaging of the postoperative spine (Djukic et al., 1990). Discitis can also be evaluated with MRI (Woodruff, 1988). MRI and conventional films are considered adequate for the preneurosurgical evaluation of cervical radiculopathy and myelopathy, with CT myelography being the follow-up procedure of choice (Brown et al., 1988).

MRI is a rapidly developing field, and the many technical advances should continue to improve its clinical utility. One such advance is the ability to decrease cerebrospinal fluid (CSF) flow artifact. This development results in better visualization of the spinal cord and the cord–CSF interface. Other advances are related to an increased variety of new imaging protocols used by radiologists. The imaging protocols of gradient-echo imaging (GRASS, FLASH, FISP, MPGR) allow for greater contrast between anatomic structures while decreasing scan time. Such gradient-echo techniques are the procedures of choice in patients with suspected cervical radiculopathy (Kricun et al., 1990), giving information of greater or equal value to that obtained from myelography or CT myelography (Hedberg, Dayer, & Flom, 1988).

Two of the primary properties of MR images are related to the various responses of different tissues to the radiofrequency applied during the MRI evaluation. These two characteristics are known as T1 and T2. Various MRI protocols can highlight either of these characteristics and thereby selectively enhance different tissues. T1-weighted images are particularly useful in the evaluation of the spinal cord and the bone marrow of vertebrae (Kricun et al., 1990; Woodruff, 1988). The discs, osteophytes, and ligaments are also well demonstrated on these images (Woodruff, 1988). Generally speaking, T1-weighted images are more valuable than T2-weighted images in the evaluation of most spinal disorders (Moffit et al., 1988).

As a result of the increased acquisition time of the second echo, the resolution of T2-weighted images is not as good as that of T1-weighted images; however, these images are the most sensitive at showing decreased signal intensity resulting from desiccation of the disc (Woodruff, 1988). Because cerebrospinal fluid has a very high signal on T2-weighted images, they also are valuable in evaluating the amount of narrowing of the subarachnoid space in cases of spinal stenosis.

The contrast medium of gadolinium (Gd-DTPA) is being used in conjunction with MRI and has been found to be safe and effective in increasing the contrast of certain pathologic conditions. Differentiation of scar formation (epidural fibrosis) from disc herniation in failed back surgery syndrome (recurrent postoperative sciatica) is improved with the use of Gd-DTPA (Hueftle et al., 1988). Gd-DTPA may also be useful in depicting disc hernia-

tions surrounded by scar tissue and free disc fragments. Gd-DTPA is also useful in the evaluation of patients with intradural tumors, but it is less useful in evaluating tumors external to the dura mater.

Ongoing research in MRI technology (Woodruff, 1988) includes developments in the hardware of the MRI unit, such as coil configurations. These changes allow large areas of the spine to be viewed at once, which is particularly useful in the evaluation of metastatic disease and syringomyelia. Other advances include three-dimensional reconstruction of spinal images with a video display that will allow images to be rotated 360° for viewing. Work is also being done with morphometry of the spine by means of MRI (Byrd et al., 1990; Cramer et al., 1992b). Morphometry means the measurement of an organism or its parts. The digital images available from MRI (and CT) scans may be used to accurately quantify certain anatomic structures of the spine. This is the first time many such measurements will be able to be made in the living. Such measurements may allow for an increased ability to study the structures influenced by a variety of therapeutic procedures.

Computed Tomography

Conventional computed tomography (CT) remains very effective in the evaluation of many conditions. It is especially valuable when accurate depiction of osseous tissues is important. Pathologic conditions including spinal stenosis, tumors of bone, congenital anomalies, degenerative changes, trauma, spondylolysis, and spondylolisthesis can all be accurately evaluated by CT (Wang, Wesolowski, & Farah, 1988). Images reformatted to the sagittal and/or coronal plane may help with the evaluation of complicated bone anatomy. Arachnoiditis ossificans, a rare ossification of the arachnoid mater as a consequence of trauma, hemorrhage, previous myelogram, or spinal anesthesia, can be better visualized on CT than MRI (Wang et al., 1988). Criteria for the diagnosis of intraspinal hemangiomas by means of CT have also been established (Salamon & Freilich, 1988). Although lumbar disc disease can be adequately evaluated by means of CT, "beam hardening" artifacts lead to inadequate evaluation of disc disease in the thoracic and, to a lesser extent, the lower cervical canal (Woodruff, 1988).

CT is especially valuable in the evaluation of lumbar spinal stenosis. Artifacts sometimes make the evaluation of cervical and thoracic spinal stenosis difficult (Wang et al., 1988). The evaluation of facet joint disease and calcification of the ligamentum flavum is currently more efficient with CT than with MRI (Wang et al., 1988).

CT is also quite effective in the evaluation of osseous changes subsequent to spinal trauma. CT is particularly good at identifying the presence of bony fragments in the spinal canal following posterior arch fracture (Wang et al., 1988). Therefore CT is considered to be the imaging method of choice in the evaluation of spine trauma, but it should be reserved for use in those patients with neurologic deficits and those whose plain radiographs are suggestive of, or demonstrate, spinal abnormality (Foster, 1988).

Intrathecal contrast-enhanced CT (CT myelography) results in a more complete depiction of the spinal canal, the IVD relative to the spinal canal, and the perimeter of the spinal cord (Woodruff, 1988). Contrast-enhanced CT and MRI are comparable in their abilities to demonstrate spinal stenosis (Schnebel et al., 1989). CT and MRI have a complementary role in the evaluation of such disorders as canal stenosis, congenital disorders, facet disorders, and acute spinal injury (Tracy, Wright, & Hanigan, 1989; Wang et al., 1988). Extraforaminal (far lateral and anterior) disc herniations can also be readily identified on both CT and MRI if scans include L2 through S1, and if the IVF and paravertebral spaces are closely examined (Osborn et al., 1988).

Other Imaging Modalities

Myelography. Myelography is the injection of radiopaque dye into the subarachnoid space of the lumbar cistern followed by spinal x-ray examinations. Myelography for the evaluation of lumbar disc herniation is rapidly being replaced by CT and MRI. However, it may be useful when the level of the lesion is clinically unclear or when the entire lumbar region and thoracolumbar junction are to be examined (Fagerlund & Thelander, 1989).

Discography. Discography is the injection of radiopaque dye into the IVD. This technique is useful as an adjunct in the evaluation of symptomatic disorders of the disc. Discography in conjunction with CT (CT/discography) allows for delineation and classification of anular disc disruption not possible with plain discography (discography used in conjunction with conventional radiographs) and, in some cases, identifies such disruption when not seen on T2-weighted MR images. Discography may be particularly useful in evaluating patients with suspected disc disorders (McFadden, 1988) when the patient's pain is at a significant level of intensity (stress discography).

Angiography. Spinal angiography is the imaging of the vasculature after the injection of a radiopaque contrast medium. This technique is used to evaluate the arterial supply of spinal tumors (e.g., aneurysmal bone cyst) to assist the surgeon in operative planning (Wang et al., 1988).

Ultrasonography. Ultrasonography (sonography) is currently being used in the evaluation of posterior arch defects in spina bifida (dysraphism), in the intraoperative and postoperative evaluation of the spinal cord, and in the evaluation of the fetal and neonate spine (Wang et al., 1988).

Three-Dimensional Computed Tomography. Three-dimensional CT uses the digital data obtained from conventional CT and reprocesses the information to create a three-dimensional display that can be rotated 360° on a video console. Although clinical utility is currently limited, this technique may be useful as an adjunct to conventional CT in the evaluation of complex spinal fractures, spondylolisthesis, postoperative fusion, and in some cases of spinal stenosis (Pate, Resnick, & Andre, 1986).

Radionuclide Imaging. Single photon emission CT (SPECT) uses tomographic slices obtained with a gamma camera to evaluate radionuclide uptake. This modality has been shown to be a useful adjunct to planar bone scintigraphy (bone scans) in the identification and localization of spinal lesions, especially those responsible for low back pain (Kricun et al., 1990). SPECT is also very effective in the evaluation of spondylolysis.

Digital Imaging. Digital imaging uses a conventional x-ray film source and a very efficient detector to digitize and immediately obtain images. This technique is currently being used in the follow-up evaluation of scoliosis because of its relatively small radiation dose. However, because of the lack of adequate spatial resolution, conventional radiographs should be used at the initial evaluation of scoliosis with osseous etiologic components (e.g., congenital anomaly) (Kricun et al., 1990; Kushner & Cleveland, 1988).

REFERENCES

Alcalay, M. et al. (1988). Traitement par nucleolyse a la chymopapaine des hernies discales a forme purement lombalgique. *Revue du Rhumatisme, 55,* 741-745.

Alexander, A. (1988). Magnetic resonance imaging of the spine and spinal cord tumors. In J.H. Bisese (Ed.), *Spine, state of the art reviews, spinal imaging: Diagnostic and therapeutic applications.* Philadelphia: Hanley & Belfus.

Amonoo-Kuofi, H.S. et al. (1988). Ligaments associated with lumbar intervertebral foramina. I. L1 to L4. *J Anat, 156,* 177-183.

Awalt, P. et al. (1989). Radiographic measurements of intervertebral foramina of cervical vertebra in forward and normal head posture. *J Craniomand Pract, 7,* 275-285.

Bachop, W. & Hilgendorf, C. (1981). Transforaminal ligaments of the human lumbar spine. *Anat Rec, 199* (abstract).

Bachop, W. & Janse, J. (1983). The corporotransverse ligament at the L5 intervertebral foramen. *Anat Rec, 205* (abstract).

Bachop, W.E. & Ro, C.S. (1984). A ligament separating the nerve from the blood vessels at the L5 intervertebral foramen. *J Bone Joint Surg, 8,* 437.

Bahk, Y.W. & Lee, J.M. (1988). Measure-set computed tomographic analysis of internal architectures of lumbar disc: Clinical and histologic studies. *Invest Radiol, 23,* 17-23.

Bakkum, B.W., & Mestan, M. (in press). The effects of transforaminal ligaments on the sizes of T11 to L5 human intervertebral foramina. *J Manipulative Physiol Ther.*

Bayliss, M. et al. (1988) Proteoglycan synthesis in the human intervertebral disc: Variation with age, region, and pathology. *Spine, 13,* 972-981.

Bogduk, N. (1981). The lumbar mamillo-accessory ligament: Its anatomical and neurosurgical significance. *Spine, 6,* 162-167.

Bogduk, N. (1991). *Clinical anatomy of the lumbar spine.* London: Churchill Livingstone.

Bogduk, N. & Engel, R. (1984). The menisci of the lumbar zygapophyseal joints. *Spine, 9,* 454-460.

Bogduk, N. & Twomey, L.T. (1991). *Clinical anatomy of the lumbar spine.* London: Churchill Livingstone.

Bodguk, N. Tynan, W., & Wilson, A. (1981). The nerve supply to the human lumbar intervertebral discs. *J Anat, 132,* 39-56.

Breger, R. et al. (1988). Truncation artifact in MR images of the intervertebral disc. *AJRN, 9,* 825-828.

Breig, A. & Troup, J. (1979). Biomechanical considerations in the straight leg raising test. *Spine, 4,* 242-250.

Brown, B.M. et al. (1988). Preoperative evaluation of cervical radiculopathy and myelopathy by surface-coil MRI imaging. *AJR, 151,* 1205-1212.

Buckwalter, J. et al. (1989). Articular cartilage and intervertebral disc proteoglycans differ in structure: An electron microscopic study. *J Orthop Res, 7,* 146-151.

Byrd, R. et al. (1990). Reliability of magnetic resonance imaging for morphometry, of the intervertebral foramen. *Proc 1990 Intrnatl Conf Spin Manip, 1,* 79-82.

Chen, K.P. et al. (1989). The depth of the epidural space. *Anaesth Sinica, 27,* 353-356.

Clarke, G.A. et al. (1985). Can infant malnutrition cause adult vertebral stenosis? *Spine, 10,* 165-170.

Coventry, M.B. (1969). Anatomy of the intervertebral disc. *Clin Orthop, 67,* 9-15.

Cramer, G. et al. (1992a.). Comparative evaluation of the lumbar intervertebral foramen by computed tomography and magnetic resonance imaging. *Clin Anat, 5,* 238.

Cramer, G. et al. (1992b.). Lumbar intervertebral foramen dimensions from thirty-seven human subjects as determined by magnetic resonance imaging. *Proc 1992 Intrnatl Conf Spin Manipulation, 1,* 3-5.

Crock, H.V. (1970). Isolated lumbar disk resorption as a cause of nerve root canal stenosis. *Clin Orthop, 115,* 109-115.

Czervionke, L. et al. (1988). Cervical neural foramina: Correlative anatomic and MR imaging study. *Radiology, 169,* 753-759.

Dabezies, E. et al. (1988). Safety and efficacy of chymopapain (discase) in the treatment of sciatica due to a herniated nucleus pulposus: Results of a double-blind study. *Spine, 13,* 561-565.

Djukic, S. et al. (1990). Magnetic resonance imaging of the postoperative lumbar spine. *Radiol Clin North Am, 28,* 341-360.

Domisse, G.F. & Louw, J.A. (1990). Anatomy of the lumbar spine. In Y. Floman (Ed.), *Disorders of the lumbar spine.* Rockville, Md, and Tel Aviv: Aspen Publishers and Freund Publishing House.

Edgar, M. & Ghadially, J. (1976). Innervation of the lumbar spine. *Clin Orthop, 115,* 35-41.

Engel, R. & Bogduk, N. (1982). The menisci of the lumbar zygapophysial joints. *J Anat, 135,* 795-809.

Fagerlund, M.K.J. & Thelander, U.E. (1989). Comparison of myelography and computed tomography in establishing lumbar disc herniation. *Acta Radiol, 30,* 241-246.

Fardon, D.F. (1988). The name of the ring. *Spine, 13,* 713-715.

Fesmire, F. & Luten, R. (1989). The pediatric cervical spine: Development anatomy and clinical aspects. *J Emerg Med, 7,* 133-142.

Foreman, S.M. & Croft, A.C.. (1988). Whiplash injuries: The cervical acceleration/deceleration syndrome. Baltimore: Williams & Wilkins.

Forristall, R., Marsh, H., & Pay, N. (1988). Magnetic resonance imaging and contrast CT of the lumbar spine: Comparison of diagnostic methods of correlation with surgical findings. *Spine, 13,* 1049-1054.

Foster, R. (1988). Computed tomography of spinal trauma. In J.H. Bisese (Ed.), *Spine, state of the art reviews, spinal imaging: Diagnostic and therapeutic applications.* Philadelphia: Hanley & Belfus.

Frocrain, L. et al. (1989). Recurrent postoperative sciatica: Evaluation with MR imaging and enhanced CT. *Radiology, 170,* 531-533.

Giles, L.G. (1992). The surface lamina of the articular cartilage of human zygapophyseal joints. *Anat Rec, 233,* 350-356.

Giles, L.G., & Taylor, J.R. (1987). Human zygapophyseal joint capsule and synovial fold innervation. *Br J Rehumatol, 26,* 93-98.

Gilsanz, V. (1988). Vertebral bone density in children: Effects of puberty. *Radiology, 166,* 847-850.

Gilsanz, V. et al. (1988). Peak trabecular vertebral density: A comparison of adolescent and adult females. *Calcif Tissue Int, 43,* 260-262.

Golub, B. & Siverman, B. (1969). Transforaminal ligaments of the lumbar spine. *J Bone Joint Surg, 51,* 947-956.

Hasue, M. et al. (1983). Anatomic study of the interrelation between lumbosacral nerve roots and their surrounding tissues. *Spine, 8,* 50-58.

Hedberg, M.C., Dayer, B.P., & Flom, R.A. (1988). Gradient echo (GRASS) MR imaging in cervical radiculopathy. *AJNR, 9,* 145-151.

Herkowitz, H.N., et al. (1992). Discussion on cigarette smoking and the prevalence of spinal procedures. *J Spin Disord, 5,* 135-136.

Hewitt, W. (1970). The intervertebral foramen. *Physiotherapy, 56,* 332-336.

Ho, P.S.P. et al. (1988). Progressive and regressive changes in the nucleus pulposus. Part I. The neonate. *Radiology, 169,* 87-91.

Holm, S. & Nachemson, A. (1983). Variations in the nutrition of the canine intervertebral disc induced by motion. *Spine, 8,* 866-874.

Hueftle, M. et al. (1988). Lumbar spine: Postoperative MR imaging with Gd-DTPA. *Radiology, 167,* 817-824.

Humzah, M.D. & Soames, R.W. (1988). Human intervertebral disc: Structure and function. *Anat Rec, 220,* 337-356.

Isherwood, I. & Antoun, N.M. (1980). CT scanning in the assessment of lumbar spine problems. In M. Jayson (Ed.) *The lumbar spine and back pain* (2nd ed.). London: Pitman Publishing.

Ito, S. et al. (1991). An observation of ruptured annulus fibrosus in lumbar discs. *J Spin Disord, 4,* 462-466.

Jackson, R. et al. (1989). The neuroradiographic diagnosis of lumbar herniated nucleus pulposes. II. A comparison of computed tomography (CT), myelography, CT-myelography, and magnetic resonance imaging. *Spine, 14,* 1362-1367.

Jayson, M. (1980). *The lumbar spine and back pain* (2nd ed.). Baltimore: Urban & Schwarzenberg and Pitman Publishing.

Jayson, M. (1992). *The lumbar spine and back pain* (4th ed). London: Churchill Livingstone.

Jeffries, B. (1988). Facet joint injections. *Spine: State of the art reviews, 2,* 409-417.

Kos, J. & Wolf, J. (1972). Les menisques intervertebraux et le role possible dans les blocages vertebraux (translation), *J Orthop Sports Phys Ther, 1,* 8-9.

Kraemer, J. et al. (1985). Water and electrolyte content of human intervertebral discs under variable load. *Spine, 0,* 69-71.

Kricun, R., Kricun, M., & Danlinka, M. (1990). Advances in spinal imaging. *Radiol Clin North Am, 28,* 321-339.

Kushner, D.C. & Cleveland, R.H. (1988). Digital imaging in scoliosis. In M.E. Kricun (Ed.). *Imaging modalities in spinal disorders.* Philadelphia. WB Saunders.

Lancourt, J.E., Glenn, W.V. & Wiltse, L.L. (1979). Multiplanar computerized tomography in the normal spine and in the diagnosis of spinal stenosis: A gross anatomic-computerized tomographic correlation. *Spine, 4,* 379-390.

LeBlanc, A.D. et al: (1988). The spine: Changes in T2 relaxation times from disuse. *Radiology, 169,* 105-107.

Leiviska, T. et al. (1985). Radiographic versus direct measurements of the spinal canal at the lumbar vertebrae L3-L5 and their relations to age and body stature. *Acta Radiol, 26*, 403-411.

Lippitt, A.B. (1984). The facet joint and its role in spine pain: Management with facet joint injections. *Spine, 9*, 746-750.

Lipson, S.J. (1988). Metaplastic proliferative fibrocartilage as an alternative concept to herniated intervertebral disc. *Spine, 13*, 1055-1060.

Louis, R. (1985). Spinal stability as defined by the three-column spine concept. *Anatomia Clinica, 7*, 33-42.

Martin, G. (1978). The role of trauma in disc protrusion. *N Z Med J, March*, 208-211.

Mayoux-Benhamou, M.A. et al. (1989). A morphometric study of the lumbar foramen: Influence of flexion-extension movements and of isolated disc colapse. *Surg Radiol Anat, 11*, 97-102.

McFadden, J.W. (1988). The stress lumbar discogram. *Spine, 13*, 931-933.

Mendel, T. et al. (1992). Neural elements in human cervical intervertebral discs. *Spine, 17*, 132-135.

Mirkovic, S. & Melany, M. (1992). A thoracolumbar epidural hematoma simulating a disc syndrome. *J Spin Disord, 5*, 112-115.

Mixter, W.J. & Barr, J.S. (1934). Rupture of the intervertebral disc with involvement of the spinal canal. *N Engl J Med, 211*, 210-215.

Moffit, B. et al. (1988). Comparison of T1 and T2 weighted images of the lumbar spine. *Computer Med Imaging Graph, 12*, 271-276.

Mooney, V. & Robertson, J. (1976). The facet syndrome. *Clin Orthop Res, 115*, 149-156.

Moroney, S. et al. (1988). Load displacement properties of lower cervical spine motion segments. *J Biomech, 21*, 769-779.

Mosekilde, L. (1989). Sex differences in age-related loss of vertebral trabecular bone mass and structure biomechanical consequences. *Bone, 10*, 425-432.

Mosekilde, L. & Mosekilde, L. (1990). Sex differences in age-related changes in vertebral body size, density and biomechanical competence in normal individuals. *Bone, 11*, 67-73.

Nathan, H., Weizenbluth, M., & Halperin, N. (1982). The lumbosacral ligament (LSL), with special emphasis on the "lumbosacral tunnel" and the entrapment of the 5th lumber nerve. *Int Orthopaedics, 6*, 197-202.

Nitobe, T. et al. (1988). Degradation and biosynthesis of proteoglycans in the nucleus pulposus of canine intervertebral disc after chymopapain treatment. *Spine, 11*, 1332-1339.

Nowicki, B.H. & Haughton, V.M. (1992a). Ligaments of the lumbar neural foramina: A sectional anatomic study. *Clin Anat, 5*, 126-135.

Nowicki, B.H. & Haughton, V.M. (1992b). Neural foraminal ligaments of the lumbar spine: Appearance at CT and MR imaging. *Radiology, 183* (1), 257-264.

Osborn, A. et al. (1988). CT/MR spectrum of far lateral and anterior lumbosacral disk herniations. *AJNR, 9*, 775-778.

Pal, G.P. et al. (1988). Trajectory architecture of the trabecular bone between the body and the neural arch in human vertebrae. *Anat Rec, 222*, 418-425.

Panjabi, M., Oxland, T., & Parks, E. (1991). Quantitative anatomy of cervical spine ligaments. II. Middle and lower cervical spine. *J Spin Disord, 4*, 277-285.

Paris, S. (1983). Anatomy as related to function and pain. Symposium on Evaluation and Care of Lumbar Spine Problems. *Orthop Clin North Am, 14*, 476-489.

Pate, D., Resnick, D., & Andre, M. (1986). Perspective: Three-dimensional imaging of the musculoskeletal system. *AJNR, 147*, 545-551.

Pfaundler, S. (1989). Pedicle origin and intervertebral compartment in the lumbar and upper sacral spine. *Acta Neurochir, 97*, 158-165.

Ribot, C. et al. (1988). Influence of the menopause and aging on spinal density in French women. *Bone Miner, 5*, 89-97.

Rydevik, B. et al. (1984). Pathoanatomy and physiology of nerve root compression. *Spine, 9*, 7-15.

Salamon, O. & Freilich, M. (1988). Calcified hemangioma of the spinal canal: Unusual CT and MR presentation. *AJNR, 9*, 799-802.

Sanders, M. & Stein, K. (1988). Conservative management of herniated nucleus pulposes: Treatment approaches. *J Manipulative Physiol Ther, 11*, 309-313.

Schnebel, B. et al. (1989). Comparison of MRI to contrast CT in the diagnosis of spinal stenosis. *Spine, 14*, 332-337.

Sei, A. et al. (1991). Cervical spinal epidural hematoma with spontaneous remission. *J Spin Disord, 4*, 234-237.

Shapiro, R. (1990). Talmudic and other concepts of the number of vertebrae in the human spine. *Spine, 15*, 246-247.

Shealy, C.N. (1975). Facet denervation in the management of back and sciatic pain. *Clin Orthop, 115*, 157-164.

Singer, K., Giles, L., & Day, R. (1990). Intra-articular synovial folds of thoracolumbar junction zygapophyseal joints. *Anat Rec, 226*, 147-152.

Taylor, J. (1990). The development and adult structure of lumbar intervertebral discs. *J Man Med, 5*, 43-47.

Theil, H.W., Clements, D.S., & Cassidy, J.D. (1992). Lumbar apophyseal ring fractures in adolescents. *J Manipulative Physiol Ther, 15*, 250-254.

Tracy, P.T., Wright, R.M., & Hanigan, W.C. (1989). Magnetic resonance imaging of spinal injury. *Spine, 14*, 292-301.

Vital, J. et al. (1989). The neurocentral vertebral cartilage: Anatomy, physiology, and physiopathology. *Surg Radiol Anat, 11*, 323-328.

Wang, A., Wesolowski, D., & Farah, J. (1988). Evaluation of posterior spinal structures by computed tomography. In J.H. Bisese (Ed.), *Spine, state of the art reviews, spinal imaging: Diagnostic and therapeutic applications.* Philadelphia: Hanley & Belfus.

Weinstein, J., Claverie, W., & Gibson, S. (1988). The pain of discography. *Spine, 13*, 1344-1348.

White, A.A., & Panjabi, M.M. (1990). *Clinical biomechanics of the spine* (2nd ed.). Philadelphia: JB Lippincott.

Williams, P.L. et al. (1989). *Gray's anatomy* (37th ed.). Edinburgh: Churchill Livingstone.

Woodruff, W., Jr. (1988). Evaluation of disc disease by magnetic resonance imaging. In J.H. Bisese (Ed.), *Spine, state of the art review, spinal imaging: Diagnostic and therapeutic applications.* Philadelphia: Hanley & Belfus.

Wyke, B. (1985). Articular neurology and manipulative therapy. In E.F. Glasgow, et al. (Eds.), *Aspects of Manipulative Therapy*, (2nd ed). London: Churchill Livingstone.

Xu, G. et al. (1991). Normal variations of the lumbar facet joint capsules. *Clin Anat, 4*, 117-122.

CHAPTER 3

General Anatomy of the Spinal Cord

Susan A. Darby

The purpose of this chapter is to describe in detail the gross anatomy of the external spinal cord, its coverings, and its vasculature. To help the reader acquire a general appreciation of the spinal cord as a complete entity, this chapter also provides a cursory description of the organization and physiology of the spinal cord's internal aspect. Subsequent chapters expand on the generalities presented here. The spinal cord's intimate relationship to the vertebral column makes the spinal cord anatomy extremely important to those who treat disorders of the spine.

OVERVIEW OF SPINAL CORD ORGANIZATION

The spinal cord, which is located in the vertebral (spinal) canal, is a cylindric-shaped structure with a tapered inferior end. The cord is well protected by the vertebrae and the ligaments associated with the vertebrae. In addition to these bones and ligaments, cerebrospinal fluid (CSF) and a group of membranes, collectively referred to as the meninges, also provide protection. It is important to realize that the cord does not lie immediately adjacent to the bone and ligaments but that fluid, meninges, fat, and a venous plexus separate the bone from the spinal cord (Fig. 3-1).

At the level of the skull's foramen magnum, the spinal cord becomes continuous with the medulla oblongata of the brain stem (Fig. 3-2). Although in cross section it is impossible to delineate the exact beginning of the cord and the end of the brain stem at that particular level, the beginning of the cord is easily distinguished by the definitive presence of the skull and vertebrae. As mentioned in Chapter 12, a period during development occurs when the spinal cord extends the length of the vertebral column. However, while the vertebral column continues to develop in length, the spinal cord lags behind so that it occupies the upper two thirds of the vertebral (spinal) canal. At birth the cord ends at approximately the level of the L3 vertebra. In adults, because of continued greater growth of the vertebral column, the spinal cord ends at the level of the disc between the L1 and L2 vertebrae. In some individuals, however, the spinal cord may end as high as the T12 vertebra or as low as the L3 vertebra. At the level of the caudal part of the T12 vertebral body, the cord tapers down to a cone, which is known as the conus medullaris (Fig. 3-3, B). The overall length of the spinal cord is approximately 42 cm in an average-sized female and 45 cm in an averaged-sized male. The spinal cord's weight is approximately 30 to 35 g. It is important to remember that in most individuals the spinal cord does not extend inferior to the L2 vertebra. Therefore a lesion such as a herniated disc or trauma occurring below the L2 vertebra does not directly affect the spinal cord.

Before discussing the external surface of the spinal cord in detail, it is pertinent to describe the cord's general function. The spinal cord and brain develop from the same embryologic structure, the neural tube,

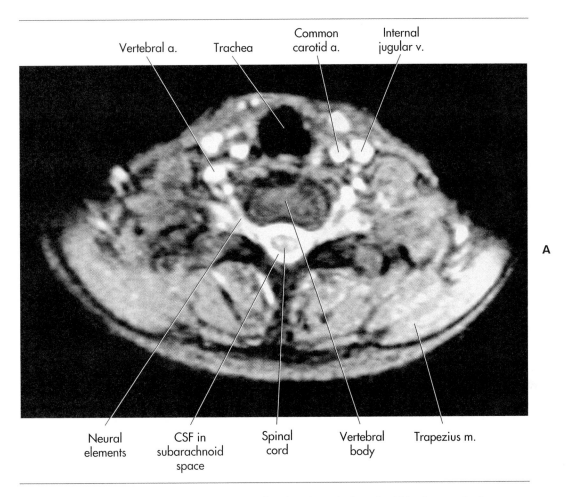

Vertebral a.   Trachea   Common carotid a.   Internal jugular v.

A

Neural elements   CSF in subarachnoid space   Spinal cord   Vertebral body   Trapezius m.

FIG. 3-1   Magnetic resonance images (MRIs) showing the spinal cord within the vertebral canal. **A,** Horizontal section through the cervical cord.   *Continued.*

and together they form the central nervous system (CNS). The obvious difference is that one end of the neural tube becomes encased in the skull, while the remainder of the neural tube becomes encased in the vertebral column. Size alone indicates that the higher centers making up the brain process information more thoroughly and complexly than the processing that occurs in the spinal cord. For the CNS to respond to the environment, it requires input from structures peripheral to the CNS and, in turn, a means to send output to structures called effectors. The sensory input begins in peripheral receptors found throughout the entire body in skin, muscles, tendons, joints, and viscera. These receptors send electrical currents (action potentials) toward the spinal cord of the CNS via the nerves that make up the peripheral nervous system (PNS). The sensory receptors respond to general sensory information such as pain, temperature, touch, or proprioception (awareness of body position and movement). The PNS also is used when the CNS sends output to the body's effectors, for example, smooth muscle, cardiac muscle, skeletal muscle, and glands. Thus the PNS is a means by which the CNS communicates with its surrounding environment.

By now it is apparent that the PNS consists of the body's nerves. Twelve pairs of these nerves are associated with the brain (10 of which are attached to the brain stem) and innervate structures primarily in the head. These nerves, called cranial nerves, also convey special sense information such as hearing, vision, and taste. In the context of this chapter, another group of peripheral nerves is more pertinent. These 31 pairs of nerves attach to the spinal cord; communicate with structures primarily located in the neck, trunk, and extremities; and are called the spinal nerves. In general, once input reaches the spinal cord via the spinal nerves, a reflex arc may be formed, and output is sent immediately back to the peripheral effectors. The spinal cord may also send the input to higher brain centers for further processing. The higher centers may then send information down to the spinal cord, which in turn relays it out to the periphery, again via spinal nerves (Fig. 3-4).

One spinal nerve is formed by the merger of two roots within the intervertebral foramen (IVF). One root, called

B

FIG. 3-1, cont'd. **B,** Midsagittal section of the thoracic cord.

the dorsal root, conveys the sensory information. The cell bodies of these sensory fibers are located in the dorsal root ganglion. The cell bodies are not found in the spinal cord because they developed from neural crest (see Chapter 12). Each sensory neuron of the PNS is pseudounipolar because two processes diverge from one common stem (Fig. 3-4). One of the processes is called the peripheral process and is attached to a peripheral receptor. The other process is the central process, which is in the dorsal root and enters the spinal cord (CNS). The dorsal root contains fibers of various diameters and conduction velocities that convey all types of sensory information. Cutaneous fibers of the dorsal root convey sensory information from a specific strip of skin called a dermatome. As the dorsal root approaches the spinal cord within the individual vertebral foramen, it divides into approximately six to eight dorsal rootlets, or filaments. These rootlets attach in a vertical row to the cord's dorsolateral sulcus. The other root, which helps form a spinal nerve, is called the ventral root and conveys motor information to the body's effectors, that

is, all muscle tissue and glands. The cell bodies of these axons are located in the spinal cord. The axons emerge from the cord's ventrolateral sulcus as ventral rootlets and unite to form one ventral root. Within the IVF the dorsal and ventral roots form the spinal nerve, which subsequently divides into its two major components: the *dorsal* and *ventral rami* (also known as the posterior primary division and anterior primary division, respectively).

From this description, it can be seen that nerves formed distal to the formation of the spinal nerve (distal to the IVF and including the rami) are mixed because they contain fibers conveying sensory input and fibers conveying motor output. However, proximal to the IVF, sensory and motor information is segregated in the form of separate dorsal and ventral roots. This segregation of dorsal and ventral root fibers and therefore root function was discussed and demonstrated by Bell and Magendie in the early 1800s and later was referred to as the law of separation of function of spinal roots (law of Bell and Magendie) (Coggeshall, 1980).

EXTERNAL MORPHOLOGY

The external surface of the spinal cord is not a smooth surface but instead shows grooves of various depths called sulci and fissures. (When discussing cord anatomy, it is important to understand that the terms *dorsal* and *ventral* can be used interchangeably with *posterior* and *anterior,* respectively.) The spinal cord's dorsal surface includes a midline dorsal median sulcus, right and left dorsal intermediate sulci (located from the midthoracic cord region superiorly), and right and left dorsolateral sulci. The cord's ventral surface includes a midline ventral median fissure (approximately 3 mm deep) and right and left ventrolateral sulci. When inspecting the cord's external surface, the dorsal and ventral rootlets are readily apparent, and the outward attachment of the paired dorsal rootlets and paired ventral rootlets to the cord defines one spinal cord segment (Fig. 3-5).

One pair of spinal nerves is therefore associated with one cord segment, and since 31 pairs of spinal nerves exist, there are also 31 spinal cord segments. These cord segments are numbered similar to numbering the spinal nerves: 8 cervical, 12 thoracic, 5 lumbar, 5 sacral, and 1 coccygeal cord segment. (Note that the first seven cervical nerves exit the IVF above their corresponding vertebra, and the remaining nerves exit below their corresponding vertebra. This allows for one more cervical spinal nerve than cervical vertebrae.) Therefore the coccygeal segment is found at the very tip of the conus medullaris, which, as mentioned previously, is usually at the level of the L1-L2 disc. This means that cord segments are not necessarily located at the same level as

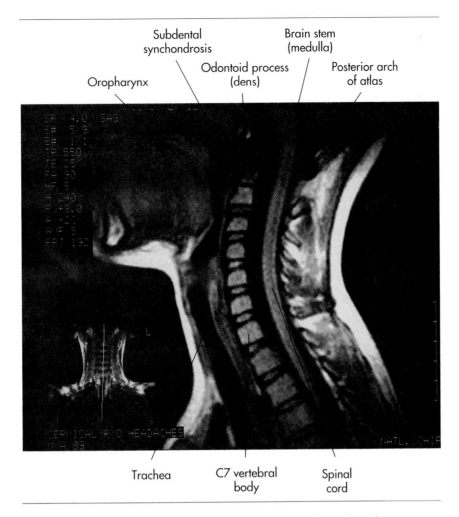

Subdental synchondrosis

Oropharynx

Odontoid process (dens)

Brain stem (medulla)

Posterior arch of atlas

Trachea

C7 vertebral body

Spinal cord

FIG. 3-2   Sagittal MR image of the brain stem and cervical spinal cord.

their corresponding vertebrae (Fig. 3-6). Since cord length may vary among individuals, the relationship between cord segments and vertebral levels is always an approximation.

Cervical cord segments and cervical vertebrae generally correspond closely to one another, but the remaining segments do not. The segment's length changes such that the L1 through coccygeal cord segments are housed by vertebrae T9 through L1. This anatomic relationship of cord segment to vertebra is important to remember for clinical reasons. For example, a patient with a fractured L1 vertebra does not experience the same lower extremity signs and symptoms as a patient with a fractured T10 vertebra, since a T10 fracture injures upper lumbar segments and an L1 fracture injures the lower sacral and coccygeal segments. Although the spinal cord ends at the L1-L2 disc, each root that corresponds to a cord segment forms a spinal nerve and exits at its corresponding IVF. This includes the IVFs below the L2 vertebra. Therefore the roots/rootlets of the more inferior cord segments need to be longer and descend to their respective IVFs at a more oblique angle than the roots/rootlets of cervical segments, which are shorter and almost at right angles to the spinal cord. The lumbosacral roots therefore become the longest and most oblique. The collection of these elongated lumbosacral roots making their way inferiorly to their corresponding IVF is called the cauda equina (Fig. 3-6; see also Fig. 3-8, *B*) because of its resemblance to a horse's tail.

In addition to the sulci and fissures, another anatomic characteristic seen on gross inspection of the spinal cord is the presence of two enlarged areas. One area is the cervical enlargement seen in cord segments C4 to T1. These cord segments are responsible for the input from and output to the upper extremities. The other cord enlargement is the lumbar enlargement, which is visible from segments L1 to S3. These segments are responsible for the input from and output to the lower extremities. Since many more structures must be innervated in the extremities than in the trunk, it is necessary to have more neuron cell bodies in the cord, and thus these two regions are enlarged (Fig. 3-7; see also Figs. 3-3, *A,* and 3-5).

MENINGES

Surrounding and providing protection and support to the spinal cord is a group of three membranes that are collectively called the meninges. The meninges surrounding the spinal cord are a continuation of the meninges surrounding the brain and consist of the dura mater, arachnoid mater, and pia mater (Figs. 3-8 and 3-9).

The dura mater, or pachymeninx, of the cord is the outermost membrane and is very tough. It is a continuation of the inner or meningeal layer of dura mater surrounding the brain and attaches to the edge of the foramen magnum, to the posterior aspect of the C2-3 vertebral bodies, and to the posterior longitudinal ligaments (Williams et al., 1989) by slips of tissue called Hofmann's ligaments (Spencer, Irwin, & Miller, 1983). The recurrent meningeal nerve (or sinuvertebral nerve of Von Luschka), which is formed outside the IVF and reenters the vertebral canal, provides a significant innervation to the anterior aspect of the spinal dura mater. Although a few nerves sparsely innervate the posterolateral dura mater, the posteromedial region appears to have no innervation, which may explain why a patient feels no pain when the dura mater is pierced during a lumbar puncture (Groen, Baljet, & Drukker, 1988). The spinal dura mater is separated from the vertebrae by the epidural space, which contains epidural fat, loose connective tissue, and an extensive epidural venous plexus (see Chapter 2).

Under the dura mater is a potential space called the subdural space. However, Haines (1991) has documented that in the cranium, this space is either artifactual or the result of some pathologic condition (e.g., subdural hematoma), and that underneath the cranial meningeal dura is a layer of dural border cells. The significance of the presence of dural border cells in the spinal meninges is unclear.

The middle layer of the meninges is the arachnoid mater. This is a nonvascular, thin, delicate, and loosely arranged membrane (Fig. 3-8, *A*). Both the dura and the arachnoid extend to the level of the S2 vertebra, well below the end of the spinal cord (conus medullaris). Also, both the dura and the arachnoid invest the roots, similar to a coat sleeve, as the roots travel distally toward the IVF, where they form their spinal nerve (Fig. 3-9). At that point the dura blends in with the epineurial connective tissue surrounding the newly formed spinal nerve. The arachnoid also merges with the connective tissue elements of the mixed spinal nerve, possibly the perineurium (Hewitt, 1970).

Under the arachnoid is the subarachnoid space (Fig. 3-9). This space is filled with CSF. Thus the cord, as with the brain, is supported and protected by floating in a fluid medium. The CSF is secreted by the choroid plexus, which is located in the ventricles within the

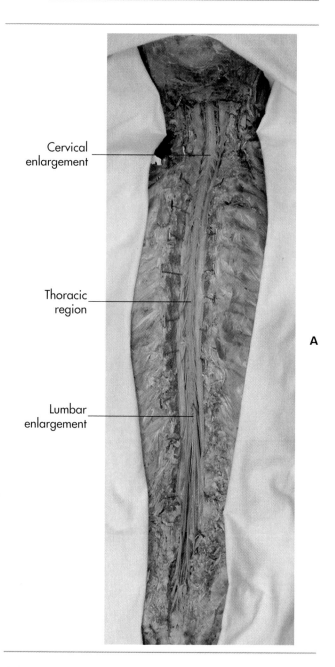

FIG. 3-3 Dorsal view of the spinal cord within the vertebral canal. The dura mater has been reflected laterally with pins. **A,** Spinal cord in its entirety.

brain. The choroid plexus, through various cellular transport mechanisms, ensures the chemical stability of CSF components. This in turn provides a constant, stable environment for the CNS.

The CSF flows in one direction within the ventricles located in the brain. At a level just rostral to the foramen magnum, most CSF leaves the most caudal (fourth) ventricle and enters the subarachnoid space surrounding the brain and the spinal cord. In addition, a very small amount of CSF remains within the cord's central canal. The subarachnoid space also contains large arteries that vascularize the cord. The pulsation of these

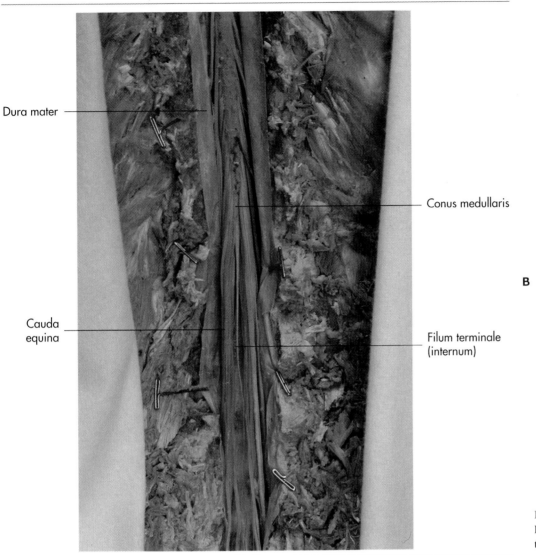

Dura mater

Conus medullaris

B

Cauda equina

Filum terminale (internum)

FIG. 3-3, cont'd. **B,** Lumbosacral region of the spinal cord.

arteries, the pressure of the CSF, and spinal movements cause the CSF surrounding the cord to flow superiorly and into the subarachnoid space surrounding the brain. Because of a pressure gradient, the CSF flows from the subarachnoid space through arachnoid granulations and into the venous sinuses of the cranial dura mater. However, at the level of the cord, some CSF is absorbed into the local venous system (Williams et al., 1989). Since the CSF ultimately flows into the systemic circulation, this one-way circulation becomes a means of removing metabolites from the CNS. At various locations throughout the CNS, the subarachnoid space may become enlarged. The enlargements are called cisterns, and the subarachnoid space below the conus medullaris is such an enlargement, called the lumbar cistern (Fig. 3-8, *B*). At this level the lumbar cistern contains not only CSF, but also the cauda equina and filum terminale (see the following discussion).

The innermost membrane of the meninges is called the pia mater. This is a thin layer of connective tissue that is subdivided into two parts: pia-glia, or pia intima, and epi-pia. The deeper pia-glia portion is avascular and intimately adheres to the cord, rootlets, and roots. The epi-pia includes blood vessels and forms a fold located in the ventral median fissure. Both layers surround the cord and follow the roots into the IVF.

Phylogenetically and embryologically (Williams et al., 1989), the pia and arachnoid of the CNS are closely related and called the leptomeninges. As they pull apart, tiny strands called trabeculae remain and can still be identified in the subarachnoid space. In the vertebral subarachnoid space the trabeculae become concentrated and form septa.

Unlike the pia surrounding the brain, the pia mater of the cord has two specializations that anchor the cord in place. One of these is a bluish white structure called the filum terminale. This slender filament of pia mater extends approximately 20 cm from the tip of the conus medullaris within the lumbar cistern (filum terminale internum) to the dorsum of the coccyx, where it blends

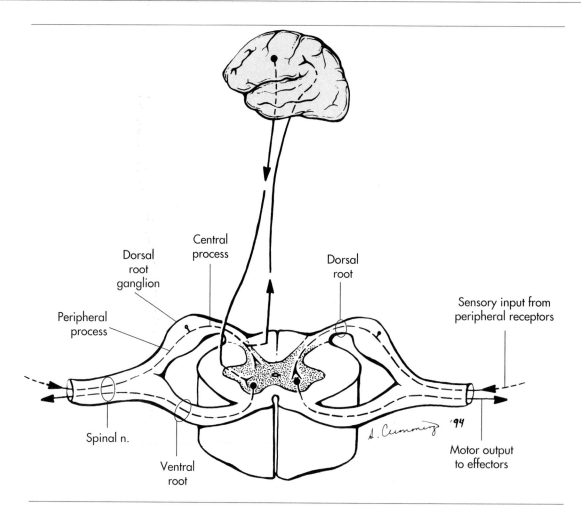

FIG. 3-4 General functions of the spinal cord. *Right,* Two-way communication between the spinal cord and the periphery. *Left,* Information within the cord traveling to and from higher centers in the brain.

into the connective tissue (Fig. 3-8, *B*). Since it must pierce the dura and arachnoid at the S2 level to reach the dorsum of the coccyx, the filum terminale picks up two additional layers (dura and arachnoid), and thus, from S2 to the coccyx, it is usually referred to as the coccygeal ligament (filum terminale externum).

The other special component of pia mater is the denticulate ligament. This is a serrated ribbon of epi-pia (Carpenter, 1991) that attaches to the dura mater at approximately 22 points on each side along the cord's length. Because of its location, the denticulate ligament forms a shelf within the vertebral canal between the dorsal and ventral roots (Figs. 3-8, *C,* and 3-9).

Since the spinal cord is usually not present below the L2 vertebra, and since the area between lumbar spinous processes is easily penetrated, a lumbar puncture (spinal tap) may be performed in this area. A long needle is inserted in the midline between the L3-4 or L4-5 vertebrae into the lumbar cistern, and 5 to 15 ml of CSF is removed. Because the cauda equina is floating in the CSF, the roots are usually avoided by the needle. A lumbar puncture is not routinely done, but when indicated, it is an important neurodiagnostic test.

The total volume of CSF ranges from 80 to 150 ml, and CSF is produced sufficiently to replace itself four to five times daily. CSF pressure ranges from 80 to 180 mm (water) and is measured on a patient lying in a curled, lateral recumbent position. CSF is normally clear, colorless, and slightly alkaline. It contains approximately six white blood cells (WBCs), usually lymphocytes, per milliliter and no red blood cells (RBCs). As with plasma, it includes sodium, potassium, magnesium, and chloride ions. It also contains glucose and protein, but the concentrations are substantially less than in plasma.

Knowing these CSF characteristics, including volume, becomes important because they may be altered as a result of a pathologic state. For example, the Monro-Kellie doctrine states that brain tissue, blood, and CSF volumes are constant, and that if one of these volumes increases,

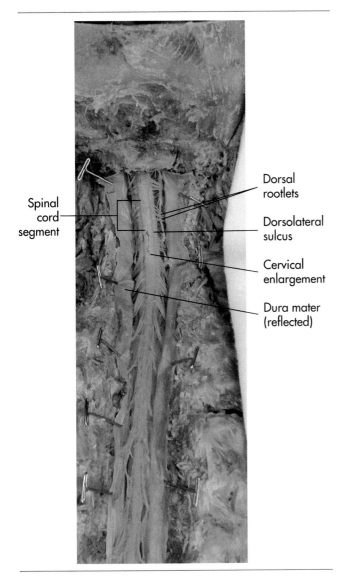

Spinal cord segment

Dorsal rootlets

Dorsolateral sulcus

Cervical enlargement

Dura mater (reflected)

FIG. 3-5 Dorsal view of the spinal cord. The cord segments are delineated by the attachment of rootlets to the spinal cord.

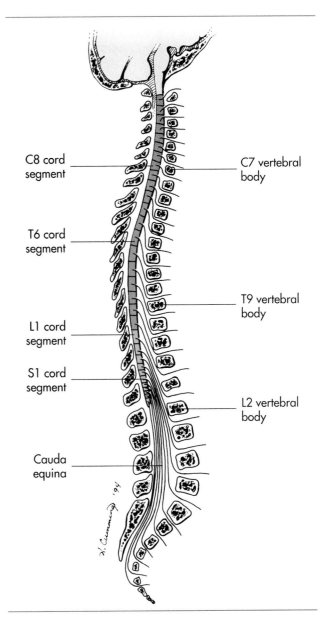

C8 cord segment

C7 vertebral body

T6 cord segment

T9 vertebral body

L1 cord segment

S1 cord segment

L2 vertebral body

Cauda equina

FIG. 3-6 Relationship of spinal cord segments and spinal nerves to vertebrae.

the other volumes must compensate because the bony confines do not. If no compensatory readjustment occurs, intracranial pressure (ICP) increases. An interference in CSF circulation in the cranium by a space-occupying lesion such as a tumor or hematoma can increase CSF pressure. If an increase in ICP is suspected, a spinal tap is contraindicated. Removal of CSF in such cases could produce a vacuum and cause herniation of the cerebellum into the foramen magnum, with serious consequences, including death. Increased CSF pressure can also cause swelling of the optic disc (papilledema) of the retina. Since the retina can easily be observed by an ophthalmoscope, papilledema could contraindicate the performance of a lumbar puncture.

In addition to pressure changes, the appearance, cell content, levels of gamma globulins (antibodies), and pro-

tein and glucose concentrations in CSF may be altered in patients with some pathologic conditions. For example, in bacterial meningitis (inflammation of the leptomeninges) the CSF is cloudy, pressure is increased, WBC count is elevated, protein concentration is increased, and glucose concentration is decreased (Daube et al., 1986). The CSF in a patient with a subarachnoid hemorrhage appears cloudy, and RBCs are present. Therefore the alterations of certain characteristics of the CSF become useful in diagnosing certain pathologic conditions.

In addition to removing CSF for analysis, agents can be injected into the region for diagnostic imaging and anesthetic purposes. In pneumoencephalography, some CSF is replaced with air via the lumbar cistern. The air

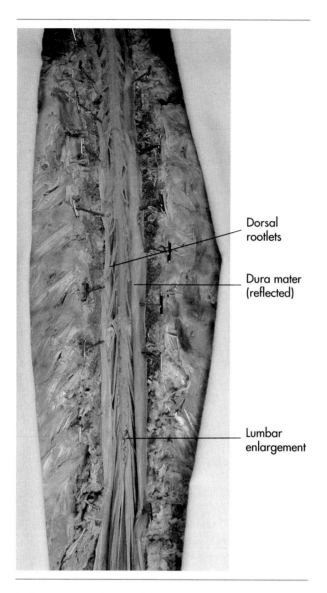

Dorsal rootlets

Dura mater (reflected)

Lumbar enlargement

FIG. 3-7 Dorsal view of the spinal cord showing the lumbar enlargement. Cervical enlargement is shown in Fig. 3-5.

travels superiorly and fills the ventricles. This allows the outline of the ventricles and the subarachnoid space to be seen on an x-ray film. In myelography, a radiopaque iodinated contrast medium is injected to outline the spinal cord and roots. Anesthetics may occasionally be injected into the subarachnoid space (spinal anesthesia) for abdominal or pelvic surgery. However, the anesthetic must be contained in that region. If it is not contained, it may travel superiorly and anesthetize the neurons of the phrenic nerve to the diaphragm (Moore, 1980). Most often, anesthetics are carefully injected into the epidural space to relieve the pain of childbirth while not anesthetizing the uterus.

INTERNAL ORGANIZATION OF THE SPINAL CORD

Having discussed the external morphology of the spinal cord and its coverings, the cord's internal morphology is now described to provide the reader with an understanding of spinal cord anatomy in its entirety. Chapter 9 provides a detailed description of the internal aspect of the spinal cord and its functions.

The overall internal organization of the spinal cord is readily seen in a transverse or horizontal cross section. This shows the spinal cord as being clearly divided into a butterfly-shaped or H-shaped central area of gray matter and a peripheral area of white myelinated axons.

Gray Matter

Each half of the H-shaped gray matter consists of a dorsal horn, a ventral horn, and an intermediate area between the horns (Fig. 3-10). In thoracic segments the intermediate zone includes a lateral horn. The crossbar of the H-shaped gray matter uniting the two laterally placed halves is composed of the dorsal and ventral commissures. These commissures surround the cord's central canal. This canal is the remnant of the lumen of the embryologic neural tube. It is lined by ependymal cells, and although it is continuous with the CSF-filled ventricles of the brain, the central canal is often filled in with cellular elements and debris, especially in the areas caudal to cervical and upper thoracic segments (Carpenter, 1991; deGroot & Chusid, 1988; Williams et al., 1989).

The cord's dense gray area consists of neurons, primarily cell bodies; neuroglia; and capillaries. Microscopically, this region appears to be a tangle of neuron processes and their synapses and neuroglial processes, all of which form the neuropil. This network forms the cord's amazingly complex circuitry. The neurons of the gray matter consist of four general types: motor, tract, interneuron, and propriospinal. The larger motor and tract neurons which have long axons, are sometimes referred to as Golgi type I cells. Interneurons and propriospinal neurons, which have shorter axons, may be referred to as Golgi type II cells (Carpenter, 1991; Williams et al., 1989).

Axons of motor neuron cell bodies leave the spinal cord, enter the ventral root, and ultimately innervate the body's effector tissues, that is, skeletal muscle, smooth muscle, cardiac muscle, and glands. Skeletal muscle is innervated by alpha and gamma motor neurons. Smooth muscle, cardiac muscle, and glands are innervated by autonomic motor fibers. Motor neuron cell bodies are located in either the ventral horn or the intermediate gray area and receive input from higher centers, incoming sensory afferent fibers, propriospinal neurons, and

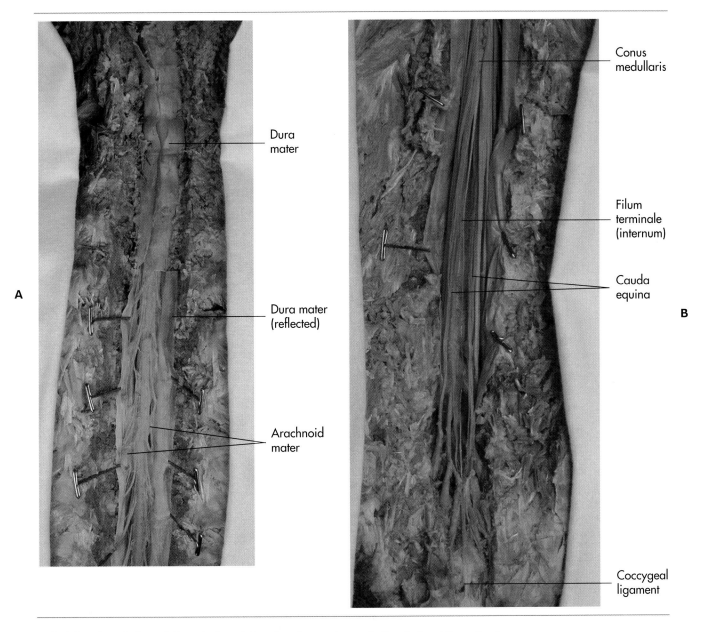

A

Dura
mater

Dura mater
(reflected)

Arachnoid
mater

B

Conus
medullaris

Filum
terminale
(internum)

Cauda
equina

Coccygeal
ligament

FIG. 3-8   Dorsal view of the spinal cord showing the meninges. **A,** Cervical and thoracic regions. **B,** Lumbar cistern and its contents.   *Continued.*

interneurons. It is believed that each of the large alpha motor neurons that innervate skeletal muscle may have 20,000 to 50,000 synapses on its surface (Barr & Kiernan, 1993; Davidoff & Hackman, 1991).

Axons of tract neurons in the gray matter emerge from the gray matter and ascend in the white matter to higher centers. These axons help to form the ascending tracts of the cord's white matter. The cell bodies of these neurons are located in the dorsal horn and in the intermediate gray area.

The third type of neuron is the interneuron. Interneurons make up the vast majority of the neuronal pop-

ulation in all parts of the gray matter. They conduct the important "business" of the CNS by forming complex connections. Although various types of interneurons exist, their processes are all relatively short, usually staying within the limits of one cord segment. The interneurons receive input from each other, from incoming sensory afferents, from propriospinal neurons, and from descending fibers from higher centers. In turn, some interneurons disseminate this input to the motor neurons. For example, some interneurons play a crucial role in motor control by their actions in motor reflexes involving peripheral proprioceptive input from neuromuscular

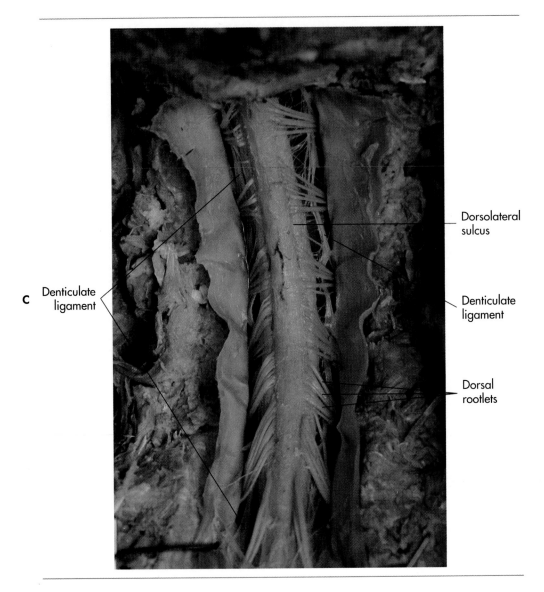

C   Denticulate ligament

Dorsolateral sulcus

Denticulate ligament

Dorsal rootlets

FIG. 3-8, cont'd.   C, Cervical cord segments.

spindles and Golgi tendon organs (see Chapter 9). Another type of "motor" interneuron called a Renshaw cell provides a negative feedback mechanism to adjacent motor neurons. This intricate circuitry may be necessary for synchronizing events such as the force, rate, timing, and coordination of contraction of muscle antagonists, synergists, and agonists that must occur in the complex motor activities performed by humans. In addition, other interneurons located in the dorsal horn are involved in the circuitry that modifies and edits pain input conveyed into the dorsal horn by afferent fibers (see Chapter 9).

The fourth type of neuron located in the gray matter is the propriospinal neuron. This neuron's axon leaves the gray matter, enters the white matter immediately adjacent to the gray, and ascends or descends to synapse on neurons in the gray matter of other cord segments. Some propriospinal neurons are short, whereas others are long enough to travel the cord's entire length. These neurons allow communication to occur among cord segments.

As mentioned, in cross section the gray matter resembles a butterfly-shaped or H-shaped area. Each half is subdivided into a dorsal horn, an intermediate area that in certain segments includes a lateral horn, and a ventral horn (Fig. 3-10). The dorsal horn functions as a receiving area for both descending information from higher centers and sensory afferents from the dorsal roots. The cell bodies of the sensory afferents are located in the dorsal root ganglia. The sensory afferents bring information from receptors in the skin (exteroceptors); muscles, tendons, and joints (proprioceptors); and the viscera (interoceptors). These afferent fibers synapse on interneurons, propriospinal neurons,

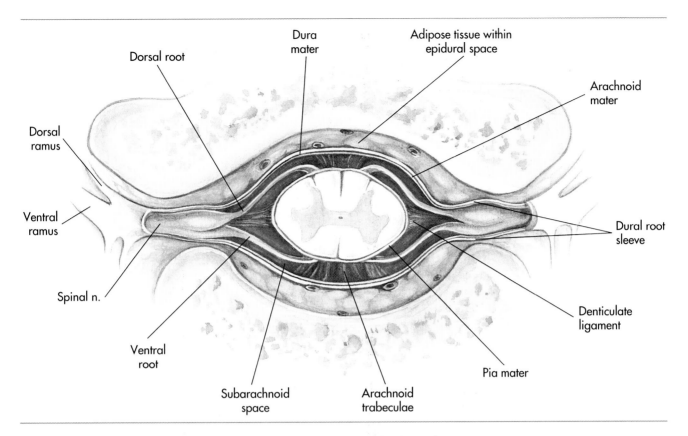

FIG. 3-9 Cross section of the spinal cord showing the meninges and dural root sleeves.

tract neurons, or motor neurons, depending on the type of information carried and the resulting action needed.

The intermediate region, which is actually the central core of each half of the gray matter, receives proprioceptive input from sensory afferents and descending input from higher centers, thus becoming an area where interaction of sensory and descending input can occur. The intermediate area also includes the cell bodies of neurons innervating smooth muscle, cardiac muscle, and glands. These cell bodies are located in cord segments T1 to L2-3 and make up the lateral horn.

The ventral horn of the gray matter includes interneurons, propriospinal neurons, terminal endings of descending tracts, and the axons of proprioceptors that are involved with monosynaptic stretch reflexes. More importantly, the cell bodies of motor neurons from which axons leave via the ventral roots to skeletal muscle (i.e., alpha and gamma motor neurons) are located here. In fact, these neurons are often called anterior horn cells.

As is the case throughout the nervous system, neurons communicate and form circuits with each other within the gray matter of the spinal cord by means of chemical substances. These chemical substances, which include neurotransmitters, are released at the synapse (i.e., the junction between two neurons). They are released from the terminal of one presynaptic neuron, cross the synaptic cleft, and bind to receptors on the postsynaptic neuron. By using techniques such as autoradiography and immunohistochemistry, chemical neuroanatomy is providing much new information concerning the neural circuitry of the spinal cord. Through labeling techniques, neurotransmitters have been localized in cell bodies in the gray matter and in axon terminals of neurons, including descending fibers and primary afferent fibers. Examples of neurotransmitters that have been found in the dorsal horn are enkephalins, somatostatin, substance P, cholecystokinin, dynorphin, gamma-aminobutyric acid (GABA), glycine, glutamate, and calcitonin gene-related peptide (CGRP). The intermediate gray matter and ventral horn include neurotransmitters such as cholecystokinin, enkephalins, serotonin, vasoactive intestinal polypeptide (VIP), glycine, and CGRP. These chemicals bind to specific receptors, some of which have also been located through labeling techniques. Examples of receptors located in various regions of the gray matter include opiate receptors, muscarinic cholinergic receptors, and receptors for GABA, CGRP, and thyrotropin-releasing hormone (Schoenen, 1991; Willis & Coggeshall, 1991).

The previous information has provided a cursory description of the three major regions of the spinal cord gray matter. In addition to the types of neurons composing gray matter, each half is also described

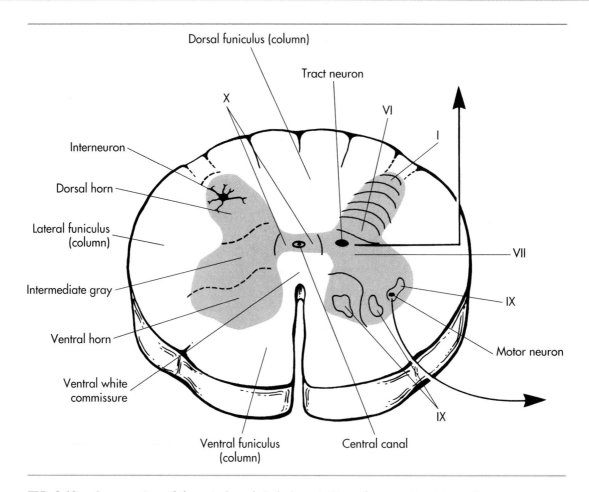

FIG. 3-10 Cross section of the spinal cord. *Left,* Organization of gray matter into regions. *Right,* Lamination of the gray matter. Motor and tract neurons and interneurons also are shown.

microscopically by its longitudinal laminar cytoarchitectural pattern. These longitudinal laminae contain nuclei. By definition, a nucleus is an aggregation of neuron cell bodies found within the CNS. The neurons of each nucleus are similar morphologically, and the axons have a common termination and function. Each nucleus may consist of interneuron, tract neuron, or motor neuron cell bodies. Numerous nuclei have been identified in the gray matter. Some are located in all cord segments, whereas others are limited to specific cord segments.

The laminar cytoarchitectural organization consists of 10 layers and was proposed by Rexed (1952) based on his studies of feline gray matter. This has since been accepted as standard in humans as well. Rexed's gray matter laminae proceed sequentially from dorsal to ventral (Fig. 3-10). Lamina I is the tip of the dorsal horn, and lamina IX is in the ventral horn. Lamina X corresponds to the dorsal and ventral gray commissures surrounding the central canal. Since the gray matter is divided into laminae, the aggregates of neurons forming nuclei are found in specific laminae. Therefore, it is important to learn what laminae house which nuclei. Chapter 9 provides a more detailed description of the laminae and nuclei.

White Matter

A cross section of the cord demonstrates that peripheral to the gray matter of the cord is a well-defined area of white matter (see Fig. 3-10). White matter includes myelinated axons, neuroglia, and blood vessels. The white matter is divided into three major areas called columns or funiculi. The dorsal funiculus or column is located between the dorsal horns, the lateral funiculus or column between each dorsal and ventral horn, and the ventral funiculus or column between the ventral horns (Fig. 3-10). The white area connecting the two halves of the cord consists of the dorsal and ventral white commissures. The ventral commissural area includes clinically important decussating axons of pain and temperature tract neurons. The neuron cell bodies of the axons that course in the funiculi are found in various locations. The cell bodies of axons that ascend in the spinal cord are located in the cord's gray matter or in the dorsal root ganglia. The cell bodies of axons that descend in the spinal cord to synapse in the gray matter are located in the brain.

The long ascending and descending axons are not randomly mixed together but are organized into bundles called tracts or fasciculi. The axons of each tract or fasciculus convey similar information to a common destination. For example, axons that are conveying impulses for pain and temperature are found in an anterolateral position in the cord. Although the tracts are well organized, they still overlap somewhat, and boundaries are often arbitrary.

Regional Characteristics

Although the characteristics of gray and white matter are generally the same in all cord segments, some identifying features are seen in cross section that distinguish the cervical, thoracic, lumbar, and sacral regions of the spinal cord (Fig. 3-11). For example, differences exist in the appearance and amount of white matter because of the presence and absence of certain tracts at different levels. Also, the gray matter changes its appearance because of regional differences in the number of somatic motor neuron cell bodies (the axons of which innervate skeletal muscles in the extremities) and autonomic motor neuron cell bodies (the axons of which innervate smooth muscle, cardiac muscle, and glands).

Cervical cord segments are large and oval shaped. At almost all levels, the transverse (side-to-side) diameter is greater than the sagittal (dorsal-to-ventral) diameter. The C1 transverse diameter is 12 mm and the C8 transverse diameter 13 to 14 mm, whereas the sagittal diameter at C8 is approximately 9 mm (Carpenter, 1991). The transverse and sagittal diameters through the junction of the C5-6 segments are 13.2 and 7 mm, respectively (Elliott, 1945). Since all ascending and descending axons to and from the brain must traverse the cervical region, the amount of white matter is greater here than in other regions. The ventral horn of gray matter found in the C4 to T1 segments is larger on its lateral aspect because of the increased number of motor neuron cell bodies, the axons of which innervate upper extremity skeletal muscles (Fig. 3-11).

Thoracic segments are most easily distinguished by their small amount of gray matter relative to white matter. Since the thoracic segments are not involved with innervating the muscles of the extremities, the lateral enlargement of the ventral horn is absent. Compared with cervical segments, both the transverse and the sagittal diameters of the thoracic spinal cord are smaller. A measurement at the junction of the T6-7 segments reveals an 8 mm transverse and 6.5 mm sagittal diameter (Elliott, 1945). One distinguishing feature of the thoracic segments is the presence of a lateral horn. This horn is located on the lateral aspect of the intermediate gray matter and is the residence of neuron cell bodies, the axons of which innervate smooth muscle, cardiac muscle, and glands. In addition, from midthoracic levels superiorly,

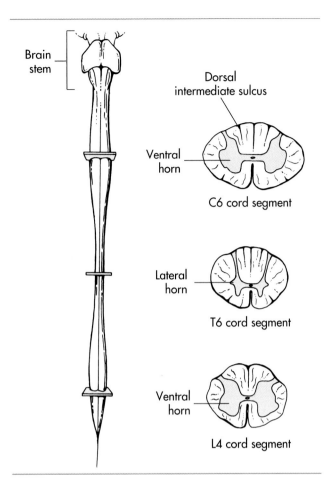

FIG. 3-11   Cross sections of the spinal cord at cervical, thoracic, and lumbar levels showing regional characteristics of gray and white matter.

the dorsal funiculus includes a dorsal intermediate sulcus (Fig. 3-11).

Lumbar segments are distinguished by their nearly round appearance. Although they contain relatively less white matter than cervical regions, the dorsal and ventral horns are very large. The ventral horns of the lumbar segments are involved with the innervation of lower extremity skeletal muscles, and the additional neuron cell bodies for the motor axons are located laterally in those ventral horns. The L3 transverse diameter is 12 mm and the sagittal diameter 8.5 mm (Carpenter, 1991). The diameters at the L5-S1 junction are 9.6 mm and 8 mm, respectively (Elliott, 1945). Although the T12 and L1 cord segments are indistinguishable, the large horns make lumbar segments easy to identify compared with cervical and thoracic segments (Fig. 3-11).

Sacral segments are recognized by their predominance of gray matter and relatively small amount of white matter. Interestingly, although cervical and lumbar segments have large transverse and sagittal diameters, the thoracic segments are the greatest in length (superior to inferior) and the sacral the shortest. The average superior-to-inferior dimensions of various cord segments are cervical, 13 mm; midthoracic, 26 mm; lumbar, 15 mm; and sacral, 5 mm (Schoenen, 1991).

Measurements of the transverse and sagittal diameters of the cord are useful clinically. Fujiwara and colleagues (1988) have shown on cadaveric cervical cord segments that measurements of the transverse and sagittal diameters and the compression ratio (sagittal diameter divided by the transverse diameter) made on computed tomography myelography (CTM) images are comparable to the actual dimensions of the gross cord segments themselves. Measurements of the transverse area and compression ratio also correlated with the severity of pathologic change in patients with cervical myelopathy. Therefore, CTM may be useful clinically in evaluating this type of pathologic condition.

ARTERIAL BLOOD SUPPLY OF THE SPINAL CORD

Spinal Arteries

The spinal cord is vascularized by branches of the vertebral artery and branches of segmental vessels. The vertebral artery, a branch of the subclavian artery, courses superiorly through the foramina of the transverse processes of the upper six cervical vertebrae to enter the posterior cranial fossa via the foramen magnum. Within the posterior fossa of the cranial cavity, one small ramus from each of the vertebral arteries anastomose in a Y-shaped configuration to form the anterior spinal artery (Fig. 3-12). Usually this occurs within 2 cm from their origin but may occur as far inferiorly as the C5 cord segment (Turnbull, Brieg, & Hassler, 1966). The anterior spinal artery courses caudally in the ventral median fissure of the medulla oblongata of the brain stem, which it helps to supply, and continues inferiorly within the pia mater at the level of the cord's ventral median fissure. This artery is usually straight, coursing inferiorly in the midline, but may alter to one side as the anterior radicular arteries anastomose with it. The anterior spinal artery is well defined in the cervical regions and largest in diameter at approximately the level of the artery of Adamkiewicz (about T9 to T12). In the thoracic region the anterior spinal artery narrows just superior to the level of the artery of Adamkiewicz and often is barely evident (Gillilan, 1958; Schoenen, 1991).

Also branching from each vertebral artery, and less frequently from the posterior inferior cerebellar artery, is the posterior spinal artery (Fig. 3-12). Each posterior spinal artery supplies the dorsolateral region of the caudal medulla oblongata. As it continues on the spinal cord, each artery forms two longitudinally irregular, anastomotic channels that course inferiorly on both sides of the dorsal rootlet attachment to the spinal cord.

The medial channel is larger than the lateral (Schoenen, 1991). The two anastomotic channels are interconnected across the midline by numerous small vessels. Small branches form a pial plexus on the cord's posterior aspect.

At the level of the conus medullaris, a loop is formed as the anterior spinal artery anastomoses with the two posterior spinal arteries (Lazorthes et al., 1971). At this location the artery of the filum terminale branches off and courses on the filum's ventral surface (Djindjian et al., 1988).

Although the spinal arteries originate in the cranial cavity, segmental vessels, which help to supply blood to the cord, originate outside the vertebral column. The segmental arteries in the cervical region include branches of the cervical part of the vertebral artery, which vascularize most of the cervical cord, and branches of ascending and deep cervical arteries. The latter arteries originate from the subclavian artery's thyrocervical and costocervical trunks, respectively. Segmental branches that help to supply the rest of the cord arise from intercostal and lumbar arteries, which are branches of the aorta, and lateral sacral arteries, which are branches of the internal iliac artery. These vessels provide spinal branches that enter the vertebral canal through the IVF; vascularize the meninges, ligaments, osseous structures, roots, and rootlets; and reinforce the spinal arteries.

As each of the 31 pairs (Lazorthes et al., 1971) of spinal branches of the segmental spinal arteries enters its respective IVF, it divides into three branches. Anterior and posterior branches vascularize the dura mater, ligaments, and osseous tissue of the vertebral canal. The third branch, called the neurospinal artery (of Kadyi) (Schoenen, 1991), courses with the spinal nerve and divides into anterior and posterior radicular arteries. The radicular arteries course on the ventral aspect of their corresponding root within the subarachnoid space. Each of the roots is vascularized by small branches (less than 0.2 mm diameter) of these radicular arteries. A variable number of the large anterior and posterior radicular arteries continue to the anterior and posterior spinal arteries that they reinforce (Figs. 3-12 and 3-13). Usually the anterior radicular artery does not reach the spinal artery at the same segmental level as the posterior radicular artery (Gillilan, 1958; Turnbull et al., 1966).

Anterior Radicular Arteries

Anterior radicular arteries (defined here as those that reach the anterior spinal artery) vary in number from 5 to 10. Since the anterior spinal artery sufficiently supplies the first two or three cervical segments, the anterior radicular arteries of the vertebral, ascending, and

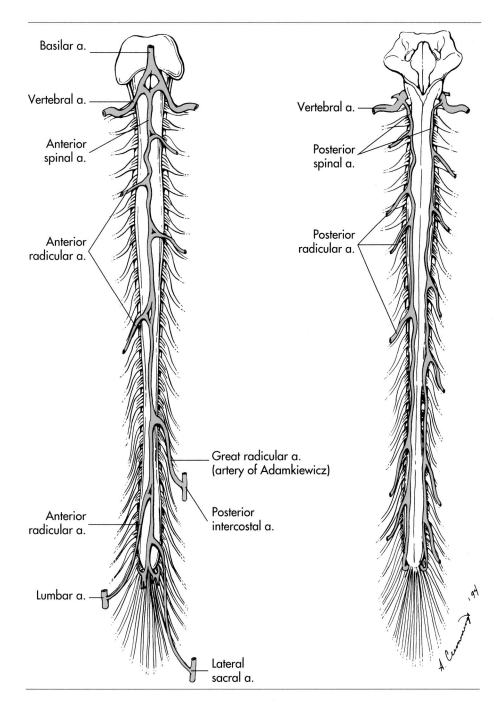

FIG. 3-12   Arterial blood supply of the spinal cord showing spinal and radicular arteries. **A,** Anterior view. **B,** Posterior view.

deep cervical arteries in general vascularize the lower cervical and upper thoracic segments, that is, the cervical enlargement (Lazorthes et al., 1971). Turnbull and colleagues (1966) did microdissection and microangiographic studies on the C3 to T1 cord segments of 43 cadavers. They discovered a range of one to six anterior radicular arteries, which were found as often on the left as on the right sides. Of the 43 spinal cords studied, 13 had a total of only two anterior radicular

arteries, and another 13 had a total of four arteries reinforcing the cord. However, 39 of 43 had at least one anterior radicular artery at the C7 or C8 segment.

Anterior radicular arteries from the intercostal and lumbar arteries are found primarily on the left side (Carpenter, 1991; Turnbull, 1973), possibly because the aorta is on the left. Although the thoracic cord segments are the longest, usually just one to four anterior radicular arteries are present. As an anterior radicular

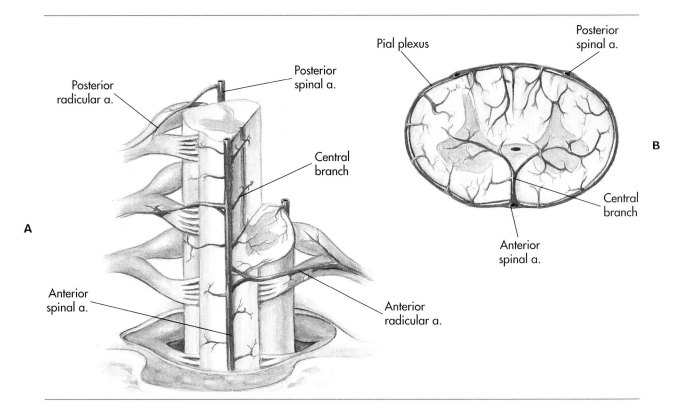

FIG. 3-13   Cross section of the spinal cord showing the arterial blood supply. **A,** Radicular arteries reinforce the spinal arteries. The anterior spinal artery gives off central branches. **B,** Note the spinal cord areas vascularized by the anterior spinal artery and by the posterior spinal arteries.

artery approaches the ventral median fissure, it often sends a branch into the pial plexus on the cord's lateral side. It then bifurcates, usually branching gently up and sharply down before uniting with the anterior spinal artery. If both right and left anterior radicular arteries join the anterior spinal artery at the same level, the anastomosis becomes diamond shaped (Turnbull et al., 1966).

The largest anterior radicular artery was first specifically described in 1882 and named "the arteria radicularis magna of Adamkiewicz." Lazorthes called it the artery of the lumbar enlargement because of its area of distribution (Turnbull, 1973). Although most anterior radicular arteries range from 0.2 to 0.8 mm in diameter, this artery is 1.0 to 1.3 mm in diameter. It arises from a posterior intercostal artery on the left side 80% of the time (Turnbull, 1973). The artery of Adamkiewicz courses with a lower (T9 to T12) thoracic root 75% of the time. However, it may be found with an L1 or L2 root (10%) or even a midthoracic T5 to T8 root (15%), in which case a lower lumbar anterior radicular artery is present. Before reaching the anterior spinal artery, the artery of Adamkiewicz supplements the posterior spinal artery by giving off a posterior branch. When it reaches the anterior spinal artery, the artery of Adamkiewicz divides into large descending and small ascending branches (Lazorthes et al., 1971; Turnbull, 1973;

Williams et al., 1989). It is possible for this artery to be the sole supply to the lumbosacral cord (Schoenen, 1991) and to even be the supplier to the lower two thirds (Williams et al., 1989) or one half of the cord (deGroot & Chusid, 1988).

Posterior Radicular Arteries

Posterior radicular arteries (defined here as those that reach the posterior spinal arteries) vary in number from 10 to 23 and outnumber the anterior radicular arteries. They range in diameter from 0.2 to 0.5 mm (Turnbull, 1973), which is generally smaller than an average anterior radicular artery. Turnbull and colleagues (1966) showed that in the C3 to T1 segments of 43 cadavers, the number of posterior radicular arteries ranged from zero to eight. Only two or three posterior radicular arteries were found in 75% of the cadavers, and of those, most were found coursing with lower cervical roots. No relationship seemed to exist between anterior and posterior radicular arteries concerning their number and position. Although posterior radicular arteries often enter on the left side, they are less prone to do so than the anterior radicular arteries (Carpenter, 1991). However, like the anterior radicular arteries, each one supplies small branches to its neighboring root. Also, as it nears the posterior spinal artery, which it reinforces, the posterior radicular artery often gives a small branch to the pial plexus on the cord's lateral side.

Arterial Supply of the Internal Cord

Having discussed the location of the spinal arteries on the external surface of the spinal cord, it is pertinent to elaborate on the vascularization of the underlying nervous tissue. The spinal cord tissue is vascularized by branches of the anterior spinal artery, posterior spinal anastomotic channels, and their interconnecting vessels. The unpaired anterior spinal artery that lies in the ventral median fissure periodically gives off a single branch, which is called the *central,* or *sulcal, branch* (Fig. 3-13). Compared with the distance between central branches in the cervical cord, the distance is greater between these branches in thoracic segments and is less between branches in lumbar and sacral segments (Hassler, 1966). The central branch comes off at right angles in the lumbar and sacral segments, but comes off at an acute superior or inferior angle in the cervical and thoracic cord (Hassler, 1966; Turnbull, 1973). Its length is approximately 4.5 mm, and the central branch courses deep into the fissure, alternately turning to the left or right.

In addition, the central branches are more numerous and larger in the cervical and lumbar regions and less frequent in the thoracic region (Barr & Kiernan, 1993; Carpenter, 1991; Gillilan, 1958; Turnbull, 1973). In the human cord these arteries number between 250 and 300 (Gillilan, 1958). The anterior spinal artery produces five to eight central branches per centimeter in the cervical region, two to six branches per centimeter in the thoracic region, and five to twelve branches per centimeter in the lumbar and sacral regions (Turnbull, 1973). The widest average diameter of the central branch is in the lumbar region (0.23 mm), followed by cervical (0.21 mm), upper sacral (0.20 mm), and thoracic (0.14 mm). As the branches of the central arteries vascularize the cord, they extend superiorly and inferiorly and overlap each other, particularly in the lumbar and sacral segments.

In addition to the vascularization of the deep tissue, an interconnecting plexus of arteriolar size vessels called the pial peripheral plexus, or vasocorona is located in the pia mater encircling the spinal cord. The dorsal and ventral aspects of the pial plexus are formed from small branches of the posterior and anterior spinal arteries, respectively. The lateral aspects of the pial plexus are formed by branches from both spinal arteries and occasionally from small branches of the radicular arteries (Barr & Kiernan, 1993; Carpenter, 1991; Gillilan, 1958; Turnbull, 1973). The pial plexus vascularizes a band of white matter on the periphery of the spinal cord. Much overlap occurs between the distributions of the central arteries and the peripheral plexus. When considering all branches, the anterior spinal artery vascularizes

approximately the ventral two thirds of the cross-sectional area of the spinal cord. This area includes the ventral horn, lateral horn, central gray matter, base of the dorsal horn, and ventral and lateral funiculi. The posterior spinal artery vascularizes the dorsal horn and dorsal funiculus (Fig. 3-13, *B*). In the C3 to T1 segments, the top of the dorsal horn is particularly well vascularized (Turnbull et al., 1966).

When studying the details of the arterial supply, it appears that at any given level of the spinal cord, a direct relationship exists between the size of the anterior spinal artery and radicular artery and the amount of gray matter, as seen in cross section (Gillilan, 1958). Since gray matter has a higher metabolic rate than white matter (Gillilan, 1958), the capillaries are denser in gray matter, especially around the top of the dorsal horn and the ventral horn cells, than in the white matter. However, the dorsal and lateral white funiculi have a better capillary supply than the ventral white funiculus (Turnbull, 1973).

The distribution of the anterior and posterior spinal arteries to the cross-sectional area of the spinal cord is clinically very important, and much research has been devoted to this topic. Any interruption of the vascular supply to the spinal cord can cause serious deficits. For example, trauma typically causes hemorrhaging of these arteries and subsequent ischemia and cell necrosis. Also, an obstruction of any vessel involved with vascularizing the spinal cord (aorta, segmental arteries and radicular branches, spinal arteries, intrinsic vessels) or a decrease in blood pressure may cause damage to the spinal cord. For example, lumbar sympathectomy, aortic surgery or injury, or a dissecting aneurysm of the aorta may interrupt intercostal and lumbar arteries. This includes the great radicular artery of Adamkiewicz, which supplies the lumbar enlargement (Carpenter, 1991; Gillilan, 1958; Moore, 1980; Morris & Phil, 1989; Turnbull, 1973). Interruption of the artery of Adamkiewicz can have serious consequences and in some cases can even result in paraplegia.

Since the spinal arteries are unable to supply the spinal cord sufficiently, the radicular supply becomes critical. In the upper thoracic segments, especially around T4, reinforcing radicular arteries originating from intercostal segmental arteries are not numerous, and therefore this area is vulnerable. For example, if one radicular artery is occluded and another is insufficient, ischemia can develop.

Although less common, occlusion of the anterior spinal artery directly may occur from thrombosis, an embolus, herniated disc compression, tumors, and other conditions. This results in an infarction of spinal cord tissue (Gillilan, 1958; Morris & Phil, 1989; Turnbull, 1973). Lesions affecting the anterior spinal arterial distribution are more common than those affecting the posterior spinal arterial region (Daube et al., 1986; Gillilan, 1958).

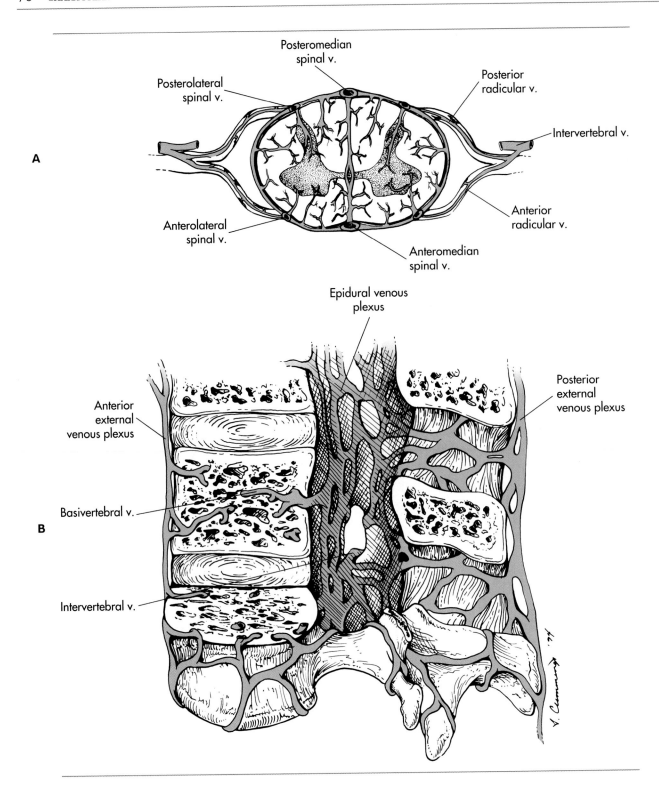

FIG. 3-14 Venous drainage of the spinal cord. **A,** Cross section of the spinal cord. **B,** Median view of the vertebral canal. The spinal cord has been removed to show the epidural venous plexus.

Thus, most spinal infarcts cause greatest damage to the areas that include cell bodies of motor neurons (ventral horn), descending motor pathways (lateral white matter), and the ascending pain and temperature pathways (ventrolateral white matter) (see Chapter 9). In these cases the posterior spinal arterial distribution to the dorsal one third of the spinal cord, which includes the pathway for vibration, position sense, and touch (dorsal white funiculus), is left intact. Several cases in the late 1800s and early 1900s established that a lesion causing insufficient vascularization to the area of distribution of the anterior spinal artery could frequently be clearly diagnosed clinically (Gillilan, 1958). This lesion has subsequently been referred to as the *anterior spinal artery syndrome* and presents with sudden bilateral loss of pain and temperature sense and motor deficits below the level of the lesion, with a preservation of vibratory and position sense.

VENOUS DRAINAGE OF THE SPINAL CORD

The venous system found within the vertebral canal consists of an epidural, or internal, vertebral venous plexus, located in the epidural space (see Chapter 2) and also an irregular venous plexus lying on the cord. This entire venous system is devoid of valves.

The venous system on the cord consists of six longitudinal veins: three anterior and three posterior (Fig. 3-14, *A*). On the anterior side of the cord in the midline, the anteromedian vein receives venous blood from both sides of the anteromedial cord via sulcal veins. Near each ventrolateral sulcus, an anterolateral vein is found receiving blood from the anterolateral cord. The anteromedian and anterolateral veins empty into one of approximately 6 to 11 anterior radicular veins that empty into the epidural venous plexus. In the lumbar region, there may be one large anterior radicular vein, the vena radicularis magna (Carpenter, 1991). The posterior aspect of the cord has a similar venous pattern. A midline posteromedian and two posterolateral veins drain the dorsal funiculus, dorsal horns, and their adjacent lateral white matter. These veins in turn become tributaries of approximately 5 to 10 posterior radicular veins that empty into the epidural venous plexus. As also seen in the arterial system, an encompassing venous vasocorona interconnects the six longitudinal veins.

The epidural venous plexus is a longitudinal plexus that is continuous with the sinuses and venous channels above the level of the foramen magnum within the skull (see Chapter 2). It also drains into intervertebral veins in the IVFs and also into another longitudinally arranged plexus, the external vertebral venous plexus (Fig. 3-14, *B*). From intervertebral veins, venous blood drains into segmental veins such as the vertebral, intercostal,

lumbar, and lateral sacral veins (Williams et al., 1989). These segmental veins lie outside the vertebral column.

A metastatic tumor in the epidural space may damage the cord by impeding venous return and cause vasogenic edema (Grant et al., 1991). These interconnecting channels also provide the opportunity for cancer to metastasize to the brain (see Chapter 2).

REFERENCES

Barr, M.L. & Kiernan, J.A. (1993). *The human nervous system* (6th ed.). Philadelphia: JB Lippincott.

Carpenter, M.B. (1991). *Core text of neuroanatomy* (4th ed.). Baltimore: Williams & Wilkins.

Coggeshall, R.E. (1980). Law of separation of function of the spinal roots. *Physiol Rev, 60*(3), 716-755.

Daube, J.R. et al. (1986). *Medical Neurosciences* (2nd ed.). Boston: Little, Brown.

Davidoff, R.A. & Hackman, J.C. (1991). Aspects of spinal cord structure and reflex function. *Neurol Clin, 9*(3), 533-550.

deGroot, J. & Chusid, J.G. (1988). *Correlative neuroanatomy* (20th ed.). East Norwalk, Conn: Appleton & Lange.

Djindjian, M. et al. (1988). The normal vascularization of the intradural filum terminale in man. *Surg Radiol Anat, 10,* 201-209.

Elliott, H.C. (1945). Cross-sectional diameters and areas of the human spinal cord. *Anat Rec, 93,* 287-293.

Fujiwara, K. et al. (1988). Morphometry of the cervical spinal cord and its relation to pathology in cases with compression myelopathy. *Spine, 13*(11), 1212-1216.

Gillilan, L.A. (1958). The arterial blood supply of the human spinal cord. *J Comp Neurol, 110*(1), 75-103.

Grant, R. et al. (1991). Changes in intracranial CSF volume after lumbar puncture and their relationship to post-LP headache. *J Neurol Neurosurg Psychiatry, 54,* 440-442.

Groen, G.J., Baljet, B., & Drukker, J. (1988). The innervation of the spinal dura mater: Anatomy and clinical implications. *Acta Neurochir (Wien), 92,* 39-46.

Haines, D.E. (1991). On the question of a subdural space. *Anat Rec, 230,* 3-21.

Hassler, O. (1966). Blood supply to the human spinal cord. *Arch Neurol, 15,* 302-307.

Hewitt, W. (1970). The intervertebral foramen. *Physiotherapy, 56,* 332-336.

Lazorthes, G. et al. (1971). Arterial vascularization of the spinal cord. *J Neurosurg, 35,* 253-262.

Moore, K.L. (1980). *Clinically oriented anatomy.* Baltimore: Williams & Wilkins.

Morris, J.H. & Phil, D. (1989). The nervous system. In R.S. Cotran, V. Kumar, & S.L. Robbins, (Eds.). *Robbins pathologic basis of disease* (4th ed.). Philadelphia: WB Saunders.

Rexed, B. (1952). The cytoarchitectonic organization of the spinal cord in the cat. *J Comp Neurol, 96,* 415-495.

Schoenen, J. (1991). Clinical anatomy of the spinal cord. *Neurol Clin, 9*(3), 503-532.

Spencer, D.L., Irwin, G.S. & Miller, J.A. (1983). Anatomy and significance of fixation of the lumbosacral nerve roots in sciatica. *Spine, 8*(6), 672-679.

Turnbull, I.M. (1973). Blood supply of the spinal cord: Normal and pathological considerations. *Clin Neurosurg, 20,* 56-84.

Turnbull, I.M., Brieg, A., & Hassler, O. (1966). Blood supply of cervical spinal cord in man. *J Neurosurg, 24,* 951-966.

Williams, P.L. et al. (1989). *Gray's anatomy* (37th ed.). Edinburgh: Churchill Livingstone.

Willis, W.D., Jr., & Coggeshall, R.E. (1991). *Sensory mechanisms of the spinal cord* (2nd ed.). New York: Plenum Press.

CHAPTER 4

Muscles That Influence the Spine

Barclay W. Bakkum
Gregory D. Cramer

Second only to the vertebral column itself, the muscles of the spine are the most important structures of the back. A thorough understanding of the back muscles is fundamental to a comprehensive understanding of the spine and its function. The purpose of this chapter is to discuss the muscles of the back and other muscles that have an indirect influence on the spine. The intercostal muscles provide an example of the latter category. These muscles do not actually attach to the spine, but their action can influence the spine by virtue of their attachment to the ribs. The abdominal wall muscles, diaphragm, hamstrings, and others can be placed into this same category. These muscles have a less direct, yet important influence on the spine. Chapter 5 discusses the sternocleidomastoid, scalene, suprahyoid, and infrahyoid muscles.

The musculature of the spine and trunk plays an important role in the normal functioning of the vertebral column. Besides their obvious ability to create the variety of spinal movements, many of these muscles also help to maintain posture. In addition, the back and trunk muscles function as shock absorbers, acting to disperse loads applied to the spine. The shear bulk of these muscles also protects the spine and viscera from outside forces.

Many muscles work together to produce a typical movement of the spine. Muscles known as prime movers are the most important. Other muscles, known as synergists, assist the prime movers. For example, during flexion of the lumbar spine from a supine position, as in the performance of a sit-up, the psoas major and the rectus abdominis muscles are prime movers of the spine. However, the erector spinae muscles also undergo an eccentric contraction toward the end of the sit-up. This contraction of the erector spinae helps to control the motion of the trunk and allows for a graceful, safe accomplishment of the movement. The erector spinae muscles are acting as synergists in this instance.

The muscles of the spine and other muscles associated with the back can, and frequently do, sustain injury. A complete understanding of the anatomy of these muscles aids in the differential diagnosis of pain arising from muscles versus pain arising from neighboring ligaments or other structures.

The back muscles are discussed from superficial to deep. This is accomplished by dividing the muscles into six layers, with layer one as the most superficial and layer six as the deepest. After a discussion of the six layers of back muscles, other important muscles of the spine are described. These include the suboccipital muscles, the anterior and lateral muscles of the cervical spine, and the iliac muscles. The muscles that have an indirect, yet important influence on the spine are discussed last.

SIX LAYERS OF BACK MUSCLES
First Layer

The first layer of back muscles consists of the trapezius and latissimus dorsi muscles (Fig. 4-1). These two muscles run from the spine (and occiput) to either the shoulder girdle (scapula and clavicle) or the humerus, respectively.

Trapezius Muscle. The trapezius muscle is the most superficial and superior back muscle (Fig. 4-1). It is a large, strong muscle that is innervated by the accessory nerve (cranial nerve XI). In addition to its innervation from the accessory nerve, the trapezius muscle receives some proprioceptive fibers from the third and fourth cervical ventral rami. Because the trapezius muscle is so large, it originates from and inserts on many structures. This muscle originates from the superior nuchal line, the external occipital protuberance, the ligamentum nuchae of the posterior neck, the spinous processes of C7 to T12, and the supraspinous ligament between C7 and T12. It inserts onto the spine of the scapula, the acromion process, and the distal third of the clavicle.

Because of its size and its many origins and insertions, the trapezius muscle also has many actions. Most of these actions result in movement of the neck and the scapula (i.e., the "shoulder girdle" as a whole). The function of the trapezius depends on which region of the muscle is contracting (upper, middle, or lower). The middle portion retracts the scapula, whereas the lower portion depresses the scapula and at the same time rotates the scapula so that its lateral angle moves superiorly. The actions of the upper part of the trapezius also depend on whether the head/neck or the scapula is stabilized. When moving the head and neck, the actions of the upper trapezius are also determined by whether the muscle is contracting unilaterally or bilaterally. Table 4-1 summarizes the actions of the trapezius muscle.

Latissimus Dorsi Muscle. The most inferior and lateral of the two muscles that make up the first layer of back muscles is the latissimus dorsi muscle (Fig. 4-1). This large muscle has an extensive origin. The origin of the latissimus dorsi includes the following:

- ◆ Spinous processes and supraspinous ligament of T6-L5 (supraspinous ligament ends between L2-L4)

- ◆ Thoracolumbar fascia
- ◆ Posterior sacrum (median sacral crest [see Chapter 8])
- ◆ Iliac crests
- ◆ Lower four ribs

The latissimus dorsi muscle derives much of its origin from the thoracolumbar fascia. This is a tough and extensive aponeurosis (see the following discussion). The latissimus dorsi muscle passes superiorly and laterally to insert into the intertubercular groove of the humerus, between the anteriorly located pectoralis major muscle and the posteriorly located teres major muscle. Contraction of the latissimus dorsi results in adduction, medial rotation, and extension of the humerus.

The latissimus dorsi is innervated by the thoracodorsal nerve (middle subscapular nerve), which is a branch of the posterior cord of the brachial plexus. The thoracodorsal nerve is derived from the anterior primary divisions of the sixth through eighth cervical nerves.

Thoracolumbar Fascia. Because of its clinical significance, the anatomy of the thoracolumbar fascia deserves further discussion. This fascia extends from the thoracic region to the sacrum. It forms a thin covering over the erector spinae muscles in the thoracic region, whereas in the lumbar region the thoracolumbar fascia is very strong and is composed of three layers. The posterior layer attaches to the lumbar spinous processes, the interspinous ligaments between these processes, and the median sacral crest. The middle layer attaches to the tips of the lumbar transverse processes and the intertransverse ligaments and extends superiorly from the iliac crest to the 12th rib. The anterior layer covers the anterior aspect of the quadratus lumborum muscle and attaches to the anterior surfaces of the lumbar transverse rocesses. Superiorly, the anterior layer forms the lateral arcuate ligament (see Diaphragm). The anterior layer continues inferiorly to the ilium and iliolumbar ligament. The posterior and middle layers surround the erector

Table 4-1 Functions of Trapezius Muscle

Region of muscle	Head and neck stabilized during muscle contraction	With scapula stabilized	
		Contraction of one side (unilateral)	Contraction of both sides (bilateral)
Upper	Elevates scapula	Extends head and neck; rotates face to opposite direction	Extends head and neck
Middle	Retracts scapula	—	—
Lower	Retracts, depresses scapula; rotates lateral angle of scapula superiorly	—	—

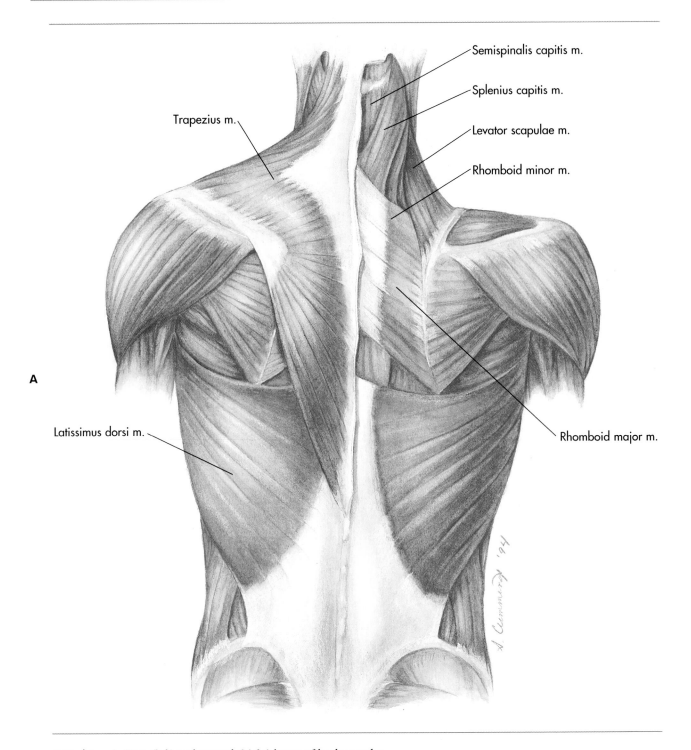

Semispinalis capitis m.

Splenius capitis m.

Levator scapulae m.

Rhomboid minor m.

Trapezius m.

Rhomboid major m.

Latissimus dorsi m.

A

FIG. 4-1   A, First *(left)* and second *(right)* layers of back muscles.

spinae muscles posteriorly and anteriorly, respectively (see Fifth Layer), and meet at the lateral edge of the erector spinae, where these two layers are joined by the anterior layer (Williams et al., 1989).

The lateral union of the three layers of the thoracolumbar fascia serves as a posterior aponeurosis for origin of the transversus abdominis muscle. Macintosh and

Bogduk (1987) found that the posterior layer of the thoracolumbar fascia is actually composed of two separate layers (laminae). The direction of the fibers within each layer of the posterior aponeurosis makes the thoracolumbar fascia stronger along its lines of greatest stress. When the thoracolumbar fascia is tractioned laterally by the action of the abdominal muscles, the distinct direc-

Trapezius m. — upper / middle / lower

Teres minor m.

Infraspinatus m.

Latissimus dorsi m.

Greater occipital n.

Splenius capitis m.

Deltoid m.

Splenius cervicis m.

Rhomboid minor m.

Rhomboid major m.

Longissimus thoracis m.

Serratus posterior inferior m.

B

FIG. 4-1, cont'd. **B,** Dissection of these same two layers.

Continued.

tion of fibers of the posterior layer's two laminae aids in extension of the spine and the maintenance of an erect posture.

Some investigators believe that because the posterior and middle layers surround the erector spinae muscles, injury to these muscles at times may lead to a "compartment" type of syndrome within these two layers of the thoracolumbar fascia (Peck et al., 1986). This syndrome results from edema within the erector spinae muscles. The edema results from injury and increases the pressure in the relatively closed compartment composed of the erector spinae muscles wrapped within the posterior and middle layers of the thoracolumbar fascia. This may result in increased pain and straightening of the lumbar lordosis (Peck et al., 1986). However, further research is necessary to determine the best approach available to diagnose this condition and the frequency with which this condition occurs.

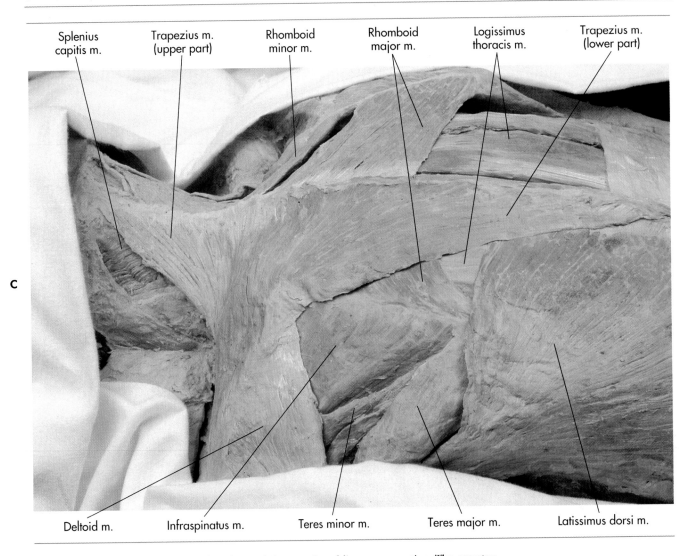

Splenius capitis m.   Trapezius m. (upper part)   Rhomboid minor m.   Rhomboid major m.   Logissimus thoracis m.   Trapezius m. (lower part)

Deltoid m.   Infraspinatus m.   Teres minor m.   Teres major m.   Latissimus dorsi m.

FIG. 4-1, cont'd. **C,** Close-up, taken from a left posterior oblique perspective. The serratus posterior inferior muscle of the third layer can also be seen in **B** and **C.**

Second Layer

The second layer of back muscles includes three muscles that, along with the first layer, connect the upper limb to the vertebral column. All three muscles lie deep to the trapezius muscle and insert onto the scapula's medial border. They include the rhomboid major, rhomboid minor, and levator scapulae muscles (Fig. 4-1).

The rhomboid major muscle originates by tendinous fibers from the spinous processes of T2 through T5 and the supraspinous ligaments at those levels. The muscle fibers run in an inferolateral direction and insert via a tendinous band on the medial border of the scapula between the root of the spine and the inferior angle.

The rhomboid minor muscle is located immediately superior to the rhomboid major, and its fibers also run in an inferolateral direction. Beginning from the lower portion of the ligamentum nuchae and the spinous processes of C7 and T1, the rhomboid minor ends on the scapula's medial border at the level of the spinal root.

Both rhomboid muscles are innervated by the dorsal scapular nerve, which arises from the anterior primary division of the C5 spinal nerve.

Since the fibers of these two muscles are parallel, their actions are similar. In addition to the other muscles that insert on the scapula, they help stabilize its position and movement during active use of the upper extremity. Specifically, the rhomboids retract and rotate the scapula so as to depress the point of the shoulder.

The levator scapulae muscle arises by tendinous slips from the transverse processes of the atlas and axis and the posterior tubercles of the transverse processes of C3 and C4. Its fibers descend and insert onto the scapula's medial border between the spinal root and the superior angle. It is innervated by branches from the ventral rami of the C3 and C4 spinal nerves and the dorsal scapular nerve (C5). If the cervical spine is fixed, the levator scapulae helps in elevating and rotating the scapula to depress the point of the shoulder. When the scapula is stabilized, contraction of this muscle laterally flexes and rotates the neck to the same side. Bilateral contraction helps in extension of the cervical spine.

Third Layer

The third layer of back muscles is sometimes referred to as the intermediate layer of back muscles. This is because the two small muscles of this group lie between layers one and two, which are frequently known as the superficial back muscles, and layers four through six, which are known as the deep back muscles.

The third layer of back muscles consists of two thin, almost quadrangular muscles: the serratus posterior superior and serratus posterior inferior (Fig. 4-2, *A* and *B*).

The serratus posterior superior muscle originates from the spinous processes of C7 through T3 and the supraspinous ligament that runs between them. It inserts onto the posterior and superior aspect of the second through the fifth ribs. This muscle is innervated by the anterior primary divisions of the second through the fifth thoracic nerves (intercostal nerves).

The serratus posterior inferior originates from the spinous processes and intervening supraspinous ligament of T11 to L2. It inserts onto the posterior and inferior surfaces of the lower four ribs and is innervated by the lower three intercostal nerves (T9 to T11) and the subcostal nerve. These nerves are all anterior primary divisions of their respective spinal nerves.

The serratus posterior superior and inferior muscles may help with respiration. More specifically, the serratus posterior superior raises the second through fourth ribs, which may aid with inspiration. The serratus posterior inferior lowers the ninth through twelfth ribs, which may help with forced expiration.

Fourth Layer

The most superficial layer of deep back muscles is the fourth layer, which consists of two muscles whose fibers ascend from spinous processes to either the occiput (splenius capitis) or the transverse processes of cervical vertebrae (splenius cervicis). This layer is composed of the splenius capitis and splenius cervicis muscles (Fig. 4-2, *C* to *E*).

The splenius capitis muscle begins from the lower half of the ligamentum nuchae and the spinous processes of C7 through T3 or T4. It attaches superiorly to the mastoid process of the temporal bone and to the occiput just inferior to the lateral third of the superior nuchal line.

The splenius cervicis muscle originates from the spinous processes of T3 through T6 and inserts onto the transverse processes of the atlas and axis and the posterior tubercles of the transverse processes of C3 and sometimes C4. These insertions are deep to the origins of the levator scapulae. The splenius capitis and cervicis are innervated by lateral branches of the posterior primary divisions of the midcervical and lower cervical spinal nerves, respectively. When the splenius muscles of both sides act together, they extend the head and neck. When the muscles of one side contract, they laterally flex the head and neck and slightly rotate the face toward the side of contraction.

Fifth Layer

The largest group of back muscles is the fifth layer. This layer is composed of the erector spinae group of muscles (Fig. 4-2, *A* and *B* and Fig. 4-3, *A*). This erector spinae group is also collectively known as the sacrospinalis muscle. The muscles that make up this group are a series of longitudinal muscles that run the length of the spine, filling a groove lateral to the spinous processes. They are covered posteriorly in the thoracic and lumbar regions by the thoracolumbar fascia. These longitudinal muscles can be divided into three groups. These three groups are, from lateral to medial, the iliocostalis, the longissimus, and the spinalis groups of muscles. Each of these groups, in turn, is made up of three subdivisions. The subdivisions are named according to the area of the spine to which they insert (e.g., lumborum, thoracis, cervicis, capitis). The erector spinae muscles are discussed from the most lateral group to the most medial, and each group is discussed from inferior to superior.

Iliocostalis Muscles. The iliocostalis (iliocostocervicalis) group of muscles is subdivided into lumborum, thoracis, and cervicis muscles (Fig. 4-3). Inferiorly, the iliocostalis muscles derive from the common origin of the erector spinae muscles.

Iliocostalis lumborum. The iliocostalis lumborum muscle is the most inferior and lateral of the erector spinae muscles. It originates from the common origin of the erector spinae muscles, which includes the following:

- Spinous processes and supraspinous ligament of T11 through L5 (supraspinous ligament ends between L2-L4)
- Median sacral crest
- Sacrotuberous ligament
- Posterior sacroiliac ligament
- Lateral sacral crest
- Posteromedial iliac crest

The iliocostalis lumborum muscle runs superiorly to insert onto the posterior and inferior surfaces of the angles of the lower six to nine ribs. This muscle has the same function as the rest of the erector spinae, which is to extend and laterally flex the spine. The erector spinae are all innervated by lateral branches of the posterior primary divisions (dorsal rami) of the nearby spinal nerves.

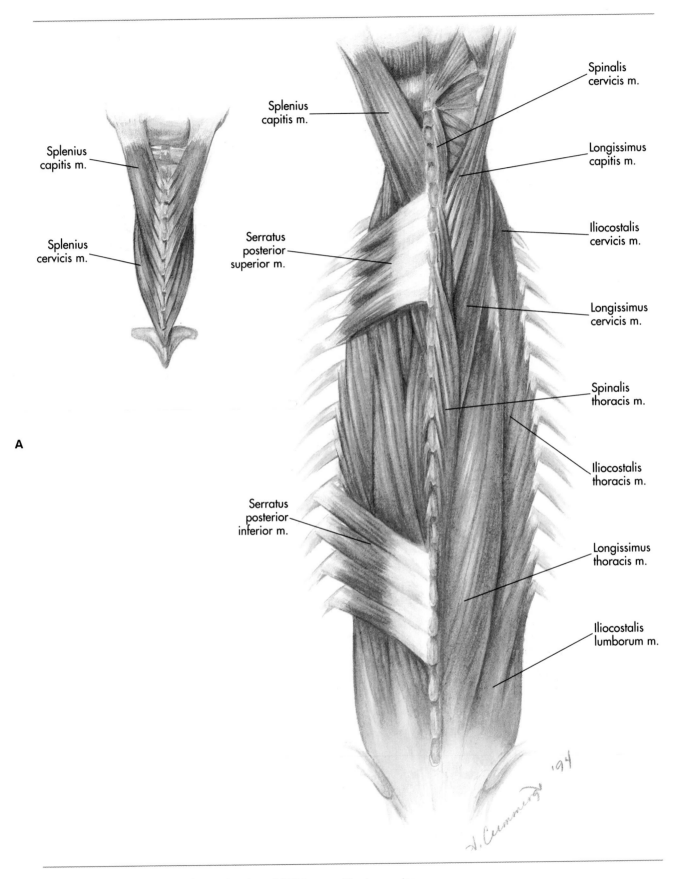

FIG. 4-2   A, Third, fourth (also see inset), and fifth layers of back muscles.

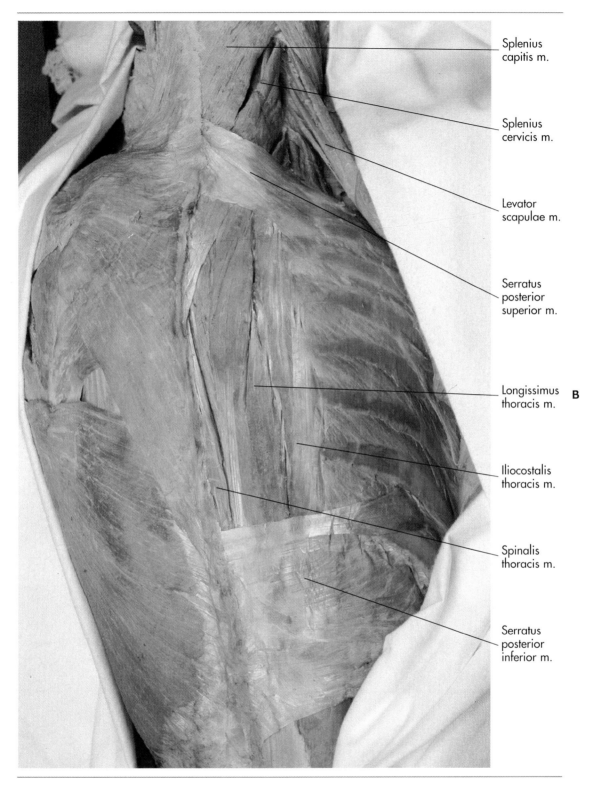

Splenius
capitis m.

Splenius
cervicis m.

Levator
scapulae m.

Serratus
posterior
superior m.

Longissimus **B**
thoracis m.

Iliocostalis
thoracis m.

Spinalis
thoracis m.

Serratus
posterior
inferior m.

FIG. 4-2, cont'd. **B,** Serratus posterior superior and inferior muscles that make up layer three. *Continued.*

Macintosh and Bogduk (1987), through a series of elegant dissections, further described the anatomy of the iliocostalis lumborum muscle. They found that part of this muscle originated from the posterior superior iliac spine and the posterior aspect of the iliac crest and inserted into the lower eight or nine ribs. They called this part the iliocostalis lumborum pars thoracis. Another part of the classically described iliocostalis lumborum was found to originate from the tips of the lumbar spinous processes and the associated middle layer of

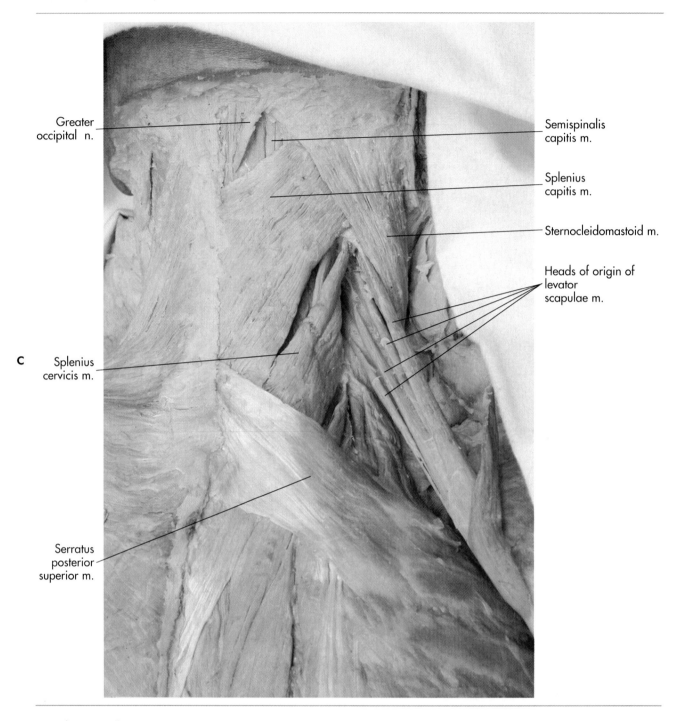

Greater occipital n.

Semispinalis capitis m.

Splenius capitis m.

Sternocleidomastoid m.

Heads of origin of levator scapulae m.

C

Splenius cervicis m.

Serratus posterior superior m.

FIG. 4-2, cont'd. **C, D,** and **E,** Splenius capitis and cervicis muscles of layer four and the levator scapulae muscle of layer three. **C,** Right posterior view.

the thoracolumbar fascia of L1 to L4 (see Thoracolumbar Fascia) and to insert onto the anterior edge of the iliac crest. They called this part the iliocostalis lumborum pars lumborum and found that it formed a considerable mass of muscle.

Iliocostalis thoracis. The iliocostalis thoracis muscle originates from the superior aspect of the angles of the lower six ribs and inserts onto the angles of approx-

imately the upper six ribs and the transverse process of the C7 vertebra. This muscle extends and laterally flexes the thoracic spine and is innervated by the lateral branches of the posterior primary divisions (dorsal rami) of the thoracic spinal nerves.

Iliocostalis cervicis. The iliocostalis cervicis originates from the superior aspect of the angle of the third through the sixth ribs and inserts onto the posterior

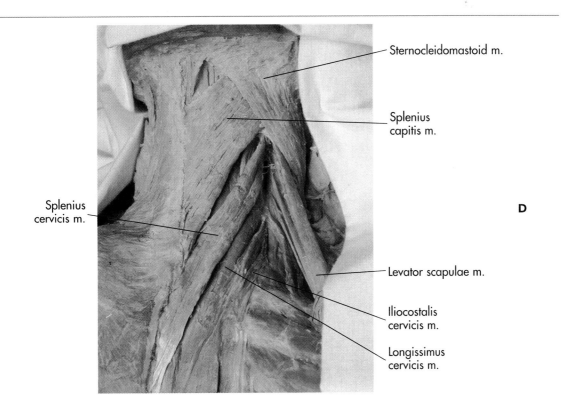

Sternocleidomastoid m.

Splenius
capitis m.

Splenius
cervicis m.

D

Levator scapulae m.

Iliocostalis
cervicis m.

Longissimus
cervicis m.

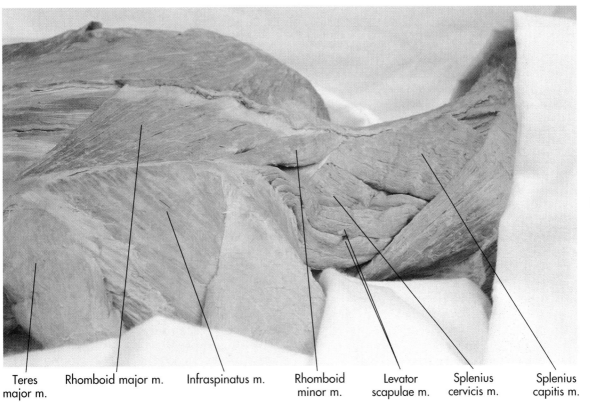

E

Teres
major m.

Rhomboid major m.

Infraspinatus m.

Rhomboid
minor m.

Levator
scapulae m.

Splenius
cervicis m.

Splenius
capitis m.

FIG. 4-2, cont'd. **D,** Right posterior view with the serratus posterior superior muscle removed. **E,** Right lateral view.

tubercles of the transverse processes of the C4 to C6 vertebrae. It laterally flexes and extends the lower cervical region and is innervated by the dorsal rami of the upper thoracic and lower cervical spinal nerves.

Longissimus Muscles. The longissimus muscles are located medial to the iliocostalis group. The longissimus group is made up of thoracis, cervicis, and capitis divisions. The lateral branches of the posterior primary divisions (dorsal rami) of the mixed spinal nerves exit the thorax and then course laterally and posteriorly between the iliocostalis muscles and the longissimus thoracis muscle (Fig. 4-3, *A*). This fact is used in the gross anatomy laboratory not only to quickly find the lateral branches of the posterior primary divisions, but also to demonstrate the separation between these two large muscle masses. After providing motor and sensory innervation to the sacrospinalis muscle, the lateral branches continue to the dermis and epidermis of the back, providing these layers with sensory innervation.

Longissimus thoracis. The longissimus thoracis is the largest of the erector spinae muscles. It arises from the common origin of the erector spinae muscles (see Iliocostalis lumborum). In addition, many fibers originate from the transverse and accessory processes of the lumbar vertebrae. This muscle is extremely long, thus the name longissimus. It inserts onto the third through the twelfth ribs, between their angles and tubercles. The longissimus thoracis also inserts onto the transverse processes of all 12 thoracic vertebrae. This muscle functions to hold the thoracic and lumbar regions erect, and when it acts unilaterally, it laterally flexes the spine. It is innervated by lateral divisions of the thoracic and lumbar posterior primary divisions.

Macintosh and Bogduk (1987) found fibers of the longissimus thoracis that are confined to the lumbar and sacral regions. These fibers originated from lumbar accessory and transverse processes and inserted onto the medial surface of the posterior superior iliac spine. The authors called these fibers the longissimus thoracis pars lumborum.

Longissimus cervicis. The longissimus cervicis muscle originates from the transverse processes of the upper thoracic vertebrae (T1 to T5) and inserts onto the posterior tubercle of the transverse processes and the articular processes of C3 through C6 and onto the posterior aspect of the transverse process and the articular process of C2. Unilateral contraction produces a combination of extension and lateral flexion of the neck to the same side. The longissimus cervicis is innervated by lateral branches of the upper thoracic and lower cervical posterior primary divisions.

Longissimus capitis. The longissimus capitis muscle derives from upper thoracic transverse processes (T1 to T5) and articular processes of C4 through C7. It inserts onto the mastoid process of the temporal bone, and its action is to extend the head. If it acts unilaterally, the longissimus capitis can laterally flex the head and rotate it to the same side. It is innervated by the posterior primary divisions of upper thoracic and cervical spinal nerves.

Spinalis Muscles. The spinalis muscle group originates from spinous processes and inserts onto spinous processes, except for the spinalis capitis muscle. This muscle group is made up of thoracis, cervicis, and capitis divisions.

Spinalis thoracis. The spinalis thoracis muscle fibers are the most highly developed of this muscle group. It originates from the lower thoracic and upper lumbar spinous processes (T11 to L2) and inserts onto the upper thoracic spinous processes (T1 to T4 and perhaps down to T8). Laterally, the fibers of this muscle blend with the fibers of the longissimus thoracis. The spinalis thoracis muscle functions to extend the thoracic spine. It is innervated by posterior primary divisions of thoracic nerves.

Spinalis cervicis. The spinalis cervicis muscle originates from upper thoracic spinous processes (T1 to T6) and inserts onto the spinous processes of C2 (occasionally C3 and C4). Maintaining the tradition of the erector spinae muscles, the spinalis cervicis functions to extend the cervical region. This muscle is usually quite small and frequently absent.

Spinalis capitis. The spinalis capitis muscle differs from the other spinalis muscles in that it does not typically originate from or insert onto spinous processes. This muscle is difficult to differentiate from the more lateral semispinalis capitis muscle (see the following discussion). Its origin is blended with that of the semispinalis capitis from the transverse processes of the C7 to the T6 or T7 vertebra, the articular processes of C4 to C6, and sometimes from the spinous processes of C7 and T1. The fibers of this muscle blend with those of the semispinalis capitis and insert with the latter muscle onto the occiput between the superior and inferior nuchal lines. The spinalis capitis muscle is sometimes called the biventor cervicis muscle because an incomplete tendinous intersection passes across it. When the left and right spinalis capitis muscles contract together, the result is extension of the head. Unilateral contraction results in lateral flexion of the head and neck and also rotation of the head away from the side of contraction. This muscle is innervated by upper thoracic and lower cervical posterior primary divisions.

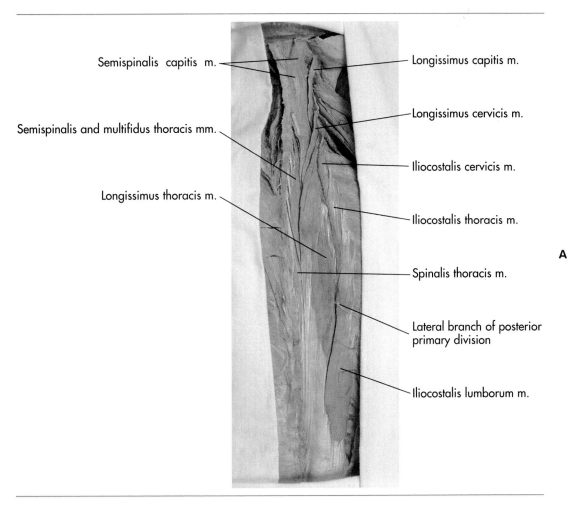

Semispinalis capitis m.

Longissimus capitis m.

Semispinalis and multifidus thoracis mm.

Longissimus cervicis m.

Iliocostalis cervicis m.

Longissimus thoracis m.

Iliocostalis thoracis m.

A

Spinalis thoracis m.

Lateral branch of posterior primary division

Iliocostalis lumborum m.

FIG. 4-3 **A,** Fifth layer of back muscles of the right side. *Continued.*

Sixth Layer

The sixth layer of back muscles includes the deep back muscles with fibers that course superiorly and medially. They are sometimes referred to as the transversospinalis group because they generally originate from transverse processes and insert onto spinous processes (Fig. 4-3, *B* to *E*). The muscles in this layer are arranged such that from superficial to deep, the length of the muscles becomes progressively shorter. Although the actions of these muscles are described separately, it must be remembered that these muscles, especially the shorter ones, function primarily in a postural role as stabilizers rather than as prime movers. This group is made up of the semispinalis, multifidus, and rotatores muscles.

Semispinalis Muscles. The semispinalis muscles are located only in the thoracic and cervical regions and are divided into three parts: semispinalis thoracis, semispinalis cervicis, and semispinalis capitis muscles (Fig. 4-3, *B* to *E*).

Semispinalis thoracis. The semispinalis thoracis consists of thin muscular fasciculi located between long tendons that attach inferiorly to the transverse processes of the lower six thoracic vertebrae and superiorly to the spinous processes of C6 to T4 (Fig. 4-3, *C*). The semispinalis thoracis is innervated by the medial branches of the posterior primary divisions of the upper six thoracic spinal nerves.

Semispinalis cervicis. The semispinalis cervicis is a thicker mass of muscle that begins from the transverse processes of the upper five or six thoracic vertebrae (Fig. 4-3, *D*). It may also arise from the articular processes of the lower four cervical vertebrae. This muscle mainly inserts onto the spinous process of the axis, but also attaches to the spinous processes of C3 to C5. It derives its innervation from the posterior primary divisions (dorsal rami) of the C6 to C8 spinal nerves.

Semispinalis capitis. The semispinalis capitis is a thick, powerful muscle and represents the best-

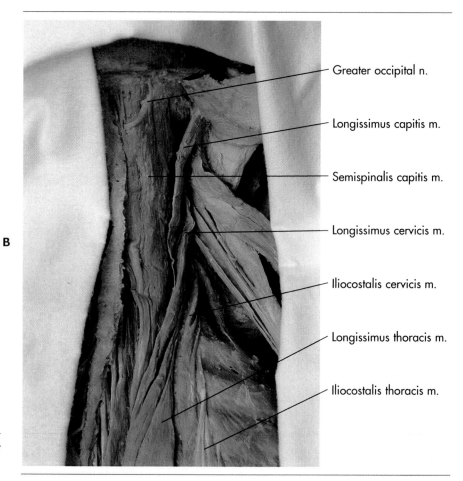

Greater occipital n.

Longissimus capitis m.

Semispinalis capitis m.

Longissimus cervicis m.

Iliocostalis cervicis m.

Longissimus thoracis m.

Iliocostalis thoracis m.

FIG. 4-3, cont'd. **B,** Right semispinalis capitis muscle of the sixth layer from a cadaveric dissection.

developed portion of the semispinalis muscle group (Fig. 4-3, *B* to *D*). It arises from the transverse processes of C7 to T6 and the articular processes of C4 to C6. The semispinalis capitis muscle inserts onto the medial part of the area between the occiput's superior and inferior nuchal lines. It is supplied by the dorsal rami of the first through sixth cervical spinal nerves.

When the muscles of both sides act together, the semispinalis thoracis and cervicis function to extend the thoracic and cervical portions of the spine, respectively, whereas unilateral contraction of these muscles rotates the vertebral bodies of those regions to the opposite side. The semispinalis capitis muscles together function to extend the head and, working separately, slightly rotate the head to the opposite side.

Multifidus Muscles

Multifidus lumborum, thoracis, and cervicis.
The multifidus muscles lie deep to the semispinalis muscles, where they fill the groove between the transverse and spinous processes of the vertebrae. This group consists of multiple muscular and tendinous fasciculi that originate from the mamillary processes of the lumbar vertebrae, the transverse processes of the thoracic ver-

tebrae, and the articular processes of the lower four cervical vertebrae. These fasciculi ascend two to four, or sometimes five, vertebral segments before inserting onto a spinous process. Multifidi insert onto all the vertebrae except the atlas.

The multifidus muscles produce extension of the vertebral column. They also produce some rotation of the vertebral bodies away from the side of contraction, and they are also active in lateral flexion of the spine. Recently, this muscle group was found to contract during axial rotation of the trunk in either direction (Oliver & Middleditch, 1991). When the oblique abdominal muscles contract to produce trunk rotation, some flexion of the trunk is also produced. The multifidus muscles oppose this flexion component and maintain a pure axial rotation, thereby acting as stabilizers during trunk rotation. The multifidus muscles are innervated segmentally by the medial branches of the posterior primary divisions of the spinal nerves.

In the lumbar spine, where the multifidus group is best developed, it is arranged into five bands, each attaching superiorly to one lumbar spinous process (Macintosh et al., 1986). In each band the deepest fascicles actually run from the mamillary process below to

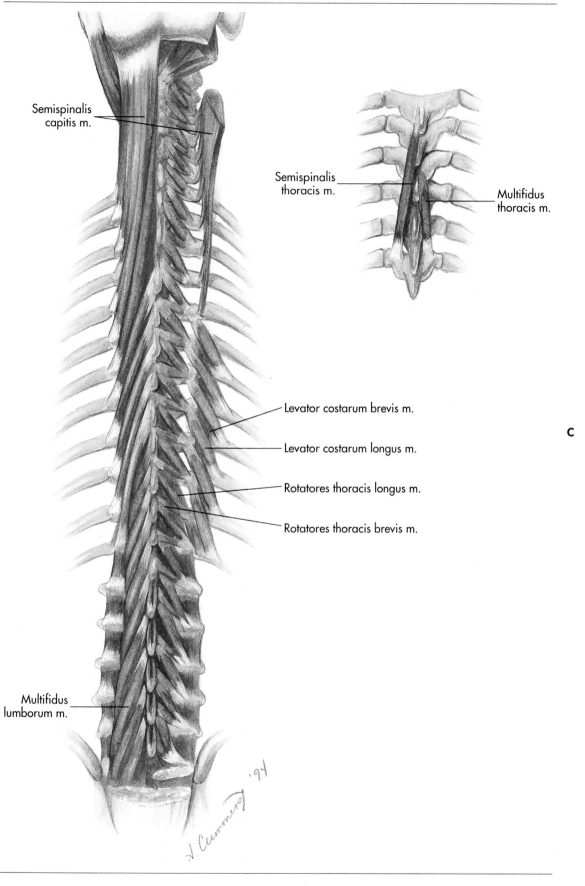

Semispinalis
capitis m.

Semispinalis
thoracis m.

Multifidus
thoracis m.

Levator costarum brevis m.

Levator costarum longus m.

Rotatores thoracis longus m.

Rotatores thoracis brevis m.

Multifidus
lumborum m.

C

FIG. 4-3, cont'd.   C, Sixth layer of back muscles. *Left,* Semispinalis capitis and thoracis and multifidus lumborum muscles. *Right,* Rotatores, intertransversarii, interspinales, and levator costarum longus and brevis muscles. *Inset,* Multifidus and rotatores muscles.

Continued.

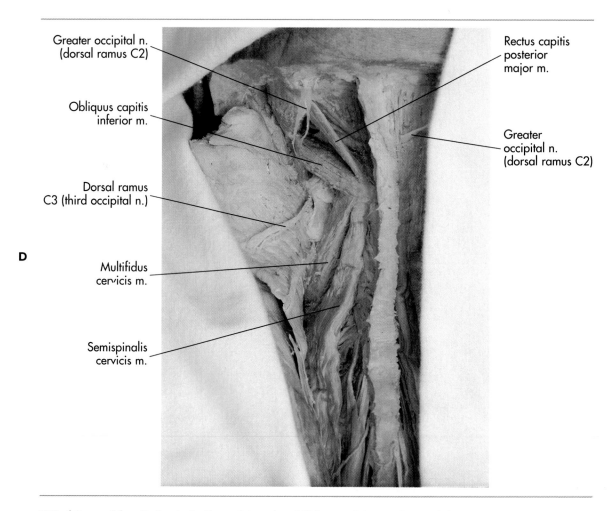

Greater occipital n. (dorsal ramus C2)

Obliquus capitis inferior m.

Dorsal ramus C3 (third occipital n.)

Multifidus cervicis m.

Semispinalis cervicis m.

Rectus capitis posterior major m.

Greater occipital n. (dorsal ramus C2)

D

FIG. 4-3, cont'd.   D, Semispinalis cervicis and multifidus cervicis muscles in a left posterior view of the upper cervical region.

the lamina of the vertebra two segments above. The more superficial fascicles are longer and run from mamillary processes to spinous processes three to five segments above. In the lower lumbar spine the inferior attachments of the fascicles include the posterior aspect of the sacrum lying adjacent to the spinous tubercles, posterior sacro-iliac ligaments, posterosuperior iliac spine, and the deep surface of the erector spinae aponeurosis.

Each band of multifidus lumborum is actually a myotome arranged such that the fibers that move a particular lumbar vertebra (i.e., those that attach superiorly to a single spinous process) are innervated by the medial branch of the dorsal ramus of that segment's spinal nerve. For example, the multifidus inserting onto the spinous process of L2 is innervated by the medial branch of the dorsal ramus (posterior primary division) of L2. Specifically in the lumbar region, the multifidus produces primarily extension (Macintosh & Bogduk, 1986). Rotation of the lumbar spine is seen only secondarily, in conjunction with extension.

Rotatores Muscles

Rotatores lumborum, thoracis, and cervicis. The rotatores muscles are located deep to the multifidus group. They constitute the deepest muscle fasciculi located in the groove between the spinous and transverse processes. This groove runs the entire length of the vertebral column from sacrum to axis. The two groups of rotatores are determined by their length. The fascicles of the rotatores brevis begin on transverse processes and attach to the root of the vertebral spinous process immediately superior. The fascicles of the rotatores longus have similar origins but insert on the root of the spinous process of the second vertebra above. The rotatores muscles are best developed in the thoracic region and are only poorly developed in the cervical and lumbar regions. Acting bilaterally, these muscles help in extension of the spine, although unilateral contraction helps produce rotation of the spine such that the vertebral bodies move away from

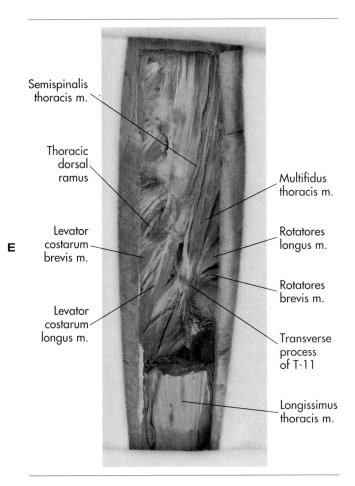

Semispinalis thoracis m.

Thoracic dorsal ramus

Levator costarum brevis m.

Levator costarum longus m.

E

Multifidus thoracis m.

Rotatores longus m.

Rotatores brevis m.

Transverse process of T-11

Longissimus thoracis m.

FIG. 4-3, cont'd.   E, Semispinalis, multifidus, and rotatores longus and brevis muscles as they arise from a single left lower thoracic transverse process (transverse process of T11).

the side contracted. The rotatores muscles' main function probably is to stabilize the vertebral column. These muscles are segmentally innervated by the medial branches of the posterior primary divisions of the spinal nerves.

The muscles of the fifth and sixth layers may be torn (strained) during hyperflexion of the spine or while lifting heavy loads. The muscles of these layers are made up of many individual strands, and these individual strands may tear near their musculotendinous junction. This tearing results in pain and tenderness, which may refer to neighboring regions (see Chapter 11). Since many attachment sites of these muscles are rather deep, localizing the torn muscle during physical examination may be difficult. However, the costal attachments of the iliocostalis lumborum and the iliac attachment of the longissimus thoracis are close to the surface, and pain from these muscles may be localized to these attachment sites during examination (Bogduk & Twomey, 1991).

OTHER MUSCLES DIRECTLY ASSOCIATED WITH THE SPINE

Suboccipital Muscles

The suboccipital muscles are a group of four small muscles located inferior to the occiput in the most superior portion of the posterior neck. They are the deepest muscles in this region, located under the trapezius, splenius capitis, and semispinalis capitis muscles. The suboccipital muscles consist of two rectus muscles, major and minor, and two obliquus muscles, superior and inferior. These muscles are concerned with extension of the head at the atlanto-occipital joint and rotation of the head at the atlanto-axial articulations. All are innervated by the posterior primary division of the C1 spinal nerve, which is also called the suboccipital nerve. The small number of muscle fibers per neuron for this group of muscles ranges from three to five (Oliver & Middleditch, 1991). This high degree of innervation allows these muscles to rapidly change tension, thus fine tuning the movements of the head and controlling head posture with a considerable degree of precision.

Rectus Capitis Posterior Major Muscle. The rectus capitis posterior major muscle (Fig. 4-4) begins at the spinous process of C2, widens as it ascends, and attaches superiorly to the lateral portion of the occiput's inferior nuchal line. When acting bilaterally, the rectus capitis posterior muscles produce extension of the head. Unilateral contraction turns the head so that the face rotates toward the side of the shortening muscle.

Rectus Capitis Posterior Minor Muscle. The rectus capitis posterior minor muscle is located just medial to and partly under the rectus capitis posterior major (Fig. 4-4). It attaches inferiorly to the posterior tubercle of the atlas and becomes broader as it ascends. It inserts on the medial portion of the occiput's inferior nuchal line and the area between that line and the foramen magnum. Contraction of this muscle produces extension of the head.

Obliquus Capitis Inferior Muscle. The obliquus capitis inferior muscle (Fig. 4-4) is the larger of the two obliquus muscles. It originates on the spinous process of the axis, passes laterally and slightly superiorly to insert onto the transverse process of C1. This muscle rotates the atlas such that the face is turned to the same side of contraction. The length of the transverse processes of the atlas gives this muscle a considerable mechanical advantage (Williams et al., 1989).

Obliquus Capitis Superior Muscle. The obliquus capitis superior arises from the transverse process of the

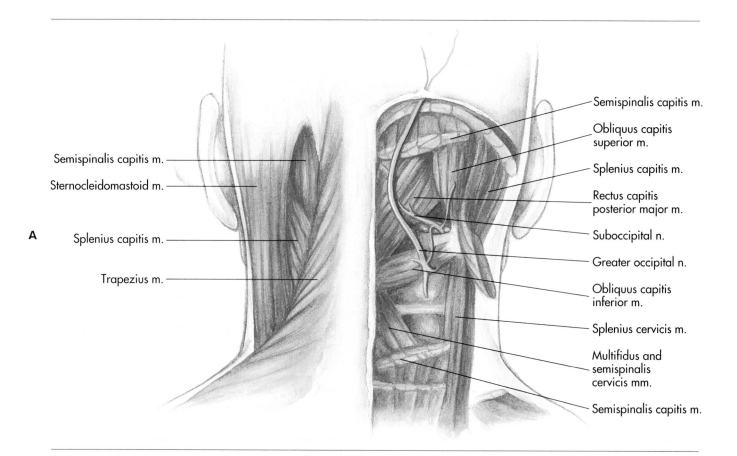

Semispinalis capitis m.

Sternocleidomastoid m.

Splenius capitis m.

Trapezius m.

Semispinalis capitis m.

Obliquus capitis superior m.

Splenius capitis m.

Rectus capitis posterior major m.

Suboccipital n.

Greater occipital n.

Obliquus capitis inferior m.

Splenius cervicis m.

Multifidus and semispinalis cervicis mm.

Semispinalis capitis m.

A

FIG. 4-4 Illustration (**A**) and photograph (**B**) of the suboccipital region. Three of the suboccipital muscles—the rectus capitis posterior major, obliquus capitis inferior, and obliquus capitis superior—form the suboccipital triangle. The remaining suboccipital muscle, the rectus capitis posterior minor, lies medial to the triangle. Notice the vertebral artery and the posterior arch of the atlas deep within the suboccipital triangle. **A** and **B**, Suboccipital muscles of the right and left sides, respectively.

atlas (Fig. 4-4). It becomes wider as it runs superiorly and posteriorly. This muscle inserts onto the occiput between the superior and inferior nuchal lines, lateral to the attachment of the semispinalis capitis, overlapping the insertion of the rectus capitis posterior major. Head extension and lateral flexion to the same side are produced by contraction of this muscle. The left and right obliquus capitis superior muscles, in conjunction with the two rectus muscles of each side, probably act more frequently as postural muscles than as prime movers (Williams et al., 1989).

Three of the four suboccipital muscles on each side of the upper cervical region form the sides of a suboccipital triangle. The boundaries of each suboccipital triangle are the (1) obliquus capitis inferior, below and laterally; (2) the obliquus capitis superior, above and laterally; and (3) the rectus capitis posterior major, medially and somewhat above. The roof of this triangle is composed of the splenius capitis laterally and the semispinalis capitis me-

dially. Deep to these muscles is a layer of dense fibrofatty tissue that also helps to form the roof. The floor of the triangle is made up of the posterior arch of the atlas and the posterior atlanto-occipital membrane. The suboccipital triangle contains the horizontal portion (third part) of the vertebral artery, the dorsal ramus of the C1 spinal nerve (suboccipital nerve), and the suboccipital plexus of veins.

Intertransversarii Muscles

The intertransversarii muscles (Fig. 4-5) extend between adjacent transverse processes. These muscles are most highly developed in the cervical region. The cervical intertransversarii usually begin at C1 (although the muscle between C1 and C2 is often absent) and continue to T1. They consist of anterior and posterior subdivisions that run between adjacent anterior and posterior tubercles, respectively. The ventral ramus of the mixed spinal

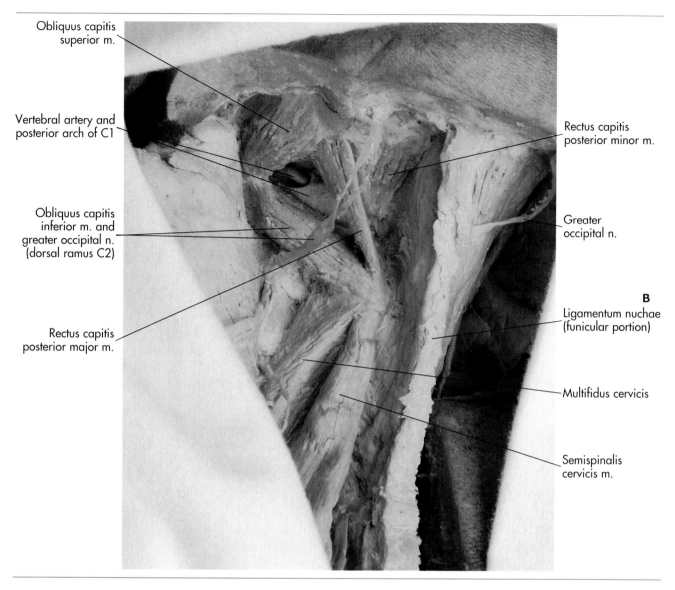

Obliquus capitis
superior m.

Vertebral artery and
posterior arch of C1

Obliquus capitis
inferior m. and
greater occipital n.
(dorsal ramus C2)

Rectus capitis
posterior major m.

Rectus capitis
posterior minor m.

Greater
occipital n.

B
Ligamentum nuchae
(funicular portion)

Multifidus cervicis

Semispinalis
cervicis m.

FIG. 4-4, cont'd.   For legend see opposite page.

nerve exits between each pair of anterior and posterior intertransversarii muscles and innervates each anterior intertransversarius muscle. Each posterior intertransversarius muscle in the cervical region is further subdivided into a medial and lateral part. The posterior primary division (dorsal ramus) of the mixed spinal nerve frequently pierces the medial part of a posterior intertransversarius muscle, and the medial branch of the posterior primary division innervates the medial part of this muscle. The anterior primary division (ventral ramus) innervates the lateral part of the posterior intertransversarius muscle and, as mentioned previously, the anterior intertransversarius muscle. The intertransversarii muscles function to flex the spine laterally by approximating adjacent transverse processes. They also help to stabilize adjacent vertebrae during large spinal movements.

The thoracic intertransversarii muscles are small and are usually only present in the lower thoracic region. They are not divided into subdivisions and are innervated by the dorsal rami (posterior primary divisions).

The lumbar intertransversarii muscles are found between all lumbar vertebrae. As with the cervical intertransversarii, the lumbar group of muscles divides into medial and lateral divisions. Each medial division passes from the accessory process, mamillo-accessory ligament, and mamillary process of the vertebra above to the mamillary process of the vertebra below (Fig. 4-5). Each

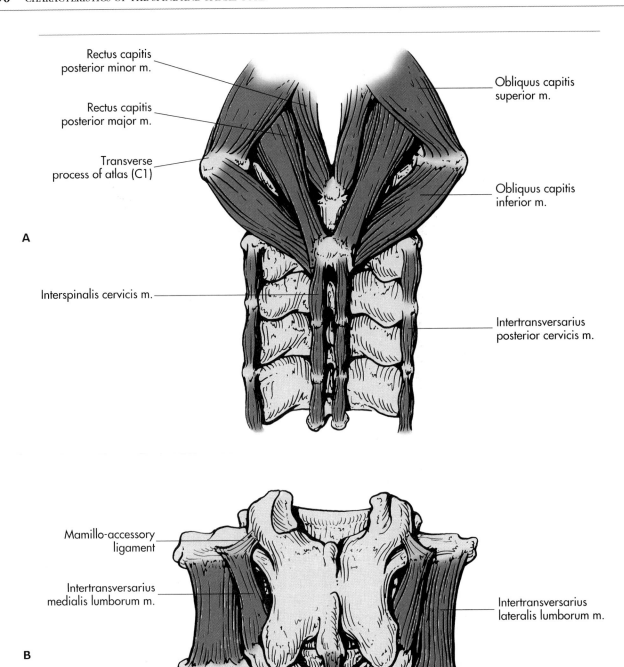

FIG. 4-5 **A,** Suboccipital, cervical interspinales, and cervical intertransversarii muscles. **B,** Lumbar interspinalis and left and right lumbar intertransversarii muscles. Also illustrated is the mamillo-accessory ligament. Notice the intertransversarii mediales lumborum muscles on each side, taking part of their origin from the left and right mamillo-accessory ligaments.

lateral intertransversarius muscle in the lumbar region can be further subdivided into an anterior and posterior division. The anterior division runs between adjacent transverse processes, and the posterior division runs from the accessory process of the vertebra above to the transverse process of the vertebra below. Both the anterior and the posterior divisions of the lateral intertransversarii muscles are innervated by lumbar anterior primary divisions (ventral rami). The medial intertransversarii muscles are innervated by lumbar posterior primary divisions.

The intertransversarii muscles are generally thought to flex the lumbar region laterally and stabilize adjacent vertebrae during spinal movement. However, the intertransversarii muscles are short and lie close to the axes of motion for lateral flexion and rotation of the spine. This places them at a considerable biomechanical disadvantage, and thus their usefulness as lateral flexors or stabilizers has been questioned (Bogduk & Twomey, 1991). In addition, the intertransversarii and interspinales muscles have been found to possess up to six times more muscle spindles than the other deep back muscles. The large number of muscle spindles in these muscles has led Bogduk and Twomey (1991) to speculate that the intertransversarii muscles function as proprioceptive transducers, providing afferent information for spinal and supraspinal circuits. By adjusting and regulating neural activity to the back muscles, these circuits help to maintain posture and to produce smooth and accurate movements of the spine.

Interspinales Muscles

The interspinales muscles (Fig. 4-5) are small muscles that extend between adjacent spinous processes. They are located on each side of the interspinous ligament. Interspinales muscles are present as small, distinct bundles of fibers throughout the cervical region, beginning at the spinous processes of C2 and continuing to the spinous process of T1. The thoracic interspinales muscles are variable and are located only in the upper and lower few segments. The lumbar region, as with the cervical region, has interspinales muscles running between all the lumbar spinous processes. They are innervated by the medial branches of the posterior primary divisions of spinal nerves. The interspinales muscles function to extend the spine and may act as proprioceptive organs.

Levator Costarum Muscles

The levator costarum (see Fig. 4-3, C) are muscular fasciculi that arise from the tips of the transverse processes of C7 to T11 and run inferiorly and laterally, parallel with the posterior borders of the external in-

tercostal muscles. The levator costarum brevis attaches to the superior surface, between the tubercle and angle, of the rib immediately inferior to its origin. Sometimes, especially in the lower thoracic levels, fasciculi attach to the second rib below. These fasciculi are known as levator costarum longus muscles and are located medial to the brevis muscle originating from the same transverse process. The levator costarum elevate the ribs and may help laterally flex and rotate the trunk to the same side. They are segmentally innervated by lateral branches of the posterior primary divisions (dorsal rami) of the spinal nerves.

Muscles Associated With the Anterior Aspect of the Cervical Vertebrae

The muscles associated with the anterior aspect of the cervical vertebrae include the longus colli, longus capitis, rectus capitis anterior, and rectus capitis lateralis (Fig. 4-6). These muscles are responsible for flexing the neck and occiput and may be injured during extension injuries of the cervical region.

Longus Colli Muscle. The left and right longus colli muscles (Fig. 4-6) are located along the anterior aspect of the cervical vertebral bodies. Each of these muscles is made up of three parts: vertical, inferior oblique, and superior oblique. Together the three parts of this muscle flex the neck. The superior and inferior oblique parts may also aid with lateral flexion. The inferior oblique part also rotates the neck to the opposite side. The longus colli muscle is innervated by branches of the anterior primary divisions of C2 to C6. This muscle is probably one of the muscles responsible for reversal of the cervical lordosis after extension injuries of the neck. The origins, insertions, and unique characteristics of the three parts of the longus colli muscle are listed next.

Vertical portion. The vertical portion of the longus colli originates from and inserts onto vertebral bodies. More specifically, this muscle originates from the anterior aspect of the vertebral bodies of C5 to T3 and inserts onto the vertebral bodies of C2 to C4.

Inferior oblique portion. The inferior oblique portion of the longus colli muscle originates from the vertebral bodies of T1 to T3 and passes superiorly and laterally to insert onto the anterior tubercles of the transverse processes of C5 and C6.

Superior oblique portion. The superior oblique portion of the longus colli muscle originates from the anterior tubercles of the transverse processes of C3 to C5.

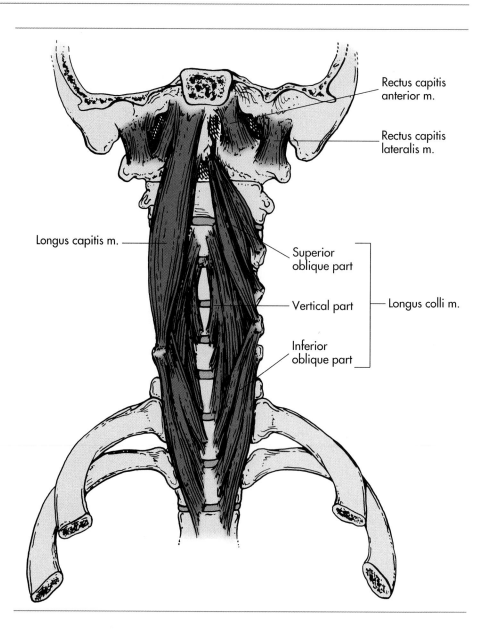

FIG. 4-6 Muscles associated with the anterior aspect of the cervical vertebrae and the occiput. *Right,* Three parts of the longus colli muscle (vertical, inferior oblique, superior oblique). *Left,* Longus capitis muscle. The rectus capitis anterior and lateralis can also be seen as they pass from the atlas to the occiput.

Its fibers course superiorly and medially and converge to insert onto the anterior tubercle of the atlas by means of a rather narrow tendon. This tendinous insertion can be torn during an extension injury of the neck. Such an injury can be followed by the deposition of calcium in the region, a condition known as retropharyngeal calcific tendonitis. The calcium may be seen on x-ray film approximately 3 weeks after injury and usually appears as an irregular and sometimes subtle region of increased radiopacity located just anterior to the atlas. The calcium is usually resorbed as the injury heals and is then no longer visible on x-ray film.

Longus Capitis Muscle. The longus capitis muscle is located anterior and slightly lateral to the longus colli muscle (Fig. 4-6). It originates as a series of thin tendons from the anterior tubercles of the transverse processes of C3 to C6. The tendinous origins unite to form a distinct muscular band that courses superiorly toward the occiput. This muscular band inserts onto the region of the occiput anterior to the foramen magnum and posterior to the pharyngeal tubercle. The longus capitis muscle functions to flex the head and is innervated by branches of the anterior primary divisions of C1 to C3.

Rectus Capitis Anterior Muscle. The rectus capitis anterior is a small muscle located deep to the inserting fibers of the longus capitis muscle (Fig. 4-6). It originates from the anterior aspect of the lateral mass and the most medial part of the transverse process of the atlas. The rectus capitis anterior muscle inserts onto the occiput just in front of the occipital condyle. This muscle functions to flex the head at the atlanto-occipital joints and is innervated by the anterior primary divisions of the first and second cervical nerves.

Rectus Capitis Lateralis Muscle. The rectus capitis lateralis muscle is another small muscle. It originates from the anterior aspect of the transverse process of the atlas and courses superiorly to insert onto the jugular process of the occiput (Fig. 4-6). It laterally flexes the occiput on the atlas and is innervated by the anterior primary division of the first and second cervical nerves.

Iliac Muscles

The muscles of the iliac region are sometimes referred to as the posterior abdominal wall muscles. However, since they all have direct action on the vertebral column and are attached to the lumbar region, they may properly be classified as spinal muscles. All three of these muscles attach inferiorly onto either the pelvis or the femur and therefore also help connect the lower limb to the spine. They are the psoas major, psoas minor, and quadratus lumborum muscles (Fig. 4-7).

Psoas Major and Iliacus Muscles. The psoas major muscle (Fig. 4-7) arises from the anterolateral portion of the bodies of T12 to L5, the intervertebral discs between these bones, and the transverse processes of all the lumbar vertebrae. It descends along the pelvic brim, passes deep to the inguinal ligament and in front of the hip capsule, and inserts via a tendon onto the femur's lesser trochanter. The lateral side of the tendon of the psoas major muscle receives the bulk of the fibers of the iliacus muscle, and together they form what is sometimes loosely referred to as the iliopsoas muscle. The iliacus originates from the inner lip of the iliac crest, the upper two thirds of the iliac fossa, and the superolateral portion of the sacrum. It inserts with the psoas major onto the femur's lesser trochanter.

The psoas major muscle, along with the iliacus muscle, functions primarily to flex the thigh at the hip. If the lower limb is stabilized, these muscles are concerned primarily with flexing the trunk and pelvis. They are important in raising the body from the supine to the sitting position. Electromyographic evidence further suggests that the psoas major is involved in balancing the trunk when in the sitting position (Williams et al., 1989). When the neck of the femur is fractured, this muscle acts as a lateral rotator of the thigh, which results in the characteristic laterally rotated position of the lower limb. Both the psoas major and the iliacus muscles are usually innervated by fibers arising from the L2 and L3 spinal cord levels. The iliacus muscle receives branches of the femoral nerve, and the psoas major muscle is supplied by direct fibers from the ventral rami of the L2-3 spinal nerves. Sometimes the L1 and L4 spinal nerves also send branches into the psoas major muscle.

Psoas Minor Muscle. The psoas minor is a variable muscle, absent in about 40% of the population (Williams et al., 1989). When present, it is located on the anterior surface of the psoas major muscle. The psoas minor muscle attaches superiorly to the lateral aspect of the bodies of T12 and L1 and the interposing intervertebral disc. It descends to attach inferiorly by a long tendon to the pecten pubis and the iliopubic eminence. The psoas minor acts as a weak trunk flexor and is innervated by fibers arising from the anterior primary division of the L1 spinal nerve.

Quadratus Lumborum Muscle. The quadratus lumborum (Fig. 4-7) lies along the tips of the transverse processes of the lumbar vertebrae and is irregularly quadrangular in shape. It attaches inferiorly to the transverse process of L5, the iliolumbar ligament, and the posterior aspect of the iliac crest adjacent to that ligament. Superiorly, the quadratus lumborum is attached to the lower border of the 12th rib and the tips of the transverse processes of L1 to L4. If the pelvis is fixed, this muscle laterally flexes the lumbar spine. When both muscles contract, they help with extension of the spine. Each quadratus lumborum muscle also depresses the 12th rib and aids in inspiration by stabilizing the origin of the diaphragm to the 12th rib. It is innervated by fibers from the ventral rami of the T12 to L3 (sometimes L4) spinal nerves.

MUSCLES THAT INDIRECTLY INFLUENCE THE SPINE
Muscles of Respiration

All the muscles of respiration have attachments to ribs. In addition to aiding respiration, all these muscles are involved to some extent with stabilizing the thoracic cage during trunk movements. The muscles of respiration are composed of the following: those that connect adjacent ribs (intercostals), those that span across more than one rib (subcostals), those that attach ribs to the sternum (transverse thoracis), those connecting ribs to vertebrae (levator costarum and serratus posterosuperior and posteroinferior), and the diaphragm. Since the levator costarum and posterior serratus muscles have vertebral attachments, they are considered true back muscles and are discussed in previous sections.

Diaphragm. The diaphragm is the principal muscle of respiration (Fig. 4-7). It is a domelike musculotendinous sheet that is convex superiorly. It completely separates the thoracic and abdominal cavities, except where it has apertures that allow for the passage of the esophagus, aorta, inferior vena cava, sympathetic trunks, and splanchnic nerves. This sheet consists of muscle fibers that attach to the entire border of the thoracic outlet. These fibers converge superiorly and medially and end as a central tendon. From anterior to posterior, muscle fibers arise from the posterior surface of the xiphoid

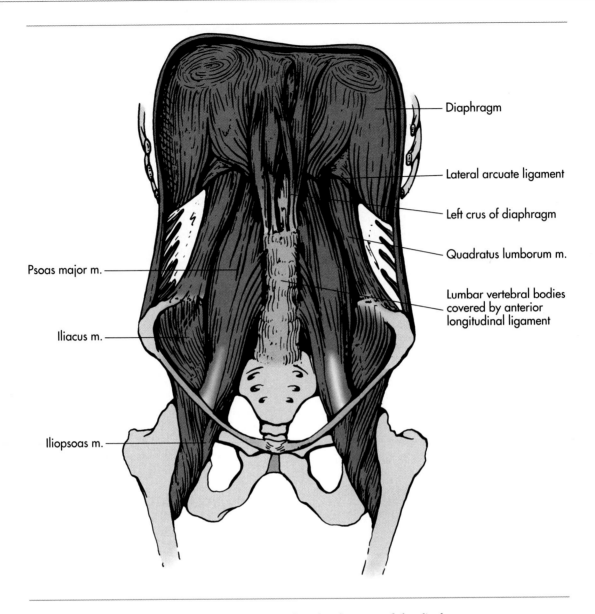

Psoas major m.

Iliacus m.

Iliopsoas m.

Diaphragm

Lateral arcuate ligament

Left crus of diaphragm

Quadratus lumborum m.

Lumbar vertebral bodies covered by anterior longitudinal ligament

FIG. 4-7   Iliac muscles and the diaphragm. The left and right crura of the diaphragm are prominently displayed. Also notice the left and right quadratus lumborum, psoas major, and iliacus muscles.

process, the deep surface of the lower six ribs and their costal cartilages, interdigitations with the origin of the transversus abdominis muscle, the lateral and medial lumbocostal arches, and the first three lumbar vertebrae. The origins from the lumbar vertebrae form the left and right crura.

The lateral lumbocostal arch, also known as the lateral arcuate ligament, is a thickening of the fascia of the quadratus lumborum muscle. It attaches medially to the transverse process of L1, arches over the upper portion of the quadratus lumborum, and ends laterally on the lower border of the 12th rib.

The medial lumbocostal arch, or medial arcuate ligament, is a similar structure, except it is associated with the psoas major muscle. This arch is also attached to the transverse process of L1, but it arches medially over the psoas major and is connected to the lateral aspect of the body of L1 or L2.

The crura of the diaphragm originate from the anterolateral surfaces of the upper two (on the left) or three (on the right) lumbar vertebrae, their discs, and the anterior longitudinal ligament. The two crura meet in the midline and arch over the aorta's anterior aspect to form what is sometimes called the median arcuate ligament.

When the diaphragm first contracts, the lower ribs are fixed; then the central tendon is drawn inferiorly and anteriorly. The abdominal contents provide resistance to further descent of the diaphragm, which leads to protrusion of the anterior abdominal wall ("abdominal" breathing) and elevation of the rib cage ("thoracic" breathing). The diaphragm is innervated by the left and right phrenic nerves, which arise from the ventral rami of C3 to C5. Also, some afferent fibers from the peripheral aspect of this muscle are carried in the lower six or seven intercostal nerves. These nerves, and the sensory fibers of the phrenic nerves, are responsible for the referred pain patterns seen with some diaphragmatic diseases.

External, Internal, and Innermost Intercostal Muscles. The intercostal muscles (Fig. 4-8, *A*) comprise three sets of superimposed muscles located between adjacent ribs. These sets of muscles consist of the external intercostal, internal intercostal, and innermost intercostal muscles.

The external intercostal muscles, 11 on each side, have attachments that extend along the shafts of the ribs from the tubercles to just lateral to the costal cartilages. More anteriorly, each is replaced by an aponeurosis, called the external intercostal membrane, which continues to the sternum. Each external intercostal originates from the lower border of one rib and inserts onto the upper border of the adjacent rib below. The fibers of each are directed obliquely; in the posterior chest, they run inferolaterally, although at the front, they course inferomedially and somewhat anteriorly.

The 11 pairs of internal intercostal muscles are located immediately deep to the external intercostals. Their attachments begin anteriorly at the sternum, or at the costal cartilages for ribs 8 through 10, and continue posteriorly to the costal angles. At that point, they are replaced by an aponeurotic layer, termed the internal intercostal membrane, which continues posteriorly to the anterior fibers of the superior costotransverse ligament. Each internal intercostal muscle attaches superiorly to the floor of the costal groove and corresponding portion of the costal cartilage and runs obliquely inferior to its attachment on the superior surface of the adjacent rib below. The fibers of the internal intercostal muscles are arranged orthogonally to those of the external intercostals.

The fibers of the innermost intercostal muscles lie just deep to and run parallel with those of the internal intercostals. They are poorly developed in the upper thoracic levels but become progressively more pronounced in the lower levels. They are attached to the deep surfaces of adjacent ribs and are best developed in the middle two fourths of the intercostal space. The intercostal veins, arteries, and nerves (from superior to inferior) can be found in the superior aspect of the intercostal space passing between the fibers of the internal and innermost intercostal muscles.

Although the intercostal muscles play a role in respiration, their exact function is still controversial (Williams et al., 1989). Conflicting evidence exists as to the actions of the various layers of the intercostals during inspiration and expiration. Results from studies using electromyography show differences in the activity of upper versus lower intercostals during the different phases of respiration. In addition, activity has been recorded in the intercostals during many trunk movements, and they appear to act as stabilizers of the thoracic cage (Oliver & Middleditch, 1991). The intercostals are innervated by branches of the adjacent intercostal nerves.

Subcostal Muscles. The subcostal muscles (Fig. 4-8, *D*) are musculotendinous fasciculi that are usually best developed only in the lower thorax. Each arises from the inferior border of one rib, near the angle, and runs obliquely inferior to the second or third rib below. The fibers of the subcostals are parallel to those of the internal intercostals. They probably help depress the ribs and are innervated by branches from adjacent intercostal nerves.

Transversus Thoracis Muscles. The transversus thoracis, or sternocostalis, muscle is located on the deep surface of the anterior thoracic wall (Fig. 4-8, *B*). It originates from the posterior surface of the inferior one third of the sternal body, posterior surface of the xiphoid process, and the posterior surfaces of the costal cartilages of the lower three or four true ribs. It inserts onto the inferior and deep surfaces of the costal cartilages of the second through sixth ribs. The fibers of the muscle form a fanlike arrangement, with the upper fibers being almost vertically oriented and the intermediate fibers more obliquely oriented. The lowermost fibers not only are horizontal, but also are continuous with the most superior fibers of the transversus abdominis muscle. The transversus thoracis pulls the costal cartilages, to which it inserts in an inferior direction. The transversus thoracis muscle is innervated by the adjacent intercostal nerves.

Anterolateral Abdominal Muscles

Although the four muscles composing the anterolateral abdominal wall do not have direct attachments to the spine, they are involved in producing several movements of the trunk, including flexion, lateral flexion, and rotation. They are also important as postural muscles and in increasing intraabdominal pressure. These muscles include the external abdominal oblique, internal abdominal oblique, rectus abdominis, and transversus abdominis muscles.

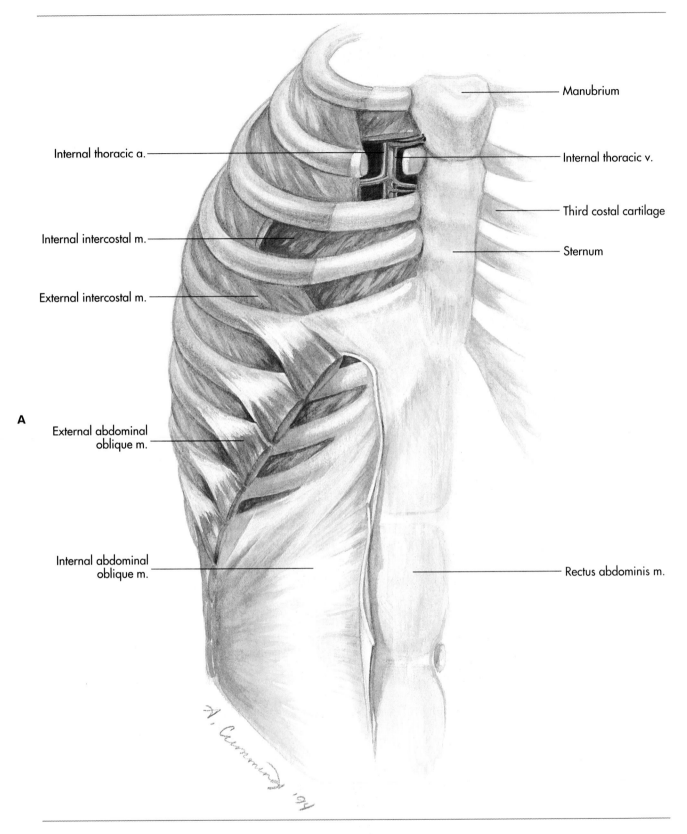

A

Internal thoracic a.

Internal intercostal m.

External intercostal m.

External abdominal
oblique m.

Internal abdominal
oblique m.

Manubrium

Internal thoracic v.

Third costal cartilage

Sternum

Rectus abdominis m.

FIG. 4-8 **A,** Anterolateral view of the thoracic and abdominal walls. *Upper aspect,* Cutaway view of the medial intercostal spaces demonstrating the internal thoracic artery and vein. The external intercostal muscle has been reflected between two ribs to show the internal intercostal muscle to best advantage. The external abdominal oblique muscle has also been reflected and cut away to reveal the internal abdominal oblique muscle.

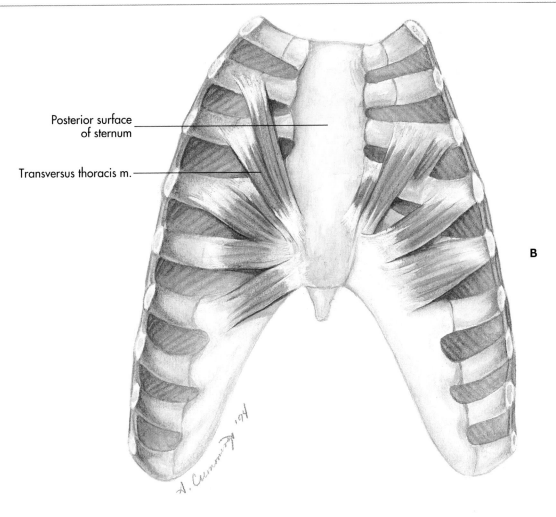

Posterior surface of sternum

Transversus thoracis m.

B

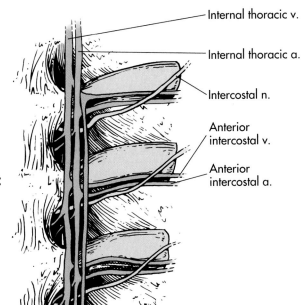

C

Internal thoracic v.

Internal thoracic a.

Intercostal n.

Anterior intercostal v.

Anterior intercostal a.

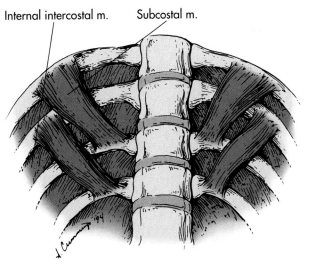

Internal intercostal m.   Subcostal m.

D

FIG. 4-8, cont'd. **B,** Internal view of the *anterior* thoracic wall showing the transversus thoracis muscle. **C,** Detail of **B** showing several intercostal spaces just lateral to the sternum. **D,** Internal view of the *posterior* thoracic wall showing several subcostal muscles.

External Abdominal Oblique Muscle. The external abdominal oblique (obliquus externus abdominis) (Fig. 4-8, *A*) is the largest and most superficial of these muscles. It originates as eight muscular slips from the inferior borders of the lower eight ribs. The upper slips attach near the cartilages of the ribs, whereas the lower ones attach at a progressively greater distance from the costal cartilages. The serratus anterior, latissimus dorsi, and sometimes the pectoralis major muscles interdigitate with these slips. The lower fibers descend almost vertically, attaching to approximately the anterior half of the outer lip of the iliac crest. The upper and middle fibers pass inferomedially and become aponeurotic by the time they pass a line connecting the umbilicus and the anterior superior iliac spine. The external oblique aponeurosis is a strong sheet of connective tissue whose fibers continue inferomedially to the midline, where they blend with the linea alba. The linea alba is a tendinous raphe running in the midline from the xiphoid process to the pubic symphysis. The inferior portion of the aponeurosis of the external oblique forms the inguinal ligament, the reflected portion of that ligament, and the lacunar ligament. It also has an opening, the superficial inguinal ring, that allows passage of the spermatic cord in the male and the round ligament of the uterus in the female. The external abdominal oblique muscle is innervated by the ventral rami of the T7 to T12 spinal nerves.

Internal Abdominal Oblique Muscle. The internal abdominal oblique (obliquus internus abdominis) (Fig. 4-8, *A*), located immediately deep to the external oblique, originates from the lateral two thirds of the inguinal ligament, anterior two thirds of the iliac crest, and the thoracolumbar fascia. The uppermost fibers insert onto the lower borders of the lower three or four ribs and are continuous with the internal intercostal muscles. The lowest fibers become tendinous and attach to the pubic crest and the medial portion of the pecten pubis. Here they are joined by the transversus abdominis aponeurosis, and together their united insertion forms the conjoint tendon, or inguinal falx. The intermediate fibers diverge from their origin and become aponeurotic. The internal oblique aponeurosis continues toward the midline, where it blends with the linea alba. In the upper two thirds of the abdomen, this aponeurosis splits into two laminae at the lateral border of the rectus abdominis. These laminae pass on either side of that muscle before reuniting at the linea alba. In the lower one third of the abdomen, the entire aponeurosis, along with the inserting aponeurosis of the transversus abdominis, passes anterior to the rectus abdominis. The internal abdominal oblique muscle is innervated by branches of the ventral rami of T7 to L1 spinal nerves.

Transversus Abdominis Muscle. The transversus abdominis muscle is located deep to the internal abdominal oblique muscle. It arises from the lateral one third of the inguinal ligament or adjacent iliac fascia, anterior two thirds of the outer lip of the iliac crest, the thoracolumbar fascia between the iliac crest and 12th rib, and the internal aspects of the lower six costal cartilages, where it blends with the diaphragm. The fibers of the transversus abdominis run basically in a horizontal direction and become aponeurotic. The lowest fibers of the transversus abdominis aponeurosis curve inferomedially and, along with the fibers from the internal oblique aponeurosis, form the conjoint tendon (see the preceding discussion). The rest of the fibers of this aponeurosis pass horizontally to the midline, where they blend with the linea alba. The upper three fourths of the fibers run posterior to the rectus abdominis, whereas the lower one fourth course anterior to this muscle. The transversus abdominis is innervated by the anterior primary divisions of the T7 to L1 spinal nerves.

Rectus Abdominis Muscle

The rectus abdominis muscle (Fig. 4-8, *A*) is a long, straplike muscle extending the entire length of the anterior abdominal wall. The linea alba forms the medial border of this muscle and separates the two (right and left). The lateral border of the rectus can usually be seen on the surface of the anterior abdominal wall and is termed the *linea semilunaris*. This muscle attaches inferiorly to the pubic crest (sometimes as far laterally as the pecten pubis) and also to ligamentous fibers anterior to the symphysis pubis. In this region the left and right rectus abdominis muscles may interlace. Superiorly, this muscle attaches to the fifth through seventh costal cartilages and the xiphoid process. Sometimes the most lateral fibers may reach the fourth or even third costal cartilages. The rectus abdominis muscle is crossed by three horizontal fibrous bands called the tendinous intersections. They are usually found at the level of the umbilicus, the inferior tip of the xiphoid process, and halfway between these two points.

The rectus abdominis muscle is enclosed by the aponeurosis of the abdominal obliques and transversus abdominis muscles. This aponeurosis is sometimes referred to as the rectus sheath. In the upper portion of the anterior abdominal wall, the external oblique and the anterior lamina of the internal oblique aponeuroses pass anterior to the rectus, whereas the posterior lamina of the internal oblique and transverse aponeuroses lie posterior to the rectus. Approximately halfway between the umbilicus and pubic symphysis, this arrangement changes, forming a curved line known as the arcuate line. Inferior to this line, all three aponeurotic layers are found anterior to the rectus, and only the transversalis fascia (the layer of fascia deep to the anterolateral abdominal muscles) separates this muscle from the parietal peritoneum. Recent data show that this traditional description of the rectus sheath may be too simplistic (Williams et al., 1989). The rectus abdominis muscle is supplied by the anterior primary divisions of the lower six or seven thoracic spinal nerves.

The abdominal muscles act to retain the abdominal viscera in place and oppose the effects of gravity on them in the erect and sitting positions. When the thorax and pelvis are fixed, these muscles, especially the obliques, increase the intraabdominal pressure. This is important for childbirth, expiration, emptying the bladder and rectum, and vomiting. It is also the basis of the Valsalva maneuver (increasing abdominal pressure for diagnostic purposes). The external abdominal oblique can further aid expiration by depressing the lower ribs. If the pelvis is fixed, these muscles, primarily the recti, bend the trunk forward and flex the lumbar spine. If the thorax is fixed, the lumbar spine still flexes, but the pelvis is brought upward. With unilateral contraction the trunk is laterally flexed to that side. In addition, the external oblique can help produce rotation of the trunk away from the side of contraction, whereas the internal oblique turns it to the same side. The transverse abdominis muscle probably has an effect only on the abdominal viscera and does not produce any appreciable movement of the vertebral column, although in light of the more recent description of the rectus sheath, rotational movements are a distinct possibility (Williams et al., 1989).

OTHER MUSCLES THAT HAVE CLINICAL RELEVANCE TO THE BACK

An important component of posture and locomotion is the tilting of the pelvis on the heads of the femurs in an anteroposterior direction. Movement of the anterior portion of the pelvis in a proximal direction (i.e., bringing the pubic symphysis toward the umbilicus) is termed *backward tilting* and involves flexion of the lumbar spine. Tilting of the pelvis in the opposite direction tends to extend the lumbar spine. This forward tilting of the pelvis is accomplished by contraction of the erector spinae and psoas major muscles. Backward tilting of the pelvis is accomplished not only by the rectus abdominis and the two oblique abdominal muscles, but also by the hamstring and gluteus maximus muscles (Fig. 4-9). Imbalance of the muscles responsible for pelvic tilt is often seen in people with low back pain. These individuals may have shortened and tight psoas major and erector spinae muscles combined with weakened gluteal and abdominal muscles (Oliver & Middleditch, 1991).

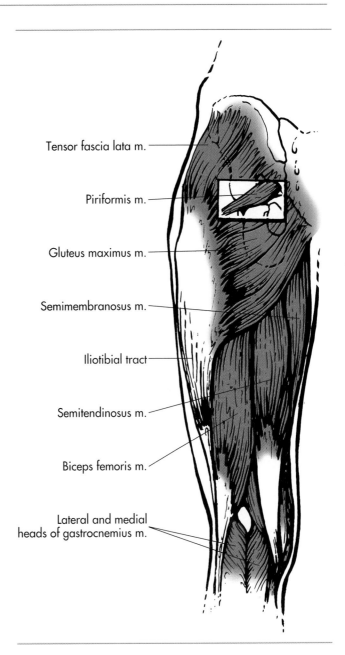

FIG. 4-9   Muscles of the posterior thigh. *Inset,* Piriformis muscle.

Hamstring Muscles

The posterior group of thigh muscles, commonly known as the hamstrings, acts to extend the hip and flex the knee joints. The three muscles in this group are the semitendinosus, semimembranosus, and biceps femoris. The latter muscle has two heads of origin, long and short (Fig. 4-9).

With the exception of the short head of the biceps femoris, all three of these muscles attach proximally to the ischial tuberosity. The short head of the biceps femoris arises from the lateral lip of the linea aspera and lateral supracondylar line of the femur. The semitendinosus and semimembranosus muscles are located posteromedial in the thigh, whereas the biceps femoris is posterolateral.

Semitendinosus Muscle. The semitendinosus, as its name implies, becomes tendinous about halfway along its course (Fig. 4-9). This long tendon curves around the medial tibial condyle, passes superficial to the tibial collateral ligament, and ends by attaching to the superior portion of the medial surface of the tibia immediately below and posterior to the attachment sites of the sartorius and gracilis muscles. This grouping of muscular insertions is sometimes known as the pes anserine. The semitendinosus muscle is innervated by the tibial portion (L5, S1, S2) of the sciatic nerve.

Semimembranosus Muscle. The semimembranosus muscle (Fig. 4-9) arises as a tendon and expands into an aponeurosis that is deep to the semitendinosus. The muscular fibers arise from this aponeurosis. The semimembranosus ends primarily on the posterior aspect of the medial tibial condyle via a short tendon. It also sends slips laterally and superiorly, some of which help form the oblique popliteal ligament. The semimembranosus muscle is innervated by the tibial portion (L5, S1, S2) of the sciatic nerve.

Biceps Femoris Muscle. The short head of the biceps femoris joins the belly of the long head of the biceps femoris on its deep surface as it descends in the thigh. After the two heads unite, the biceps femoris muscle gradually narrows to a tendon that attaches to the head of the fibula, the fibular collateral ligament, and the lateral tibial condyle (Fig. 4-9).

◆ ◆ ◆

When these muscles contract, they produce flexion at the knee and extension at the hip. When the thigh is flexed, the hamstring muscles, especially the biceps femoris, help tilt the pelvis backward. Tight hamstrings are sometimes associated with low back pain. The long head of the biceps femoris muscle is innervated by the tibial portion (L5, S1, S2) and the short head by the peroneal portion (L5, S1, S2) of the sciatic nerve.

Gluteus Maximus Muscle

The most superficial muscle in the gluteal region is the gluteus maximus (Fig. 4-9). It is considered the body's largest muscle. Its large size is a characteristic feature of the human musculature and is thought to be a result of its role in attaining an upright posture (Williams et al., 1989). It originates from the area of the ilium posterior to the posterior gluteal line. It also takes origin from the erector spinae aponeurosis, posterior and inferior

sacrum, lateral coccyx, sacrotuberous ligament, and the fascial covering of the gluteus medius. The fibers of the gluteus maximus run inferolaterally and attach distally to the iliotibial tract and gluteal tuberosity of the femur between the attachment sites of the vastus lateralis and adductor magnus.

When the pelvis is fixed, the gluteus maximus can extend the thigh from a flexed position. It also helps in strong lateral rotation of the thigh. Its upper fibers are active in strong abduction at the hip. If the thigh is stabilized, this muscle, along with the hamstrings, helps rotate the pelvis posteriorly on the femur heads, as in rising from a stooped position. By virtue of its attachment to the iliotibial tract, the gluteus maximus aids in stabilizing the femur on the tibia. It is also important for its intermittent action in various phases of normal gait. This muscle is innervated by the inferior gluteal nerve (L5 to S2).

Piriformis Muscle

The piriformis is a pear-shaped muscle lying deep to the gluteus medius (Fig. 4-9). It arises from the anterolateral sacrum by three musculotendinous slips. It also originates from the gluteal surface of the ilium (in proximity to the posterior inferior iliac spine), the capsule of the adjacent sacro-iliac joint, and sometimes from the anterior surface of the sacrotuberous ligament. The piriformis exits the pelvis via the greater sciatic foramen. The piriformis is the largest structure within the foramen. It attaches distally by a tendon to the upper border of the femur's greater trochanter. Normally, this muscle lies immediately superior to the sciatic nerve as it exits the greater sciatic foramen, but sometimes the common peroneal portion of the sciatic nerve pierces the piriformis and splits it. Entrapment of the nerve at this location is sometimes termed *piriformis syndrome.* With contraction, this muscle produces lateral rotation of the extended thigh. If the thigh is flexed, abduction at the hip occurs. It is innervated by branches from the ventral rami of the L5 to S2 spinal nerves.

Rectus Femoris Muscle

The quadriceps femoris is the great extensor muscle of the leg. This muscle consists of four parts: vastus lateralis, vastus interemedius, vastus medialis, and rectus femoris muscles. Three parts of this muscle, the vasti muscles, originate on the femur, but the rectus femoris arises from the pelvis. The rectus femoris muscle begins as two (or three) heads. The straight head attaches to the anterior inferior iliac spine, and the reflected head attaches to the superior rim of the acetabulum and capsule of the hip. Sometimes a recurrent head that arises from the anterosuperior angle of the femur's

Text continued on p. 107

Table 4-2 Summary of Muscles Affecting the Spine

Muscle	Origin	Insertion	Action	Innervation
Layer one				
Trapezius	Superior nuchal line, external occipital protuberance, ligamentum nuchae, spinous processes and supraspinous ligament of C7-T12	Spine of the scapula, acromion process, distal third of clavicle	See Table 4-1	Motor: spinal portion of accessory (spinal accessory [cranial nerve XI]) Sensory (proprioception): ventral rami of C3-4
Latissimus dorsi	Spinous processes and supraspinous ligament of T6-L5, thoracolumbar fascia, median sacral crest, iliac crests, lower four ribs	Intertubercular groove of the humerus (between insertions of pectoralis major and teres major)	Adduction, internal rotation, and extension of the humerus	Thoracodorsal (C6-8)
Layer two				
Rhomboid major	Spinous processes and supraspinous ligaments (T2-5)	Medial border of scapula inferior to root of scapular spine	Retract scapula, rotate point of shoulder down	Dorsal scapular (C5)
Rhomboid minor	Lower portion of ligamentum nuchae, spinous processes (C7 and T1)	Medial border of scapula at level of root of scapular spine	Retract scapula, rotate point of shoulder down	Dorsal scapular (C5)
Levator scapulae	Transverse processes (C1-4)	Medial border of scapula above root of scapular spine	If neck stabilized: elevate scapula, rotate point of shoulder down If scapula stabilized: bilaterally—extend neck; unilaterally—lateral flex and rotate neck to same side	Ventral rami of C3-4, dorsal scapular (C5)
Layer three				
Serratus posterior superior	Spinous processes and supraspinous ligament (C7-T3)	Posterior and superior aspect of second through fifth ribs	Aids respiration, raises second through fifth ribs	Ventral rami of T2-5 (intercostal nerves)
Serratus posterior inferior	Spinous processes and supraspinous ligament of T11-L2(3)	Posterior and inferior surfaces of lower four ribs (9-12)	Aids respiration, lowers ninth through twelfth ribs	Ventral rami of T9-12 (lower three intercostal nerves and subcostal nerve)
Layer four				
Splenius capitis	Lower part of ligamentum nuchae and spinous processes of C7-T3(4)	Mastoid process, temporal bone, and occiput below lateral part of superior nuchal line	Bilaterally: extend head Unilaterally: lateral flex and rotate face to same side	Lateral branches of dorsal rami of midcervical spinal nerves (C3-5)
Splenius cervicis	Spinous processes (T3-6)	Transverse processes of C1-3(4)	Bilaterally: extend neck Unilaterally: lateral flex and rotate neck toward same side	Lateral branches of dorsal rami of lower cervical spinal nerves (C5-7)

Continued.

Table 4-2 Summary of Muscles Affecting the Spine—cont'd

Muscle	Origin	Insertion	Action	Innervation
Layer five				
Iliocostalis lumborum	Common origin of erector spinae muscles: spinous processes and supraspinous ligament of T11-L5, median sacral crest, sacrotuberous ligament, posterior sacroiliac ligament, lateral sacral crest, posteromedial iliac crest	Angles of lower six to nine ribs	Extend and laterally flex spine	Lateral branches of dorsal rami of nearby spinal nerves
Iliocostalis thoracis	Angles of lower six ribs	Angles of upper six ribs and transverse process of C7	Extend and laterally flex spine	Lateral branches of dorsal rami of nearby spinal nerves
Iliocostalis cervicis	Angles of third through sixth ribs	Posterior tubercles of transverse processes of C4-6	Extend and laterally flex spine	Dorsal rami of nearby spinal nerves
Longissimus thoracis	Common origin of erector spinae muscles (see iliocostalis lumborum), also transverse and accessory processes of all lumbar vertebrae	Third through twelfth ribs, transverse processes of all 12 thoracic vertebrae	Extend and laterally flex spine	Lateral branches of dorsal rami of nearby spinal nerves
Longissimus cervicis	Transverse processes of upper thoracic vertebrae (T1-5)	Transverse processes and articular processes of C2-6	Extend and laterally flex spine	Lateral branches of dorsal rami of nearby spinal nerves
Longissimus capitis	Upper thoracic transverse processes (T1-5) and articular processes C4-7	Mastoid process temporal bone	Extend and laterally flex head	Lateral branches of dorsal rami of nearby spinal nerves
Spinalis thoracis	Lower thoracic and upper lumbar spinous processes (T11-L2)	Upper thoracic spinous processes (T1-4, sometimes down to T8)	Extend spine	Dorsal rami of nearby spinal nerves
Spinalis cervicis	Upper thoracic spinous processes (T1-6)	Spinous processes of C2 (occasionally C3 and C4)	Extend spine	Dorsal rami of nearby spinal nerves
Spinalis capitis	Transverse processes of C7-T6(7), articular processes of C4-6, sometimes spinous processes of C7 and T1	Occiput between superior and inferior nuchal lines	Extend head	Dorsal rami of upper thoracic and lower cervical spinal nerves
Layer six				
Semispinalis thoracis	Transverse processes (T7-12)	Spinous processes of four to six vertebrae above (C6-T4)	Bilaterally: extend thoracic spine Unilaterally: extend, laterally flex, and rotate vertebral bodies of thoracic spine to opposite side	Medial branches of dorsal rami of T1-6

Table 4-2 Summary of Muscles Affecting the Spine—cont'd

Muscle	Origin	Insertion	Action	Innervation
Semispinalis cervicis	Transverse processes (T1-5), articular processes (C4-7)	Spinous processes of four to six vertebrae above (C2-3)	Bilaterally: extend neck Unilaterally: extend, laterally flex, and rotate neck to opposite side	Dorsal rami of C6-8
Semispinalis capitis	Transverse processes (C7-T6), articular processes (C4-6)	Occiput between medial portions of superior and inferior nuchal lines	Bilaterally: extend head Unilaterally: slight rotation of face to opposite side	Dorsal rami of C1-6
Multifidus	Posterior sacrum, L1-5 mamillary processes, T1-12 transverse processes, C4-7 articular processes*	Spinous processes two to four segments above (C2-L5)*	Bilaterally: extend spine Unilaterally: extend, laterally flex, and rotate vertebral bodies to opposite side	Medial branches of dorsal rami of spinal nerves
Rotatores (lumborum, thoracis, cervicis)	Transverse processes	Spinous processes; longus ascends two vertebral segments, brevis ascends one vertebral segment	Bilaterally: extend spine Unilaterally: rotate vertebral bodies to opposite side	Medial branches of dorsal rami of spinal nerves

Suboccipital muscles

Muscle	Origin	Insertion	Action	Innervation
Rectus capitis posterior major	Spinous process (C2)	Lateral portion of inferior nuchal line	Bilaterally: extend head Unilaterally: rotate face toward same side	Suboccipital (dorsal ramus of C1)
Rectus capitis posterior minor	Posterior tubercle (C1)	Medial portion of inferior nuchal line	Extend head	Suboccipital (dorsal ramus of C1)
Obliquus capitis inferior	Spinous process (C2)	Transverse process (C1)	Rotate face toward same side	Suboccipital (dorsal ramus of C1)
Obliquus capitis superior	Transverse process (C1)	Occiput between lateral portions of superior and inferior nuchal lines	Bilaterally: extend head Unilaterally: lateral flex head to same side	Suboccipital (dorsal ramus of C1)

Small muscles of the spine

Muscle	Origin	Insertion	Action	Innervation
Intertransversarius*	Transverse process	Transverse process of adjacent vertebra	Lateral flexion of vertebra (approximates transverse processes)	Medial part of posterior intertransversarius: dorsal ramus of spinal nerve Anterior intertransversarius and lateral part of posterior intertransversarius: ventral ramus
Interspinalis	Spinous process	Spinous process	Extend spine (approximate spinous processes)	Medial branch of dorsal rami
Levator costarum (longus and brevis)	Lateral aspect of transverse processes (C7-T11)	Brevis: rib immediately below Longus: second rib below	Elevate ribs, may help laterally flex and rotate trunk to same side	Segmentally innervated by lateral branches of dorsal rami of spinal nerves

*See text for further details.

Continued.

Table 4-2   Summary of Muscles Affecting the Spine—cont'd

Muscle	Origin	Insertion	Action	Innervation
Muscles of the anterior aspect of the cervical vertebrae				
Longus colli (vertical part)	Anterior aspect vertebral bodies (C5-T3)	Anterior aspect vertebral bodies (C2-4)	Flex neck	Ventral rami of C2-6 spinal nerves
Longus colli (inferior oblique part)	Vertebral bodies (T1-3)	Anterior tubercles of transverse processes (C5 and C6)	Flex neck, aid with lateral flexion of neck to same side, rotate neck to opposite side	Ventral rami of lower cervical spinal nerves
Longus colli (superior oblique part)	Anterior tubercles of transverse processes (C3-5)	Anterior tubercle (C1)	Flex neck, aid with lateral flexion of neck to same side	Ventral rami of upper cervical spinal nerves
Longus capitis	Anterior tubercles of transverse processes (C3-6)	Anterior occiput	Flex head	Ventral rami of C1-3
Rectus capitis anterior	Anterior aspect of lateral mass of atlas	Occiput (anterior to occipital condyle)	Flex head at atlanto-occipital joints	Ventral rami of C1 and C2
Rectus capitis lateralis	Anterior aspect of transverse process (C1)	Occiput (jugular process)	Laterally flex occiput on atlas	Ventral rami of C1 and C2
Iliac muscles				
Psoas major	Anterolateral bodies (T12-L5), discs (T12-L4), transverse processes (L1-5)	Lesser trochanter (with iliacus)	If spine stabilized: flex thigh If thigh stabilized: flex trunk, tilt pelvis forward	Ventral rami of L2-3
Iliacus	Medial lip of iliac crest, iliac fossa, superolateral sacrum	Lesser trochanter (with psoas major)	See psoas major	Femoral (L2-3)
Psoas minor	Bodies (T12-L1), disc (T12)	Pecten pubis, iliopubic eminence	Flex trunk	Ventral ramus of L1
Quadratus lumborum	Transverse process (L5), iliolumbar ligament, posterior portion of iliac crest	Lower border of 12th rib, transverse processes (L1-4)	Bilaterally: extend spine, depress 12th rib, stabilize origin of diaphragm to 12th rib Unilaterally: lateral flex spine	Ventral rami of T12-L3
Muscles of respiration				
Diaphragm	Xiphoid process, deep surface of lower six ribs and their costal cartilages, lateral and medial lumbocostal arches and bodies (L1-3)	Central tendon	Inspiration, stabilize thorax	Phrenic (C3-5), lower six intercostals (afferent only)
External intercostals	Lower border ribs (1-11) from tubercles to costal cartilages	Upper border of adjacent rib below from tubercles to costal cartilages	Respiration, stabilize thorax	Adjacent intercostals
Internal intercostals	Lower border ribs (1-11) from sternum/costal cartilage to angle	Upper border of adjacent rib below from sternum/costal cartilage to angle	Respiration, stabilize thorax	Adjacent intercostals

Table 4-2   Summary of Muscles Affecting the Spine—cont'd

Muscle	Origin	Insertion	Action	Innervation
Innermost intercostals	Lower border ribs (1-11) in middle two fourths of intercostal space	Upper border of adjacent rib below in middle two fourths of intercostal space	Respiration, stabilize thorax	Adjacent intercostals
Subcostal	Inferior border ribs (1-10) near angle	Superior border of second rib below	Depress ribs	Adjacent intercostals
Transversus thoracis	Deep surface of inferior sternal body, xiphoid process, costal cartilages (4-7)	Deep surface of costal cartilages (2-6)	Depress costal cartilages	Adjacent intercostals
Anterolateral abdominal muscles				
External abdominal oblique	Inferior borders of lower eight ribs*	Linea alba, iliac crest*	Bilaterally: flex spine, tilt pelvis backward Unilaterally: lateral flex spine to same side, rotate spine to opposite side	Ventral rami of T7-12
Internal abdominal oblique	Lateral two thirds of inguinal ligament, anterior iliac crest, thoracolumbar fascia	Pecten pubis, pubic crest, linea alba*	Bilaterally: flex spine, tilt pelvis backward Unilaterally: lateral flex and rotate spine to same side	Ventral rami of T7-L1
Transversus abdominis	Lateral two thirds of inguinal ligament, anterior iliac crest, thoracolumbar fascia, lower six costal cartilages	Linea alba*	Unilaterally: rotate spine to same side	Ventral rami of T7-L1
Rectus abdominis	Pubic crest, symphysis pubis	Costal cartilages (5-7), xiphoid process	Bilaterally: flex spine, tilt pelvis backward Unilaterally: lateral flex spine	Ventral rami of T7-12
Hamstring muscles				
Semitendinosus	Ischial tuberosity	Medial tibia (pes anserine)	If leg stabilized: extend thigh, tilt pelvis backward If thigh stabilized: flex leg	Tibial division of sciatic nerve (L5, S1, S2)
Semimembranosus	Ischial tuberosity	Posterior aspect of medial tibial condyle*	If leg stabilized: extend thigh, tilt pelvis backward If thigh stabilized: flex leg	Tibial division of sciatic nerve (L5, S1, S2)
Biceps femoris	Long head: ischial tuberosity Short head: linea aspera, lateral supracondylar line of femur	Fibular head, fibular collateral ligament, lateral tibial condyle	Long head: if leg stabilized—extend thigh, tilt pelvis backward Both heads: if thigh stabilized—flex leg	Long head: tibial division of sciatic nerve (L5, S1, S2), Short head: peroneal division of sciatic nerve (L5, S1, S2)

*See text for further details.

Continued.

Table 4-2   Summary of Muscles Affecting the Spine—cont'd

Muscle	Origin	Insertion	Action	Innervation
Muscles attaching to the sacrum and ilium				
Gluteus maximus	Ilium, posterior-to-posterior gluteal line, aponeurosis of erector spinae, posterior sacrum, lateral coccyx, sacrotuberous ligament	Gluteal tuberosity, iliotibial tract	If pelvis stabilized: extend, abduct, and laterally rotate thigh If thigh stabilized: tilt pelvis backward, stabilize knee	Inferior gluteal (L5-S2)
Rectus femoris	Straight head: anteroinferior iliac spine Reflected head: acetabulum, capsule of hip*	Base of patella	If thigh stabilized: extend leg, tilt pelvis forward If pelvis stabilized: flex hip	Femoral (L2-4)
Piriformis	Anterolateral sacrum, gluteal surface of ilium, capsule of sacroiliac joint	Greater trochanter	If thigh extended: laterally rotate hip If thigh flexed: abduct hip	Ventral rami of L5-S2

*See text for further details.

SUMMARY OF ACTIONS OF SPINAL MUSCLES

MUSCLES ACTING ON THE HEAD AT THE ATLANTOAXIAL AND ATLANTOOCCIPITAL JOINTS

Extension

Trapezius
Semispinalis capitis
(Spinalis capitis)
Rectus capitis posterior major
Rectus capitis posterior minor
Obliquus capitis superior
Splenius capitis
Longissimus capitis

Flexion

Longus capitis
Rectus capitis anterior
Sternocleidomastoid

Lateral flexion

Trapezius
Sternocleidomastoid
Splenius capitis
Longissimus capitis
Semispinalis capitis
Rectus capitis lateralis
Obliquus capitis superior

Rotation

Splenius capitis, same side
Longissimus capitis, same side
Obliquus capitis inferior, same side
Longus capitis, same side
Rectus capitis posterior major, same side
Trapezius, opposite side
Sternocleidomastoid, opposite side

MUSCLES ACTING ON THE CERVICAL REGION

Extension

Levator scapulae
Splenius capitis
Splenius cervicis
Longissimus capitis
Longissimus cervicis
(Spinalis capitis)
(Spinalis cervicis)
Iliocostalis cervicis
Semispinalis capitis
Semispinalis cervicis
Multifidus
Interspinales

Flexion

Sternocleidomastoid
Longus capitis
Longus colli
Scalenus anterior

SUMMARY OF ACTIONS OF SPINAL MUSCLES—cont'd

MUSCLES ACTING ON THE CERVICAL REGION—cont'd

Lateral flexion
Sternocleidomastoid
Scalenus anterior
Scalenus medius
Scalenus posterior
Splenius capitis
Splenius cervicis
Levator scapulae
Longissimus capitis
Longissimus cervicis
Iliocostalis cervicis
Semispinalis cervicis
Trapezius
Intertransversarii

Rotation
Splenius capitis, same side
Splenius cervicis, same side
Longissimus cervicis, same side
Iliocostalis cervicis, same side
Sternocleidomastoid, opposite side
Semispinalis cervicis, opposite side
Multifidus, opposite side
Rotatores, opposite side
Scalenus anterior, opposite side
Trapezius, opposite side

MUSCLES ACTING ON THE TRUNK

Flexion
Psoas major
Psoas minor
Rectus abdominis
External abdominal oblique
Internal abdominal oblique

Extension
Quadratus lumborum
Multifidus
Rotatores
Semispinalis thoracis
Spinalis thoracis
Longissimus thoracis
Iliocostalis thoracis
Iliocostalis lumborum
Interspinales

Lateral flexion
External abdominal oblique
Internal abdominal oblique
Rectus abdominis
Iliocostalis lumborum
Iliocostalis thoracis
Longissimus thoracis
Semispinalis thoracis
Multifidus
Quadratus lumborum
Intertransversarii
Psoas major

Rotation
Internal abdominal oblique, same side
Iliocostalis thoracis, same side
Iliocostalis lumborum, same side
External abdominal oblique, opposite side
Multifidus, opposite side
Rotatores, opposite side

MUSCLES PRODUCING ANTEROPOSTERIOR TILTING OF THE PELVIS

Forward tilting
Erector spinae
Psoas major
Rectus femoris

Backward tilting
Rectus abdominis
External abdominal oblique
Internal abdominal oblique
Gluteus maximus
Biceps femoris (long head)
Semitendinosus
Semimembranosus

greater trochanter is described (Segal & Jacob, 1983). All the heads join, and the belly of the muscle then runs down the anterior thigh to attach by a broad aponeurosis to the base of the patella. By virtue of its proximal attachment sites, the rectus femoris muscle not only extends the knee, but also flexes the hip. If the thigh is fixed, contraction of this muscle helps to tilt the pelvis forward. The rectus femoris, along with the rest of the quadriceps femoris, is innervated by the femoral nerve (L2 to L4).

SUMMARY OF MUSCLES AFFECTING THE SPINE

Table 4-2 provides a summary of the muscles that influence the spine. This table does not give a complete account of all the points of origin and insertion of some of the more complex muscles. A more detailed description of each muscle appears in the text of this chapter. The box on pp. 106-107 organizes the muscles that influence the spine according to the motion produced by their contraction.

REFERENCES

Bogduk, N. & Twomey, L.T. (1991). *Clinical anatomy of the lumbar spine.* London: Churchill Livingstone.

Macintosh, J.E. & Bogduk, N. (1986). The biomechanics of the lumbar multifidus. *Clin Biomech, 1,* 205-213.

Macintosh, J.E. & Bogduk, N. (1987). The biomechanics of the thoracolumbar fascia. *Clin Biomech, 2,* 78-83.

Macintosh, J.E. & Bogduk, N. (1987). The morphology of the lumbar erector spinae. *Spine, 12,* 658-668.

Macintosh, J.E. et al. (1986). The morphology of the human lumbar multifidus. *Clin Biomech, 1,* 196-204.

Oliver, J. & Middleditch, A. (1991). *Functional anatomy of the spine.* Oxford: Butterworth-Heinemann.

Peck, D. et al. (1986). Are there compartment syndromes in some patients with idiopathic back pain? *Spine, 11,* 468-475.

Segal, P. & Jacob, M. (1983). *The knee.* Chicago: Year Book.

Williams, P.L. et al. (Eds.). (1989). *Gray's anatomy* (37th ed.). Edinburgh: Churchill Livingstone.

CHAPTER 5

The Cervical Region

Gregory D. Cramer

The cervical region is possibly the most distinct region of the spine. The fact that so many structures, spinal and otherwise, are "packed" into such a small cylinder, connecting the head to the thorax, makes the entire neck an outstanding feat of efficient design. The cervical spine is the most complicated articular system in the body, comprising 37 separate joints (Bland, 1989). It allows for more movement than any other spinal region and is surrounded by a myriad of nerves, vessels, and many other vital structures. All clinicians who have spent significant time working with patients suffering from pain of cervical origin have been challenged and sometimes frustrated with this region of immense clinical importance. Understanding the detailed anatomy of this area helps clinicians make more accurate assessments of their patients, which in turn, results in the establishment of more effective treatment protocols.

This chapter begins by covering the general characteristics of the cervical spine as a whole. This is followed by a discussion of the region's typical and atypical vertebrae. The external aspect of the occiput is included because of its intimate relationship with the upper two cervical segments. The ligaments of the cervical region are then covered, followed by a discussion of the cervical spine's ranges of motion. The most important structures of the anterior neck and the cervical viscera are also included.

CHARACTERISTICS OF THE CERVICAL SPINE AS A WHOLE
Cervical Curve (Lordosis)

The cervical curve is the least distinct of the spinal curves. It is convex anteriorly (lordosis) and is a secondary (compensatory) curvature (see Chapter 2). The cervical curve begins to develop before birth and as early as 9 weeks of prenatal life. Onset of fetal movements plays an important role in the early development of the cervical lordosis (Bagnall, Harris, & Jones, 1977; Williams et al., 1989). However, the curve becomes much more marked when the child begins to lift the head at about 3 to 4 months after birth, and the curve increases as the child begins to sit upright at about 9 months of age (Williams et al., 1989).

Some authors state that the cervical curve is actually composed of two curves, upper and lower (Kapandji, 1974; Oliver & Middleditch, 1991). The upper cervical curve is described as a distinct primary curve that extends from the occiput to the axis and is concave anteriorly (kyphotic). The lower cervical curve is the classically described lordosis, but in this case begins at C2 rather than C1. This description helps to describe the dramatic differences seen between the upper and lower cervical vertebrae, such as the independent movements that can occur in the two regions (e.g., flexion of the lower cervicals and simultaneous extension of occiput on atlas and atlas on axis).

The lack of a normal cervical lordosis is a rather frequent finding in children and adolescents under age 17, but a lack of cervical lordosis in the adult may be a sign of ligamentous injury (Fesmire & Luten, 1989) or anterior cervical muscular hypertonicity. However, some controversy exists on this topic. Some authors (G. Schultz, personal communication, June 8, 1994) consider a hypolordotic, or even kyphotic, cervical curve to be clinically insignificant, especially if a tendency toward the establishment of a lordosis can be demonstrated during extension of the cervical region. Methods used to evaluate such a tendency include palpation at the spinous processes during extension, lateral projection x-ray films taken with the patient holding the neck in extension, and cineradiography studies in which a series of x-ray films are taken while the patient moves the neck.

Typical Cervical Vertebrae

The typical cervical vertebrae are C3 through C6. These are some of the smallest but most distinct vertebrae of any vertebral region. C1 and C2 are considered to be atypical vertebrae, and C7 is unique. These three vertebrae are discussed later in this chapter.

The individual components of the typical cervical vertebrae are discussed in the following section. Special emphasis is placed on those characteristics that distinguish typical cervical vertebrae from the other spinal vertebrae.

Vertebral Bodies. Each cervical vertebra is made up of a vertebral body and a posterior arch (Fig. 5-1). The vertebral bodies of the cervical spine are rather small and are more or less rectangular in shape when viewed from above. Their transverse (side to side) diameter increases from C2 to C7. This allows the lower vertebrae to support the greater weights they are required to carry. The anterior surface of the cervical vertebral body is convex from side to side and ridged at the superior and inferior borders (discal margins) by the attachment sites of the anterior longitudinal ligaments. Indentations seen on the left and right of the anterior midline of the vertebral bodies are for attachment of the vertical fibers of the longus colli muscle.

The anterior aspects of the vertebral bodies can develop bony spurs (osteophytes). Asymptomatic osteophytes may occur in 20% to 30% of the population. Pressure on the more anteriorly located esophagus or trachea from osteophytes may rarely lead to difficulty with swallowing (dysphagia) and difficulty with speech (dysphonia) (Kissel & Youmans, 1992).

The posterior surface of the cervical vertebral body is flat and possesses two or more foramina for exit of the basivertebral veins (Williams et al., 1989). The posterior longitudinal ligament attaches to the superior and inferior margins of the posterior aspect of the cervical vertebral bodies.

The superior and inferior surfaces of the vertebral bodies are typically described as being sellar, or saddle shaped. More specifically, the superior surface is concave from left to right as a result of the raised lateral lips. The superior surface is also convex from front to back because of the beveling of the anterior surface. The inferior surface is convex from left to right and concave from anterior to posterior. Much of the concavity is created by the anterior lip of the inferior surface.

The anteroinferior aspect of each vertebral body usually protrudes inferiorly to overlap the anterior portion of the intervertebral disc (IVD) and occasionally the vertebra below. When this occurs, the anterosuperior aspect of the vertebra below is more beveled than would otherwise be the case. This increased beveling allows the vertebra to receive the projecting portion of the body above during flexion of the cervical spine.

Raised Lips at the Superior Aspect of the Vertebral Bodies and the Uncovertebral Joints. When viewed from the lateral or anterior aspect, several unique characteristics of the vertebral bodies become apparent (Fig. 5-1, *B*). Lateral lips (uncinate processes) project from the superior surface of each typical cervical vertebra. These structures arise as elevations of the lateral and posterior rims on the top surface of the vertebral bodies (Dupuis et al., 1985). The posterior components of the uncinate processes tend to become more prominent in the lower cervical vertebrae. Normally, the uncinate processes allow for flexion and extension of the cervical spine and help to limit lateral flexion. In addition, the uncinate processes serve as barriers to posterior and lateral IVD protrusion. The relationship of the left and right uncinate processes to the IVD has led at least one investigator to state that IVD herniation in the cervical region may occur less frequently than previously thought (Bland, 1989).

The uncinate processes of one vertebra may articulate with the small indentations found on the inferior surface of the vertebra above by means of small synovial joints. These joints are sometimes referred to as the uncovertebral joints (of Luschka). They consist of oblique clefts

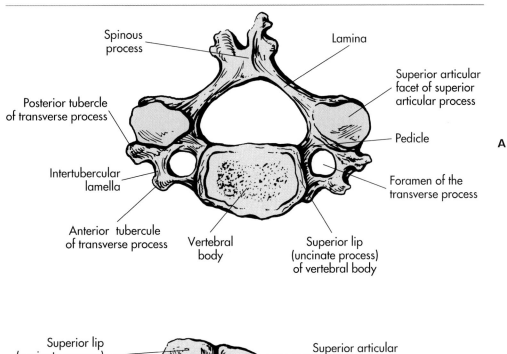

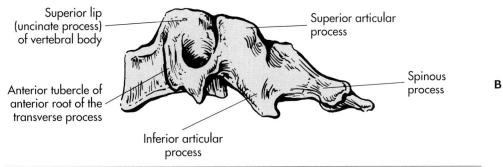

FIG. 5-1   Superior (**A**) and lateral (**B**) views of a typical cervical vertebra.

that develop at approximately 9 to 10 years of age. The clefts are limited medially by the IVD and laterally by capsular ligaments (Williams et al., 1989), the latter being derived from the annulus fibrosus of the IVD. Some investigators do not believe that the uncovertebral joints can be classified as synovial joints (Bland, 1989; Orofino, Sherman, & Schecter, 1960; Tondury, 1943), whereas others believe they do possess a synovial lining (Cave, 1955). Regardless of their true classification, the uncovertebral "joints" frequently undergo degeneration with resulting bony outgrowth, which may encroach on neighboring structures such as the vertebral artery and the exiting cervical spinal nerves (Bland, 1989).

Injury to the Vertebral Bodies.   Injury to the vertebral bodies frequently, but not always, results in swelling of the prevertebral soft tissues (Miles & Finlay, 1988). Therefore, swelling of the prevertebral tissues seen on standard x-ray films after trauma is an indication for further diagnostic studies such as computed tomography.

Pedicles.   The left and right pedicles of a typical cervical vertebra (Fig. 5-1) are quite small, project posterolaterally from the vertebral bodies, and form the medial boundary of the left and right foramina of the transverse processes, respectively. They are placed more or less midway between the superior and inferior margins of the vertebral body. Therefore the superior and inferior vertebral notches are of approximately equal size (Williams et al., 1989). The mixed spinal nerve, surrounded by a sleeve of dura, courses just above (superior to) the pedicle of each typical cervical vertebra.

The central compact bone of the cervical pedicles is continuous with that of the articular processes. This allows for transfer of loads from the vertebral body to the articular pillar (discussed later in this chapter) during flexion and from the articular pillar to the vertebral body during extension (Pal et al., 1988).

Transverse Processes.   The left and right transverse processes (TPs) of a typical cervical vertebra are each composed of two roots, or bars, one anterior and one posterior (Fig. 5-1). The two roots end laterally as tubercles (anterior and posterior). The two tubercles are joined to one another by an intertubercular lamella, which is less correctly known as a costotransverse lamella (bar) (Williams et al., 1989). The distance between the tips of the tubercles of the left and right TPs is greatest at C1, and this same distance, although smaller, remains relatively constant from C2 through C6, then increases greatly at C7.

A gutter, or groove, for the spinal nerve is formed between the anterior and posterior roots of each TP (Fig. 5-2). This groove serves as a passage for exit of the mixed spinal nerve and its largest branch, the anterior primary division (ventral ramus). The gutters for the mixed spinal nerves of C4 to C6 are the deepest. The intertubercular lamellae of C3 and C4 have a rather oblique course, descending from the anterior root and passing laterally as they reach the posterior root of the TP. Therefore the anterior tubercles (roots) of these vertebrae are shorter than the posterior ones, and the grooves for the spinal nerves are deeper posteriorly than anteriorly. The left and right intertubercular lamellae of C6 are wide (from left to right) and shallow (from superior to inferior) (Williams et al., 1989).

A dural root sleeve, which surrounds each mixed spinal nerve, and its continuation as the epineurium of the ventral ramus (anterior primary division) are held to the gutter of the TP by fibrous tissue. This strong attachment to the TP is unique to the cervical region (Sunderland, 1974). A dorsal ramus leaves each mixed spinal nerve shortly after its formation. The dorsal ramus (posterior primary division) runs posteriorly and laterally along the zygapophyseal joint (see next section), supplying the joint with sensory innervation. The ramus then passes posteriorly to supply the cervical parts of the deep back muscles with motor, nociceptive, and proprioceptive innervation and then continues posteriorly to reach the dermal and epidermal layers of the back to supply them with sensory innervation. The nerves of the cervical region are discussed in more detail later in this chapter.

The anterior aspect of the TPs of C4 to C6 end in roughened tubercles that serve as attachments for the tendons of the scalenus anterior, longus colli (superior and inferior oblique fibers), and longus capitis muscles. The posterior tubercles extend further laterally and slightly more inferiorly than their anterior counterparts (except for C6, where they are level). The splenius cervicis, longissimus cervicis, iliocostalis cervicis, levator scapulae, and scalenus medius and posterior muscles attach to the posterior tubercles.

As the name implies, the foramen of the TP is an opening within the TP. This foramen is present in the left and right TPs of all cervical vertebrae. It was previously called the foramen transversarium, but the currently preferred term is simply *foramen of the transverse process*. The boundaries of this foramen are formed by four structures: the pedicle, the anterior root of the TP, the posterior root of the TP, and the intertubercular lamella. The left and right foramina of the TPs of a single vertebra frequently are asymmetric. Occasionally the foramen of a single TP are double (Taitz et al., 1978). The vertebral artery normally enters the foramen of the TP of C6 and continues superiorly through the corresponding foramina of C5 through C1. The vertebral artery of each side loops posteriorly and then medially around the superior articular process of the atlas on the corresponding side. The artery then continues superiorly to pass through the foramen magnum. The ventral rami of the C3 to C7 spinal nerves pass posterior to the vertebral artery as they exit the gutter (groove) for the spinal nerve of the TP (Fig. 5-2).

Several vertebral veins on each side also pass through the foramina of the TPs. These veins begin in the atlanto-occipital region and continue inferiorly through the foramina of the TPs of C1 through C7 and then enter the subclavian vein. The vertebral veins receive branches from both the epidural venous plexus and the external vertebral venous plexus. In addition to the veins, a plexus of sympathetic nerves also accompanies the vertebral artery as it passes through the foramina of the TPs of C1 through C6 (see Fig. 5-19). The vertebral artery and the sympathetic plexus associated with it are discussed in more detail later in this chapter.

As mentioned in Chapter 2, the vertebrae of each region of the spine possess specific sites that are capable of developing ribs. Such regions are known as costal elements, costal processes, or pleurapophyses. The cervical region is no exception. The costal process of a typical cervical vertebra makes up the majority of its TP. In fact, all but the most medial aspect of the posterior root of the TP participates in the formation of the costal process. The costal processes may develop into cervical ribs in some individuals (Williams et al., 1989). This occurs most frequently at the level of C7. A cervical rib at C7 may be present and may compress portions of the brachial plexus and the subclavian artery. The symptom complex that results from compression of these structures is known as the thoracic outlet syndrome, and a cervical rib is one cause of this syndrome (Bland, 1987). A cervical rib may develop as a very small projection of the TP or may be a complete rib that attaches to the manubrium of the sternum or the first thoracic rib. However, the cervical rib is usually incomplete, and a bridge of fibrous tissue connects the tip of the cervical rib to either the manubrium or the first thoracic rib. The osseous extension of the cervical TP can be frequently detected on standard x-ray films, but the fibrous band is much more difficult to evaluate radiographically.

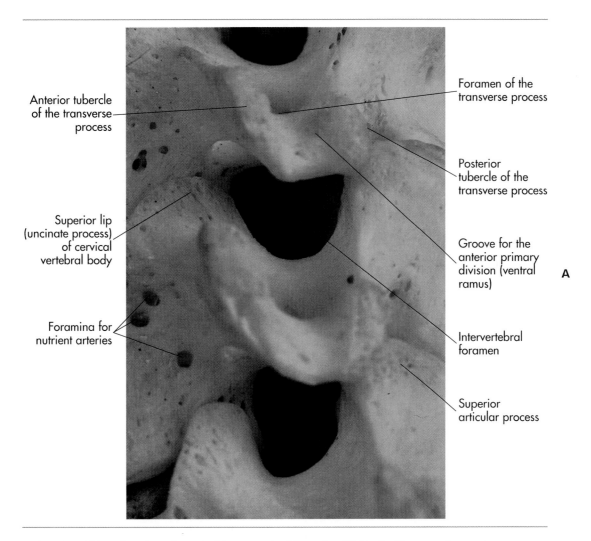

Anterior tubercle of the transverse process

Superior lip (uncinate process) of cervical vertebral body

Foramina for nutrient arteries

Foramen of the transverse process

Posterior tubercle of the transverse process

Groove for the anterior primary division (ventral ramus)

Intervertebral foramen

Superior articular process

A

FIG. 5-2 Obliquely oriented cervical intervertebral foramina (IVFs). **A,** Close-up of several cervical IVFs. Notice that the superior lip (uncinate process) of a typical cervical vertebral body helps to form the anterior border of the IVF. *Continued.*

Articular Processes and Zygapophyseal Joints. The general characteristics of the articular processes and the zygapophyseal joints (Z joints) are discussed in Chapter 2. The unique characteristics of the cervical Z joints are discussed here. The superior articular processes and their hyaline cartilage–lined facets face posteriorly, superiorly, and slightly medially (see Fig. 5-1). The cervical Z joints lie approximately 45° to the horizontal plane (Panjabi et al., 1991; White & Panjabi, 1990). More specifically, the facet joints of the upper cervical spine lie at approximately a 35° angle to the horizontal plane, and the lower cervical Z joints form a 65° angle to the horizontal plane (Oliver & Middleditch, 1991).

The appearance of the cervical Z joints changes significantly with age. Before age 20 the articular cartilage is smooth and approximately 1.0 to 1.3 mm thick, and the subarticular bone is regular in thickness. The articular cartilage thins with age, and most adult cervical

Z joints possess an extremely thin layer of cartilage with irregularly thickened subarticular cortical bone. These changes of articular cartilage and the subchondral bone usually go undetected on computed tomography (CT) and magnetic resonance imaging (MRI) scans. Osteophytes (bony spurs) projecting from the articular processes and sclerosis (thickening) of the bone within the articular processes occur quite often in adult cervical Z joints (Fletcher et al., 1990).

The articular capsules of the cervical region are quite thin (Panjabi et al., 1991) and are longer and looser than those of the thoracic and lumbar regions. The collagen fibers, which make up the capsules, run from the region immediately surrounding the articular facet of the inferior articular process of the vertebra above to the corresponding region of the superior articular process of the vertebra below (Figs. 5-3, 5-11, and 5-15). The bands of collagen fibers are approximately 9 mm long and run

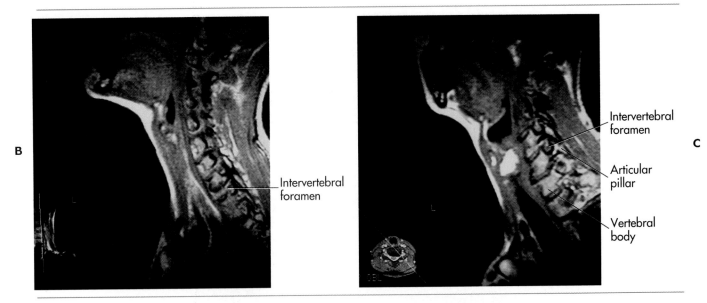

B, Intervertebral foramen

C, Intervertebral foramen / Articular pillar / Vertebral body

FIG. 5-2, cont'd.   **B,** Standard parasagittal magnetic resonance imaging (MRI) scans of the cervical region frequently show only the lower cervical IVFs. **C,** Because the cervical IVFs face anteriorly as well as laterally, MRI scans taken at a 40° to 45° angle to a sagittal plane show the cervical IVFs to better advantage. The insets of the two MRI scans show the plane in which each scan was taken.

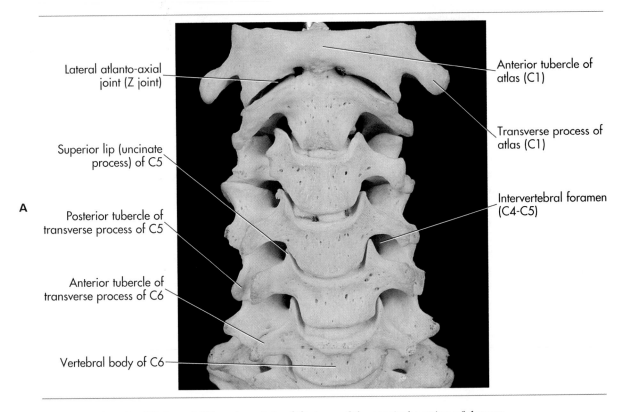

Labels: Lateral atlanto-axial joint (Z joint); Superior lip (uncinate process) of C5; Posterior tubercle of transverse process of C5; Anterior tubercle of transverse process of C6; Vertebral body of C6; Anterior tubercle of atlas (C1); Transverse process of atlas (C1); Intervertebral foramen (C4-C5)

FIG. 5-3   Anterior **(A),** lateral **(B),** and posterior **(C)** views of the cervical portion of the vertebral column. **A,** Superior lips (uncinate processes) of the C3 to C6 vertebral bodies to advantage.

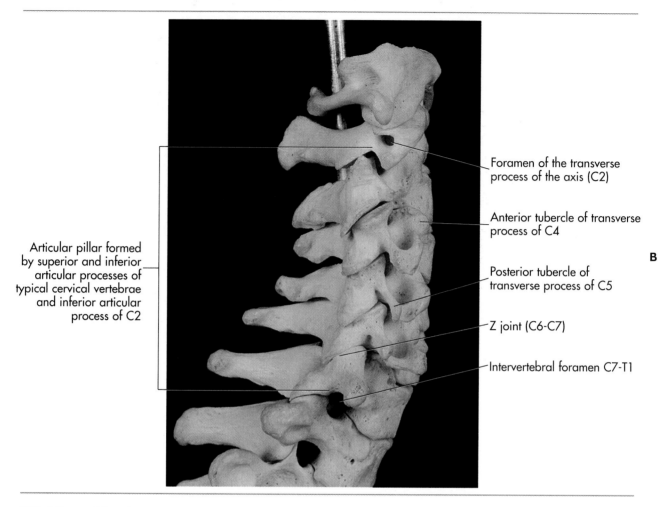

Articular pillar formed by superior and inferior articular processes of typical cervical vertebrae and inferior articular process of C2

Foramen of the transverse process of the axis (C2)

Anterior tubercle of transverse process of C4

Posterior tubercle of transverse process of C5

Z joint (C6-C7)

Intervertebral foramen C7-T1

B

FIG. 5-3, cont'd. **B,** Note the articular pillar, formed by the C3 through C6 superior and inferior articular processes. *Continued.*

perpendicular to the plane created by the Z joint (Panjabi et al., 1991).

Z joint synovial folds (menisci) project into the Z joints at all levels of the cervical spine. Yu, Sether, and Haughton (1987) found four distinct types of cervical Z joint menisci (Fig. 5-4). Type I menisci are thin and protrude far into the Z joints, covering approximately 50% of the joint surface. They are found only in children. Type II menisci are relatively large wedges that protrude a significant distance into the joint space and are found almost exclusively at the lateral C1-2 Z joints. Type III folds are rather small nubs and are found throughout the C2-3 to C6-7 cervical Z joints of most healthy adults. Type IV menisci are quite large and thick and are usually only found in degenerative Z joints. Types II and IV have been seen on MRI scans.

When the individual vertebrae are united, the articular processes of each side of the cervical spine form an articular pillar that bulges laterally at the pediculolaminar junction (Williams et al., 1989). This pillar is conspicuous on lateral x-ray films. The cervical articular pillars

(left and right) help to support the weight of the head and neck (Pal et al., 1988). Therefore, weight bearing in the cervical region is carried out by a series of three longitudinal columns: one anterior column, which runs through the vertebral bodies, and two posterior columns, which run through the right and left articular pillars (Louis, 1985; Pal et al., 1988).

Articular pillar fracture is fairly common in the cervical spine and frequently goes undetected (Renaudin & Snyder, 1978). This type of fracture is usually a chip fracture of a superior articular facet. The patient often experiences transient radicular pain (see Chapter 11), which is usually followed by mild to intense neck pain. Persistent radiculopathy in such patients indicates displacement of the fractured facet onto the dorsal root as it exits the intervertebral foramen (Czervionke et al., 1988) (Fig. 5-2).

Pain arising from pathologic conditions or dysfunction of the cervical Z joints can refer to regions quite distant from the affected joint (Bogduk, 1989b; Dwyer, Aprill, & Bogduk, 1990). The two most common types of pain

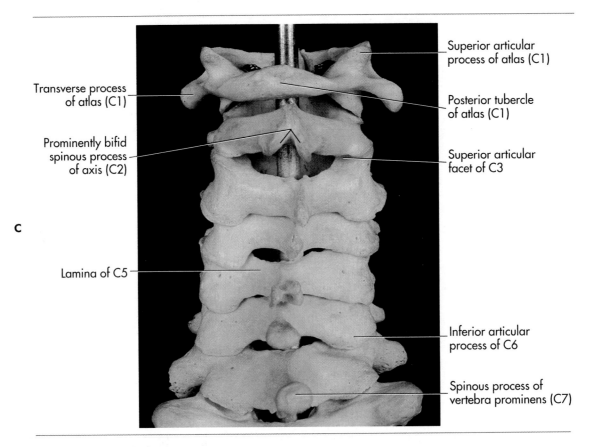

C

Transverse process of atlas (C1)

Prominently bifid spinous process of axis (C2)

Lamina of C5

Superior articular process of atlas (C1)

Posterior tubercle of atlas (C1)

Superior articular facet of C3

Inferior articular process of C6

Spinous process of vertebra prominens (C7)

FIG. 5-3, cont'd. **C,** Posterior view of the cervical portion of the vertebral column.

referral are neck pain and head pain (headache) arising from the C2-3 Z joints, and neck pain and shoulder pain arising from the C5-6 Z joints (Bogduk & Marsland, 1988).

Laminae. The laminae of the cervical region are fairly narrow from superior to inferior. Therefore, in a dried specimen, a gap can be seen between the laminae of adjacent vertebrae (Fig. 5-3, *C*). However, this gap is filled by the ligamentum flavum in the living (see Fig. 7-20). The upper border of each cervical lamina is thin, and the anterior surface of the inferior border is roughened by the attachment of the ligamentum flavum. The ligamentum flavum is discussed in detail later in this chapter.

Vertebral Canal. A vertebral foramen of a typical cervical vertebra is rather triangular (trefoil) in shape (see Fig. 5-1). It is also rather large, allowing it to accommodate the cervical enlargement of the spinal cord.

Recall that the collection of all the vertebral foramina is known as the vertebral (spinal) canal. Therefore the IVDs and ligamenta flava also participate in the formation of the vertebral canal.

The vertebral canal is fairly large in the upper cervical region but narrows from C3 to C6. In fact, the spinal cord makes up 75% of the vertebral canal at the C6 level. Table 5-1 summarizes the general characteristics of the cervical vertebral canal. A variety of pathologic conditions can compromise the spinal cord within the vertebral canal, including IVD protrusion, spinal cord tumor, posterior spondylosis of the vertebral body, Z joint hypertrophy, ossification of the posterior longitudinal ligament, buckling of a ligamentum flavum in a congenitally narrow vertebral canal, and a displaced fracture of a lamina, pedicle, or vertebral body.

The critical anteroposterior dimension of the cervical vertebral canal, before symptoms occur, is approximately 12 to 13 mm. A vertebral canal this narrow is usually the result of one of the previously mentioned pathologic conditions combined with a congenitally narrow canal. Narrowing of the vertebral canal can lead to compression of the cervical spinal cord, a condition known as cervical myelopathy. Increased bone formation (spondylosis) of the articular processes close to the Z joint or to the uncovertebral "joints" can contribute to this condition. When this is the case, the term *cervical spondylotic myelopathy* is appropriate. Cervical myelopathy usually is associated with diffuse neck pain accompanied by varying degrees of neurologic deficit (Cusick, 1988). Metrizamide myelography (injection of radiopaque dye followed by x-ray examination)

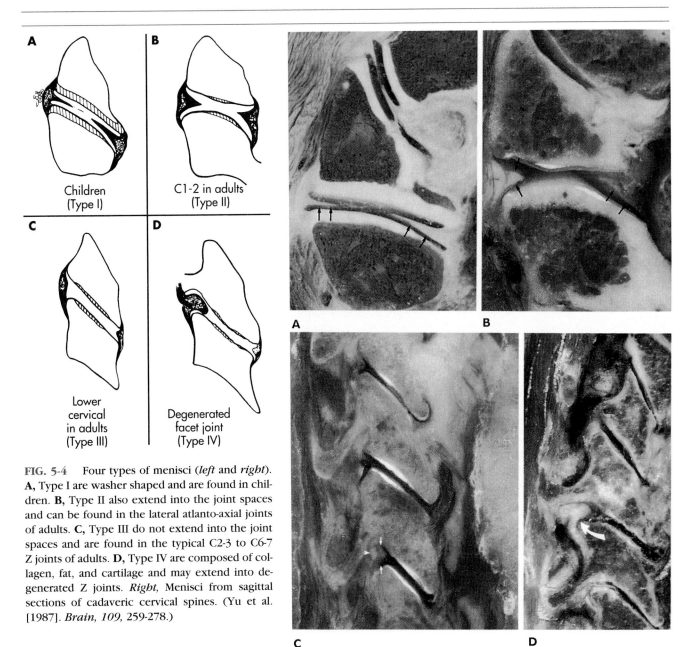

FIG. 5-4 Four types of menisci (*left* and *right*). **A,** Type I are washer shaped and are found in children. **B,** Type II also extend into the joint spaces and can be found in the lateral atlanto-axial joints of adults. **C,** Type III do not extend into the joint spaces and are found in the typical C2-3 to C6-7 Z joints of adults. **D,** Type IV are composed of collagen, fat, and cartilage and may extend into degenerated Z joints. *Right,* Menisci from sagittal sections of cadaveric cervical spines. (Yu et al. [1987]. *Brain, 109,* 259-278.)

and computer-assisted myelography (injection of dye followed by CT scanning) have been shown to be useful in the evaluation of cervical spondylotic myelopathy (Yu, Sether, & Haughton, 1987). Measurement (morphometry) of the cervical cord by means of MRI has been shown to correlate well with the severity of cord compression (Fujiwara et al., 1988).

Spinous Process. The spinous process of a typical cervical vertebra is short and bifid posteriorly. It is bifid because it develops from two separate secondary centers of ossification. This morphology is unique to cervical spinous processes. "Terminal tubercles" of unequal size allow for attachment of the ligamentum nuchae (Williams et al., 1989) and many of the deep extensors of the spine (semispinalis thoracis and cervicis, multifidi

cervicis, spinalis cervicis, and interspinalis cervicis muscles).

Cervical spinous processes, as with spinous processes throughout the spine, may deviate from the midline, making the determination of structural defects, fractures, and dislocations more challenging (Williams et al., 1989). The length of the spinous processes decreases from C2 to C4 and then increases from C4 to C7 (Panjabi et al., 1991).

Intervertebral Foramina. The left and right intervertebral foramina (IVFs) in the cervical region lie between the superior and inferior vertebral notches of adjacent cervical vertebrae (Fig. 5-2). They face obliquely anteriorly at approximately a 45° angle from the midsagittal plane. IVFs are also directed inferiorly at

Table 5-1   General Characteristics of the Cervical Vertebral Canal

Region	Dimensions
Upper cervical vertebral canal	Upper canal is infundibular in shape, wider superiorly than inferiorly; less than half the available space is occupied by the spinal cord at C1.
C4	Narrowing of the vertebral canal begins.
C6	Cord occupies 75% of the vertebral canal.
C1-C7	Critical anteroposterior dimension is 12-13 mm.

approximately a 10° angle to a horizontal plane passing through the superior vertebral end plate. The specific borders and contents of the IVF are discussed in Chapter 2. However, unique to the cervical region are the uncinate processes, which help to form the anterior border of the IVFs. The cervical IVFs, as with those of the thoracic and lumbar regions, can best be considered as neural canals since they are 4 to 6 mm in length. They are almost oval in shape. The vertical diameter of each foramen is approximately 10 mm and the anteroposterior diameter 5 mm, although these dimensions change during spinal movement (the anteroposterior diameter decreases during extension).

Approximately one fifth of the IVF in the cervical region is filled by the dorsal and ventral roots (medially) or the spinal nerve (laterally). When the spine is in the neutral position, the dorsal and ventral roots are located in the inferior portion of the IVF at or below the disc level (Pech et al., 1985). Epidural fat and blood vessels are found in the superior aspect of the IVF. The dorsal root and dorsal root ganglion are located posterior to and slightly above the ventral root. The dorsal root is also in contact with the superior articular process. The dorsal root ganglion is associated with a small notch on the anterior surface of the superior articular process. The ventral root contacts the uncinate process, and the dorsal and ventral roots are separated from each other by adipose tissue (Pech et al., 1985). This adipose-filled region between the dorsal and ventral roots has been called the interradicular foramen or cleft and can be seen on MRI (Yenerich & Haughton, 1986). Hypertrophy of the superior and inferior articular processes secondary to degeneration (osteoarthritis) of the Z joints may result in compression of the dorsal rootlets, dorsal root, or dorsal root ganglion (Bland, 1989).

Kinalski and Kostro (1971) found the area of the cervical IVFs (as recorded from plain oblique radiographs) to correlate with age and patient symptoms. Individuals 20 to 40 years of age had larger IVFs than those older than 40. Also, a smaller IVF size was found among patients with chronic neck pain.

An IVF may enlarge as a result of various pathologic conditions. The most common cause of significant pathologic enlargement of the IVF is the presence of a neurofibroma. Less frequently, enlargement may be caused by meningioma, fibroma, lipoma, herniated meningocele, a tortuous vertebral artery (Danziger & Bloch, 1975), congenital absence of the pedicle with malformation of the TP (Schimmel, Newton, & Mani, 1976), and chordoma (Wang et al., 1984).

EXTERNAL ASPECT OF THE OCCIPITAL BONE

The external surface of the occipital bone is so intimately related to the spine (direct articulation and ligamentous attachments with the atlas and ligamentous attachments with the axis) that it is included in this section on the cervical region.

The external aspect of the occipital bone consists of three different regions: squamous, left and right lateral, and basilar. These three regions are discussed separately.

Squamous Part

The squamous part of the occipital bone (occipital squama) is located posterior to the foramen magnum (Fig. 5-5). The most prominent aspect of the occipital squama is the external occipital protuberance (EOP). This mound, whose summit is known as the inion, serves as the attachment site for the medial insertion of the trapezius muscle. The external occipital crest extends inferiorly from the EOP.

The squamous part of the occipital bone also has several markings formed by muscular and ligamentous attachments. Extending laterally from the EOP are two pairs of nuchal lines. The first is only occasionally present and is known as the highest (supreme) nuchal line. The second is almost always present and is known as the superior nuchal line. The highest nuchal line, when present, extends superiorly and laterally from the EOP. It is formed by attachment of the occipital belly of the occipitofrontalis (epicranius) muscle. The superior nuchal line extends almost directly laterally from the EOP and is formed by the attachment of the trapezius and the sternocleidomastoid muscles. A third nuchal line called the inferior nuchal line extends laterally from the external occipital crest about midway between the EOP and the foramen magnum. Several muscles attach above and below the inferior nuchal line (Table 5-2), and the posterior atlanto-occipital membrane attaches to the most inferior aspect of the occipital squama, which is the posterior border of the foramen magnum.

Lateral Parts

The left and right lateral portions of the occipital bone are located to the sides of the foramen magnum. They

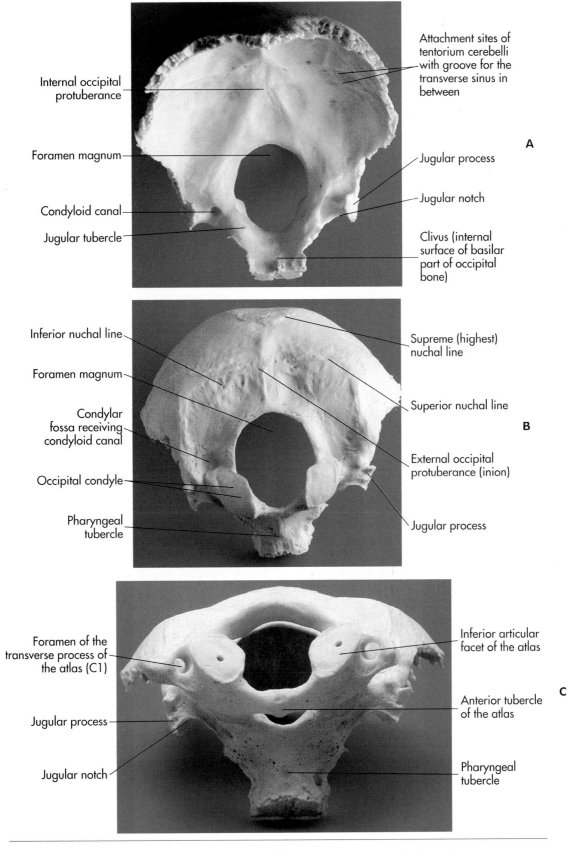

FIG. 5-5 Superior **(A)**, or internal, and inferior **(B)**, or external, views of the occiput. **C,** Atlas articulating with the occiput.

Table 5-2 Attachments to the Occiput

Region	Muscles Attached
Squamous	Trapezius
	Sternocleidomastoid
	Occipital belly of occipitofrontalis
	Splenius capitis
	Semispinalis capitis
	Obliquus capitis superior
	Rectus capitis posterior major and minor
	Posterior atlanto-occipital membrane
Lateral	Rectus capitis lateralis
Basilar	Rectus capitis anterior
	Longus capitis
	Superior constrictor
	Anterior atlanto-occipital membrane
	Apical ligament of the odontoid process
	Superior (upper) band of the cruciform ligament
	Tectorial membrane

include the left and right occipital condyles, jugular processes, and jugular notches.

The two occipital condyles are convex structures located on each side of the foramen magnum. Each condyle follows the contour of the large foramen and protrudes anteriorly and medially (Fig. 5-5). Each possesses a hyaline cartilage lined articular facet, which may be constricted in the center and occasionally is completely divided. The left and right occipital condyles fit snugly into the superior articular facets of the atlas, and the left and right atlanto-occipital articulations allow for flexion, extension, and lateral flexion of the occiput on the atlas.

The jugular notch is a groove along the lateral margin of each side of the occiput. This groove helps to form the large jugular foramen of the same side by lying in register with the jugular fossa of the temporal bone.

The jugular notch is bounded laterally by the jugular process. The jugular process is an anterior projection on the lateral aspect of each side of the occiput. Each one helps to form the posterolateral margin of the jugular foramen of the same side. The rectus capitis lateralis muscle, which helps to laterally flex the occiput on the atlas, attaches to this process.

Basilar Part

The basilar region of the occipital bone extends anteriorly from the foramen magnum. It meets the basilar portion of the sphenoid bone, and together the two basilar processes are known as the clivus.

The superior constrictor muscle of the pharynx attaches to the distinct pharyngeal tubercle, which is located in the center of the external surface of the basiocciput. The rectus capitis anterior muscle attaches just in

front of the occipital condyle, and the longus capitis muscle attaches anterior and lateral to the pharyngeal tubercle. The anterior atlanto-occipital membrane attaches just in front of the foramen magnum. The apical ligament of the odontoid process attaches to the rim of the foramen magnum, and the superior (upper) band of the cruciform ligament attaches to the inner surface of the clivus, covered posteriorly by the tectorial membrane. The transition of the spinal dura to the meningeal layer of the cranial dura occurs just posterior to the tectorial membrane.

ATYPICAL AND UNIQUE CERVICAL VERTEBRAE

The atypical cervical vertebrae are C1 and C7. C2 is unique. C6 is considered to have unique characteristics but remains typical. The distinctive features of these vertebrae are discussed in the following sections.

Atlas (First Cervical Vertebra)

The most superior atypical vertebra of the spine is the first cervical vertebra (Fig. 5-6). Given the name atlas, after the Greek god, this vertebra also functions to support a round sphere (the head). It develops from three primary centers of ossification, one in each lateral mass and one in the anterior arch. The centers located in the lateral masses are the first to appear, being formed by approximately the seventh week after conception. These centers develop posteriorly into the future posterior arch of the atlas, where they usually unite with one another by approximately the third or fourth year of life. Occasionally, these ossification centers fail to unite posteriorly, leaving a cartilaginous bridge. This cartilaginous bridge appears as a radiolucency on standard x-ray films. Such a radiolucency must be differentiated from a fracture in trauma patients.

The fully developed atlas comprises two arches (anterior and posterior) separated by two laterally placed pieces of bone known as the lateral masses. The lateral masses, in turn, have a TP projecting from their sides.

Anterior Arch. The anterior arch of the atlas develops from a bridge of tissue that connects the two lateral masses of the atlas in the embryo. This bridge is known as the hypochordal arch, and although the hypochordal arch is found throughout the spine embryologically, the anterior arch of the atlas is the only place where it persists into adulthood. The primary ossification center of the anterior arch usually appears by the end of the first year of postnatal life and fuses with the left and right lateral masses between the ages of 6 and 8 years.

The anterior arch is the smaller of the two atlantal arches (Fig. 5-6). It possesses an elevation on its anterior

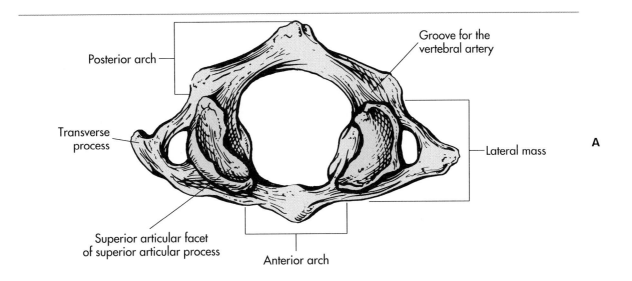

Posterior arch

Groove for the
vertebral artery

Transverse
process

Lateral mass

A

Superior articular facet
of superior articular process

Anterior arch

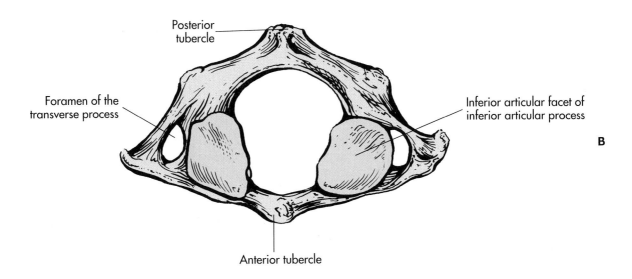

Posterior
tubercle

Foramen of the
transverse process

Inferior articular facet of
inferior articular process

B

Anterior tubercle

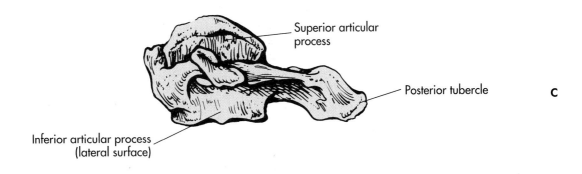

Superior articular
process

Posterior tubercle

C

Inferior articular process
(lateral surface)

FIG. 5-6 Superior **(A)**, inferior **(B)**, and lateral **(C)** views of the first cervical vertebra, the atlas.

surface known as the anterior tubercle. This tubercle serves as the attachment site for the anterior longitudinal ligament centrally and the superior oblique fibers of the longus colli muscle slightly laterally.

The posterior surface of the anterior arch (Fig. 5-6) contains a smooth articulating surface known as the facet for the dens (odontoid). This facet is covered with hyaline cartilage and articulates with the anterior surface of the odontoid process as a diarthrodial joint. Since the atlas has no vertebral body, the odontoid process of the axis occupies the region homologous to the body of the atlas. Therefore the atlas is oval in shape and can easily pivot around the odontoid process at the diarthrodial joint between this process and the anterior arch of C1.

Posterior Arch. The posterior arch is larger than the anterior arch and forms approximately two thirds of the ring of the atlas. The larger posterior arch contains an elevation on its posterior surface known as the posterior tubercle. This tubercle may be palpated in some individuals. It serves centrally as an attachment site for the ligamentum nuchae (Williams et al., 1989) and also as the origin for the rectus capitis posterior minor muscle.

The first left and right ligamenta flava attach to the lower border of the posterior arch of the atlas. The ligamenta flava are discussed in more detail later in this chapter. The lateral aspects of the superior surface posterior arch are extremely thin and "dug out." These dug-out regions are known as the left and right grooves for the vertebral arteries. Each groove allows passage of the vertebral artery, vertebral veins, and the suboccipital nerve of the same side. The suboccipital nerve is the dorsal ramus of C1 and is located between the vertebral artery and the posterior arch. The groove for the vertebral artery has been found to be covered by bone in approximately 32% to 37% of subjects studied (Taitz & Nathan, 1986; Williams et al., 1989). This results in the formation of a foramen, sometimes referred to as the arcuate or arcuale foramen. Each vertebral artery forms its respective groove as it courses around the superior articular process and comes to lie on top of the posterior arch. The posterior atlanto-occipital membrane attaches to each side of the groove, and it is the lateral edge of this membrane that may ossify to create an arcuate foramen (see Fig. 5-10). When ossification occurs, the bone bridge that is created is known as a posterior ponticle. A study of 672 atlas vertebrae found that 25.9% had a partial posterior ponticle and 7.9% had a complete posterior ponticle (Taitz & Nathan, 1986). Interestingly, these authors reported that a much higher number of atlases (57%) from a Middle Eastern population showed partial or complete ponticle formation, possibly because this population customarily carried heavy loads on their heads. However, these authors stated that further study

is necessary to determine with certainty the cause of the high incidence of posterior ponticles in this population.

Occasionally a bone bridge for the vertebral artery develops laterally between the superior articular process of the atlas and the TP. Such a process is known as a lateral ponticle (ponticulus lateralis) (Buna et al., 1984). Taitz and Nathan (1986) found such a ponticle in 3.8% of the atlases they studied. Regardless of whether the ponticle is posteriorly or laterally placed, they are usually more than 12 mm in length and are usually thicker than 1 mm. Some controversy surrounds whether posterior and lateral ponticles are congenital or are a part of the aging process. Taitz and Nathan (1986) found that partial ponticles were predominant in the specimens of 10 to 30-year-old individuals, and complete posterior ponticles were usually found in specimens from individuals 30 to 80 years of age. This would indicate that posterior ponticles are created by ossification of the lateral-most portion of the posterior atlanto-occipital membrane as some people age. Even though these ponticles have been implicated in some cases of vertebrobasilar arterial insufficiency (Buna et al., 1984), their clinical significance remains a matter of debate.

Lateral Masses. Located between the anterior and posterior arches are the left and right lateral masses. Each mass consists of a superior articular process and an inferior articular process and is oriented so that the anterior aspect is more medially positioned than the posterior aspect. The medial surface of each lateral mass has a small tubercle for attachment of the transverse atlantal ligament. The anterior aspect of each lateral mass serves as origin for the rectus capitis anterior muscle.

The superior articular process of each lateral mass is irregular in shape. In fact, the hyaline-lined superior articular facet has the appearance of a peanut. That is, it is narrow centrally and may occasionally be completely divided into two (Williams et al., 1989). The superior articular process is quite concave superiorly and faces slightly medially to accommodate the convex occipital condyle of the corresponding side. The joint between the occiput and the atlas is categorized as a condyloid, diarthrodial joint, although some authors describe it as being ellipsoidal in type because of its shape (Williams et al., 1989). The primary motion at this joint is anteroposterior rocking (flexion and extension). In addition, a small amount of lateral flexion occurs at this articulation.

The inferior articular process of each lateral mass of the atlas presents as a regularly shaped oval. In fact, in many cases it is almost circular. This process is flat or slightly concave (Williams et al., 1989) and faces slightly medially. Hyaline cartilage lines the slightly smaller inferior articular facet of the articular process, which articulates with the superior articular facet of C2. A loose articular capsule attaches to the rim of the corresponding articular facets, surrounding the lateral C1-2 joint. This loose capsule allows for 45° of unilateral rotation to occur at each atlanto-occipital joint. This joint is categorized as a planar diarthrodial articulation (typical joint type for Z joints).

The large vertebral foramen of C1 usually has a greater anteroposterior diameter than transverse diameter (Le Minor, Kahn, & Di Paola, 1989). The anteroposterior dimensions of the C1 vertebral foramen can be divided into thirds, with one third filled with the odontoid process of C2, one third filled with the spinal cord and one third being "free space." The free space is actually filled with epidural adipose tissue, vessels, ligaments, the meninges, and the subarachnoid space. This division of the vertebral foramen of the atlas into three parts is sometimes known as Steele's rule of thirds (Foreman & Croft, 1992).

Transverse Processes. The left and right TPs of the atlas are quite large and may be palpated between the mastoid process and the angle of the mandible. Each projects laterally from the lateral mass and acts as a lever by which the muscles that attach to it may rotate the head. Because of the large size of the TPs, the atlas is wider than all the cervical vertebrae, except for C7. The width ranges from approximately 65 to 76 mm in females and 74 to 90 mm in males (Williams et al., 1989). Although they are composed of only a single lateral process (rather than having anterior and posterior tubercles, as is the case with typical cervical vertebrae), the atlantal transverse processes are almost completely homologous to the posterior roots, or bars, of the other cervical vertebrae. In fact, the TP of the atlas can be considered to be composed of a posterior root and a small portion of the intertubercular lamella (Williams et al., 1989). A foramen for the vertebral artery, which also provides passage for the vertebral veins and the vertebral artery sympathetic nerve plexus, is also found within each transverse process. This foramen of the TP of C1 is the largest of the cervical spine (Taitz et al., 1978).

In addition to its relationship with the vertebral vessels, each TP of the atlas is also the site of muscle attachments. These muscles include the rectus capitis lateralis, obliquus capitis superior, obliquus capitis inferior, levator scapulae, splenius cervicis, and scalenus medius muscles. Each TP is also related to the C1 spinal nerve. Although the dorsal ramus of this spinal nerve (the suboccipital nerve) provides motor innervation to the suboccipital muscles, the ventral ramus passes laterally around the lateral mass, remaining medial to the vertebral artery and the rectus capitis lateralis muscle. It courses between the rectus capitis lateralis and anterior muscles and then descends anterior to the atlas and is joined by the ascending branch of the ventral

ramus of C2. The nerves of the cervical region are discussed in more detail later in this chapter.

Axis (Second Cervical Vertebra)

The second cervical vertebra, the axis or epistropheus, is also atypical. This vertebra develops from five primary and two secondary centers of ossification (Williams et al., 1989). The primary centers are distributed as follows: one in the vertebral body, two in the neural arch (one on each side), and two in the dens (odontoid process, see the following section). One secondary center of ossification is associated with the odontoid process and another is associated with the inferior aspect of the vertebral body.

The major distinguishing features of the axis are the prominent odontoid process, the superior articular processes, and the transverse processes (Fig. 5-7). In addition, the vertebral foramen of C2 is very large. These distinguishing features are discussed in the following sections.

Dens (Odontoid Process). Also known as the odontoid process, the dens develops from two laterally placed primary centers of ossification and an apical secondary center of ossification. The two primary centers appear in utero and usually fuse in the midline by the seventh fetal month (Fesmire & Luten, 1989). The united primary ossification centers then normally fuse along their inferior outer rim to the vertebral body of C2 by approximately age 3 to 6 years. The fusion line between the odontoid and the body of C2 is usually visible on x-ray film until about age 11, and one third of individuals retain the line of fusion throughout life. This line is frequently confused with a fracture (Fesmire & Luten, 1989). Inside the rim of attachment between the dens and the body of C2 a small disc is present, which persists until late in life. This disc can frequently be seen on sagittal MRI scans. This area of fusion between the odontoid and the body of C2 is known as the subdental synchondrosis. Rarely, the odontoid does not fuse with the body of C2 or it may be united by only a rim of cartilage. Therefore its appearance on x-ray film is that of a free and unattached odontoid. This unfused odontoid is known as an os odontoideum.

The apical secondary center of ossification first appears at 3 to 6 years of age. It is V or cuneiform in shape, forming a deep cleft between the primary centers of ossification. This secondary center unites with the remainder of the odontoid process usually by age 12. When seen on x-ray film before fusion occurs or if fusion does not occur, the small bone fragment is known as an ossiculum terminale and can also be difficult to distinguish from a fracture.

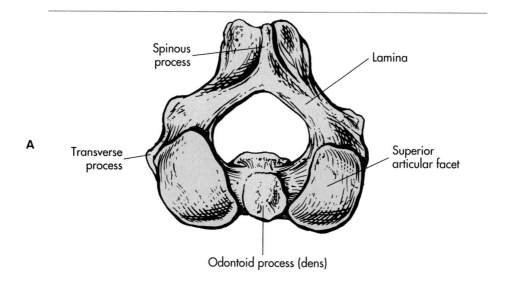

A

Spinous process

Lamina

Transverse process

Superior articular facet

Odontoid process (dens)

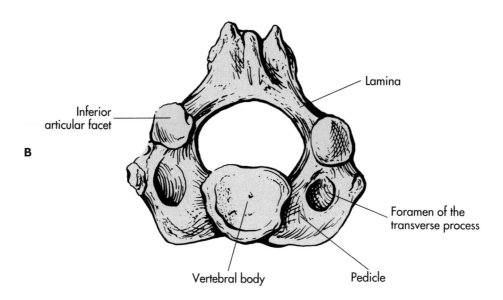

B

Inferior articular facet

Lamina

Vertebral body

Foramen of the transverse process

Pedicle

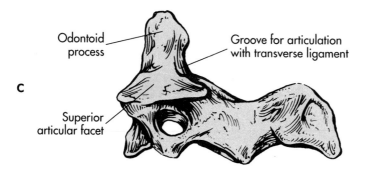

C

Odontoid process

Groove for articulation with transverse ligament

Superior articular facet

FIG. 5-7   Superior **(A)**, inferior **(B)**, and lateral **(C)** views of the second cervical vertebra, the axis.

The fully developed odontoid process (dens) is peg shaped with a curved superior surface. It is approximately 1.5 cm in height (Williams et al., 1989). The dens has a hyaline-lined articular facet on its anterior surface. This facet articulates with the corresponding facet on the posterior surface of the anterior arch of the atlas. The posterior surface of the dens has a groove at its base formed by the transverse atlantal ligament (transverse portion of the cruciform ligament). The transverse ligament forms a synovial joint with the groove on the posterior surface of the dens. Together the complex of anterior and posterior joints between the atlas, odontoid, and transverse ligament is classified as a trochoid (pivot) diarthrodial joint. This joint allows the atlas to rotate on the axis through approximately 45° of motion in each direction (left and right). The sides of the odontoid process above the groove formed by the transverse ligament are flat and serve as attachment sites for the left and right alar ligaments. The apical odontoid ligament attaches to the top of the odontoid process. The ligaments of the cervical spine are discussed later in this chapter.

The body of C2 contains less compact bone than the dens (Williams et al., 1989). The anterior surface of the body is hollowed out because of the attachment of the longus colli muscle. As occurs throughout the cervical spine, the anterior longitudinal ligament attaches to the inferior border of the vertebral body of C2 in close association with the attachment of the anterior fibers of the anulus fibrosus. Another similarity of the inferior, or discal border of C2 with the same border of the other cervical vertebrae is that its anterior aspect projects inferiorly. The posterior aspect of the vertebral body serves as an important attachment for the posterior longitudinal ligament and its superior continuation as the tectorial membrane. Specifically, these structures attach to the posterior and inferior borders of the vertebral body. Also associated with the vertebral body is the first IVD of the spine, which is found between the inferior surface of the vertebral body of C2 and the superior surface of the vertebral body of C3.

Pedicles. The pedicles of the axis are thick from anterior to posterior and from superior to inferior (Fig. 5-7, *B*). The inferior vertebral notch is large, whereas the superior vertebral notch is almost nonexistent.

Superior Articular Processes. The superior articular processes of the axis can be thought of as smoothed out regions of the left and right pedicles of C2. That is, the superior articular processes do not project superiorly from the pediculolaminar junction, as occurs with the typical cervical vertebrae. Instead, they lie almost flush with the pedicle (Fig. 5-7). This configuration, along with the very loose articular capsule at this level, allows for much axial rotation (approximately

45° unilaterally) to occur between C1 and C2. The articular cartilage of the superior articular process of C2 is convex superiorly, with a transverse ridge running from medial to lateral along the central region of the process. This ridge allows the anterior and posterior aspects of the facet to slope inferiorly, aiding in more effective rotation between C1 and C2 (Koebke & Brade, 1982) (see Atlanto-Axial Articulations). The articulation between the superior articular facet of C2 with the inferior articular facet of C1 is located anterior to the rest of the Z joints of the cervical spine. Therefore the superior articular processes of C2 and the inferior articular processes of C1 are not a part of the articular pillars, as is the case with the lower cervical spine's articular processes.

Laminae. The laminae of C2 are taller and thicker than those found in the rest of the cervical vertebrae. Because of the distinct architecture of the axis, the forces applied to it from above (by carrying the head) are transmitted from the superior articular processes to both the inferior articular processes and the vertebral body via the pedicle. Because the superior and inferior facets of the axis are arranged in different planes, the forces transmitted to the inferior articular processes are, by necessity, transferred through the laminae. This is accomplished by a rather complex arrangement of bony trabeculae (Pal et al., 1988). The laminae of the axis are therefore quite strong compared with the laminae of the rest of the cervical vertebrae.

Transverse Processes. The TPs of C2 are quite small and, like the TPs of C1 but unlike those of the rest of the cervical spine, do *not* possess distinct anterior and posterior tubercles. Developmentally, they are considered to be homologues of the posterior roots, or bars, of the TPs, although minute homologues of the anterior tubercles are associated with the junction of the anterior aspect of the TPs with the vertebral body of C2.

The small left and right transverse processes of C2 face obliquely superiorly and laterally. Each has a foramen of the TP that, at C2, is an angular canal with two openings, one inferior and one lateral (Taitz et al., 1978). Therefore the vertebral artery courses laterally from the foramen of the TP of C2 to proceed to the more lateral foramen of the TP of C1.

Even though they are very small, the TPs of the axis serve as attachment sites for many muscles. Table 5-3 lists the muscles that attach to the transverse and spinous processes of C2.

Spinous Process and Inferior Articular Processes. The spinous process of C2 is more prominently bifid than the other spinous processes of the cervical vertebrae because of the many muscles attaching to it (Table 5-3). The inferior articular processes of C2 are typical for the cervical region. They arise from the junction of the pedicle and lamina and face anteriorly, inferiorly, and laterally.

Vertebra Prominens (Seventh Cervical Vertebra)

Spinous Process. The seventh cervical vertebra is known as the vertebra prominens because of its very prominent spinous process (Fig. 5-8). The spinous process of C7 is the most prominent of the cervical region, although occasionally C6 is more prominent (C6 is the last cervical vertebra with palpable movement in flexion and extension). Also, the spinous process of T1 may be more prominent than that of C7 in some individuals. The spinous process of C7 usually projects directly posteriorly. Unlike typical cervical vertebrae, the spinous process of C7 is not bifid. The funicular portion of the ligamentum nuchae attaches to the single posterior tip of the spinous process of C7. This ligament is discussed in more detail later in this chapter.

Because of its large spinous process and its location at the base of the neck, C7 serves as an attachment site for many muscles. Table 5-4 lists the muscular attachments of C7.

Transverse Processes. The TPs of C7 are also unique. The anterior tubercle of each TP of C7 is small and short. The posterior tubercle is quite large, making the entire TP large. The anterior tubercle is the costal element of C7. The anterior tubercle is unique because it develops from an independent primary center of ossification. This center usually unites with the TP by the fifth or sixth year of life. However, it may remain distinct and develop into a cervical rib. The formation of a cervical rib may also occur at C4 to C6 by the same mechanism, although this is less common. The intertubercular lamella is usually grooved by the ventral ramus of C7 anterior and lateral to the foramen of the TP (Williams

Table 5-3 Muscular Attachments to the Axis

Region	Muscles Attached
Transverse processes	Levator scapula
	Scalenus medius
	Splenius cervicis
	Intertransversarii (to upper and lower surfaces)
Spinous process	Obliquus capitis inferior
	Rectus capitis posterior major
Notch of spinous process	Semispinalis cervicis
	Spinalis cervicis
	Interspinalis cervicis
	Multifidus (also ligamentum nuchae, when present)

Table 5-4 Muscular Attachments of C7

Region	Muscles Attached
Spinous process	Trapezius
	Rhomboid minor
	Serratus posterior superior
	Splenius capitis
	Spinalis cervicis
	Semispinalis thoracis
	Multifidus thoracis
	Interspinales
Transverse process	Middle scalene
	Levator costarum (1st pair) (also the suprapleural membrane [cupola])

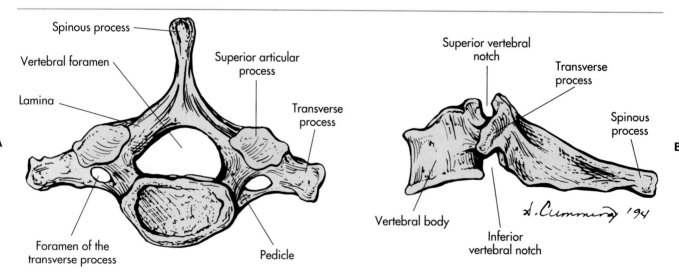

FIG. 5-8 Superior **(A)** and lateral **(B)** views of the seventh cervical vertebra, the vertebra prominens.

et al., 1989). The suprapleural membrane, or cupola, which is the protective layer of connective tissue that reinforces the apical pleura of each lung, is attached to the posterior tubercle of the C7 TP.

Similar to the rest of the cervical region, the left and right C7 TPs contain a foramen. This foramen is usually the smallest of the cervical spine. Occasionally a double foramen is found in one of the TPs of C7 (Taitz et al., 1978). Frequently, branches of the stellate ganglion run through the foramen of the TP of C7, although normally the only structures that course through this opening are accessory arteries and veins (Jovanovic, 1990). The accessory vessels comprise branches of the deep or ascending cervical arteries and their accompanying veins. The remainder of the C7 TP foramen is filled with areolar connective tissue. Recall that the vertebral artery and its associated sympathetic plexus run with the vertebral veins through the C6 TP foramen and the more superior vertebrae. Approximately 5% of the time, the vertebral artery and vein(s) traverse the foramen of the C7 TP (Jovanovic, 1990).

Carotid Tubercles (Sixth Cervical Vertebra)

Although the C6 vertebra is considered typical, its left and right anterior tubercles of the TPs are unique. These tubercles are very prominent and are known as the carotid tubercles. This is because each is so closely related to the overlying common carotid artery of the corresponding side. The common carotid artery may be compressed in the groove between the carotid tubercle and the vertebral body of C6 (Wiliams et al., 1989).

ARTICULATIONS OF THE UPPER CERVICAL REGION

The Z joints of the cervical region are covered earlier in this chapter. The atlanto-occipital and atlanto-axial joints are discussed here.

The articulations (joints) of the upper cervical spine are extremely important. These joints allow much of the flexion and extension that occurs in the cervical region and at least one half of the axial (left and right) rotation of the cervical spine. In addition, the proprioceptive input from the atlanto-occipital and atlanto-axial joints, as well as proprioception from the suboccipital muscles, is responsible for the control of head posture (Panjabi et al., 1991).

Left and Right Atlanto-Occipital Articulations

The joints between the left and right superior articular surfaces of the atlas and the corresponding occipital condyles have been described as ellipsoidal (Williams et al., 1989) and condylar (Gates, 1980) in shape and type.

The superior articular processes of the atlas are concave superiorly and face medially (Fig. 5-6). Recall that the facets are narrow in their center, resulting in their peanut shape. The occiput and the atlas are connected by articular capsules and the anterior and posterior atlanto-occipital membranes (Figs. 5-10 and 5-14). The fibrous capsules surround the occipital condyles and the superior articular facets of the atlas. These capsules are thickest posterolaterally. Each capsule is further reinforced in the posterolateral region by a ligamentous band that passes between the jugular processes of the occiput and the lateral mass of the atlas. This band has been referred to as the lateral atlanto-occipital ligament (Oliver & Middleditch, 1991). The atlanto-occipital joint capsules are thin and sometimes completely nonexistent medially. When present, this medial deficiency frequently allows the synovial cavity of the atlanto-occipital joint to connect with the bursa or joint cavity between the dens and the transverse atlantal ligament (Cave, 1934; Williams et al., 1989).

Atlanto-Axial Articulations. The atlas and axis articulate with one another at three synovial joints: two lateral joints and a single median joint complex (Fig. 5-9, *B*).

Lateral atlanto-axial joints. The lateral atlanto-axial joints are planar joints that are oval in shape. The atlantal surfaces are concave, and the axial surfaces are convex. The fibrous capsule of each lateral joint is thin and loose and attaches to the outermost rim of the articular margins of the atlas and axis (inferior and superior articular facets of the axis). Each capsule is lined by a synovial membrane. A posteromedial accessory ligament attaches inferiorly to the body of the axis near the base of the dens and courses superiorly to the lateral mass of the atlas near the attachment site of the transverse ligament. This ligament is known as the accessory atlanto-axial ligament (see Ligaments of the Cervical Region).

Median atlanto-axial joint. The median atlanto-axial joint is a pivot (or trochoid) joint between the dens and a ring of structures that encircles the dens. These structures are the anterior arch of the atlas anteriorly and the transverse ligament posteriorly. The joint possesses two synovial cavities, one anterior and one posterior, which act together to allow movement. The facet on the anterior surface of the dens articulates with the posterior aspect of the anterior arch of the atlas. This articulation has a weak, loose capsule lined by a synovial membrane. The posterior joint cavity is the larger of the two. It is frequently described as a synovial cavity, although sometimes as a bursa. In either case it is located between the anterior surface of the transverse ligament and the posterior grooved surface of the odontoid process. This

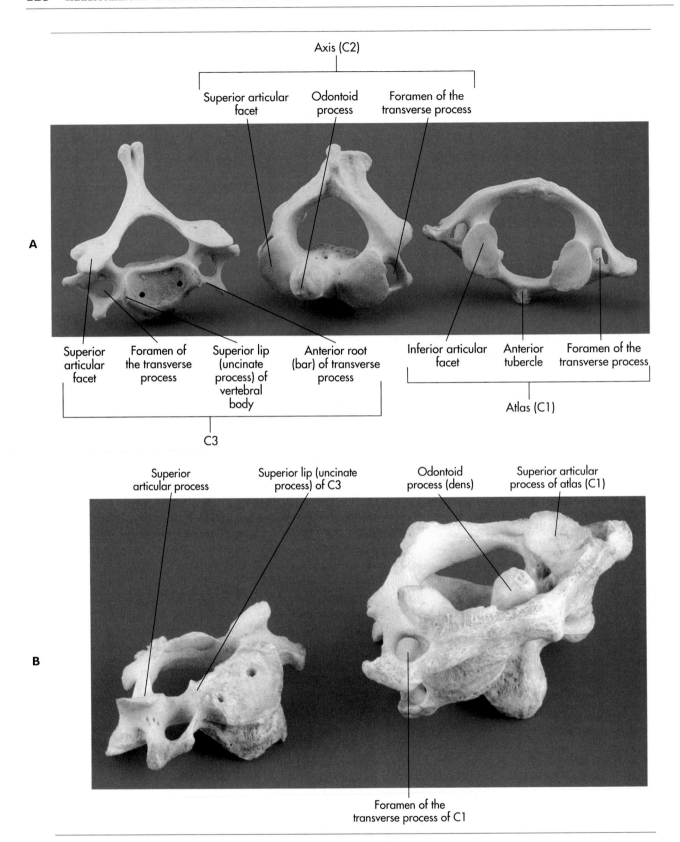

FIG. 5-9 **A,** Inferior view of the atlas and a superior view of the axis and third cervical vertebra. **B,** Atlas and axis in typical anatomic relationship, with C3 to the side.

posterior joint is often continuous with one of the atlanto-occipital joints (Williams et al., 1989).

CLINICAL APPLICATIONS

Children frequently have increased ligamentous laxity, which leads to increased spinal motion. This occurs most often in the cervical region. Increased motion seen during physical or x-ray examination should be differentiated from pathologic subluxation (Fesmire & Luten, 1989). For example, the space between the anterior arch of the atlas and the odontoid process, known as the predental space, usually should not exceed 3 mm. A predental space greater than 3 mm is generally considered to indicate a tear of the transverse ligament (see later discussion) or pathologic subluxation of C1 on C2. However, a 3 mm or greater predental space has been found in 20% of normal patients less than 8 years of age (Fesmire & Luten, 1989). Although a space of greater than 3.5 mm is usually considered abnormal in children, spaces of up to 5 mm have been seen in normal children (Fesmire & Luten, 1989). Therefore, x-ray evaluation of atlanto-axial stability in children should be tempered with sound clinical judgment.

Pathologic subluxation of the atlas on the axis resulting in compromise of the spinal cord (compressive myelopathy) has been frequently associated with rheumatoid arthritis (Kaufman & Glenn, 1983) and less frequently with ankylosing spondylitis. Displacement of the atlas on the axis has also been found in 9% of Down syndrome patients ages 5 to 21. In addition, significant degeneration of the entire cervical spine with osteophyte formation, narrowing of foramina, and narrowing of the disc space has been found with increasing incidence in the adult Down syndrome population. The premature aging process that occurs in individuals with this syndrome may be one possible explanation for this latter finding (Van Dyke & Gahagan, 1988).

LIGAMENTS OF THE CERVICAL REGION

The ligaments of the cervical region can be divided into upper and lower cervical ligaments. The upper ligaments are those associated with the occiput, atlas, and the anterior and lateral aspect of the axis. The lower cervical ligaments encompass all other ligaments of the cervical region. The ligaments of both categories are discussed in the following sections. The points of insertion and the function of each are discussed, beginning with those located most posteriorly and progressing to those located most anteriorly.

Upper Cervical Ligaments

Posterior Atlanto-Occipital Membrane. The posterior atlanto-occipital membrane is a rather thin structure that attaches to the posterior arch of the atlas and the posterior rim of the foramen magnum (Fig. 5-10). The

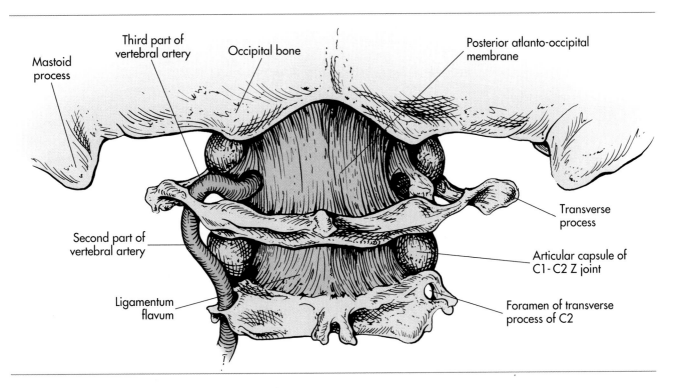

FIG. 5-10 Posterior ligaments of the upper cervical region.

posterior atlanto-occipital membrane functions to limit flexion of the occiput on the atlas. The ligament is so broad from left to right that the term *membrane* applies. It spans the distance between the left and right lateral masses. Laterally this ligament arches over the left and right grooves for the vertebral artery on the posterior arch of the atlas (Fig. 5-10). This allows for passage of the vertebral artery, vertebral veins, and the suboccipital nerve. These structures are covered in more detail later in this chapter. This lateral arch of the posterior atlanto-occipital membrane occasionally ossifies, creating a foramen for the previously mentioned structures. (See previous section on the atlas for elaboration on the arcuate, or arcuale, foramen created by the ossified posterior atlanto-occipital membrane.)

Tectorial Membrane. The tectorial membrane is the superior extension of the posterior longitudinal ligament (Fig. 5-11). It begins by attaching to the posterior aspect of the vertebral body of C2. It then crosses over the odontoid process and inserts onto the anterior rim of the foramen magnum (specifically, the upper region of the basilar part of the occipital bone). The tectorial membrane has superficial and deep fibers. The deep fibers have a median band that extends all the way to the basilar portion of the occipital bone. Two lateral bands of deep fibers pass medial to the atlanto-occipital joints before attaching to the occiput. The superficial fibers extend even more superiorly than the deep fibers and blend with the cranial dura mater at the upper region of the basilar part of the occipital bone. This ligament limits both flexion and extension of the atlas and occiput (Williams et al., 1989).

Accessory Atlanto-Axial Ligaments. Each of the accessory atlanto-axial ligaments (left and right) course from the base of the odontoid process to the inferomedial surface of the lateral mass of the atlas on the same side (Figs. 5-11 and 5-12). They help to strengthen the posteromedial aspect of the capsule of the lateral atlanto-axial joints. They are considered to be deep fibers of the tectorial membrane.

Cruciform Ligament. The cruciform ligament is named such because of its cross shape. It may actually be divided into several parts: a large transverse ligament, a

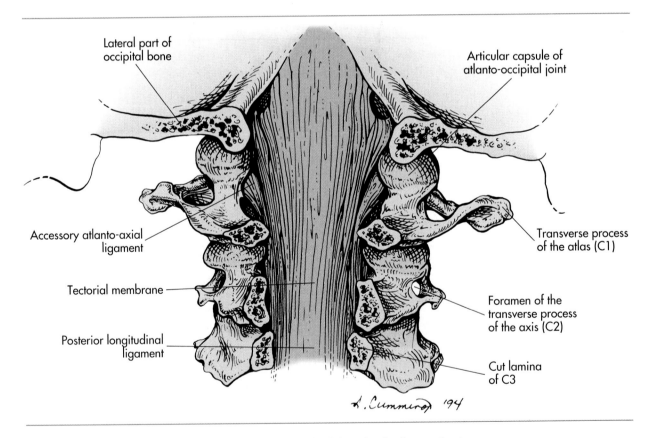

FIG. 5-11 Posterior aspect of the occiput, posterior arch of the atlas, laminae and spinous processes of C2 and C3, neural elements, and meninges have all been removed to show the ligaments covering the anterior aspect of the upper cervical vertebral canal and foramen magnum.

superior band, and an inferior band (Fig. 5-12). Each portion is discussed next.

Transverse ligament. The transverse ligament has been called the most important ligament of the occiput–C1-2 complex of joints (White & Panjabi, 1990). It is a strong ligament that runs from a small medial tubercle of one lateral mass of the atlas to a similar tubercle on the opposite side. The transverse ligament lies in the horizontal plane. However, approximately a 21° angle with the frontal (coronal) plane is created from the origin of the transverse ligament to the region where it passes behind the odontoid process (Panjabi, Oxland, & Parks, 1991a). The superoinferior width of this ligament is greatest at its center, where it passes posterior to the odontoid process. Anteriorly, the transverse ligament is lined by a thin layer of cartilage (Williams et al., 1989). This enables it to form a diarthrodial joint with the odontoid as it passes posterior to this structure.

The transverse ligament allows the atlas to pivot on the axis. It also holds the atlas in its proper position, thereby preventing compression of the spinal cord during flexion of the head and neck. Because the transverse

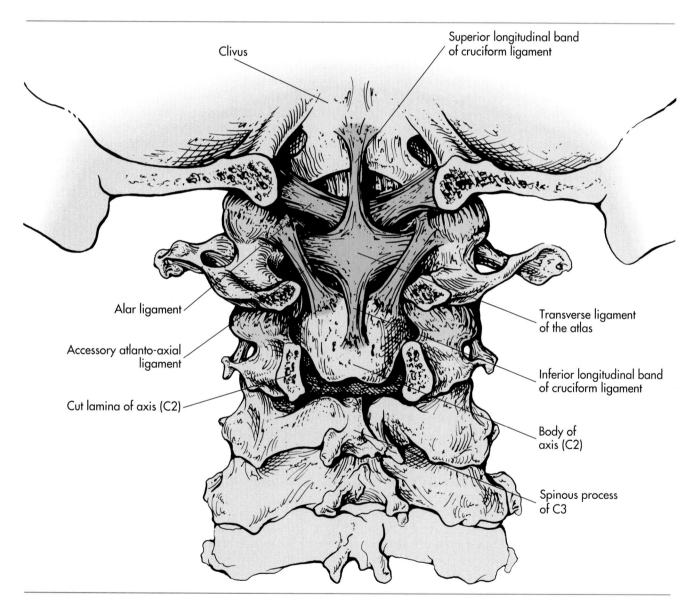

FIG. 5-12 Anterior aspect of the vertebral canal and foramen magnum as seen from behind. The tectorial membrane has been removed, and many of the upper cervical ligaments can be seen. Notice the centrally located cruciform ligament with its narrow superior and inferior longitudinal bands and its stout transverse ligament. The alar and accessory atlanto-axial ligaments can also be seen.

ligament fits into the groove on the posterior surface of the odontoid, it holds the atlas in proper position even when all other ligaments are severed (Williams et al., 1989). Panjabi and colleagues (1991a) found that this ligament appears to exist in two distinct layers, superficial and deep.

Superior longitudinal band. The superior longitudinal band of the cruciform ligament runs from the transverse ligament to the anterior lip of the foramen magnum (Fig. 5-12). More specifically it attaches to the superior aspect of the basilar part of the occipital bone. It is interposed between the apical ligament of the odontoid process, which is anterior to it, and the tectorial membrane, which is posterior to it. Although it may limit both flexion and extension of the occiput, its primary function may be to hold the transverse ligament in its proper position, thus aiding the transverse ligament in holding the atlas against the odontoid process.

Inferior longitudinal band. The inferior longitudinal band of the cruciform ligament attaches the transverse ligament to the body of C2, preventing the transverse ligament from riding too far superiorly (Fig. 5-12). It also helps to limit (with the aid of the superior band and the transverse ligament) flexion of the occiput and atlas on the axis.

Alar Ligaments. The left and right alar ligaments originate from the posterior and lateral aspect of the odontoid process with some of the fibers covering the entire posterior surface of the dens (Panjabi et al., 1991a). Each alar ligament passes anteriorly and superiorly to insert onto a roughened region of the medial surface of the occipital condyle of the same side (Figs. 5-12 and 5-13). The alar ligaments are about the width of a pencil and are very strong.

The functions of the alar ligaments are rather complex and are not completely understood. However, each alar ligament limits contralateral axial rotation (Dvorak & Panjabi, 1987). For example, the left alar ligament primarily limits right rotation. More specifically, the fibers of the left alar ligament, which attach to the odontoid process posterior to the axis of movement, act in concert with those fibers of the right alar ligament, which attach to the odontoid in front of the axis of movement. Both of these segments of the alar ligaments act together to limit right axial rotation. The opposite is also true: right posterior odontal fibers and left anterior odontal fibers limit left rotation (Williams et al., 1989). Because the alar ligaments limit or check rotation, they are also known as the check ligaments.

The alar ligaments also limit flexion of the upper cervical spine after the tectorial membrane and cruciform ligaments have torn. The alar ligaments are themselves most vulnerable to tearing during the combined

movements of axial rotation and flexion. This combination of movements may occur during a motor vehicle accident (hit from the front while looking in the rearview mirror) (Foreman & Croft, 1992). Injury as a result of this same pair of movements can also irreparably stretch the alar ligaments while sparing the cruciform ligament. When an alar ligament is torn or stretched, increased rotation occurs at the occipito-atlantal and atlanto-axial joint complexes, and increased lateral displacement occurs between the atlas and the axis during lateral flexion (Dvorak & Panjabi, 1987).

Dvorak and Panjabi (1987) found that in addition to attaching to the occipital condyle of the same side, a portion of each alar ligament usually attaches to the lateral mass of the atlas on the same side (Fig. 5-13). They also occasionally found fibers running from the odontoid process to the anterior arch of the atlas. They named these latter fibers the anterior atlanto-dental ligament and believed that this ligament, when present, would give functional support to the transverse ligament. They stated that the alar ligaments also help to limit lateral flexion at the atlanto-occipital joint. The atlantal fibers of the alar ligament on the side of lateral flexion tighten first during this motion, followed by tightening of the occipital fibers of the alar ligament on the opposite side.

Apical Ligament of the Odontoid Process. The apical ligament of the odontoid process is thin, approximately 1 inch in length and runs from the posterior and superior aspects of the odontoid process to the anterior wall of the foramen magnum (Fig. 5-13). Its fibers of insertion blend with the deep fibers of the superior band of the cruciform ligament. Its course from the odontoid to the clivus results in approximately a 20° anterior tilt of the apical odontoid ligament. Its insertion is wider than its origin, giving it a V shape (Panjabi et al., 1991a). Embryologically, this ligament develops from the core of the centrum of the proatlas (see Chapter 12) and contains traces of the notochord (Williams et al., 1989). The apical odontoid ligament probably functions to prevent some vertical translation and anterior shear of the occiput (Panjabi et al., 1991a).

Anterior Atlanto-Occipital Membrane. The anterior atlanto-occipital membrane is located in front of the apical odontoid ligament and runs from the superior aspect of the anterior arch of the atlas to the anterior margin of the foramen magnum (Fig. 5-14). It is composed of densely woven fibers (Williams et al., 1989) and is so broad that it can best be described as a membrane. The anterior atlanto-occipital membrane blends laterally with the capsular ligaments of the atlanto-occipital articulation (Fig. 5-14). It functions to limit extension of the occiput on C1. Fibers continuous with the anterior longitudinal ligament strengthen the anterior atlanto-occipital

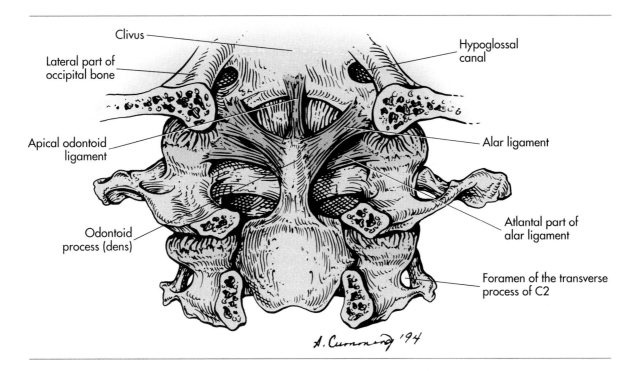

FIG. 5-13 Alar and apical odontoid ligaments. This is the same view as that of Figs. 5-11 and 5-12. The tectorial membrane and cruciform ligament have been removed. Notice that some fibers of each alar ligament attach to the lateral mass of the atlas. These fibers have been described by Dvorak and Panjabi (1987).

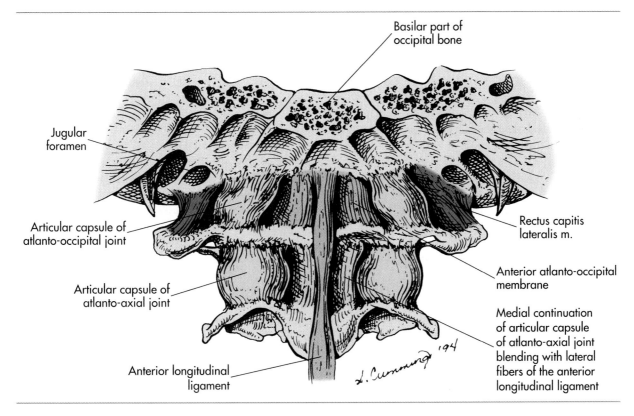

FIG. 5-14 Anterior view of the occiput, atlas, axis, and related ligaments. The anterior longitudinal ligament narrows considerably between the atlas and the occipital bone and blends with the anterior atlanto-occipital membrane. The articular capsules of the atlanto-occipital and lateral atlanto-axial joints are also clearly seen in this figure.

ligament medially and form a tough central band between the anterior tubercle of the atlas and the occiput (Williams et al., 1989) (Fig. 5-14). The anterior longitudinal ligament is discussed in more detail in the following section.

Lower Cervical Ligaments

Anterior Longitudinal Ligament. The anterior longitudinal ligament (ALL) is quite wide and covers the anterior aspect of the vertebral bodies and IVDs from the occiput to the sacrum. Superiorly the ALL thickens medially to form a cord that attaches to the body of the axis and the anterior tubercle of the atlas (Fig. 5-14). Some of the atlantal fibers diverge laterally as the ALL fibers attach to the inferior aspect of the anterior arch of the atlas. Further superiorly the ALL becomes continuous with the medial portion of the anterior atlanto-occipital membrane (see previous discussion). The ALL is approximately 3.8 mm wide at C1-2, is somewhat wider at C2-3, and increases in width to 7.5 mm from C3 to T1. Panjabi, Oxland, and Parks (1991b) state the ALL has a rather strong attachment to both the vertebral bodies and the IVDs, whereas Bland (1989) states the discal attachment is weak. Laterally, this ligament is sometimes difficult to distinguish from the anterolateral fibers of the anulus fibrosus.

The ALL has several layers associated with it. The superficial fibers span several vertebrae, whereas the deep fibers run from one vertebra to the next. This ligament tends to be thicker from anterior to posterior in the regions of the vertebral bodies rather than the areas over the IVDs. Therefore the ALL helps to smooth the contour of the anterior surface of the vertebral bodies by filling the natural concavity of the anterior vertebral bodies. The ALL functions to limit extension and is frequently damaged in extension injuries to the cervical region (Bogduk, 1986b).

Posterior Longitudinal Ligament. The posterior longitudinal ligament (PLL) is the inferior continuation of the tectorial membrane (see Fig. 5-11). It runs from the posterior aspect of the body of C2, inferiorly to the sacrum, and possibly to the coccyx (Behrsin & Briggs, 1988). The PLL is quite wide and regularly shaped in the cervical and upper thoracic regions and is also three to four times thicker, from anterior to posterior, in the cervical region than in the thoracic or lumbar regions (Bland, 1989). Its superficial fibers span several vertebrae, and its deep fibers run between adjacent vertebrae. Panjabi and colleagues (1991b) found the cervical PLL to be firmly attached to both the vertebral bodies and the IVDs, whereas Bland (1989) found the PLL to have a stronger discal attachment. In either case, the PLL probably functions to help prevent posterior IVD protrusion. The PLL is more loosely attached to the central region of

the vertebral bodies to allow the exit of the basivertebral veins from the vertebral bodies (Williams et al., 1989). The PLL in the middle and lower thoracic and lumbar regions differs from the PLL in the cervical region in that it becomes narrow over the vertebral bodies and then widens considerably over the IVDs in the thoracic and lumbar areas.

The PLL may occasionally ossify. This occurs most frequently in the cervical region and occasionally occurs in the lumbar region. (Do not confuse this with ossification of the ligamenta flava, which occurs most frequently in the thoracic region.) Ossification of the PLL is clinically relevant because it may be a source of compression of the spinal cord in the cervical region, and it has been associated with radicular symptoms in the lumbar region (Hasue et al., 1983).

Ligamenta Flava. The ligamenta flava (*sing.,* ligamentum flavum) are paired ligaments (left and right) that run between the laminae of adjacent vertebrae (see Fig. 5-10). They are found throughout the spine beginning with C1-2 superiorly and ending with L5-S1 inferiorly. The posterior atlanto-occipital membrane is the homologue of the ligamenta flava at the level of occiput-C1. Each ligamentum flavum is approximately 5 mm thick from anterior to posterior (Panjabi et al., 1991b). These ligaments are thinnest in the cervical region, become thicker in the thoracic region, and are thickest in the lumbar region.

Each ligament runs from the anterior and inferior aspect of the lamina of the vertebra above to the posterior and superior aspect of the lamina of the vertebra below. The ligamenta flava increase in length from C2-3 to C7-T1. This implies that the distance between the laminae also increases in a similar manner. Laterally, each ligamentum flavum helps to support the anterior aspect of the Z joint capsule. Although each ligament is considered to be distinct, a ligamentum flavum frequently blends with the ligamentum flavum of the opposite side (Panjabi et al., 1991b) and also blends with the interspinous ligament. Small gaps exist between the left and right ligamenta flava, allowing for the passage of veins that unite the posterior internal (epidural) vertebral venous plexus with the posterior external vertebral venous plexus.

The ligamentum flavum between C1 and C2 is usually thin and membranous and is pierced by the C2 spinal nerve. In fact, Panjabi and colleagues (1991b) were unable to find ligamenta flava between C1 and C2 in their study of six cervical spines.

The ligamentum flavum is unique in that it contains yellow-colored elastin, which causes it to constrict naturally. Therefore, this ligament may actually do work; that is, it may aid in extension of the spine. It also slows the last few degrees of spinal flexion. However, the most important function of the elastin may be to prevent buckling of the ligamentum flavum into the spinal canal during extension.

The ligamentum flavum may undergo degeneration with age or after trauma. Under such circumstances, it usually increases in thickness and may calcify or become infiltrated with fat (Ho et al., 1988). These changes may cause the ligament to lose its elastic characteristics, which can result in buckling of the thickened ligamentum flavum into the vertebral canal or medial aspect of the IVF. This further results in narrowing of these regions, which can compromise the neural elements running within them (spinal cord, cauda equina [lumbar region], or exiting nerve roots). Ossification of the ligamentum flavum is reported to occur most often in the thoracic and thoracolumbar regions of the spine, where it may compress either the posterior aspect of the spinal cord or the exiting nerve roots (Hasue et al., 1983).

Interspinous Ligaments. The interspinous ligaments are a series of ligaments that run between the spinous processes of each pair of vertebrae from C2-3 to L4-5. Some authors consider this ligament to be the anterior aspect of the ligamentum nuchae in the cervical region (see following discussion). The interspinous ligaments are poorly developed in the cervical region, consisting of a thin, membranous, translucent septum (Panjabi et al., 1991). They are short from superior to inferior and broad from anterior to posterior in the thoracic region and more rectangular in shape in the lumbar region (Williams et al., 1989). Because these ligaments are more fully developed in the thoracic region, they are discussed in more detail in Chapter 6.

Ligamentum Nuchae. The ligamentum nuchae is a flat, membranous structure that runs from the region between the cervical spinous processes anteriorly to the skin of the back of the neck posteriorly (Fig. 5-15) and spans the region between the occiput superiorly to the spinous process of C7 inferiorly. The posterior portion is its thickest and most distinct part and is sometimes referred to as the funicular portion of the ligamentum nuchae. This funicular part extends from the external occipital protuberance to the spinous process of C7. The thinner, larger, and more membranous anterior portion of this ligament can be extremely thin and, in some instances, is no more than an intermuscular septum between the left and right semispinalis capitis muscles. This thinner anterior part is sometimes known as the lamellar portion. The ligamentum nuchae is considered to be the homologue of the supraspinous and interspinous ligaments of the thoracic and lumbar regions.

Intertransverse Ligaments. Each intertransverse ligament runs from one transverse process to the transverse process of the vertebra below. These ligaments are not well defined in the cervical region and are frequently replaced by the posterior intertransverse muscles. The thoracic intertransverse ligaments are rounded cords closely related to the deep back muscles (Williams et al., 1989). Some authors describe the lumbar intertransverse ligaments as being thin membranous bands. Others consider them to be rather discrete and well defined. Still others consider them to consist of two distinct lamellae (Bogduk & Twomey, 1991) (see Chapter 7).

CERVICAL INTERVERTEBRAL DISCS

The IVDs of the cervical spine make up more than 25% of the superior-to-inferior length of the cervical spine. These important structures help to allow the large amount of motion that occurs in this region. Recall that there are no IVDs between the occiput and atlas and between the atlas and axis. The C2-3 interbody joint is the first such joint to possess an IVD. Therefore the C3 spinal nerve is the most superior nerve capable of being affected by IVD protrusion.

Mendel and colleagues (1992) studied the innervation of the cervical IVDs and found sensory nerve fibers throughout the anulus fibrosus. No nerves were found in the nucleus pulposus. The sensory fibers were most numerous in the middle third (from superior to inferior) of the anulus. The structure of many of the nerve fibers and their end receptors was consistent with those that transmit pain. In addition, pacinian corpuscles and Golgi tendon organs were found in the posterolateral aspect of the disc. These authors' findings help to confirm that the anulus fibrosus is a pain-sensitive structure. Further, their findings indicate that the cervical discs are involved in proprioception, thereby enabling the central nervous system to monitor the mechanical status of the IVDs. These authors hypothesized that the arrangement of the sensory receptors may allow the IVD to sense peripheral compression or deformation and also alignment between adjacent vertebrae.

The IVDs in the cervical region become thinner with age, whereas the uncinate processes continue to enlarge. As a result, by age 40 the uncinate processes create a substantial barrier that prevents lateral and posterolateral herniation of the IVD (Bland, 1989).

Bland (1989) believes that the cervical IVDs dehydrate earlier in life than those of the thoracic and lumbar regions. He states that virtually no nucleus pulposus exists in the cervical spine beyond age 45, and therefore believes that IVD protrusion has been overdiagnosed in the cervical region. However, this stance is somewhat controversial, and further investigation of the incidence of cervical IVD protrusion is necessary.

MRI has been shown to be effective in evaluating the status of the IVD (Forristall, Marsh, & Pay, 1988). Viikari-Juntara and colleagues (1989) also found that ultra-low-field MRI is useful in identifying posterior disc displacement below the level of C4. These MRI units are less expensive, and as resolution improves, they may be more frequently used in place of standard x-ray procedures.

The basic anatomy of the cervical IVDs is similar to that of IVDs throughout the spine. Those interested in the detailed anatomy of the IVDs should refer to the sections of Chapters 2 and 13 devoted to the gross and microscopic anatomy of these clinically relevant structures.

RANGES OF MOTION OF THE CERVICAL SPINE

Atlanto-Occipital Joint. The right and left atlanto-occipital joints together form an ellipsoidal joint that allows movement in flexion, extension, and to a lesser extent, left and right lateral flexion (see Table 5-5). A little rotation also occurs between occiput and atlas (Williams et al., 1989). Extension is limited by the opposition of the posterior aspect of the superior articular

Table 5-5   Approximate Ranges of Motion at the Atlanto-Occipital Joints

Direction	Amount
Combined flexion and extension	25°
Unilateral lateral flexion	5°
Unilateral axial rotation	5°

From White & Panjabi (1990). *Clinical biomechanics of the spine.* Philadelphia: JB Lippincott.

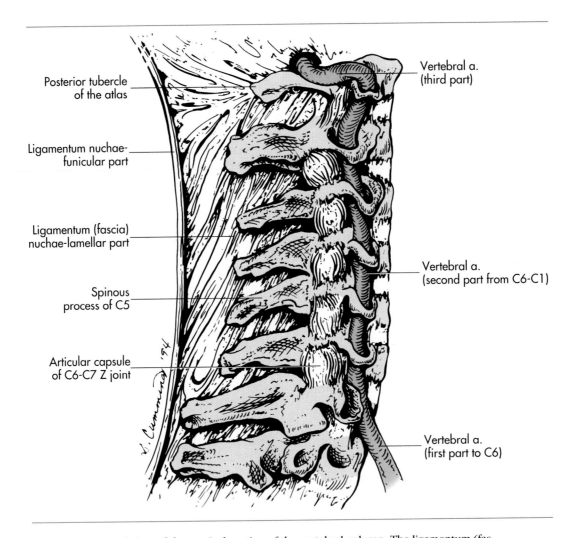

FIG. 5-15   Lateral view of the cervical portion of the vertebral column. The ligamentum (fascia) nuchae and the articular capsules of the C1-2 through C6-7 Z joints are seen. The vertebral artery can be seen entering the foramen of the transverse process (TP) of C6 and ascending through the remaining foramina of the TPs of C5 through C1. It can then be seen passing around the superior articular process of C1. The vertebral artery disappears from view as it courses beneath the posterior atlanto-occipital membrane.

processes of the atlas with the bone of the occiput's condylar fossa. Flexion is limited by soft tissue "stops," such as the posterior atlanto-occipital membrane.

Table 5-6 lists the muscles that produce the most flexion, extension, and lateral flexion between the occiput and atlas and between the atlas and axis.

Atlanto-Axial Joints. Motion occurs at all three (median and left and right lateral) atlanto-axial joints simultaneously. Most motion is axial rotation (see Table 5-7), which is limited by the alar ligaments (see earlier discussion). Since the superior articular process of C2 is convex superiorly and the inferior articular facet of C1 is slightly concave inferiorly, anterior and posterior gliding is accompanied by descent of the atlas. This moves the upper joint surface inferiorly, which conserves the amount of capsule necessary to accommodate the large amount of unilateral axial rotation that can occur at this joint. In addition, the descent of the atlas, as its inferior articular processes move along the superior articular processes of the axis, allows for added rotation to occur between the two segments (Williams et al., 1989).

Muscles that produce rotation at this joint include the following: obliquus capitis inferior, rectus capitis posterior major, splenius capitis, and the contralateral sternocleidomastoid.

Lower Cervicals. The ranges of motion for the cervical region from C2-3 through C7-T1 are given in Table 5-8.

Usually, extension is somewhat greater than flexion. Extension is limited below by the inferior articular processes of C7 entering a groove below the superior articular processes of T1. Flexion is limited by the lip on the anterior and inferior aspects of the cervical vertebrae

pressing against the beveled surface of the anterior and superior aspects of the vertebral bodies immediately below (Williams et al., 1989).

Rotation with Lateral Flexion

Lateral flexion of the cervical spine is accompanied by rotation of the vertebral bodies into the concavity formed by the lateral flexion (vertebral body rotation to the same side as lateral flexion). For example, right lateral flexion of the cervical region is accompanied by right rotation of the vertebral bodies. This phenomenon is known as *coupled motion* and occurs because the superior articular processes of cervical vertebrae face not only superiorly, but also are angled slightly medially. This arrangement forces some rotation with any attempt at lateral flexion.

NERVES, VESSELS, ANTERIOR NECK MUSCLES, AND VISCERA OF THE CERVICAL REGION

Vertebral Artery

The vertebral artery is so closely related to the cervical spine that it is discussed before the nerves of the neck. The remaining arteries of the neck are covered later in this chapter.

The vertebral artery is the first branch of the subclavian artery. It enters the foramen of the TP of C6 and ascends through the remaining foramina of the TPs of the cervical vertebrae (Figs. 5-15 and 5-16). Continuing, it passes through the foramen of the TP of C1, winds

Table 5-6	Muscles Producing Flexion, Extension, and Lateral Flexion at Occiput–C1-2
Movement	**Muscles**
Flexion	Longus capitis
	Rectus capitis anterior
Extension	Rectus capitis posterior major and minor
	Obliquus capitis superior
	Semispinalis and spinalis capitis
	Longissimus capitis
	Splenius capitis
	Trapezius
	Sternocleidomastoid
Lateral flexion	Rectus capitis lateralis
	Semispinalis capitis
	Longissimus capitis
	Splenius capitis
	Sternocleidomastoid
	Trapezius

Table 5-7	Approximate Ranges of Motion at the Atlanto-Axial Joint	
Direction		**Amount**
Combined flexion and extension		20°
Unilateral lateral flexion		5°
Unilateral axial rotation		40°

From White & Panjabi (1990). *Clinical biomechanics of the spine.* Philadelphia: JB Lippincott.

Table 5-8	Total Range of Motion of Cervical Vertebrae (C2-T1)*	
Direction		**Amount**
Flexion/extension		91°
Lateral/flexion		51° (unilateral)
Axial rotation		33° (unilateral)

Values calculated from White & Panjabi (1990). *Clinical biomechanics of the spine.* Philadelphia: JB Lippincott.
*Ranges are for C2-3 through C7-T1 and do not include occiput-C1 and C1-2 (see Tables 5-5 and 5-7 for upper cervical ranges of motion).

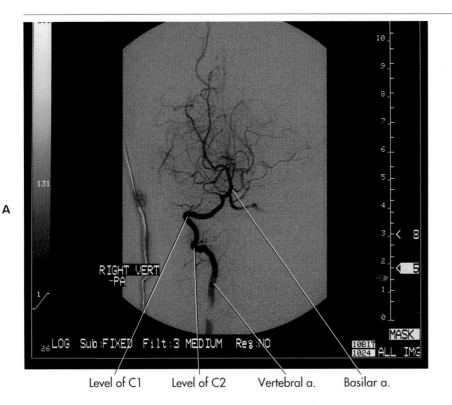

Level of C1   Level of C2   Vertebral a.   Basilar a.

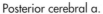

Posterior cerebral a.

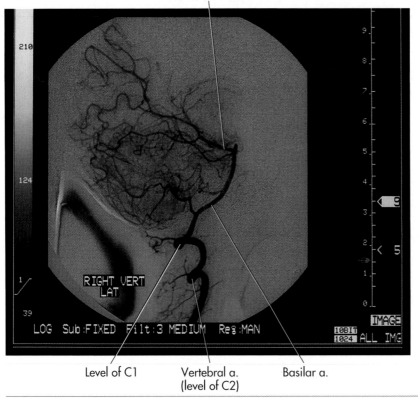

Level of C1   Vertebral a.   Basilar a.
(level of C2)

FIG. 5-16 Posteroanterior **(A)** and lateral **(B)** angiograms of the right vertebral artery. A radiopaque dye has been injected into the vertebral artery, and x-ray films have been taken. The vertebral artery can be seen as it courses superiorly through the foramina of the TPs of C6 through C1. Notice the normal tortuosity seen as the vertebral artery passes laterally at C2 to reach the foramen of the TP of C1. The vertebral artery is also quite tortuous as it passes around the superior articular process of C1 and then passes superiorly to enter the foramen magnum. It then unites with the vertebral artery of the opposite side to form the basilar artery. Several branches of the basilar artery can be seen, and its termination as the posterior cerebral arteries can also be seen.

medially around the superior articular process of the atlas, and passes beneath the posterior atlanto-occipital membrane (see Fig. 5-10). The vertebral artery then pierces the dura and arachnoid and courses superiorly through the foramen magnum to unite with the vertebral artery of the opposite side. The union of the two vertebral arteries forms the basilar artery.

The vertebral artery can be divided into four parts (Williams et al., 1989). The first part of the vertebral artery begins at the artery's origin from the subclavian artery and continues until it passes through the foramen of the TP of C6. The first part courses between the longus colli and scalenus anterior muscles before reaching the TP of C6. In a study of 36 vertebral arteries, Taitz and Arensburg (1989) found that 18 (50%) were tortuous to some degree in the first segment. Currently there is debate as to whether or not tortuosity of a vertebral artery may cause a decrease in flow to the structures supplied by it. However, to date no clinical significance has been ascribed to mild-to-moderate tortuosity of the vertebral artery.

The first part of the vertebral artery is joined by several venous branches that become the vertebral vein in the lower cervical region. It is also joined by a large branch and several small branches from the more posteriorly located inferior cervical ganglion or, when present, the cervicothoracic ganglion (present 80% of the time). These branches form a plexus of nerves around the vertebral artery. This plexus is discussed in more detail later in this chapter.

The second part of the vertebral artery is the region that passes superiorly through the foramina of the transverse processes of C6 to C1 (Figs. 5-15, 5-16, and 5-17). This part is accompanied by the vertebral veins and the nerve plexus derived from the sympathetic chain. The second part of the vertebral artery passes anteriorly to the C2 to C6 cervical ventral rami, which course from medial to lateral in the grooves (gutters) for the spinal nerves of their respective cervical TPs (see Fig. 5-20). The vertebral artery makes a rather dramatic lateral curve (45°) after passing through the transverse foramen of the axis (Figs. 5-10 and 5-17). This allows the artery to reach the more laterally placed TP of the atlas. Taitz and Arensburg (1989) found that 4 of 36 vertebral arteries (11%) showed marked kinking or tortuosity at the foramen of the TP of the axis. The vertebral artery can be quite tortuous in some individuals. Whether this tortuosity is congenital, acquired (secondary to atherosclerosis), or a combination of both has yet to be determined (Taitz & Arensburg, 1989).

Extension combined with rotation of the head to one side normally impairs blood flow through the second part of the vertebral artery of the opposite side. The constriction occurs between the axis and atlas (Taitz et al., 1978).

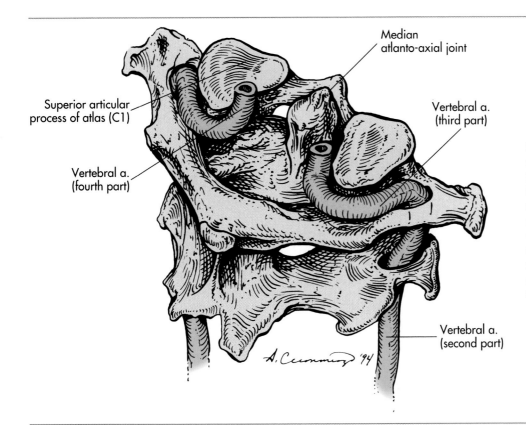

Median atlanto-axial joint

Superior articular process of atlas (C1)

Vertebral a. (third part)

Vertebral a. (fourth part)

Vertebral a. (second part)

FIG. 5-17 The second, third, and fourth parts of the left and right vertebral arteries. Notice that each vertebral artery courses laterally between C2 and C1. It then courses posteriorly and medially at the level of C1, and finally passes superiorly and medially to reach the foramen magnum.

The third part of the vertebral artery begins as the artery passes through the foramen of the TP of the atlas (Fig. 5-17). Here it is located posterior and medial to the rectus capitis lateralis. Immediately the vertebral artery curves farther posteriorly and medially around the superior articular process of C1. It reaches the posterior arch of the atlas, where it lies in the groove for the vertebral artery of the posterior arch. The dorsal ramus of the first cervical nerve (suboccipital nerve) passes between the vertebral artery and the posterior arch of the atlas in this region. The artery then passes inferior to the posterior atlanto-occipital membrane (see Fig. 5-10). This membrane may form an ossified bridge for the artery, which, when present, runs from the posterior arch of the atlas to the lateral mass. This bony bridge is known as a posterior ponticle and is discussed earlier in this chapter.

The fourth part of the vertebral artery begins as the artery passes beneath the bridge of the posterior atlanto-occipital membrane. The artery then runs medially to pierce the dura mater and arachnoid mater and courses superiorly to pass through the foramen magnum. Once above the foramen magnum, it courses within the subarachnoid space along the clivus until it meets the vertebral artery of the opposite side to form the basilar artery. The basilar artery is formed in the region of the inferior pons (Williams et al., 1989).

The fourth part of the vertebral artery has several branches. Each vertebral artery gives off a branch that unites with its pair from the opposite side to form a single anterior spinal artery. The anterior spinal artery supplies the anterior aspect of the spinal cord throughout its length. Each vertebral artery then gives off a posterior spinal artery. The left and right posterior spinal arteries remain separate as they course along the posterior aspect of the spinal cord (see Chapter 3 for both anterior and posterior spinal arteries). Each vertebral artery then gives off a posterior inferior cerebellar artery that supplies the inferior aspect of the cerebellum and a portion of the medulla.

The right and left vertebral arteries unite at the level of the pons to form the basilar artery. The basilar artery gives off anterior inferior cerebellar, labyrinthine (internal auditory), pontine, and superior cerebellar arteries before ending by dividing into the posterior cerebral arteries. The posterior cerebral arteries participate in the cerebral arterial circle (of Willis) and then continue posteriorly to supply the occipital lobes of the cerebral cortex and the inferior portion of the temporal lobes.

Nerves of the Cervical Region

A thorough understanding of patients presenting with neck pain can only be achieved if clinicians know those structures capable of nociception (pain perception). Also, clinicians first must understand how pathologic conditions, aberrant movement, or pressure affecting these structures can result in nociception, and then how the patient perceives that nociception. A knowledge of the innervation of the cervical region gives clinicians an understanding of the structures that are pain sensitive and the way in which this nociceptive information is transmitted to the central nervous system. This topic is of significance to clinicians dealing with pain of cervical origin.

Rootlets, Roots, Dorsal Root Ganglia, Mixed Spinal Nerves, and Rami. The dorsal and ventral rootlets of the cervical region leave the spinal cord and unite into dorsal and ventral roots (see Chapter 3). The dorsal and ventral roots unite within the region of the IVF to form the mixed spinal nerve (Fig. 5-18). The mixed spinal nerve is short and almost immediately divides into a dorsal ramus (posterior primary division) and a ventral ramus (anterior primary division).

Unique rootlets, roots, and dorsal root ganglia. The posterior rootlets of C1 are unique. They are so thin that they are frequently mistaken for arachnoidal strands during dissection (Edmeads, 1978). Stimulation of the C1 rootlets has been found to cause orbital pain (superior rootlets of C1), frontal pain (middle rootlets), and vertex pain (lower rootlets). Conditions such as tumors of the posterior cranial fossa, herniations of the cerebellar tonsils through the foramen magnum, bony anomalies of the craniovertebral junction, and possibly prolonged muscle tightness can cause irritation of the sensory rootlets or root of C1. Irritation of these rootlets or root may, in turn, refer pain to the regions just mentioned (Darby & Cramer, 1994; Edmeads, 1978).

Great variation exists in the distribution of rootlets in the cervical region. More specifically, anastomoses frequently exist between rootlets of adjacent spinal cord segments. These anastomoses occur 61% of the time in the cervical spinal cord, compared with 7% in the thoracic region and 22% in the lumbar cord (Moriishi, Otani, Tanaka, & Inoue, 1989). This is clinically significant because sensory impulses conducting nociceptive (pain) sensations through the dorsal root ganglion at one vertebral level may enter the spinal cord at the next spinal cord segment above or below. The pain sensations in such cases may be perceived one segment "off," adding to the body's already difficult task of pain localization (Darby & Cramer, 1994). These anastomoses would also complicate the presentation of radicular pain by disrupting the normal dermatomal pattern of innervation by dorsal roots and dorsal root ganglia (see Chapter 11).

Recall that the cell bodies of all afferent nerve fibers are located in the dorsal root ganglia (DRG), which are also known as the spinal ganglia. These ganglia, with the exception of those of the C1 and C2 cord segments, are located within the IVFs. The C1 DRG may be absent;

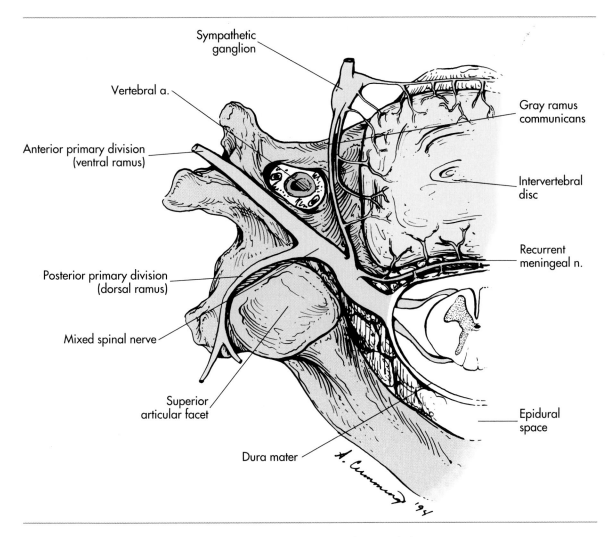

Sympathetic ganglion

Vertebral a.

Anterior primary division (ventral ramus)

Posterior primary division (dorsal ramus)

Mixed spinal nerve

Superior articular facet

Dura mater

Gray ramus communicans

Intervertebral disc

Recurrent meningeal n.

Epidural space

FIG. 5-18 Superior view of a typical cervical segment showing the neural elements. Notice the dorsal and ventral roots, the mixed spinal nerve, and the posterior and anterior primary divisions (dorsal and ventral rami). The posterior primary division can be seen dividing into a medial and a lateral branch. The recurrent meningeal nerve is shown entering the intervertebral foramen. Fibers arising from the middle cervical ganglion and the gray communicating ramus are also shown. Notice that these fibers supply the anterior and lateral aspects of the intervertebral disc, the vertebral body, and the anterior longitudinal ligament. The sympathetic plexus that surrounds the vertebral artery is shown in Fig. 5-19.

however, when present, it usually is found lying on the posterior arch of the atlas (Williams et al., 1989). The C2 DRG is located between the posterior arch of the atlas and the lamina of C2; more exactly, it is located posterior and medial to the lateral atlanto-axial joint. It contains the cell bodies of sensory fibers innervating the median atlanto-axial joint, the lateral atlanto-axial joint, and a large part of the neck and scalp, extending from the posterior occipital region to the vertex and occasionally even to the coronal suture of the skull (Bogduk, 1982). Another unique characteristic of the C2 DRG is that it is the only such ganglion normally located outside the dura. Its prominent and predictable location has enabled investigators to study the effects of localized anesthesia on the C2 DRG (Bogduk, 1989a), allowing for a

better understanding of the importance of the second cervical nerve in suboccipital headaches.

Dorsal rami. The dorsal rami (posterior primary divisions) are generally smaller than the ventral rami (anterior primary divisions). Recall that each dorsal ramus exits the mixed spinal nerve just lateral to the IVF (Fig. 5-18). After exiting the IVF, the dorsal ramus curves posteriorly, close to the anterolateral aspect of the articular pillar. In fact, the dorsal rami of C4 and C5 produce a groove on the lateral aspect of the articular pillars of the C4 and C5 vertebrae. On reaching the posterior and lateral aspect of the superior articular process, each dorsal ramus quickly divides into a medial and lateral branch (Fig. 5-18).

Some of the most important structures innervated by the dorsal rami are the deep back muscles. The deeper and more segmentally oriented transversospinalis muscles receive innervation from the medial branch of the dorsal rami. The longer and more superficial erector spinae muscles are innervated by the lateral branch of the dorsal rami. Other structures innervated by the medial branch include the Z joints and the interspinous ligaments. The lateral branch of the dorsal rami of the upper cervical nerves (except C1) continue posteriorly, after innervating the erector spinae and splenius capitis and cervicis muscles, to supply sensory innervation to the skin of the neck. The dorsal rami of C6, C7, and C8 usually do not have cutaneous branches (Kasai et al., 1989).

The dorsal ramus of the C1 spinal nerve is unique. The C1 nerve exits the vertebral canal by passing above the posterior arch of the atlas. It quickly divides into a ventral and dorsal ramus. The dorsal ramus (suboccipital nerve) runs between the posterior arch of the atlas and the vertebral artery. It does not divide into a medial and lateral branch, but rather curves superiorly for a short distance (about 1 cm) and terminates by providing motor innervation to the suboccipital muscles. It also sends a communicating branch to the dorsal ramus of C2. Some authors have described an inconsistent cutaneous branch that runs to the posterolateral scalp (Williams et al., 1989), although other detailed studies have not reproduced this finding (Bogduk, 1982).

The C2 spinal nerve branches into a dorsal and ventral ramus posterior to the lateral atlanto-axial joint. The dorsal ramus loops superiorly around the inferior border of the obliquus capitis inferior muscle and then divides into medial, lateral, superior communicating, inferior communicating, and a branch to the obliquus capitis inferior. The lateral branch of the dorsal ramus of C2 helps to supply motor innervation to the longissimus capitis, splenius capitis, and semispinalis capitis muscles (Bogduk, 1982). The medial branch of the dorsal ramus of C2 is large and is known as the greater occipital nerve. This nerve receives a communicating branch from the third occipital nerve before piercing the large semispinalis capitis muscle. The greater occipital nerve, accompanied by the occipital artery, reaches the scalp by passing through a protective aponeurotic sling. This sling is associated with the insertions of the trapezius and sternocleidomastoid muscles onto the superior nuchal line (Bogduk, 1982). The aponeurotic sling actually prevents the greater occipital nerve from being compressed during contraction of these muscles. After passage through the sling, the greater occipital nerve courses superiorly and divides into several terminal branches. These branches provide a broad area of sensory innervation extending from the occipital region medially to the region superior to the mastoid process and posterior to the ear laterally. Superiorly, they supply sensory innervation to the scalp from the region of the posterior occiput to as far as the skull's coronal suture (Bogduk, 1982). Terminal branches of the greater occipital nerve also provide sensory branches to the occipital and transverse facial arteries.

Disorders of the upper cervical spine, including irritation of the greater occipital nerve or the C2 ganglion, can definitely cause headaches (Bogduk, 1986c; Bogduk, 1989a; Bogduk et al., 1985; Edmeads, 1978). Causes of irritation to the nerve or ganglion include direct trauma to the posterior occiput and entrapment between traumatized or hypertonic cervical muscles, particularly the semispinalis capitis (Edmeads, 1978). Hyperextension injuries to the neck, especially during rotation, can also compress the C2 ganglion between the posterior arch of the atlas and the lamina of the axis.

The C3 spinal nerve is the most superior nerve to pass through an IVF. Within the lateral aspect of the IVF the C3 nerve branches into a dorsal and ventral ramus. The dorsal ramus of C3 passes posteriorly between the C2 and C3 TPs, where it divides into deep and superficial medial branches, a lateral branch, and a communicating branch with the C2 dorsal ramus (Bogduk, 1982). The superficial medial branch of the dorsal ramus is known as the third occipital nerve. This nerve courses around the lower part of the C2-3 Z joint from anterior to posterior. The deep surface of the third occipital nerve provides articular branches to the C2-3 Z joint (Bogduk & Marsland, 1986). Because of its close relationships with the bony elements of the C2-3 IVF, the third occipital nerve has been implicated by one investigator as the cause of the headaches that frequently accompany generalized osteoarthritis of the cervical spine (Trevor-Jones, 1964). After supplying the C2-3 Z joint, the third occipital nerve courses superiorly; pierces the semispinalis capitis, splenius capitis, and trapezius muscles; then assists the greater occipital nerve (C2) in its sensory innervation of the suboccipital region (Bogduk, 1982).

The deep medial branch of the C3 dorsal ramus helps to supply the uppermost multifidus muscles. The lateral branch of the C3 dorsal ramus helps supply the more superficial neck muscles (longissimus capitis, splenius capitis, semispinalis capitis). In addition, the C3 dorsal ramus also helps to supply the C2-3 (via dorsal ramus itself, the third occipital nerve, or a communicating branch) and the C3-4 (via the deep medial branch) Z joints. The atlanto-occipital joints and the median and lateral atlanto-axial joints are innervated by the C1 and C2 ventral rami, respectively (Bogduk, 1982). Bogduk and Marsland (1986) reported on the relief of occipital and suboccipital headaches by local anesthetic block of the third occipital nerve in 10 consecutive patients with headaches of suspected cervical origin. They suggested that the cause of the headaches was traumatic arthropathy or degenerative joint disease of the C2-3 Z joints and stated that their findings "may reflect an actual high incidence in the community of a condition that has remained unrecognized by specialists dealing with headache, and perhaps misdiagnosed as tension headache." They also mentioned that C1-2 joints may be another cause of cervical headache but thought further investigation was required before differentiation between C1-2 and C2-3 headaches could be accurately performed.

Injury to structures of the upper cervical spine can result in pain referral to the occipital regions innervated by the dorsal rami of the upper three cervical nerves. Upper cervical injury can also refer to regions of the head innervated by the trigeminal nerve. This is possible because the central processes of the upper three cervical sensory nerves enter the upper cervical spinal cord and converge on neurons of the spinal tract and spinal nucleus of the trigeminal nerve. This region has been called the trigemino-cervical nucleus (Bogduk et al., 1985). The specific location of pain referral depends on the central neurons stimulated by the incoming cervical fibers. Therefore, after injury to the upper cervical region, pain can be interpreted as arising from as far away as the anterior aspect of the head (trigeminal nerve, C2 ventral ramus) or the suboccipital region to the scalp above the vertex of the skull (region innervated by [C1] C2 and C3 dorsal rami).

The spinal nerves of C4 through C8 exit through their respective IVFs (e.g., C4 through the C3-4 IVF, C8 through the C7-T1 IVF). The dorsal rami are quickly given off and pass posteriorly, medial to the posterior intertransversarii muscles, which they supply. They then divide into medial and lateral branches. The medial branches of C4 and C5 (occasionally C6) divide into a superficial and deep branch. The dorsal rami of (C6) C7 and C8 do not divide and only have deep medial branches. The superficial branches help to supply the semispinalis cervicis and capitis muscles and then send cutaneous fibers to provide sensory innervation to the skin of the posterior neck. The deep medial branches of the dorsal rami run to the multifi muscles, where they provide a very specific innervation. Each nerve supplies those muscle fibers that attach to the spinous process of a segmental level numbered one less than the nerve. Therefore the C5 deep medial branch supplies those multifidus fibers that insert onto the C4 spinous process (Bogduk, 1982). The deep medial branches of C4 to C8 also supply the Z joints. Each deep medial branch sends a rostral branch to the Z joint above and a caudal branch to the Z joint below. These branches run along the dorsal aspect of the joints within the pericapsular fibrous tissue (Bogduk, 1982). The lateral branches of the C4 to C8 dorsal rami help to supply the semispinalis capitis, longissimus cervicis, splenius cervicis, and iliocostalis cervicis muscles (C8).

Since many structures of the cervical region that can produce pain receive their sensory supply from dorsal rami, certain diagnostic procedures and therapies for neck and head pain have been directed specifically at these nerves (Bogduk, 1989a; Bogduk, 1989b).

Ventral rami. Each ventral ramus of the cervical region leaves its mixed spinal nerve of origin and then exits the spine by passing posterior to the vertebral artery and then between the anterior and posterior intertransversarii muscles. The cervical ventral rami innervate the anterior muscles of the cervical spine, including the longus capitis, longus colli, and rectus capitis anterior and lateralis muscles. The atlanto-occipital joints and the median and lateral atlanto-axial joints are innervated by the C1 and C2 ventral rami, respectively (Bogduk, 1982).

Bogduk (1986a) stated that abnormal position (subluxation) of a lateral atlanto-axial joint, compressing the C2 ventral ramus, is the most likely cause of neck-tongue syndrome. This syndrome includes suboccipital pain with simultaneous numbness of the tongue on the same side. The author explained the tongue numbness by the fact that some proprioceptive fibers to the tongue accompany the hypoglossal nerve and then pass through the ventral ramus of C2. Such "numbness" is analogous to that reported in Bell's palsy, in which the proprioceptive fibers of the seventh cranial nerve give the sensation of numbness over a region of the face that receives its sensory innervation from the trigeminal nerve.

The cervical ventral rami also help to supply the vertebral bodies, anterior longitudinal ligament, and anterior aspect of the IVD with sensory innervation. These latter structures also receive sensory innervation from fibers arising from the sympathetic chain (Fig. 5-18) and from the autonomic fibers associated with the vertebral artery (Bogduk et al., 1988; Groen, Baljet, & Drukker, 1990). A thorough understanding of the specific sensory innervation to the anterior structures of the spine is important because these structures can be damaged during an extension injury or during the acceleration portion of an acceleration/deceleration injury (Foreman & Croft, 1992). Therefore the autonomic fibers associated with the recurrent meningeal nerve, the sympathetic chain itself, and the vertebral artery are listed in the following discussion.

The ventral rami of cervical spinal nerves also form the cervical and brachial plexuses, which innervate the anterior neck and upper extremities. These neural elements are discussed at the end of this section.

Recurrent Meningeal Nerve. The recurrent meningeal nerves are also known as the sinuvertebral nerves. In the cervical region, each nerve originates from the ventral ramus and then receives a contribution from the gray communicating ramus and other sympathetic nerves that run with the vertebral artery (Groen et al., 1990) (Figs. 5-18 and 5-19). The recurrent meningeal nerve then courses medially, through the medial aspect of the IVF and anterior to the spinal dura. This nerve supplies the posterior aspect of the IVD, the posterior longitudinal ligament, the anterior spinal dura mater (Williams et al., 1989), the posterior vertebral bodies, and the uncovertebral joints (Xiuqing, Bo, & Shizhen, 1988). Usually the recurrent meningeal nerve supplies these structures at the level where it enters the vertebral canal and then continues superiorly to innervate the same structures at the vertebral level above, although the distribution varies (Groen et al., 1990).

More than one recurrent meningeal nerve is usually present at each vertebral level (Groen et al., 1990). The recurrent meningeal nerves of the cervical region probably carry both vasomotor fibers, derived from the sympathetic contribution, and general somatic afferent fibers (including nociceptive fibers), arising from the ventral rami (Bogduk et al., 1988).

The recurrent meningeal nerves of C1, C2, and C3 have relatively large meningeal branches that ascend to the posterior cranial fossa. As they course superiorly to reach the posterior cranial fossa, they supply the atlanto-axial joint complex (also supplied by the ventral ramus of C2), the tectorial membrane, components of the cruciate ligament, and the alar ligaments (Bogduk et al., 1988). Once in the posterior cranial fossa, they help to supply the cranial dura mater, including the region of the clivus, which is supplied by the recurrent meningeal nerve of C3 (Bogduk et al., 1988). These meningeal branches probably are related to the pain referral patterns associated with disorders of the upper cervical spine and occipital headache (Williams et al., 1989).

Cervical Sympathetics. This section focuses on those aspects of the sympathetic nervous system most closely related to the general anatomy of the cervical spine. The specific anatomy of the cervical sympathetics is discussed in Chapter 10. The cervical sympathetic chain lies anterior to the longus capitis muscle. It is composed of three ganglia: superior, middle, and inferior. The superior ganglion is by far the largest, and it is positioned inferior to the occiput and anterior to the TPs of C2 and C3. The middle cervical ganglion is not always present. When it is present, it lies anterior to the TP of C6. Usually the inferior ganglion unites with the first thoracic ganglion to form the cervicothoracic (stellate) ganglion, located just inferior to the TP of C7.

The relationships at the sympathetic plexus surrounding the vertebral artery are rather complex (Fig. 5-19). Because of the intimate relationship of this plexus with the vertebral artery and the spinal structures innervated by this plexus, it is discussed here. Chapter 10 also discusses this plexus in the context of the entire autonomic nervous system.

The plexus surrounding the vertebral artery has been referred to as the vertebral nerve (Edmeads, 1978). Other authors (Gayral & Neuwirth, 1954; Xiuqing et al.,

1988) state that of the nerves surrounding the vertebral artery, the vertebral nerve is the largest of the several branches that arise from the cervicothoracic (stellate) ganglion to follow the vertebral artery through the foramen of the TP of C6. This discussion uses the term *vertebral nerve* only when discussing the previously mentioned large branch of the stellate ganglion. The term *vertebral plexus of nerves* is used to refer to the neural network surrounding the vertebral artery.

In addition to the branches of the cervicothoracic ganglion that reach the vertebral artery, a branch (or branches) from the middle cervical ganglion and sometimes branches from intermediate ganglia join the vertebral plexus of nerves above the level of C6 (Xiuqing et al., 1988). The branch from the middle cervical ganglion runs lateral to either the C5-6 or C4-5 uncovertebral joint before reaching the vertebral artery. The superior part of the plexus surrounding the vertebral artery is joined by branches directly from the ventral rami of C1 and C2 (Bogduk, Lambert, & Duckworth, 1981) and C3 (Xiuqing et al., 1988). Most of the large nerves accompanying the vertebral artery are gray rami communicantes that follow the artery superiorly to join the ventral rami of C3 to C6 (Fig. 5-19). Other branches of the vertebral artery nerve plexus supply sensory innervation to the lateral aspects of the cervical IVDs (Bogduk, Windsor, & Inglis, 1988). A deeper and more dense plexus of nerves also surrounds the vertebral artery. This deeper plexus is derived from smaller branches of the vertebral nerve, the stellate, middle and intermediate cervical ganglia, and cervical ventral rami. These fibers form vascular branches that create a dense neural plexus around the vertebral artery. The vertebral arteries themselves have been found to be capable of producing pain. The afferents for their nociceptive sensation run with the autonomic fibers. Therefore, irritation of these fibers by degenerative spur formation of the upper cervical uncovertebral or Z joints may be a cause of headaches (Edmeads, 1978).

Nerves of the Anterior Neck. This section and the sections that follow discuss the neural, muscular, vascular, and visceral structures of the anterior neck. Even though an extensive description of the anatomy of this region is beyond the scope of this text, the previously mentioned structures of the neck are so intimately related to the cervical spine that covering them in adequate detail is important. Also, flexion and extension injuries to the cervical region, commonly known as "whiplash injuries," are quite prevalent (Foreman & Croft, 1992). Such injuries vary considerably in severity and can result in damage to a variety of anatomic structures. Injury to the anterior longitudinal ligament, posterior longitudinal ligament, interspinous ligament (ligamentum nuchae), IVDs, vertebral end plates, odontoid process, spinous processes, Z joints, muscles,

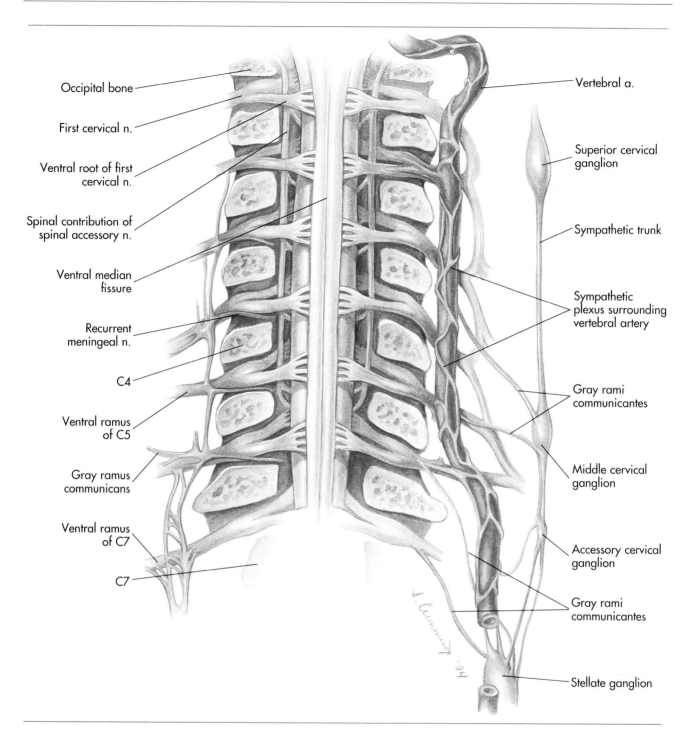

FIG. 5-19 Sympathetic plexus surrounding the vertebral artery. The pedicles have been cut coronally, and the vertebral bodies and transverse processes have been removed to reveal an anterior view of the neural elements. *Right,* One vertebral artery was spared. Notice several branches from the stellate ganglion coursing to this vertebral artery. The largest of these branches is sometimes known as the vertebral nerve. Also, notice several gray communicating rami (GR) contributing to the vertebral artery sympathetic plexus. *Left,* Components of this plexus after the vertebral artery has been removed. Notice that the GR branch considerably and send twigs to join branches of adjacent GR. In addition, the GR sends twigs to ventral rami of the same level, the level above, and the level below. Other twigs of the plexus unite with branches of the ventral rami to form recurrent meningeal nerves. The recurrent meningeal nerves, in turn, course medially to enter the vertebral canal. Branches of the plexus also innervate the vertebral artery itself by passing into the arterial walls (see text for further details). The ventral rami of the mixed spinal nerves can be seen uniting to form the cervical and brachial plexuses on the right side of the illustration. Notice that the vertebral artery is sending a small arterial branch to the C2 spinal nerve. This branch can be seen dividing into anterior and posterior radicular arteries. These branches, which are normally found at each vertebral level, have been removed from the remaining levels to display the neural elements more clearly.

esophagus, sympathetic trunk, temporomandibular joint, cranium, and brain have all been reported, either through experimental studies or during clinical examination, after flexion and extension injury to the cervical region (Bogduk, 1986b). In addition, proper examination of the cervical region includes an examination of the anterior neck. Therefore the following sections describe the most clinically relevant relationships of the anterior neck, beginning with the nerves.

The nerves of the anterior neck include the ventral rami of the cervical nerves. These ventral rami make up the cervical and brachial (including T1) plexuses (Fig. 5-20). Also, several cranial nerves (CNs) are found in the anterior neck. These include the glossopharyngeal (CN IX), the vagus (CN X), the accessory (CN XI), and the hypoglossal (CN XII) nerves. The cervical and brachial plexuses are discussed in modest detail, and the most relevant points of CNs IX through XII are covered.

Ventral ramus of C1. This ramus passes laterally around the superior articular process of the atlas. It lies anterior to the vertebral artery in this region and runs medial to the artery as the nerve passes medial to the rectus capitis lateralis muscle (which it supplies) to exit above the TP of the atlas. The ventral ramus of C1 receives some fibers from the ventral ramus of C2, and together these fibers join the hypoglossal nerve. Some fibers of the ventral ramus of C1 follow the hypoglossal nerve proximally and help provide sensory innervation to the dura mater of the posterior cranial fossa. (Agur, 1991). However, most fibers of the ventral ramus of C1 continue distally along CN XII and then give several branches that leave CN XII. The first such branch participates in the ansa cervicalis and is known as the superior (upper) root of the ansa cervicalis (descendens hypoglossi). The next branch is the nerve to the thyrohyoid, which innervates the thyrohyoid muscle. The nerve to the geniohyoid is the last branch. It innervates the muscle of the same name.

Cervical plexus. The cervical plexus can be divided into a sensory and motor portion. The sensory portion of the cervical plexus is more superficially placed than the motor portion. The named nerves of the sensory portion (Fig. 5-20) are formed deep to the sternocleidomastoid muscle (SCM) by the union of individual C2 to C4 ventral rami. The named nerves course around the posterior surface of the SCM and emerge from behind its midpoint in proximity to one another. They then proceed in different directions to reach their respective destinations. The named nerves of the sensory (superficial) part of the cervical plexus and their ventral rami of origin are reviewed in Table 5-9 (and Fig. 5-20).

The motor portion of the cervical plexus lies deep to the sensory portion and is located within the anterior triangle. The motor portion makes up the ansa cervicalis

(Fig. 5-20). The two limbs (roots) of the ansa cervicalis are the following:

- ◆ C1 ventral ramus (see preceding discussion): provides separate motor innervation to the thyrohyoid and geniohyoid muscles and also forms the superior root of the ansa cervicalis (descendens hypoglossi)
- ◆ C2 and C3 rami: combine to form the inferior root of the ansa cervicalis (descendens cervicalis)

Together the superior and inferior roots combine to form the ansa cervicalis. Branches of this neural loop provide motor innervation to all of the infrahyoid (strap) muscles (i.e., both bellies of the omohyoid, the sternohyoid, and the sternothyroid), except the thyrohyoid muscle, which is supplied by the ventral ramus of C1.

The phrenic nerve is also considered to be a part of the cervical plexus. It arises from the ventral rami of C3, C4, and C5, with C4 providing the most significant contribution. The phrenic nerve provides motor and sensory innervation to the diaphragm. Occasionally an accessory phrenic nerve arises from the ventral rami of C5 and C6. When present, the accessory phrenic nerve branches from the nerve to the subclavius and courses to the diaphragm.

Brachial plexus. The brachial plexus (Fig. 5-20) is formed by the ventral rami of C5 through T1. The ventral rami that participate in forming the brachial plexus are referred to as the "roots" of the brachial plexus. The ventral rami (or roots of the plexus) form trunks, the trunks form anterior and posterior divisions, the divisions form cords, and the cords end as terminal branches. The brachial plexus is discussed in more detail in the following section. Where appropriate, the spinal cord segments that contribute to the formation of the individual named nerves are included in parentheses following the named nerves, for example, radial nerve (C5,6,7,8,T1).

The ventral rami of C5 and C6 form the upper trunk of the brachial plexus. The ventral ramus of C7 remains free of the complex relationships seen in the other rami and forms the middle trunk by itself. The C8 and T1 ventral rami converge to form the lower trunk. A few

Table 5-9 Sensory Portion of Cervical Plexus

Nerve	Cord segments	Destination
Lesser occipital nerve	C2 (C3)	Mastoid region and superior aspect of ear
Great auricular nerve	C2, C3	Ear and region overlying angle of mandible
Transverse cervical nerve	C2, C3	Anterior neck
Supraclavicular nerve	C3, C4	Medial, intermediate, and lateral branches to skin over clavicle and deltoid muscle

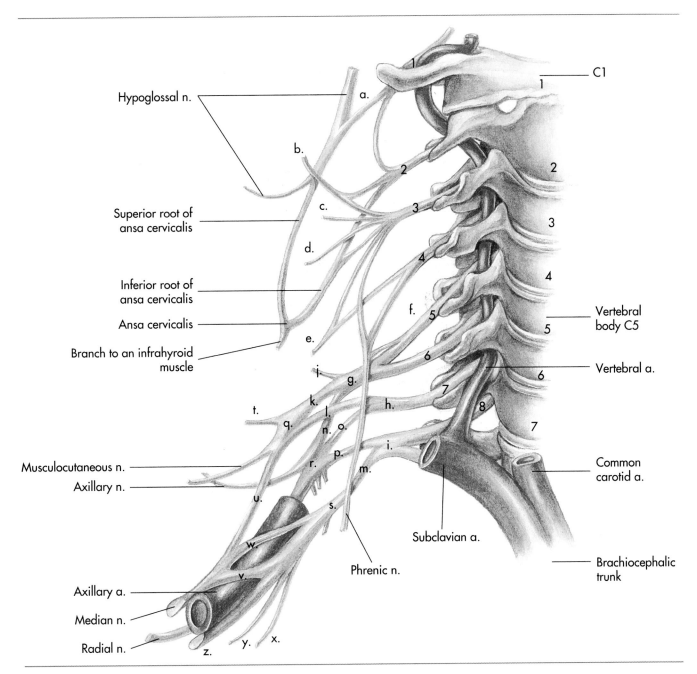

FIG. 5-20 Nerves of the cervical region, including the cervical plexus and the brachial plexus. Notice that the anterior primary divisions (ventral rami) exit posterior to the vertebral artery. The anterior primary divisions of C1 through C4 (with a contribution from C5 to the phrenic nerve) form the cervical plexus, and the anterior primary divisions of C5 through T1 form the roots of the brachial plexus. The following structures are identified: *a*, anterior primary division (ventral ramus) of C1, uniting with the hypoglossal nerve; *b*, lesser occipital nerve; *c*, great auricular nerve (receives contributions from both C2 and C3 ventral rami); *d*, transverse cervical nerve, also known as the transverse cutaneous nerve of the neck (also receives contributions from both C2 and C3 ventral rami); *e*, supraclavicular nerve (common trunk of origin for lateral, intermediate, and medial supraclavicular nerves); *f*, dorsal scapular nerve from C5 ventral ramus would be given off here; *g*, upper trunk of the brachial plexus; *h*, middle trunk; *i*, lower trunk; *j*, suprascapular nerve; *k*, anterior division of upper trunk of the brachial plexus; *l*, anterior division of middle trunk; *m*, anterior division of lower trunk; *n*, posterior division of upper trunk of the brachial plexus; *o*, posterior division of middle trunk; *p*, posterior division of lower trunk; *q*, lateral cord of the brachial plexus; *r*, posterior cord; *s*, medial cord; *t*, lateral pectoral nerve; *u*, contribution of the lateral cord to the median nerve; *v*, contribution of the medial cord to the median nerve; *w*, variant additional contribution of medial cord to the median nerve; *x*, medial brachial cutaneous nerve (medial cutaneous nerve of the arm); *y*, medial antebrachial cutaneous nerve (medial cutaneous nerve of the forearm); *z*, ulnar nerve. The medial pectoral nerve is shown arising from the inferior aspect of the medial cord *(s)*. From proximal to distal, the upper subscapular, thoracodorsal, and lower subscapular nerves are shown arising from the posterior cord *(r)*. The long thoracic nerve, which arises from the ventral rami of C5, C6, and C7, is not shown in this illustration.

important branches arise from the ventral rami before they form trunks. The first is the dorsal scapular nerve, which branches from the C5 ramus and provides motor innervation to the rhomboid major and minor muscles and occasionally to the levator scapulae muscle. Branches of the fifth, sixth, and seventh ventral rami form the long thoracic nerve (of Charles Bell), which innervates the serratus anterior muscle.

The suprascapular nerve branches from the upper trunk (it is therefore derived from C5 and C6). It courses through the scapular notch (beneath the superior transverse scapular ligament) to innervate the supraspinatus and infraspinatus muscles. The suprascapular nerve also sends articular twigs to the shoulder joint and the acromioclavicular joint. The nerve to subclavius muscle (C5,6), which also branches from the upper trunk (C5 and C6), supplies the small muscle of the same name. The nerve to the subclavius usually sends a communicating branch to the phrenic nerve (usually from the C5 contribution).

The trunks divide into anterior and posterior divisions. The anterior divisions of the upper and middle trunks unite to form the lateral cord. The anterior division of the lower trunk remains alone to form the medial cord, and all the posterior divisions unite to form the posterior cord.

The cords of the brachial plexus are named according to their anatomic relationship to the axillary artery (i.e., lateral cord is lateral to artery, etc.). The cords themselves have branches. The lateral cord has a branch called the lateral pectoral nerve (C5,6,7), which innervates both the pectoralis major and minor muscles. The medial cord gives off the medial pectoral nerve (C8,T1), which innervates the pectoralis minor muscle, and a few branches may help to supply the pectoralis major (Williams et al., 1989). The posterior cord gives off the superior or upper (C5,6) and inferior or lower (C5,6) subscapular nerves and the thoracodorsal (middle subscapular) nerve (C6,7,8). The upper subscapular nerve supplies the subscapularis muscle. The thoracodorsal nerve supplies the latissimus dorsi muscle, and the inferior subscapular nerve supplies the teres major muscle and helps to supply the subscapularis muscle.

The cords end as terminal branches of the brachial plexus. The lateral cord divides into the musculocutaneous nerve (C5,6,7) and a large contributing branch to the median nerve (C[5],6,7). The musculocutaneous nerve provides motor innervation to the flexor muscles of the arm and sensory innervation to the lateral forearm. The median nerve is discussed in more detail in the following section.

The medial cord provides the medial brachial (C8,T1) and medial antebrachial (C8,T1) cutaneous nerves (sensory to arm and forearm, respectively) before dividing into the ulnar nerve (C[7],8,T1) and the medial cord

contribution to the median (C8,T1) nerve. The ulnar nerve sends articular branches to the elbow and wrist, motor fibers to one and a half muscles of the forearm, and the majority of the intrinsic muscles of the palm. The ulnar nerve is also sensory to the medial distal forearm and medial band (medial palm, fifth digit, ulnar side of the fourth digit).

Recall that both the lateral and the medial cords participate in the formation of the median nerve (C[5],6,7,8,T1). This nerve provides articular branches to the elbow and wrist joints, motor innervation to the majority of the muscles of the anterior forearm, and innervation to five muscles of the palm (three thenar muscles, first two lumbricals). In addition, the median nerve provides sensory innervation to the lateral aspect (radial side) of the palm, the anterior aspect of the first three and a half digits, and the distal aspect of the posterior surface of the first three and a half digits. However, the sensory innervation to the hand is subject to significant variation.

The posterior cord ends by dividing into the axillary (C5,6) and radial nerves (C5,6,7,8,T1). The axillary nerve courses through the quadrangular space (space between the teres minor, teres major, long head of the triceps muscles, and surgical neck of the humerus), supplying motor innervation to the teres minor and the deltoid muscles. In addition, the axillary nerve provides sensory innervation to the upper lateral aspect of the arm.

The radial nerve provides motor and sensory innervation to the posterior arm and forearm. It also gives articular branches to the elbow and wrist joints. In addition, the radial nerve provides sensory innervation to the lateral aspect of the dorsum of the hand and the dorsal aspect of the first two and a half digits (except for the distal portions of these digits that are innervated by the median nerve). Chapter 9 provides additional information on the large terminal branches of the brachial plexus.

Vagus nerve. The vagus nerve exits the jugular foramen of the posterior cranial fossa and courses inferiorly throughout the entire length of the neck. Accompanying the vagus nerve in its course through the neck are the internal jugular vein and the internal and common carotid arteries. These structures are wrapped in a fibrous tissue sheath known as the carotid sheath. The vagus nerve is located within the posterior aspect of the carotid sheath between the internal jugular vein, which is lateral to it, and the internal carotid artery, which is medial to it. Inferiorly, the vagus nerve lies between the internal jugular vein and the common carotid artery.

The vagus nerve has several branches in the neck:
◆ *Pharyngeal branch.* This nerve participates in the pharyngeal plexus, which supplies motor and sensory innervation to the pharynx.

◆ *Superior laryngeal nerve.* This nerve divides into two branches. The first, the internal laryngeal nerve, pierces the thyrohyoid membrane to provide sensory innervation to laryngeal structures above the true vocal folds. The second branch, the external laryngeal nerve, runs inferiorly to innervate the cricothyroid muscle and also helps to supply the inferior constrictor muscle with motor innervation.

◆ *Nerve to the carotid body.* This nerve supplies sensory innervation to the chemoreceptor of the same name. It also may help to innervate the carotid sinus, the baroreceptor located at the bifurcation of the common carotid artery into the internal and external carotid arteries.

◆ *Cardiac nerves.* Several cardiac nerves enter the thorax and participate in the cardiac plexus of nerves. The cervical cardiac nerves of the vagus provide parasympathetic innervation to the heart.

◆ *Recurrent laryngeal nerve.* This nerve loops around the subclavian artery (from anterior to posterior) on the right to run in the groove between the trachea and the esophagus (tracheo-esophageal groove). It provides motor innervation to all the muscles of vocalization with the exception of the cricothyroid muscle, which is innervated by the external laryngeal nerve. The left recurrent laryngeal nerve wraps around the arch of the aorta (from anterior to posterior) just lateral to the ligamentum arteriosum and continues superiorly in the left tracheo-esophageal groove.

Cranial nerves IX, XI, XII. As with the vagus nerve, the glossopharyngeal nerve (CN IX) exits the posterior cranial fossa by passing through the jugular foramen. It courses along the posterior pharynx just lateral to the stylopharyngeus muscle, which it supplies. CN IX enters the pharynx together with the stylopharyngeus muscle by passing between the superior and middle constrictor muscles and terminates on the posterior third of the tongue. This branch supplies both general sensation and taste sensation to this region of the tongue. The glossopharyngeal nerve also participates in the pharyngeal plexus of nerves. This plexus supplies both motor and sensory innervation to the pharynx. In addition, CN IX with the vagus supplies sensory fibers to the carotid body and sinus. It also provides the parasympathetic fibers that eventually become the lesser petrosal nerve. This nerve synapses in the otic ganglion, and the postganglionic fibers supply secretomotor fibers to the parotid gland.

The accessory and hypoglossal nerves (CNs XI and XII) are located in the superior neck just behind the posterior belly of the digastric muscle. The accessory (spinal accessory) nerve enters the carotid triangle by coursing behind the posterior belly of the digastric and enters the posterior aspect of the SCM. It innervates this muscle before continuing posteriorly to supply the trapezius muscle.

The hypoglossal nerve (CN XII) enters the neck dorsal to the posterior belly of the digastric, courses anteriorly and slightly inferiorly, and then exits the neck by passing medial to the intermediate tendon of the digastric muscle. It continues deep to the mylohyoid muscle and supplies the intrinsic and extrinsic (except the palatoglossus muscle, supplied by CN X-pharyngeal branch) muscles of the tongue.

Muscles of the Anterior Neck

The muscles of the anterior neck (Fig. 5-21) can conveniently be divided into those below the hyoid bone (**infrahyoid muscles**) and those above the hyoid bone (**suprahyoid muscles**). The salient features of these two groups of muscles are listed in Table 5-10 and Table 5-11 for easy reference.

In addition to the infrahyoid and suprahyoid muscles, the SCM and the scalene muscles are also associated with the anterior aspect of the cervical spine and neck. The principal features of the scalene muscles are listed

Table 5-10	Infrahyoid Muscles and SCM				
Muscle	Origin	Insertion	Nerve	Function	Notes
Sternocleidomastoid	Manubrium, proximal clavicle	Mastoid process	Accessory (CN XI), ventral rami (C2,3[4])	Bilaterally flex neck, extend head	Unilaterally, laterally flex same side, rotate head to opposite side
Omohyoid	Scapular notch	Hyoid bone	Ansa cervicalis (C1-C3)	Depress hyoid bone	Superior and inferior bellies divided by intermediate tendon
Sternohyoid	Posterior manubrium	Hyoid bone	Ansa cervicalis (C1-C3)	Depress or stabilize hyoid bone	—
Sternothyroid	Posterior manubrium	Thyroid cartilage	Ansa cervicalis (C1-C3)	Depress or stabilize thyroid cartilage	—
Thyrohyoid	Thyroid cartilage	Hyoid bone	C1	Elevate thyroid cartilage, depress hyoid bone	—

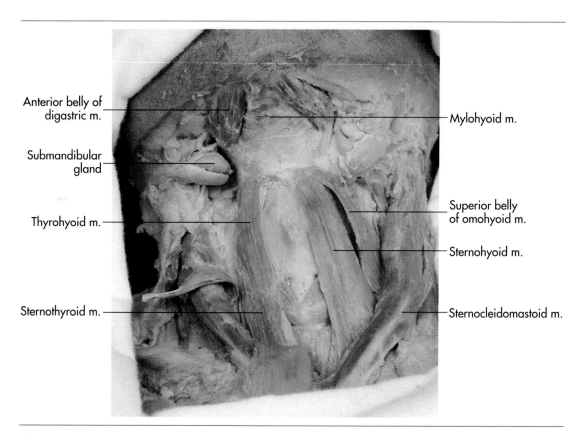

FIG. 5-21 Anterior dissection of the neck. The suprahyoid and infrahyoid muscles are shown. The sternohyoid muscle has been removed on the right side of the cadaver to demonstrate the sternothyroid and thyrohyoid muscles more clearly.

Table 5-11 Suprahyoid Muscles

Muscle	Origin	Insertion	Nerve	Function	Notes
Digastric	Mastoid process	Digastric fossa of mandible	Posterior belly-CN VII; anterior belly-CN V3 (nerve to mylohyoid)	Elevate hyoid, move hyoid anteriorly or posteriorly	Anterior and posterior bellies separated by an intermediate tendon
Mylohyoid	Mylohyoid line of mandible	Median raphe, hyoid bone	CN V3 (nerve to mylohyoid)	Elevate hyoid and floor of oral cavity	—
Geniohyoid	Genial spine of mandible	Hyoid bone	Ventral ramus C1	Elevate hyoid bone	—

in Table 5-12. Because of its importance, the SCM is discussed next.

Sternocleidomastoid Muscle. The sternocleidomastoid (SCM), or sternomastoid muscle is a prominent and important muscle of the cervical region. Its origin, insertion, innervation, and function are listed in Table 5-10. As shown in the table, when it contracts unilaterally, the SCM laterally flexes the neck to the same side and rotates the face to the opposite side. Occasionally this muscle becomes abnormally tight, holding the neck in the laterally flexed and contralaterally rotated position. This is

known as torticollis, or "wry neck." Torticollis is caused by a variety of factors, including prolonged exposure (e.g., a night of sleep) in the presence of a cool breeze, congenital torticollis, neurologic torticollis, and unknown causes (idiopathic).

In addition to its innervation from the accessory nerve (CN XI), the SCM receives some fibers of innervation from the ventral rami of C2-C4. These are thought to be primarily proprioceptive, although some authors believe that a small proportion of motor fibers may also be present. The presence of motor fibers from cervical ventral rami would explain reports of individuals

Table 5-12   Scalene Muscles

Origin	Insertion	Nerve	Function	Notes
Anterior scalene				
Anterior tubercles of C3-C6 TPs	Anterior aspect of first rib (scalene tubercle)	Anterior primary divisions of C4-C6	Combination of flexion and lateral flexion of neck, rotate neck to opposite side, elevate first rib	Subclavian vein passes anterior to this muscle
Middle scalene				
TP of C2 (sometimes C1), posterior tubercles of C3-C7 TPs	Anterior aspect of first rib, posterior to insertion of anterior scalene	Anterior primary divisions of C3-C8	Combination of flexion and lateral flexion of neck, rotate neck to opposite side, elevate first rib	Largest of scalene muscles; subclavian artery and roots of brachial plexus pass between this muscle and anterior scalene
Posterior scalene				
Posterior tubercles of C4-C6 TPs	Lateral aspect of second rib	Anterior primary divisions of C6-C8	Lateral flexion of neck, elevate second rib	Smallest of scalene muscles

TPs, Transverse processes

retaining some SCM function after their CN XI had been severed.

Vascular Structures of the Anterior Neck

Lymphatics of the Head and Neck. Lymphatics of the face and head drain inferiorly into the pericervical lymphatic collar. This collar consists of a series of connected lymph nodes, which form a chain that encircles the junction of the head and the neck. The collar consists of the following groups of nodes (from posterior to anterior): occipital, postauricular (retroauricular), preauricular, submandibular, and submental. These lymph nodes are drained by lymphatic channels, which eventually drain into the deep cervical lymph nodes, located along the internal jugular vein. The deep cervical lymph nodes empty into the thoracic duct on the left side and the right lymphatic duct on the right side.

Major Arteries of the Anterior Neck. The major arteries of the anterior neck (Fig. 5-22) begin in the base (root) of the neck. The root of the neck lies between the neck and the thorax. This region is bounded by the first thoracic vertebra, the first rib, and the manubrium of the sternum. The principal arteries of this region are the right and left subclavian and the right and left common carotid. The right subclavian and right common carotid arteries are branches of the brachiocephalic trunk from the aortic arch. The left subclavian and left common carotid arteries branch directly from the aortic arch.

Subclavian arteries. The branches of the first part of the subclavian artery (from its origin to the medial border of the anterior scalene muscle) are listed next.
1. *Vertebral artery.* This artery enters the foramen of the TP of C6 and ascends the cervical region through the foramina of the TPs of the remaining five cervical vertebrae. This artery is discussed in detail earlier in this chapter.
2. *Internal thoracic artery.* This artery passes inferiorly into the thorax along the posterior aspect of the anterior thoracic wall.
3. *Thyrocervical trunk.* This artery has several branches:
   a. *Inferior thyroid artery.* This branch provides the ascending cervical artery before supplying the inferior aspect of the thyroid gland. The ascending cervical artery helps to supply the neck musculature and the posterior elements of the cervical vertebrae.
   b. *Superficial (transverse) cervical artery.* This artery supplies the superficial and deep back muscles of the cervical and upper thoracic regions.
   c. *Suprascapular artery.* This artery supplies several muscles of the scapula.
The following are branches of the second part of the subclavian artery (between the medial and lateral borders of the anterior scalene muscle).
4. *Costocervical trunk.* This short artery divides into two branches:
   a. *Deep cervical artery.* This branch helps to supply the posterior neck musculature and the posterior

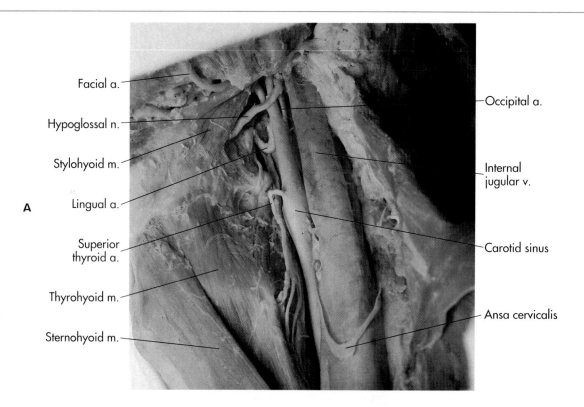

Facial a.

Hypoglossal n.

Stylohyoid m.

Lingual a.

A

Superior thyroid a.

Thyrohyoid m.

Sternohyoid m.

Occipital a.

Internal jugular v.

Carotid sinus

Ansa cervicalis

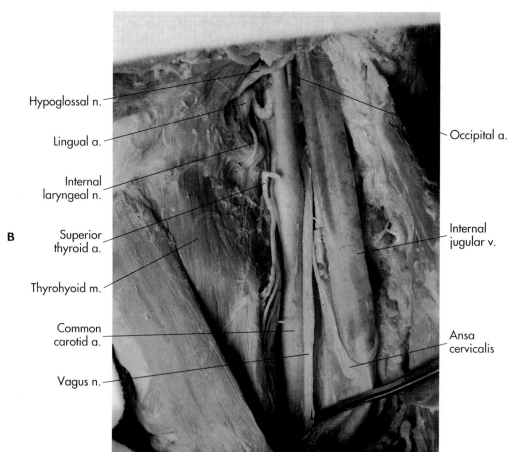

Hypoglossal n.

Lingual a.

Internal laryngeal n.

B

Superior thyroid a.

Thyrohyoid m.

Common carotid a.

Vagus n.

Occipital a.

Internal jugular v.

Ansa cervicalis

FIG. 5-22 Anterolateral dissection of the neck showing the internal jugular vein, common carotid artery, and external carotid artery and several of its branches. The internal jugular vein has been moved laterally in **B** to reveal the left vagus nerve, which lies between the internal jugular vein and the common carotid artery. Superior to the bifurcation of the common carotid artery, the vagus nerve lies between the internal jugular vein and the internal carotid artery. The ansa cervicalis can be seen looping across the internal jugular vein in both **A** and **B**.

arches of the cervical vertebrae.
   b. *Highest intercostal artery.* This branch runs to the first two intercostal spaces.
5. *Dorsal scapular artery.* This is a branch from the third part of the subclavian (between the lateral aspect of the anterior scalene muscle and the first rib) and is only present when there is no deep branch of the superficial (transverse) scapular artery. It supplies the superficial and deep back muscles of the upper thoracic region.

Carotid arteries. The common carotid artery divides into the internal and external carotid arteries (Fig. 5-22). Before its bifurcation, the common carotid artery expands to form the carotid sinus, which contains baroreceptors to monitor blood pressure. At the bifurcation of the common carotid artery into its internal and external branches, the carotid body is found. The carotid body is responsible for monitoring oxygen and carbon dioxide concentration in the blood. The carotid sinus and body are innervated by CNs IX and X.

Each internal carotid artery ascends the neck to enter the cranial cavity via the carotid foramen (canal). The internal carotid artery then supplies the orbit, pituitary gland, and a large part of the frontal, parietal, and temporal lobes of each cerebral hemisphere.

The external carotid artery is responsible for the blood supply to the neck and face (both the superficial and deep face) (Fig. 5-22). The branches of the external carotid artery are listed next.
1. *Superior thyroid artery.* This artery courses to the thyroid gland. The superior laryngeal artery branches from the superior thyroid artery. This artery pierces the thyrohyoid membrane with the internal laryngeal nerve and helps supply the larynx.
2. *Ascending pharyngeal artery.* This is a long artery of small diameter that ascends between the internal and external carotid arteries and supplies the pharynx.
3. *Lingual artery.* This is a tortuous artery that runs to the tongue by passing deep to the mylohyoid and hyoglossus muscle.
4. *Facial artery.* This is another tortuous artery that courses to the anterior face; it runs deep to the submandibular gland. (*Note:* Sometimes the lingual and facial arteries arise from a common faciolingual [linguofacial] trunk.)
5. *Occipital artery.* This branch courses to the occiput. It is "held" against the external carotid artery by the hypoglossal nerve (CN XII).
6. *Posterior auricular artery.* This artery runs to and supplies the region posterior to the ear.
The external carotid artery ends by dividing into the:
7. *Superficial temporal artery.* This large artery courses superiorly to the temporal region and divides into frontal and parietal branches.

8. *Maxillary artery.* This artery supplies the structures within the infratemporal fossa (deep face), nasal cavity, palate, maxilla, and superior aspect of the pharynx.

Major Veins of the Anterior Neck. A large part of the scalp and the superior and lateral face is drained by the external jugular vein. This vein is formed by the union of the posterior auricular vein and the posterior division of the retromandibular vein. The external jugular vein empties into the subclavian vein.

The central region of the face and the deep structures of the head and neck drain into the internal jugular vein (Fig. 5-22). This vein is formed at the jugular foramen by the union of the sigmoidal and the inferior petrosal dura mater venous sinuses of the cranial cavity.

More specifically, the central region of the face is drained by the facial vein (anterior facial vein). This vein ends by passing in front of the submandibular gland to join the anterior branch of the retromandibular vein (posterior facial vein). The union of these two veins forms the common facial vein. The common facial vein, in turn, empties into the internal jugular vein. The internal jugular vein joins the subclavian vein to form the brachiocephalic vein. The right and left brachiocephalic veins then unite to form the superior vena cava, which empties into the right atrium.

The anterior jugular veins (right and left) drain the anterior neck. They may communicate in the midline low in the neck close to the region between the left and right clavicular heads (the jugular fossa). The anterior jugular vein drains into either the external jugular or the subclavian vein.

Viscera of the Anterior Neck

The pharynx and esophagus lie in the midline and allow for passage of food from the oral cavity through the thorax and eventually to the abdomen. The larynx and trachea lie anterior to the esophagus and function in vocalization and passage of air to and from the lungs.

The thyroid gland lies in contact with the anterolateral aspect of the inferior larynx and the superior trachea. This gland has two lobes, a right and a left, which are united in the midline by the isthmus. The isthmus covers the anterior aspect of the second to fourth tracheal rings. The superior and inferior thyroid arteries provide the blood supply to the thyroid gland. Sympathetics (vasomotor) reach the gland via the middle cervical ganglion. Parasympathetics (uncertain function) are supplied by the laryngeal branches of the vagus nerve.

The small parathyroid glands, four in number (two on each side), are located on the posterior aspect of the thyroid gland.

REFERENCES

Agur, A.M. (1991). *Grant's atlas of anatomy* (9th ed.). Philadelphia: Williams & Wilkins.

Bagnall, K.M., Harris, P.F., & Jones, P.R.M. (1977). A radiographic study of the human fetal spine. 2. The sequence of development of ossification centres in the vertebral column. *J Anat, 124,* 791-802.

Behrsin, J. & Briggs, C. (1988). Ligaments of the lumbar spine: A review. *Surg Radiol Anat, 10,* 211-219.

Bland, J. (1987). *Disorders of the cervical spine.* Philadelphia: WB Saunders.

Bland, J. (1989). The cervical spine: From anatomy to clinical care. *Med Times, 117,* 15-33.

Bogduk, N. (1982). The clinical anatomy of the cervical dorsal rami. *Spine, 7,* 319-330.

Bogduk, N. (1986a). An anatomical basis for the neck-tongue syndrome. *J Neurol Neurosurg Psychiatry, 44,* 202-208.

Bogduk, N. (1986b). The anatomy and pathophysiology of whiplash. *Clin Biomech, 1,* 92-101.

Bogduk, N. (1986c). Headaches and the cervical spine (editorial). *Cephalalgia 4,* 7-8.

Bogduk, N. (1989a). Local anesthetic blocks of the second cervical ganglion: A technique with application in occipital headache. *Cephalalgia, 1,* 41-50.

Bogduk, N. (1989b). The rationale for patterns of neck and back pain. *Patient Management, 13,* 17-28.

Bogduk, N. & Marsland, A. (1986). On the concept of third occipital headache. *J Neurol Neurosurg Psychiatry, 49,* 775-780.

Bogduk, N. & Marsland, A. (1988). The cervical zygapophysial joints as a source of neck pain. *Spine, 13,* 610-617.

Bogduk, N. & Twomey, L.T. (1991). *Clinical anatomy of the lumbar spine.* London: Churchill Livingstone.

Bogduk, N., Lambert G., & Duckworth, J. (1981). The anatomy and physiology of the vertebral nerve in relation to cervical migraine. *Cephalalgia, 1,* 11-24.

Bogduk, N., Windsor, M., & Inglis, A. (1988). The innervation of the cervical intervertebral discs. *Spine, 13,* 2-8.

Bogduk, N. et al. (1985). Cervical headache. *Med J Aust, 143,* 202-207.

Buna, M. et al. (1984). Ponticles of the atlas: A review and clinical perspective. *J Manipulative Physiol Ther, 7,* 261-266.

Cave, A.J.E. (1934). On the occipito-atlanto-axial articulations. *J Anat, 68,* 416-423.

Cave, A.J.E., Griffiths, J.D., & Whiteley, M.M. (1955). Osteo-arthritis deformans of Luschka joints. *Lancet, 1,* 176-179.

Cusick, J. (1988). Monitoring of cervical spondylotic myelopathy. *Spine, 13,* 877-880.

Czervionke, L. et al. (1988). Cervical neural foramina: Correlative anatomic and MR imaging study. *Radiology, 169,* 753-759.

Danziger, J. & Bloch, S. (1975). The widened cervical intervertebral foramen. *Radiology, 116,* 671-674.

Darby, S. & Cramer, G. (1994). Pain generators and pain pathways of the head and neck. In D. Curl (Ed.), *Chiropractic approach to head pain.* Baltimore: Williams & Wilkins.

Dupuis, P.R., et al. (1985). Radiologic diagnosis of degenerative lumbar spinal instability. *Spine, 10,* 262-276.

Dvorak, J. & Panjabi, M. (1987). Functional anatomy of the alar ligament. *Spine, 12,* 183-189.

Dwyer, A., Aprill, C., & Bogduk, N. (1990). Cervical zygapophyseal joint pain patterns. I. A study in normal volunteers. *Spine, 15,* 453-457.

Edmeads, J. (1978). Headaches and head pains associated with diseases of the cervical spine. *Med Clin North Am, 62,* 533-544.

Fesmire, F. & Luten, R. (1989). The pediatric cervical spine: Developmental anatomy and clinical aspects. *J Emerg Med, 7,* 133-142.

Fletcher, G. et al. (1990). Age-related changes in the cervical facet joints: Studies with cryomicrotomy, MR and CT. *AJNR, 11,* 27-30.

Foreman, S.M. & Croft, A.C. (1992). *Whiplash injuries: The cervical acceleration/deceleration syndrome.* Baltimore: Williams & Wilkins.

Forristall, R., Marsh, H., & Pay, N. (1988). Magnetic resonance imaging and contrast CT of the lumbar spine: Comparison of diagnostic methods of correlation with surgical findings. *Spine, 13,* 1049-1054.

Fujiwara, K. et al. (1988). Morphometry of the cervical spinal cord and its relation to pathology in cases with compression myelopathy. *Spine, 13,* 1212-1216.

Gates, D. (1980). *Correlative spinal anatomy.* Lakemont, Ga: CHB Printing and Binding.

Gayral, L. & Neuwirth, E. (1954). Oto-neuro-ophthalmologic manifestations of cervical origin, posterior cervical sympathetic syndrome of Barré-Lieou. *NY State J Med, 54,* 1920-1926.

Groen, G., Baljet, B., & Drukker, J. (1990). Nerves and nerve plexuses of the human vertebral column. *Am J Anat, 188,* 282-296.

Hasue, M. et al. (1983). Anatomic study of the interrelation between lumbosacral nerve roots and their surrounding tissues. *Spine, 8,* 50-58.

Ho, P.S. et al. (1988). Ligamentum flavum: Appearance on sagittal and coronal MR images. *Radiology, 168,* 469-472.

Jovanovic, M. (1990). A comparative study of the foramen transversarium of the sixth and seventh cervical vertebrae. *Surg Radiol Anat, 12,* 167-172.

Kapandji, I.A. (1974). *The physiology of the joints. Annotated diagrams of the mechanics of the human joints* (2nd ed.). Edinburgh: Churchill Livingstone.

Kasai, T. et al. (1989). Cutaneous branches from the dorsal rami of the cervical nerves, with emphasis on their positional relations to the semispinalis cervicis. *Okajimas Folia Anat Jpn, 66,* 153-160.

Kaufman, R. & Glenn, W. (1983). Rheumatoid cervical myelopathy evaluation by computerized tomography with multiplanar reconstruction. *J Rheumatol, 10,* 42-54.

Kinalski, R. & Kostro, B. (1971). Planimetric measurements of intervertebral foramina in cervical spondylosis. *Polish Med J, 10,* 737-742.

Kissel, P. & Youmans, J. (1992). Post-traumatic anterior cervical osteophyte and dysphagia: Surgical report and literature review. *J Spin Disorders, 5,* 104-107.

Koebke, J. & Brade, H. (1982). Morphological and functional studies on the lateral joints of the first and second cervical vertebrae in man. *Anat Embryol, 161,* 265-275.

Le Minor, J., Kahn, E., & Di Paola, R. (1989). Osteometry by computer aided image analysis: Application to the human atlas. *Gegenbaurs morphol. jahrb. Leipzig, 135,* 865-874.

Louis, R. (1985). Spinal stability as defined by the three column spine concept. *Anat Clin, 7,* 33-42.

Mendel, T. et al. (1992). Neural elements in human cervical intervertebral discs. *Spine, 17,* 132-135.

Miles, K.A. & Finlay, D. (1988). Is prevertebral soft tissue swelling a useful sign in injury of the cervical spine? *Injury, 19,* 177-179.

Moriishi, J., Otani, K., Tanaka, K., & Inoue, S. (1989). The intersegmental anastomoses between spinal nerve roots. *Anat Rec, 224,* 110-116.

Oliver, J. & Middleditch, A. (1991). *Functional anatomy of the spine.* Oxford: Butterworth Heinemann.

Orofino, C., Sherman, M.S., & Schecter, D. (1960). Luschka's joint: A degenerative phenomenon. *J Bone Joint Surg, 42A,* 853-858.

Pal, G.P. et al. (1988). Trajectory architecture of the trabecular bone between the body and the neural arch in human vertebrae. *Anat Rec, 222,* 418-425.

Panjabi, M., Oxland, T., & Parks, E. (1991a). Quantitative anatomy of cervical spine ligaments. Part I. Upper cervical spine. *J Spin Disorders, 4,* 270-276.

Panjabi, M., Oxland, T., & Parks, E. (1991b). Quantitative anatomy of cervical spine ligaments. Part II. Middle and lower cervical spine. *J Spin Disorders, 4,* 277-285.

Panjabi, M. et al. (1991). Flexion, extension, and lateral bending of the upper cervical spine in response to alar ligament transections. *J Spin Disorders, 4,* 157-167.

Pech, P. et al. (1985). The cervical neural foramina: Correlation on microtomy and CT anatomy. *Radiology, 155,* 143-146.

Renaudin, J. & Snyder, M. (1978). Chip fracture through the superior articular facet with compressive cervical radiculopathy. *J Trauma, 18,* 66-67.

Schimmel, D., Newton, T., & Mani, J. (1976). Widening of the cervical intervertebral foramen. *Neuroradiology, 12,* 3-10.

Schultz, G. Personal communication, 1994.

Sunderland, S. (1974). Meningeal neural relations in the intervertebral foramen. *J Neurosurg, 40,* 756-763.

Taitz, C., Nathan, H., & Arensburg, B. (1978). Anatomical observations of the foramina transversaria. *J Neurol Neurosurg Psychiatry, 41,* 170-176.

Taitz, C. & Arensburg, B. (1989). Erosion of the foramen transversarium of the axis. *Acta Anat, 134,* 12-17.

Taitz, C. & Nathan, H. (1986). Some observations on the posterior and lateral bridge of the atlas. *Acta Anat, 127,* 212-217.

Tondury, G. (1943). Zur anatomie der Halswirbelsaule. Gibt es Uncovertebralgelenke? *Z Anat EntwGesch, 112,* 448-459.

Trevor-Jones, R. (1964). Osteo-arthritis of the paravertebral joints of the second and third cervical vertebrae as a cause of occipital headaches. *S Afr Med J, May,* 392-394.

Van Dyke, D. & Gahagan, C. (1988). Down's syndrome cervical spine abnormalities and problems. *Clin Pediatr, 27,* 415-418.

Viikari-Juntara, E. et al. (1989). Evaluation of cervical disc degeneration with ultralow field MRI and discogrophy: An experimental study on cadavers. *Spine, 14,* 616-619.

Wang, A. et al. (1984). Cervical chordoma presenting with intervertebral foramen enlargement mimicking neurofibroma CT findings. *J Comput Assist Tomogr, 8,* 529-532.

White & Panjabi. (1990). Clinical biomechanics of the spine. Philadelphia: JB Lippincott.

Williams, P.L. et al. (1989). *Gray's anatomy* (37th ed.). Edinburgh: Churchill Livingstone.

Xiuqing, C., Bo, S., & Shizhen, Z. (1988). Nerves accompanying the vertebral artery and their clinical relevance. *Spine, 13,* 1360-1364.

Yenerich, D.O. & Haughton, V.M. (1986). Oblique plane MR imaging of the cervical spine. *J Comput Assist Tomogr, 5,* 823-826.

Yu, S., Sether, L., & Haughton, V.M. (1987). Facet joint menisci of the cervical spine: Correlative MR imaging and cryomicrotomy study. *Radiology, 164,* 79-82.

Yu, Y. et al. (1986). Computer-assisted myelography in cervical spondylotic myelopathy and radiculopathy: Clinical correlations and pathogenetic mechanisms. *Brain, 109,* 259-278.

CHAPTER 6

The Thoracic Region

Gregory D. Cramer

The thoracic region contains the most vertebrae (12) of any of the movable regions of the spine. Consequently, it is the longest region of the spine. However, because of its relationship with the ribs, which attach anteriorly to the sternum, the thoracic region has relatively little movement. Many of the unique characteristics of the thoracic region result from its anatomic relationship with the ribs. The typical thoracic vertebrae are T2 through T8. T1, T9 (occasionally), T10, T11, and T12 can perhaps best be described as unique rather than "atypical." The size of the thoracic vertebrae generally increases from the superior vertebrae to the inferior ones, just as the load they are required to carry increases from superior to inferior.

This chapter first discusses the typical thoracic vertebrae, ribs, and sternum. This is followed by a discussion of the thoracic vertebrae that have unique features (T1, T9 to T12). Next, ligaments with distinctive features in the thoracic region are covered. Many ligaments are described with the cervical region in Chapter 5 and are not covered again here. This chapter also includes a brief discussion of lateral curves that may develop in the thoracic region (scoliosis). The last section is devoted to nerves, vessels, and visceral structures associated with the thoracic vertebrae and the thoracic cage.

THORACIC CURVE (KYPHOSIS)

As stated in Chapter 2, the normal thoracic curve is a rather prominent kyphosis, which extends from T2 to T12. It is created by the larger superior-to-inferior dimensions of the posterior portion of the thoracic vertebrae. Occasionally the thoracic kyphosis is almost completely absent. This is logically referred to as the straight back syndrome. This syndrome is associated with systolic heart murmurs and a distorted cardiac silhouette on x-ray film, and as a result, it can simulate organic heart disease. The straightening of the thoracic kyphosis results in a narrowing of the anterior-to-posterior dimension of the thoracic cage, which decreases the space available for the heart. The heart is forced to shift to the left, which leads to kinking of the great vessels. This results in a variety of heart murmurs. The straight back syndrome has also been associated with idiopathic mitral valve prolapse, a potentially life-threatening condition (Spapen et al., 1990).

TYPICAL THORACIC VERTEBRAE, RIBS, AND STERNUM
Typical Thoracic Vertebrae

Vertebral Bodies. The vertebral bodies of the typical thoracic vertebrae (T2 to T8) are larger than those of the cervical region (Fig. 6-1). They appear to be heart shaped when viewed from above, and their anteroposterior dimensions are approximately equal to their lateral dimensions. Dupuis and colleagues (1985) report that the posterior edge of the superior surface of upper thoracic vertebral bodies exhibit small remnants of the cervical uncinate processes.

The T2 vertebral body is somewhat cervical in appearance, being slightly larger in transverse diameter than in anteroposterior diameter. The body of the T3 vertebra is the smallest of the thoracic region, and below this level the vertebral bodies gradually increase in size. The vertebral bodies of T5 through T8 become more and more heart shaped. This means that the concavity of the posterior aspect of the vertebral bodies becomes more

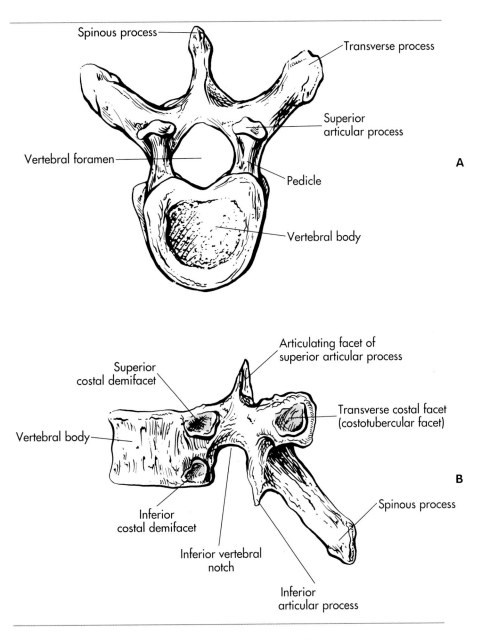

FIG. 6-1   Typical thoracic vertebra. **A,** Superior view. **B,** Lateral view.

prominent. The heart-shaped appearance is also accentuated because the anteroposterior dimension of the vertebral bodies increases, whereas the transverse dimension remains about the same. Typical thoracic vertebrae are also more flattened on their left surfaces than on their right because of pressure from the thoracic aorta. The T9 through T12 vertebral bodies begin to acquire lumbar characteristics (see following discussion) and to enlarge more in their transverse diameter than in the anteroposterior dimension. The T12 vertebral body is similar in shape to that of a lumbar vertebra. Experimental studies have shown that the vertebral bodies of the thoracic vertebrae become stronger from upper to lower thoracic vertebrae. This is an increase in bone density. The increase in bone density is probably a response to the increase in compressive forces placed on the successively lower vertebral bodies (Humzah & Soames, 1988).

Typical thoracic vertebral bodies have four small facets, two on each side, for articulation with the heads of two adjacent ribs. These facets are known as costal demifacets (literally, "half-facets") because the head of each rib articulates with both the superior demifacet of the vertebra with the same number and the inferior demifacet of the vertebra above (Fig. 6-5). For example, the head of the sixth rib articulates with the superior demifacet of T6 and the inferior demifacet of T5. A ridge on the head of each rib, known as the crest of the head, is located between the two articular surfaces of the rib head. The crest of the head of each rib has a ligamentous attachment (intraarticular ligament) to the intervertebral disc (IVD) between adjacent thoracic vertebrae. A fibrous capsule surrounds each vertebral demifacet and continues to the rib surrounding the articular surface on the corresponding half of the rib head. The capsule is lined by synovium, making the costovertebral joint (costocorporeal joint) a synovial joint (diarthrosis). The radiate ligaments extend from the head of each rib to the adjoining vertebral bodies and the surface of the intervening IVD (see Ligaments of the costocorporeal articulation).

Many structures attach to the thoracic vertebral bodies. Table 6-1 summarizes these attachments.

Pedicles. The pedicles of the thoracic spine are rather long and stout. They become larger on their inferior surface from T1 to T12. Unlike the cervical pedicles, which attach at a significant lateral angle with the cervical vertebral bodies, the thoracic pedicles form only a slight lateral angle in the transverse plane with the thoracic vertebral bodies (with the exception of T12, which forms no angle with the vertebral body in this plane). The thoracic pedicles incline slightly superiorly in the sagittal plane (Marchesi et al., 1988). They also attach very high on their respective vertebral bodies, and as a result, no superior vertebral notch is associated with typical thoracic vertebrae. T1, which is atypical, does have a

superior vertebrae notch (see following discussion). On the other hand, the inferior vertebral notches of the typical thoracic vertebrae are very prominent.

Transverse Processes. The transverse processes (TPs) of typical thoracic vertebrae project obliquely posteriorly (see Chapter 2). They also lie in a more posterior plane than those of the cervical or lumbar regions, being located behind the pedicles, intervertebral foramina, and articular processes of the thoracic vertebrae (Williams et al., 1989). The TPs also become progressively shorter from T1 to T12.

Each thoracic TP possesses a facet for articulation with the articular tubercle of the corresponding rib (e.g., the TP of T6 articulates with the sixth rib). This facet is appropriately named the transverse costal facet, or costal facet of the transverse process, and is located on the anterior surface of the TP.

The first six transverse costal facets are rather concave and face not only *anteriorly* but also slightly *laterally*. The transverse costal facets inferior to T6 are more planar (flatter) in shape, and they face *anteriorly, laterally,* and *superiorly.* The forces applied to the ribs during movements, load carrying, or muscular contraction are transmitted through the TPs to the laminae of the thoracic vertebrae (Pal et al., 1988).

The TPs serve as attachment sites for many muscles and ligaments. Table 6-2 lists the most important attachments to the TPs of thoracic vertebrae.

The distance between the tips of the left and right TPs is the greatest at T1 and then decreases incrementally until T12, where the TPs are quite small. This distance then increases in the lumbar region (see Chapter 7).

Articular Processes. The superior articular processes of the thoracic spine are small superior projections of bone oriented in a plane that lies approximately 60° to the horizontal plane (White & Panjabi, 1990). This makes them much more vertically oriented than the cervical superior articular processes. The superior thoracic processes face posteriorly, slightly superiorly, and laterally (Fig. 6-1). The inferior articular processes and their facets face anteriorly, slightly inferiorly, and medially. The orientation of the thoracic articular processes and their articulating facets allows for a significant amount of

Table 6-1 Attachments to Thoracic Vertebral Bodies

Region	Structure(s) attached
Anterior surface	Anterior longitudinal ligament, origin of longus colli muscle (T1, T2, T3, lateral to anterior longitudinal ligament)
Posterior surface	Posterior longitudinal ligament
Lateral surface	Origin of psoas major and minor muscles from T12

rotation to occur in this region (see section on ranges of motions). Flexion, extension, and lateral flexion are all quite limited, partly because of the orientation of the thoracic facets. However, the firm attachment of the thoracic vertebrae to the relatively immobile thoracic cage, by means of the costocorporeal and costotransverse articulations, is the primary reason movement of the thoracic spine is so limited.

Laminae. The laminae in the thoracic region are short from medial to lateral, broad from superior to inferior, and thick from anterior to posterior. They completely protect the vertebral canal from behind. Therefore no space exists between the laminae of adjacent vertebrae in a dried preparation. This is unique to thoracic vertebrae. The rotators longus and brevis muscles partially insert on the laminae of the thoracic vertebrae.

Vertebral Canal. The vertebral canal in the thoracic region is more smoothly rounded in shape than any other region. It is also smaller in the thoracic region than either the cervical or the lumbar regions. The thoracic spinal cord is also smaller than the other regions of the spinal cord.

Spinous Processes. The spinous processes of thoracic vertebrae are generally quite large. The upper four thoracic spinous processes project almost directly posteriorly. The next four (T5 through T8) project dramatically inferiorly. The spinous process of T8 is the longest of this group. The last four thoracic spinous processes begin to acquire the characteristics of lumbar spinous processes by projecting more directly posteriorly and being larger in their superior-to-inferior dimension (see Unique Thoracic Vertebrae). The spinous processes of thoracic vertebrae serve as attachment sites for many muscles and ligaments. Because of the length of the thoracic region, attachments vary somewhat from the upper to lower thoracic vertebrae. Table 6-3 lists the attachments to the spinous processes of the upper and lower thoracic spinous processes.

Intervertebral Foramina. The intervertebral foramina (IVFs) are covered in detail in Chapter 2. The IVFs in the thoracic region differ from those of the cervical region by facing directly laterally rather than facing obliquely anterolaterally. The lateral orientation of the thoracic IVFs is similar to that found in the lumbar region.

Unique to the thoracic region is that the T1 through T10 IVFs are associated with the ribs. The eleventh and twelfth ribs are not directly associated with IVFs. More precisely, the following structures are associated with the T1 through T10 IVFs: the head of the closest rib (e.g., T5-6 IVF associated with head of sixth rib), the articulation for the rib with the demifacets of the vertebral bodies, and the associated ligamentous and capsular attachments with the vertebral bodies and the interposed IVD (see Costocorporeal Articulations). All these structures help to form the anterior and inferior boundary of the first 10 thoracic IVFs. Pathologic conditions of these articulations may compromise the contents of the thoracic IVFs (Williams et al., 1989).

About one twelfth of the IVF contains spinal nerve in the thoracic region, whereas approximately one fifth of the IVF contains spinal nerve in the cervical region, and approximately one third of the IVF is filled with spinal nerve in the lumbar region. This may be one reason why radiculopathy as a result of IVD protrusion is much less common in the thoracic region than in the lumbar or cervical areas. Thoracic disc protrusion is also less common than cervical or lumbar disc protrusion. One reason may be that the thoracic spine is rendered less movable than the cervical and lumbar regions. This is because the

Table 6-2	Attachments to Thoracic Transverse Processes
Region	**Structure(s) attached**
Anterior surface (medial to transverse costal facet)	Costotransverse ligament
Apex	Lateral costotransverse ligament
Posterior apex	Levator costarum muscle
Inferior surface	Superior costotransverse ligament
Superior border	Intertransversarius muscle (or remnant)
Inferior border	Intertransversarius muscle (or remnant)
Posterior surface	Deep back muscles (longissimus thoracis, semispinalis thoracis and cervicis, multifidus thoracis, rotatores thoracis longus and brevis)

Data from Williams et al. (1989). *Gray's anatomy* (37th ed.). Edinburgh: Churchill Livingstone.

Table 6-3	Attachments to Thoracic Spinous Processes
Region	**Structure(s) attached**
Upper thoracic region	Ligaments: supraspinous, interspinous
	Muscles: trapezius, rhomboid major and minor, serratus posterior superior, deep back muscles (erector spinae and transversospinalis)
Lower thoracic region	Ligaments: supraspinous, interspinous
	Muscles: trapezius, latissimus dorsi, serratus posterior inferior, deep back muscles (erector spinae and transversospinalis)

Data from Williams et al. (1989). *Gray's anatomy* (37th ed.). Edinburgh: Churchill Livingstone.

thoracic region is strongly supported by the ribs and sternum. The reduced motion may result in a reduction of stress on the thoracic IVDs.

Thoracic Cage

Since the bony elements of the thoracic cage are so intimately involved with the thoracic vertebrae, it is appropriate to discuss them here. However, because the primary focus of this book is the spine, the ribs and sternum are not discussed in as much detail as the vertebrae. The intercostal muscles of the thoracic wall are covered in Chapter 4.

Components of the Thoracic Cage. The components of the thoracic cage (Fig. 6-2) include the following:
- Anteriorly: sternum, costal cartilages
- Laterally: ribs
- Posteriorly: T1 through T12

Thoracic Inlet. The thoracic cage is bounded superiorly by the superior thoracic aperture and inferiorly by the inferior thoracic aperture. The superior thoracic aperture (thoracic inlet) is bounded by the following: T1, first ribs (left and right), and superior aspect of the sternum. The superior thoracic aperture allows anatomic structures of the thorax and the neck to connect.

Clinically, the term *thoracic inlet* has a slightly different meaning. It refers to the superior thoracic aperture, the region just above the first rib, and the opening between the clavicle and the first rib. Ironically, the term *thoracic outlet syndrome* is frequently used to describe symptoms and signs arising from compromise of the neural or vascular structures as they pass through the region of the thoracic *inlet.* The symptoms associated with this syndrome are typically felt in the distal aspect of the upper extremity rather than the area of neurovascular compromise (Bland, 1987). The occurrence of thoracic outlet syndrome remains a matter of clinical debate, with some authorities stating that true compression of these structures is extremely rare. Others are convinced that such compression is rather common. This section discusses the areas and structures typically associated with the thoracic outlet syndrome.

The right and left subclavian arteries and veins pass through the superior thoracic aperture. These vessels may be compromised by pathologic conditions of the lower cervical or upper thoracic viscera. Examples include lymphosarcoma affecting the lymphatics of the thoracic inlet (Moore, 1992) and tumors of the apex of the lung (Pancoast tumor), the esophagus, and the thyroid gland.

As the subclavian arteries and veins exit the superior thoracic aperture, they are met by the inferior structures of the brachial plexus. These neural structures include the anterior primary divisions of C8 and T1 and their union as the inferior trunk of the brachial plexus. All these vascular and neural structures pass over the first rib. The subclavian artery and the inferior trunk of the brachial plexus course directly across the first rib between the insertions of the anterior and middle scalene muscles. The subclavian vein passes over the first rib anterior to the anterior scalene muscle. The inferior trunk of the brachial plexus and the subclavian artery are thought to be vulnerable in this region. Anomalous insertion of the scalenes or an inferior trunk of the brachial plexus, which pierces either the anterior or the middle scalene muscles, may provide the means by which these structures may become entrapped. Extension of the neck and rotation to the same side closes the interval between the anterior and middle scalene muscles, providing another possible mechanism of compromise. An elongated TP of C7 or a cervical rib (see Chapter 5) can dramatically crowd this region, and many believe that either one is a significant contributor to thoracic outlet syndrome (Bland, 1987; Foreman & Crofts, 1988). Cervical ribs range considerably in size, and even the smallest cervical rib can be associated with fibrous bands running from the cervical rib to the first rib or sternum. Any or all of these structures could restrict the subclavian vessels and the inferior trunk of the brachial plexus.

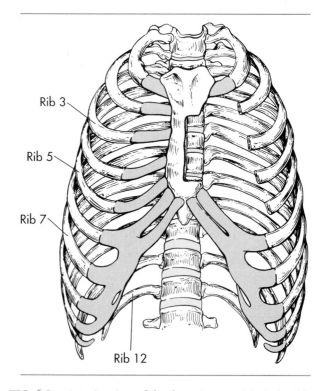

FIG. 6-2 Anterior view of the thoracic cage. A "window" has been removed (left side of thorax) to show to better advantage the relationship between the ribs and vertebrae.

The subclavian artery becomes the axillary artery at the lateral border of the first rib. Surrounding the transition region of the subclavian artery to the axillary artery are the divisions of the brachial plexus, which soon combine into the cords of the plexus. The divisions and cords pass beneath the clavicle and can be compressed between the clavicle and the first rib.

The axillary artery is surrounded by the cords of the brachial plexus as the artery passes beneath the coracoid process of the scapula. The axillary vein accompanies the artery in this region. The pectoralis minor muscle passes anterior to these structures as it inserts onto the coracoid process. The axillary artery, axillary vein, and the cords of the brachial plexus may be compressed against the coracoid process and the tendon of the pectoralis minor muscle during abduction and lateral rotation of the arm.

Inferior Thoracic Aperture. The inferior thoracic aperture (thoracic outlet) is bounded by the following: T12, 12th ribs, anterior costal margins, and the xiphisternal joint. The inferior thoracic aperture contains the diaphragm, which serves as the boundary between the thorax and the abdomen.

General Characteristics of the Thoracic Cage. The thoracic cage functions to protect underlying structures, support underlying structures (e.g., pericardium via sternopericardial ligaments), support overlying muscles and skin, and assist in respiration.

The adult thorax is wider from side to side than front to back. During inspiration the anteroposterior diameter increases. This is quite different than a child's thorax, which is circular in shape and therefore does not allow change to occur during inspiration. In contrast to adults, children rely almost completely on the excursions of the diaphragm for respiration.

Ribs

Certain groups of cells throughout the spine, known as the costal elements, have the ability to develop into ribs (see Chapter 2) and do so in the thoracic region. These thoracic costal elements push through the ventral myotomal plates, which form the intercostal muscles. The costal elements further develop to become precartilaginous ribs, which, after undergoing chondrification and then ossification, become the ribs themselves. The TPs of the thoracic vertebrae grow behind the proximal ends of the developing ribs and are united to them by mesenchyme. This mesenchyme forms the articulations and the ligaments of the costocorporeal and the costotransverse joints. The fully developed ribs serve to protect the underlying thoracic viscera while at the same time they provide attachment sites for a wide variety of muscles (Table 6-4).

Typical Ribs. The typical ribs are ribs three through nine. Each consists of a head, neck, tubercle, and shaft (Fig. 6-3).

Table 6-4 Relationships of the Thoracic Cage

Region	Structure(s) attached
Superiorly	Sternocleidomastoid, sternohyoid, sternothyroid, and anterior, middle, and posterior scalene muscles
Anteriorly	Pectoralis major and minor muscles, mammary glands
Posteriorly	Serratus posterior superior and inferior, and deep back muscles; trapezius, rhomboid minor and major, scapula and all muscles related to it rest against the thoracic cage
Laterally	Serratus anterior muscles
Inferiorly	Abdominal muscles attaching to thoracic cage (i.e., rectus abdominis, external and internal abdominal oblique, transversus abdominis)

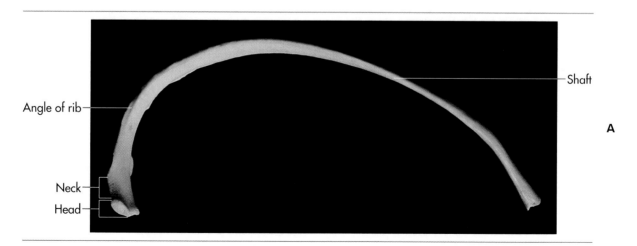

FIG. 6-3   Three views of a typical rib. **A,** Superior view.   *Continued.*

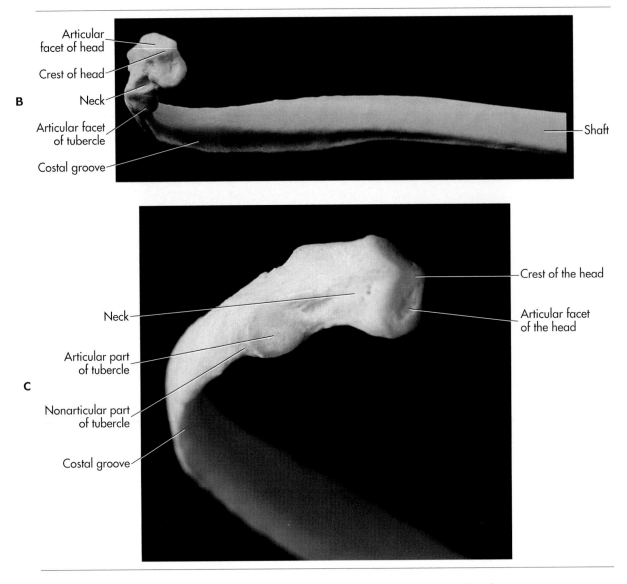

FIG. 6-3, cont'd.   **B,** The head, angle, and shaft of a rib. **C,** Close-up of the head and neck.

The head of a typical rib articulates with two adjacent vertebral bodies (see Vertebral Bodies). Inferior and superior articular facets of the rib head articulate with the superior costal demifacet of the same-number vertebra as the rib and with the inferior costal demifacet of the vertebra above, respectively. The crest of the head is a ridge that runs between the two articular surfaces of the rib head. The crest is joined by the intraarticular ligament to the adjacent IVD. This creates the two separate components of the costocorporeal joints, one superior to the crest of the head of the rib, and one inferior to the crest (see Costocorporeal Articulations and Fig. 6-5).

The neck of a typical rib is located between its head and tubercle. The neck serves as the attachment site for the costotransverse ligament and the superior costotransverse ligament.

The tubercle of a rib is a process that forms the lateral boundary of the neck and the beginning of the shaft. It possesses an articular facet (articular portion) for articulation with the transverse costal facet on the TP of a typical thoracic vertebra. The tubercle of a rib articulates with the same-number vertebra as the rib (e.g., fourth rib articulates with TP of T4). The tubercle also contains a nonarticular part lateral to the articular portion. The nonarticular region serves as an attachment site for the lateral costotransverse ligament.

The shaft of a rib begins at the articular tubercle and extends distally to the end of the rib at its articulation with the costal cartilage. The typical ribs curve inferiorly and anteriorly. Much of this anterior curve is achieved at the angle of the rib. The angle of the rib is located a few centimeters distal to the articular tubercle and is where the shaft makes the sharpest anterior bend.

A costal depression or groove, located on the inferior aspect of each rib, shelters (from superior to inferior) the intercostal vein, artery, and nerve.

Anteriorly, each typical rib attaches to the costal cartilage. The costal cartilage, in turn, joins each of the first through seventh ribs with the sternum. The eighth through tenth costal cartilages articulate with the costal cartilage immediately above. The xiphoid process, seventh costal cartilage, and the union of the eighth through tenth costal cartilages together form the substernal angle.

Atypical Ribs. The first, second, tenth, eleventh, and twelfth ribs all have special features (Williams et al., 1989). The first rib is short, flat, and strong. It lies almost completely in the horizontal plane and does not angle inferiorly as do typical ribs. Its superior surface is marked by a scalene tubercle (for insertion of the anterior scalene muscle). The subclavian vein runs anterior to the scalene tubercle (and the anterior scalene muscle), and the subclavian artery and inferior trunk of the brachial plexus run posterior to this tubercle. The first rib usually articulates with only one vertebra (T1). Occasionally the head also articulates with the body of C7.

The second rib is much more typical than the first and is almost twice its size. The major distinguishing characteristic of the second rib is a tuberosity on its superior surface, which serves as the partial origin of the serratus anterior muscle.

The tenth rib has only a single facet, and no crest, on its head. The head articulates with the large, single costal facet on the lateral aspect of the body (close to the pedicle) of T10. Sometimes the head of the tenth rib also articulates with the IVD between T9 and T10.

The eleventh and twelfth ribs are quite short, and neither possesses a neck or tubercle. They are considered to be free, or floating ribs because they do not attach to costal cartilage anteriorly. As with the first and tenth ribs, the eleventh and twelfth each articulate with only one vertebra (T11 and T12, respectively).

Sternum

The sternum develops from left and right bars of mesenchyme that migrate to the midline and eventually fuse. The fully developed sternum is composed of a manubrium, body, and xiphoid process. The superior aspect of the manubrium is at the level of the T2-3 IVD. The manubrium possesses a superior concavity known as the jugular notch (Fig. 6-2). Lateral to the jugular notch is the clavicular notch, which projects superolaterally, allowing its concavity to articulate with the clavicle. The apex of the lung extends above the sternoclavicular joint and the clavicle. The lung is vulnerable here

and may be punctured from the anterior in this region. Inferior to the clavicular notch, on the lateral aspect of the manubrium, is the articulation with the first costal cartilage (Fig. 6-2).

The inferior margin of the manubrium joins the body of the sternum. The manubriosternal joint is usually a symphysis, although occasionally it may develop a joint cavity, giving it characteristics of a synovial joint. The sternal angle (of Lewis) is formed by the angle between the manubrium and the body of the sternum at the manubriosternal symphysis (Fig. 6-2). This angle makes the sternum slightly convex anteriorly. The second costal cartilage articulates with the sternum at this angle. The sternal angle is located on a horizontal plane that posteriorly passes approximately through the level of the T4-5 IVD (this level varies from the vertebral bodies of T4 to T6; see Chapter 1). Other anatomic structures are present at the general level of this plane. These include the bifurcation of the trachea into primary (mainstem) bronchi, the hilus of the lung, and the superior extent of the aortic arch.

The body of the sternum is formed by the union of four segments known as sternebrae. The lateral margin is notched for articulation with costal cartilages of ribs. The inferior process of the sternum is the xiphoid process. It is joined with the body of the sternum by a symphysis that usually ossifies by 40 years of age. The xiphoid process also articulates with the costal cartilage of the seventh rib.

◆ ◆ ◆

The thoracic cage serves as an attachment site for a variety of structures. See Table 6-4 for structures associated with various regions of the thoracic cage.

UNIQUE THORACIC VERTEBRAE

Several thoracic vertebrae have distinct characteristics: T1, T9 (occasionally), T10, T11, and T12. They can best be considered as unique, not atypical, thoracic vertebrae.

First Thoracic Vertebra

T1 possesses two characteristics associated with cervical vertebrae but not normally found on typical thoracic vertebrae: the presence of uncinate processes on T1 and the presence of superior vertebral notches above the pedicles of T1. In addition, the vertebral body of T1 resembles that of a cervical vertebra, being rectangular in shape instead of heart shaped, with the transverse diameter greater than the anteroposterior diameter.

The superior facet on the vertebral body for articulation with the head of the first rib is usually a full facet (not a demifacet). Occasionally the superior facet is a demifacet, allowing the first rib to attach to both T1 and C7 vertebral bodies and the intervening IVD. Frequently a deep depression can be found on the vertebral body just inferior to the superior costal facet of T1 (Williams et al., 1989). The inferior demifacet of T1 is typical. The spinous process of T1 is quite large, projects directly posteriorly, and is often as long and sometimes longer than the spinous process of C7.

Ninth Thoracic Vertebra

Occasionally the tenth rib does not articulate with the T9, resulting in the absence of an inferior demifacet on T9. The other characteristics of T9 conform to those of typical thoracic vertebrae.

Tenth Thoracic Vertebra

The vertebral body of T10 contains only a single facet on each side for articulation with the head of each tenth rib. As stated previously, typical thoracic vertebrae possess two demifacets on each side for articulation with the rib of the same number and with the rib below. The single facet is usually oval or semilunar in shape. The precise shape depends on whether the tenth rib articulates with just the body of T10 or also with the body of T9 and the IVD between the two. The former results in an oval-shaped facet, and the latter results in a semilunar-shaped facet. The TP of T10 does not always have a facet for articulation with the articular tubercle of the tenth rib.

Eleventh Thoracic Vertebra

T11 also has only a single facet on each side for articulation with the head of the eleventh rib. However, each facet is located on the pedicle. There is also no articular facet on the TP for articulation with the articular tubercle of the rib. Therefore the eleventh rib does not articulate with the TP of T11. The vertebral body of T11 also resembles that of a lumbar vertebra. The spinous process of T11 is almost triangular in shape with a blunt apex (Williams et al., 1989).

The superior articular processes of T11 resemble those of other thoracic vertebrae. However, usually T11 represents the transition of thoracic-type articular processes to the lumbar type. Therefore the inferior articular processes are usually convex and face anteriorly and laterally. The articular processes of thoracic vertebrae allow for rotation to be the primary movement, whereas the lumbar articular processes limit rotation but encourage flexion and some extension. This transition of facet type can also occur at T12 or occasionally T10.

Twelfth Thoracic Vertebra

The vertebral body of T12 is quite large, but the TPs are quite small. In fact, each TP is actually replaced by three smaller processes (Williams et al., 1989). One process projects laterally and is the equivalent of a thoracic TP except it is small. The largest of the three processes projects posteriorly and superiorly and is the homologue of the mamillary process of a lumbar vertebra. However, this mamillary process is not as closely related to the superior articular process as it is in the lumbar region. Finally, a small process that is homologous to the accessory process of lumbar vertebrae projects posteriorly and slightly inferiorly. T12 also has a single facet on each side for articulation with the head of the corresponding twelfth rib. The facet is circular and is located primarily on the pedicle but may extend onto the vertebral body. The small TP has no facet for articulation with the twelfth rib.

Thoracolumbar Junction

The left and right zygapophyseal (Z) joints between the T12 vertebra and the L1 vertebra are unique. At this joint the mamillary process (see Chapter 7) of each side overlaps the posterior aspect of the inferior articular process of T12. This usually occurs to a greater degree between these two vertebrae than at any other level. The result is that each inferior articular process of T12 fits closely into the superior articular process and overlying mamillary process of L1, much like a well made carpenter's joint (e.g., mortice and tenon joint). This prevents almost any movement except flexion from occurring at this articulation (Singer & Giles, 1990; Singer, Giles & Day, 1990). Singer and colleagues (1990) have shown large Z joint synovial folds (Chapter 2) protruding into this joint (Fig. 6-4). They also emphasize that normally almost no rotation occurs at this articulation.

LIGAMENTS AND JOINTS OF THE THORACIC REGION

Several ligaments found in the thoracic spine are also present in the cervical spine and are discussed in Chapter 5. These include the ligamenta flava, the anterior longitudinal ligament, the posterior longitudinal ligament, and the interspinous ligaments. The anterior longitudinal ligament in the thoracic region (see Figs. 6-7, 6-8, and 6-9, B) is thicker from anterior to posterior and thinner from side to side than in either the cervical or the lumbar regions. Also, the ligamenta flava in the thoracic region and the thoracolumbar junction may ossify in rare instances. Such ossification may result in compression of the spinal cord from behind (Hasue et al., 1983).

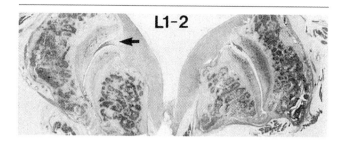

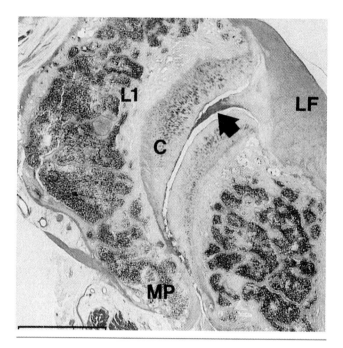

FIG. 6-4 Photomicrograph of the left Z joint at the thoracolumbar junction. L1 represents the superior articular process of L1. Notice that the mamillary process of L1 *(MP)* protrudes medially to overlap the inferior articular process of T12. Also notice the Z joint synovial fold *(arrow)* protruding into the joint space from the ligamentum flavum *(LF)*. (Courtesy of Singer et al., 1990).

Since the interspinous ligaments in the thoracic region are somewhat different than those in the cervical region, they are discussed in this section. The supraspinous ligament and thoracic intervertebral discs are also discussed here. Since the joints between the thoracic vertebrae and the ribs are unique to this region, much of this section on ligaments and joints of the thoracic region is devoted to these interesting and important articulations and the ligaments that support them. This section concludes with a discussion of the sternocostal and interchondral articulations.

Interspinous Ligaments

These ligaments run between adjacent spinous processes, filling the gap along the length of these pro-

cesses. Anteriorly each interspinous ligament is continuous with the ligamenta flava, and posteriorly each is continuous with the supraspinous ligament. Even though the thoracic interspinous ligaments are rather thin and membranous in structure, they are more fully developed in the thoracic region than in the cervical region. Some authors dispute their existence in the cervical region altogether, stating that they are simply thin, fascial, anterior extensions of the ligamentum nuchae (Williams et al., 1989). Controversy also surrounds the precise orientation of these ligaments (Behrsin & Briggs, 1988; Williams et al., 1989). Some authors believe the fibers of the interspinous ligament run from anterosuperior to posteroinferior, and others believe the fibers making up this ligament run from posterosuperior to anteroinferior (Paris, 1983; Scapinelli, 1989). The latter scenario is more likely. These interspinous ligaments have been studied more fully in the lumbar region, where they are better developed (see Chapter 7).

Supraspinous Ligament

The supraspinous ligament limits flexion of the spine. It is classically described as forming a continuous band that passes from the spinous process of C7 to the sacrum (Williams et al., 1989). However, disagreement exists as to whether or not it extends all the way to the sacrum. Some investigators believe it is almost nonexistent in the lumbar region (Behrsin & Briggs, 1988). Some authors state that it is divided into layers, with the deeper fibers running between adjacent vertebrae and the more superficial fibers spanning several (up to four) vertebrae (Williams et al., 1989). All the authors seem to agree that the deepest fibers of the thoracic supraspinous ligament become continuous with the interspinous ligaments. The supraspinous ligament seems to warrant further investigation.

Thoracic Intervertebral Discs

The thoracic IVDs have the thinnest superior-to-inferior dimension of the spine. Also, the discs of the upper thoracic region are narrower than those of the lower thoracic region. The upper thoracic region is also the least movable area of the thoracic spine. In contrast to the cervical and lumbar IVDs, which are thicker anteriorly than posteriorly, the thoracic IVDs are of more equal thickness in their anterior and posterior regions.

Calcification of the IVD is found with greater frequency in the thoracolumbar region than in any other region of the spine. Radiographic surveys have found thoracolumbar IVD calcification in 5% to 6% of adults. Postmortem examinations have found such calcification in up to 70% of adults. Disc calcification is usually asymptomatic unless it is associated with protrusion into the vertebral canal, in which case neurologic compression symptoms result (Lipson & O'Connell, 1991).

Thoracic IVD protrusion is rather infrequent, accounting for only 0.15% to 1.8% of all disc protrusions (Alvarez, Roque, & Pampati, 1988; Bauduin et al., 1989). However, they may be more common than previously believed (Vernon, Dooley, & Acusta, 1993). When present, this condition usually affects the lower thoracic discs of individuals primarily between 30 and 60 years of age (Otani et al., 1988). Symptoms vary dramatically from none at all to motor and sensory deficits resulting from spinal cord compression (myelopathy). Pain, muscle weakness, and spinal cord dysfunction are the most common clinical symptoms. Computed tomography (CT), in conjunction with contrast enhancement of the subarachnoid space (CT myelography), and magnetic resonance imaging (MRI) are useful in the detection of these rare but significant lesions (Alvarez et al., 1988;

Bauduin et al., 1989; Vernon et al., 1993). These modalities may allow for more frequent detection of thoracic IVD protrusion in the future.

Costovertebral Articulations

The ribs and vertebrae articulate in two locations. The first is the joint complex between the head of a rib and the adjacent vertebral bodies, known as the costocorporeal articulation. The second costovertebral articulation is between one rib and the TP, known as the costotransverse articulation.

Costocorporeal Articulations. The joint between the head of a rib and the adjoining typical thoracic vertebrae consists of articulations with the two adjacent vertebral bodies and the interposed IVD (Fig. 6-5). The rib head articulates with the superior demifacet of the

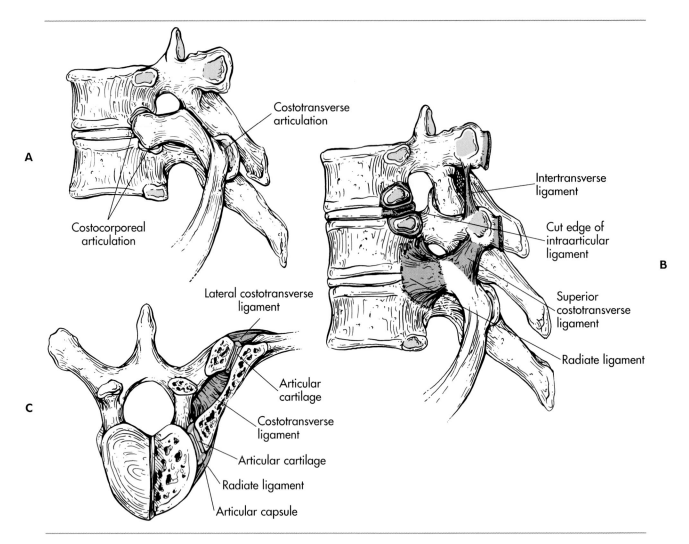

FIG. 6-5 Costovertebral articulations. **A,** Bony costocorporeal and costotransverse articulations. **B,** Ligamentous attachments of these joints. **C,** Superior view. The vertebra and rib have been horizontally sectioned on the right half of the illustration to demonstrate further the costocorporeal and costotransverse articulations.

same-number vertebra and with the inferior demifacet of the vertebra above (e.g., seventh rib articulates with superior demifacet of T7 and inferior demifacet of T6). The crest of the rib head is attached to the adjacent IVD by an intraarticular ligament. This short, flat ligament creates two distinct articular compartments (upper and lower) within the costocorporeal articulation. Both of these compartments are surrounded by a fibrous articular capsule lined with a synovial membrane. These synovial joints can best be classified as having ovoid articular surfaces, and the fibrous capsule extends around the ovoid articular surfaces of both the demifacet and the adjacent articular half of the rib head (Fig. 6-5). The capsule extends to the intraarticular ligament between the upper and lower compartments. The inferomedial fibers of the fibrous capsule blend with the IVD, and the posterior fibers blend with the costotransverse ligament. The heads of the first, tenth (occasionally), eleventh, and twelfth ribs form single ovoid synovial articulations with their respective ribs.

The ligaments of this compound joint include the capsular, intraarticular (both described previously), and radiate. Each radiate ligament (Fig. 6-5) associated with typical vertebrae attaches to the anterior aspect of the head of the articulating rib and the two vertebrae to which the head attaches. In addition, the radiate ligament attaches by horizontal fibers to the IVD between the two vertebrae. The superior fibers attach just above the superior demifacet and ascend to the vertebral body of the superior vertebra. Likewise, the inferior fibers attach just below the inferior demifacet and descend to the inferior vertebral body. The radiate ligament of the first rib has some superior fibers that attach to C7. The radiate ligaments of the tenth through twelfth ribs attach to only the vertebra with which the rib head articulates.

Costotransverse Articulation. This joint is composed of the costal (articular) tubercle of the rib articulating with the transverse costal facet (Fig. 6-5). Exceptions to this are the eleventh and twelfth ribs, which do not articulate with the TPs of their respective vertebrae. The joint surfaces of the upper five or six costotransverse joints are curved, with the transverse costal facet being concave and the articular tubercle convex. The remaining joints are more planar in configuration (Williams et al., 1989). A thin, fibrous capsule lined by a synovial membrane attaches to the two adjacent articular surfaces. A costotransverse foramen is found between the TP and the rib between the costotransverse and costocorporeal articulations. This foramen is filled by the costotransverse ligament. The costotransverse ligament passes from the posterior aspect of the rib neck to the anterior aspect of the adjacent TP (Fig. 6-5). For example, the costotransverse ligament of the sixth rib attaches to the posterior aspect of the sixth rib and to the anterior aspect of the TP of T6.

The ligaments of the costotransverse articulation include the articular capsule, costotransverse ligament (both described previously), superior costotransverse ligament, and lateral costotransverse ligament (Fig. 6-5). The strong but short lateral costotransverse ligament runs directly laterally from the lateral margin of the TP to the nonarticular region of the costal tubercle of the adjacent rib (Fig. 6-5). This ligament is found at every thoracic segment. The ligaments of the upper thoracic vertebrae run slightly superiorly, as well as laterally, whereas the lower ones run slightly inferiorly, as well as laterally.

A superior costotransverse ligament courses between the neck of each rib, except for the first, and the TP of the vertebra above. This ligament is divided into two parts, anterior and posterior. Both parts course superiorly from a rib neck to the inferior border of the TP immediately above. The anterior layer angles slightly laterally as it ascends and blends with the posterior intercostal membrane (see Fig. 6-8, *B*). The posterior layer angles slightly medially. Because it is more posteriorly placed, this ligament blends with the external intercostal muscle laterally. The intercostal vein, artery, and nerve run across the anterior surface of these ligaments. An accessory ligament is normally found medial to the superior costotransverse ligament. This accessory ligament is separated from the superior costotransverse ligament by a gap that is filled by the posterior primary division as it leaves the mixed spinal nerve to reach the more posterior structures of the spine. More specifically, the accessory ligament originates medial to the costal tubercle and runs superiorly to the inferior articular process of the vertebra above, although some fibers reach the TP. A lumbocostal ligament runs from the inferior border of the twelfth rib shaft to the superior surface of the TP of L1.

Sternocostal and Interchondral Articulations

The costal cartilages of the first through seventh ribs articulate directly with the sternum at the sternocostal joints (see Fig. 6-2). The costal cartilages of the eighth through tenth ribs attach to the costal cartilage of the rib above at articulations known as the interchondral joints.

Sternocostal Joints. A rather complex type of synarthrosis exists between the first costal cartilage and the manubrium. A thin piece of fibrocartilage is interposed between the two surfaces and is tightly adherent to both (Williams et al., 1989). A radiate ligament also unites the two surfaces. The joint between the second costal cartilage and the sternum is synovial and is separated into two compartments by an intraarticular ligament. Small synovial joints are located between the costal cartilages of the third through seventh ribs and the sternum. The costal cartilages and the sternum are united by the fibrous capsules of the joints and radiate ligaments that run from the anterior and posterior surface of each costal cartilage to the sternum. A small amount of rotation occurs at these joints. This rotation allows for the thorax to expand and contract during inspiration and expiration, respectively.

Interchondral Joints. As mentioned, the eighth through tenth costal cartilages articulate with the costal cartilage immediately above. Small synovial joints are formed at the attachment sites for the eighth and ninth ribs. The costal cartilage of the tenth rib is usually continuous with the costal cartilage of the ninth rib, and no true joint unites the two. Occasionally, no attachment exists between the tenth rib and the costal cartilage of the ninth rib. Although both the sixth and the seventh costal cartilages attach directly to the sternum, their most distal portions also contact one another. Small synovial joints are also located where these cartilages are in contact with one another.

RANGES OF MOTION IN THE THORACIC SPINE

Vertebral Motion

As stated previously, the facets of the thoracic vertebrae are oriented 60° to the horizontal plane. Therefore they are more vertically oriented than the articular processes of the cervical region. This vertical orientation dramatically limits forward flexion. Extension is limited by the inferior articular processes contacting the laminae of the vertebrae below and also by contact between adjacent spinous processes. Rotation is the dominant movement in the thoracic region. However, the vertebrae are a part of the entire thoracic cage and even this motion is limited considerably. This may help to explain why the lower thoracic region, with its relation to floating ribs and ribs with only an indirect attachment to the sternum, is the most mobile part of the thoracic spine. Ranges of motion of the thoracic spine include the following:

Combined flexion and extension	34°
Unilateral lateral flexion	15°
Unilateral axial rotation	35°

Motion of the Ribs

Motion of the ribs at the costocorporeal and costotransverse articulations is primarily one of rotation with a slight gliding motion. Motion is quite limited because of the strong ligamentous attachments. Upward and downward rotation is the primary movement of the upper six ribs, accompanied by slight superior and inferior gliding. Rotation of the seventh through tenth ribs is accompanied by more gliding than in the ribs above. This is because the transverse costal facets of T7 through T10 are more flat than those of the vertebrae above and also because the facets face upward, anteriorly, and laterally. Upward rotation of these lower ribs is accompanied by posterior and medial gliding, and downward rotation is accompanied by anterior and slightly lateral gliding. These movements tend to open and close the substernal angle, respectively (Williams et al., 1989).

LATERAL CURVATURE OF THE SPINE

Lateral curvature or lateral deviation of the spine is known as scoliosis (Fig. 6-6). A slight lateral curve with the convexity on the same side as handedness (i.e., convexity to the left in left-handed individuals) is normally found in the upper thoracic region (see Chapter 2). This is a result of the pull of the stronger musculature on the side of handedness. Lateral curves other than this mild upper thoracic curve are considered to be a variation from normal spinal structure. These scolioses range from being barely perceptible and insignificant deviations to extremely dramatic curvatures.

Scoliosis can be found in any spinal region, but the thoracic region is usually the most prominently affected, partly because of its length and central location. The thoracic region is the most noticeably affected primarily because the attachment of the rest of the thoracic cage to the thoracic vertebrae can result in deformation of the entire thorax. In addition, curvatures of the thoracic spine are more or less "held in place" by the remainder of the thoracic cage (ribs and sternum). In fact, with full forward flexion of the spine, posterior elevation on one side of the thorax ("rib hump") of 6 mm or greater has been used as one of the primary indicators of scoliosis. The incidence of such posterior thoracic elevation has been reported as 4.1% in fourth-grade schoolchildren with an average age of 10.8 years (Nissinen et al., 1989). Occasionally, scoliosis is so severe that serious compromise of lung capacity and cardiac output may result. A detailed discussion of this important clinical topic is beyond the scope of this book. However, a brief description of the most important anatomic components of scoliosis is appropriate.

Scoliosis has many causes, ranging from developmental and anatomic, such as cuneiform vertebrae (hemivertebra; see Chapter 2), to unknown causes (idiopathic). Idiopathic scoliosis is typically characterized by the presence of a concomitant lordosis at the apex of the lateral curve (Deacon, Archer, & Dickson, 1987). Idiopathic scoliosis is probably multifactorial in origin and may involve genetic, biomechanic, metabolic, growth, and central nervous system factors (Cook et al., 1986). A lesion of the posterior column pathway, above the level of the lower cervical region, resulting in hypersensitivity of proprioception and vibration sense has been implicated as a major factor in scoliosis (Wyatt et al., 1986). Other

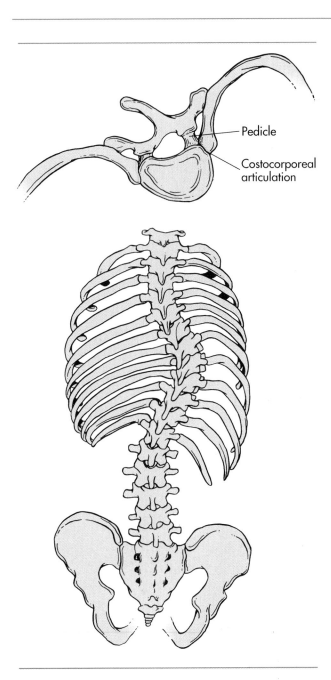

- Pedicle
- Costocorporeal articulation

FIG. 6-6 *Bottom,* Posterior view of a scoliotic spine. *Top,* Superior view of a single vertebra and the articulating ribs. Notice the asymmetry between the left and right costocorporeal and costovertebral articulations (compare with Fig. 6-5). (Modified from Netter, 1990.)

neurologic differences have been found between scoliotic patients and control subjects. These include differences in labyrinthine, visual, and vestibular functions (Cook et al., 1986).

The posterior elements of scoliotic spines have been found to be smaller in their superior-to-inferior dimensions than the posterior elements of normal spines (Deane & Duthie, 1973). Vital and colleagues (1989) found that the neurocentral vertebral cartilage (synchondrosis) of scoliotic spines was more open on the

side of concavity. This suggested to the authors that this cartilage may have undergone early closure on the opposite side. Since part of the function of the neurocentral cartilage is to ensure growth of the posterior arch of the vertebra (see Chapter 2), early closure of one cartilage could result in asymmetric vertebral growth. The authors thought further investigation was necessary to determine if the neurocentral synchondrosis was a primary cause of lateral curvature or if it was simply influenced by other causes (e.g., asymmetric muscular or neurologic activity).

NERVES, VESSELS, AND VISCERA RELATED TO THE THORACIC SPINE

The thoracic spine and the ribs are intimately related to many neural, vascular, and visceral structures (Figs. 6-7 and 6-8). The structures most closely related to the spine and ribs include posterior primary divisions; the intercostal arteries, veins, and nerves; azygos, hemiazygos, and accessory hemiazygos veins; thoracic duct and thoracic lymphatics; thoracic aorta; esophagus; trachea; vagus nerves; thoracic sympathetic chain; and splanchnic nerves. These structures are discussed briefly in this section. Chapter 1 and Table 1-1 relate many of the most important visceral structures to vertebral body levels to aid in the interpretation of scans presenting cross-sectional anatomy (CT, MRI). The intercostal muscles are discussed in Chapter 4.

Posterior Primary Divisions (Dorsal Rami)

The thoracic mixed spinal nerves are formed within the IVF by the union of the thoracic dorsal and ventral roots. The roots in the upper thoracic region descend only slightly before entering the IVF, whereas the roots of the lower thoracic region may descend as much as two vertebral levels before entering the IVF. Once formed, the mixed spinal nerves contain both sensory and motor fibers. Each mixed spinal nerve then divides into a posterior primary division (dorsal ramus) and an anterior primary division (ventral ramus) as it exits the IVF (Fig. 6-8, *B*). The anterior primary division of a thoracic nerve becomes an intercostal nerve and the subcostal nerve at the level of T12 (see following discussion). The posterior primary division (dorsal ramus) passes posteriorly across the lateral aspect of the Z joint, to which it sends fine branches. It then passes through a small but adequate opening bounded superiorly by the TP, inferiorly by the rib of the vertebra below (e.g., T5 nerve exits between T5 and T6 vertebrae and above sixth rib), medially by the Z joint, and laterally by the superior costotransverse ligament, which attaches to the rib below. This opening is known as the costotransverse foramen of Cruveilhier. The dorsal ramus then divides into medial and lateral branches. The lateral

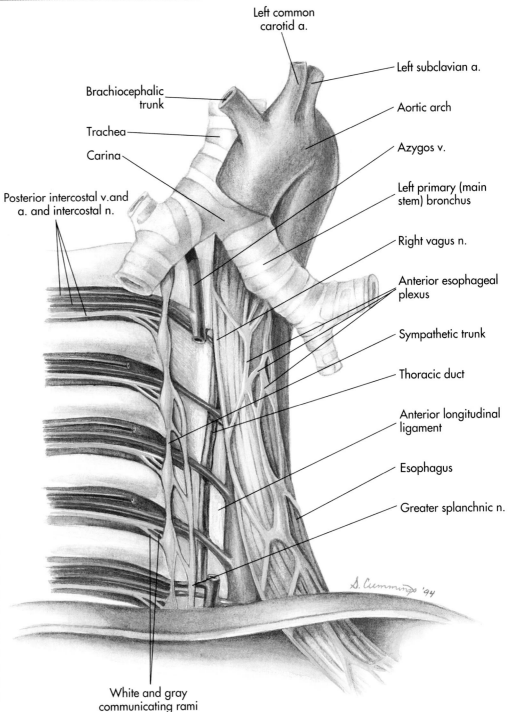

Left common
carotid a.

Left subclavian a.

Brachiocephalic
trunk

Aortic arch

Trachea

Azygos v.

Carina

Left primary (main
stem) bronchus

Posterior intercostal v.and
a. and intercostal n.

Right vagus n.

Anterior esophageal
plexus

Sympathetic trunk

Thoracic duct

Anterior longitudinal
ligament

Esophagus

Greater splanchnic n.

S. Cummings '94

White and gray
communicating rami

FIG. 6-7 Posterior thoracic wall showing the relationship of the vertebrae and ribs to the vessels and nerves of the thorax. The right vagus nerve is shown sending a few branches to the anterior esophageal plexus. The more abundant and important contributions to the posterior esophageal plexus cannot be seen from this perspective.

branch supplies the erector spinae muscles in the region and continues to provide sensory innervation to the skin of the back.

Not all of the first six lateral branches of the posterior primary divisions reach the skin. However, the lower six lateral branches all have significant cutaneous distributions. They supply the skin superficial to the spinous processes via medial cutaneous branches (of the lateral branches of the posterior primary divisions) and supply sensory innervation to the skin several inches lateral to the midline via lateral cutaneous branches (of the lateral branches of the posterior primary divisions). The lateral cutaneous branches may descend as far as four ribs before reaching the skin. The lateral cutaneous branch of the posterior primary division of T12 reaches the upper border of the iliac crest.

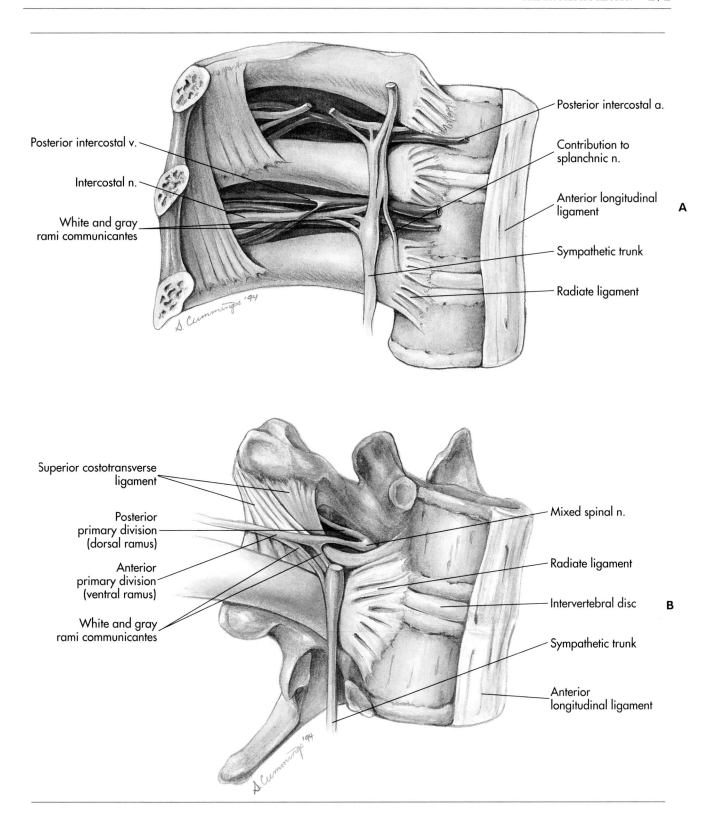

Posterior intercostal v.

Intercostal n.

White and gray rami communicantes

Posterior intercostal a.

Contribution to splanchnic n.

Anterior longitudinal ligament

Sympathetic trunk

Radiate ligament

A

Superior costotransverse ligament

Posterior primary division (dorsal ramus)

Anterior primary division (ventral ramus)

White and gray rami communicantes

Mixed spinal n.

Radiate ligament

Intervertebral disc

Sympathetic trunk

Anterior longitudinal ligament

B

FIG. 6-8   A, Nerves and vessels related to three adjacent thoracic vertebrae and the ribs that articulate with them. **B,** Close-up of the nerves associated with a single thoracic motion segment (two adjacent thoracic vertebrae).

A typical medial branch of a posterior primary division runs a rather tortuous course between the multifidus muscle on its medial surface and the levator costarum muscle on its lateral side (Maigne, Maigne, & Guerin-Surville, 1991). It then continues posteromedially and slightly inferiorly, running medial to most of the longissimus thoracis muscle fibers. The dorsal rami of the second, third, and fourth thoracic nerves then pass through the tendon of the splenius cervicis muscle, continue through the rhomboid muscles, pierce the trapezius muscle, and then reach the skin adjacent to the spinous process of its vertebra of origin (e.g., T3 nerve innervating region of T3 spinous process). The medial branches of the fifth and sixth thoracic nerves also reach the skin of the back.

Maigne and colleagues (1991) found that the upper thoracic medial branches of the dorsal rami frequently appeared to be entrapped in tendons of the erector spinae or splenius cervicis muscle. They believed this helped to explain localized areas of thoracic discomfort with associated hypesthesia and paresthesia frequently seen in their clinical practice. Also, in 1 of the 16 cadavers studied, the authors found a bilateral anastomosis between the medial branch of the dorsal ramus of T2 and the accessory nerve. They thought this may explain the occasional lack of paralysis of the trapezius muscle among certain individuals after transection of the accessory nerve during neck surgery.

The medial branches of the posterior primary divisions of the lower six thoracic nerves pass posteriorly to innervate primarily the multifidi, rotatores, and longissimus thoracis muscles; they only occasionally reach the skin of the back (Williams et al., 1989).

Intercostal Nerves, Arteries, and Veins

Intercostal Nerves. The anterior primary divisions of the T1 to T11 nerves are the intercostal nerves (Figs. 6-7 and 6-8). The ventral ramus of the T1 nerve splits, and the larger branch joins the ventral ramus of C8 to form the inferior trunk of the brachial plexus. The smaller branch of the ventral ramus of T1 forms the first intercostal nerve. The anterior primary division of the T12 nerve is the subcostal nerve.

Very close to its origin, each intercostal nerve (and the subcostal and upper two lumbar nerves) sends a white ramus communicans to the sympathetic ganglion of the same level. These ganglia are located anterior to the intercostal nerves and lie along the lateral aspect of the vertebral bodies.

The intercostal nerves also receive gray rami communicantes from the neighboring sympathetic ganglia (Fig. 6-8). This is similar to all other anterior primary divisions. The intercostal nerve then continues laterally along the subcostal groove, inferior to the intercostal vein and artery (Figs. 6-7 and 6-9). The lateral course of the intercostal nerve, within the posterior intercostal space, is subject to a rather wide degree of variation. The intercostal nerve frequently runs within the middle of the intercostal space (73% of the time) and may occasionally run along the inferior aspect of the intercostal space just above the subjacent rib (Hardy, 1988).

Each intercostal nerve provides sensory, motor (somatic motor), and sympathetic (visceral motor to blood vessels and sweat glands) innervation to the thoracic or abdominal wall. This is accomplished by means of posterior, lateral, and anterior branches.

Posterior Intercostal Arteries. The third through eleventh intercostal arteries originate from the thoracic aorta and course laterally along the inferior aspect of the corresponding rib (Fig. 6-7 and 6-9, A). The artery that runs below the twelfth rib is known as the subcostal artery because it lies inferior to the twelfth rib and not between two ribs. The first two intercostal arteries arise from the highest intercostal artery. The highest intercostal artery is a branch of the costocervical trunk, which arises from the subclavian artery.

The intercostal arteries run between the intercostal vein superiorly and the intercostal nerve inferiorly. Since the thoracic aorta lies to the left of the thoracic spine, the right intercostal arteries must cross over the thoracic vertebral bodies to reach the right intercostal spaces. This results in the right intercostal arteries being longer than the left ones.

Each posterior intercostal artery gives rise to dorsal and lateral branches that supply the dorsal (including deep back muscles) and lateral aspects of the intercostal spaces, respectively.

Anterior Intercostal Arteries. The upper six anterior intercostal arteries arise from the internal thoracic artery. The internal thoracic artery arises from the subclavian artery, then courses inferiorly, behind and lateral to the sternocostal articulations, and divides into the superior epigastric artery and the musculophrenic artery. The musculophrenic artery, in turn, supplies the seventh, eighth, and ninth anterior intercostal arteries. The nine anterior intercostal arteries supply the intercostal muscles anteriorly, as well as the muscles of the anterior thoracic wall and breast.

Intercostal Veins and the Azygos System of Veins. Venous drainage of the thoracic cage is accomplished primarily by the intercostal veins. The intercostal venous blood generally courses in the opposite direction of the arterial supply and drains into the azygos system of veins (Figs. 6-7 and 6-9, A).

The azygos vein originates from one or more of the following: inferior vena cava, right renal vein, and right ascending lumbar vein. The azygos vein passes through the diaphragm by means of the aortic hiatus.

It then courses along the right anterior aspect of the thoracic vertebral bodies. Along its course this vein receives the right lower eight intercostal veins, the right superior intercostal vein, and the hemiazygos veins. In addition, the accessory hemiazygos vein is frequently a direct tributary of the azygos vein. The right superior intercostal vein drains the upper two to three intercostal spaces and can empty into either the azygos vein or the right brachiocephalic vein. Other tributaries of the azygos vein include esophageal, bronchial, mediastinal, and pericardial veins. The azygos vein courses superiorly and arches (from posterior to anterior) around the superior aspect of the right primary bronchus. It then terminates by entering the superior vena cava.

The hemiazygos vein originates from the left ascending lumbar vein, the left renal vein, or both. The hemiazygos vein enters the thorax through the aortic hiatus. It then continues superiorly along the left anterior aspect of the vertebral bodies. Along its path the hemiazygos vein receives the lower four or five left intercostal veins. It also frequently receives the accessory hemiazygos vein. The hemiazygos helps to drain the left mediastinum and left lower esophagus. The hemiazygos vein crosses from left to right at approximately the level of T9 and terminates by emptying into the azygos vein.

The accessory hemiazygos vein connects the middle three or four intercostal veins. It occasionally receives the left superior intercostal vein, which drains the upper two to three intercostal spaces. However, the left superior intercostal vein normally is a tributary of the left brachiocephalic vein. The accessory hemiazygos ends by either draining into the hemiazygos vein or by crossing the vertebral column from left to right, just above the hemiazygos vein, to drain into the azygos vein.

Thoracic Duct

The thoracic duct is the largest and most important lymphatic channel of the body (Figs. 6-7 and 6-9). The thoracic duct drains both lower extremities, the pelvis, the abdomen, the left side of the thorax, the left upper extremity, and the left side of the head and neck. It originates at the cisterna chyli (when present) and terminates at the junction of the left subclavian and left internal jugular veins. The cisterna chyli is a large midline lymphatic collecting structure located just inferior to the aortic hiatus of the diaphragm. It collects lymphatics from the lower extremities via left and right lateral branches and from the intestinal tract via an intestinal branch. The cisterna chyli tapers at its superior aspect and becomes the thoracic duct. Most frequently the cisterna chyli is replaced by a confluence of lymph trunks in the abdominal region. The thoracic duct subsequently enters the thorax through the aortic hiatus just to the right of the aorta. On entering the thorax, the thoracic duct continues superiorly along the anterior aspect of the thoracic vertebral bodies. Between T7 and T5 it passes to the left side of the anterior aspect of the vertebral bodies. The thoracic duct continues superiorly and empties into the junction of the left subclavian and internal jugular veins.

The right lymphatic duct drains the right side of the thorax, the right upper extremity, and the right side of the neck and head. It usually empties into the right subclavian vein, the internal jugular vein, or the union of the two.

The lymphatics of the thoracic cage drain into mediastinal nodes, which in turn drain into either the right lymphatic duct or the thoracic duct. The lymphatics of the mediastinum are very abundant and can be divided into four major groups: superior mediastinal nodes, diaphragmatic nodes, posterior mediastinal nodes, and tracheobronchial nodes. These lymph nodes drain into nearby lymphatic channels. Those of the right side drain into the right lymphatic duct, and those of the left side drain into the thoracic duct.

Aortic Arch and Thoracic Aorta

Aortic Arch. The aortic arch begins at the heart as the outflow path of the left ventricle. It extends in front of the trachea, swings around the left primary bronchus, and comes to lie to the left of the midthoracic vertebrae (Fig. 6-7). The arch then continues inferiorly as the descending thoracic aorta. There are three large branches from the aortic arch: the brachiocephalic (innominate) artery, the left common carotid artery, and the left subclavian artery.

Descending Thoracic Aorta. The descending thoracic aorta is the continuation of the aortic arch (Figs. 6-7 and 6-9). It begins at approximately the T4-5 disc and continues inferiorly along the left side of the thoracic vertebrae. The thoracic aorta shifts to the midline in the lower thorax, lying on the anterior aspect of the lower thoracic vertebrae. The thoracic aorta gives off bronchial arteries (which supply the lungs) and all the intercostal arteries except the first two on each side (supplied by the highest intercostal artery of the costocervical trunk). The descending thoracic aorta also gives off the left and right subcostal arteries.

Esophagus

The esophagus (Fig. 6-7) originates posterior to the cricoid cartilage (approximately at the level of C6) and terminates at the cardia of the stomach (at the T11 vertebral body level). Therefore the esophagus has cervical, thoracic, and abdominal regions. It is approximately 10 inches in length. The esophagus lies approximately in

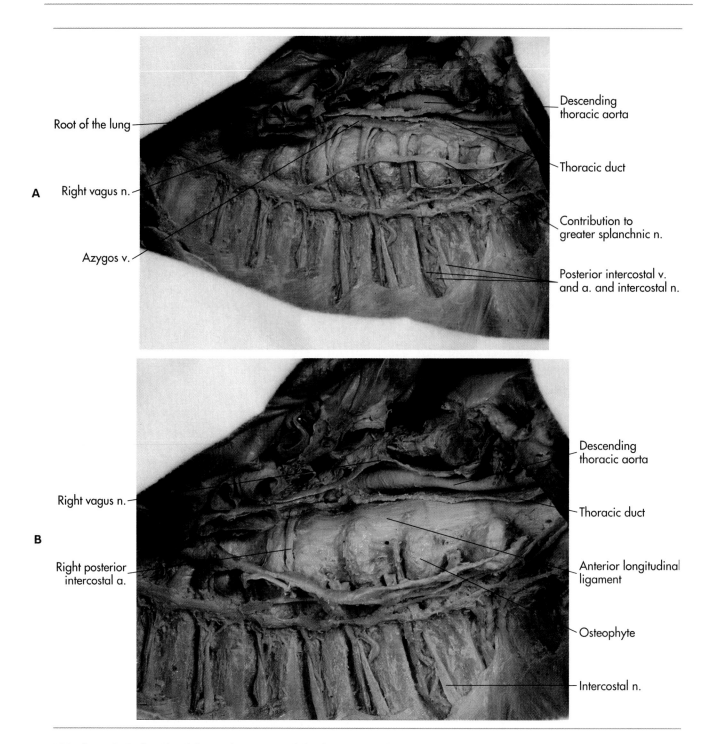

Root of the lung

Right vagus n.

Azygos v.

A

Descending thoracic aorta

Thoracic duct

Contribution to greater splanchnic n.

Posterior intercostal v. and a. and intercostal n.

Right vagus n.

Right posterior intercostal a.

B

Descending thoracic aorta

Thoracic duct

Anterior longitudinal ligament

Osteophyte

Intercostal n.

FIG. 6-9   A, Right side of the mediastinum and the thoracic vertebrae, ribs, and intercostal spaces associated with this region. **B,** Same specimen with the azygos vein and related intercostal veins retracted. This was done to show more clearly the anterior longitudinal ligament. Notice the large osteophytes extending from the anterolateral aspects of the thoracic vertebrae. Such osteophytes are typically seen in dissections of this region.

the midline in the upper and middle thorax, where it is located posterior to the left atrium. It curves left at the esophageal hiatus (approximately T10 vertebral body level), where it lies anterior and slightly to the left of the thoracic aorta and its hiatus.

Trachea

The trachea (Fig. 6-7) is a rigid tubular organ that lies anterior to the esophagus, between the brachiocephalic artery (on the right) and the left common carotid artery (on the left). The brachiocephalic veins lie anterior to the trachea. The trachea begins at the cricoid cartilage (approximately the level of C6) and ends by bifurcating into the left and right primary bronchi at approximately the level of the T4-5 disc (Fig. 6-7). The trachea is kept rigid and held open by 16 to 20 cartilaginous tracheal rings. These rings are C shaped with the open end facing posteriorly. Fibro-elastic tissue and smooth muscle (tracheal or trachealis muscle) span the posterior opening. The less rigid posterior surface allows for the passage of food through the posteriorly located esophagus. Helping to form the tracheal bifurcation is the carina, the inverted V-shaped inferior border of the last tracheal cartilage.

The trachea receives innervation from sympathetic and parasympathetic autonomic fibers. The parasympathetics arise from the vagus nerves and their recurrent laryngeal branches. Stimulation of these nerves results in constriction of the trachea and increased secretion of the mucus cells of the tracheal epithelium. Sympathetic innervation of the trachea is derived from branches of the thoracic sympathetic trunk. Stimulation of these nerves results in dilation of the trachea and decreased mucus secretions.

Vagus Nerves

The vagus nerves (right and left) run within the carotid sheath in the neck and enter the thorax medial to the phrenic nerves (right and left). Each vagus nerve is responsible for carrying preganglionic parasympathetic fibers to all the thoracic viscera. These fibers synapse in the walls of the organs they supply. General visceral afferent fibers from these same viscera also travel within the left and right vagus nerves. The parasympathetic nervous system is described in detail in Chapter 10.

Left Vagus Nerve. The left vagus nerve enters the thorax between the left common carotid and left subclavian arteries. It continues inferiorly by crossing the aortic arch, where it gives off the rather large left recurrent laryngeal nerve. This nerve loops around the aortic arch from anterior to posterior just lateral to the ligamentum arteriosum. It then runs superiorly in a groove between the esophagus and trachea (tracheo-esophageal groove) to supply eight of the nine laryngeal muscles on the left side. The main trunk of the vagus nerve continues inferiorly from the arch of the aorta (giving branches to the cardiac plexus) and follows the aorta posteriorly, passing behind the root of the left lung, where it participates in the pulmonary plexus. The vagus nerve then courses medially and comes to lie on the anterior aspect of the esophagus, where it helps to form the anterior esophageal plexus. The anterior esophageal plexus coalesces inferiorly to form the anterior vagal trunk. This trunk exits the thorax by traveling along the anterior aspect of the esophagus through the esophageal hiatus of the diaphragm.

Right Vagus Nerve. The right vagus nerve enters the thorax by crossing the right subclavian artery. The right recurrent laryngeal nerve is given off at this point. This nerve loops around the right subclavian artery and continues superiorly in the right tracheo-esophageal groove to supply eight of the nine muscles of the larynx on the right side. The right vagus nerve continues inferiorly in the thorax, contributing to the superficial and deep cardiac plexuses, and runs posterior to the root of the right lung. Here it sends several branches to the posterior pulmonary plexus. The right vagus then travels medially to the posterior aspect of the esophagus, where it forms the posterior esophageal plexus (Figs. 6-7 and 6-9). The nerves of the posterior esophageal plexus coalesce to form the posterior vagal trunk. The posterior vagal trunk exits the thorax by traveling along the posterior aspect of the esophagus through the esophageal hiatus of the diaphragm.

Thoracic Sympathetic Chain

The sympathetic nervous system is discussed in detail in Chapter 10. Because of the close anatomic relationship between the sympathetic trunk and the thoracic vertebrae, it also is discussed briefly here.

The sympathetic trunk in the thoracic region extends from superior to inferior across the heads of the ribs and is covered by the costal pleura (see Figs. 6-7, 6-8, and 10-7, B). As it reaches the inferior aspect of the thorax, the trunk courses medially to be positioned along the lateral aspect of the lower thoracic vertebral bodies. The sympathetic trunk is composed of axons of neurons whose cell bodies are located in the intermediolateral cell column of the thoracic spinal cord. These axons exit the cord via a ventral root that unites with a dorsal root, forming a mixed spinal nerve. This nerve exits the vertebral canal through the IVF. These preganglionic sympathetic fibers leave the ventral ramus close to its origin and enter a white ramus communicans, which connects to the sympathetic ganglion. Once in the sympathetic ganglion, the preganglionic sympathetic fibers have several options to reach their destinations (effector organs). (see Chapter 10). One option is to help form the splanchnic nerves, which supply a large part of the abdominal viscera with sympathetic innervation.

Splanchnic Nerves

The thorax contains three splanchnic nerves: the greater, the lesser (see Figs. 6-7, 10-4, and 10-10), and the least. Each is formed from branches of the sympathetic chain. The splanchnic nerves course along the lateral aspects of the middle and lower thoracic vertebral bodies and exit the thorax by piercing the posterior aspect of the diaphragm. They then synapse in one of several prevertebral ganglia. The postganglionic fibers from these prevertebral ganglia provide sympathetic innervation to the vast majority of the abdominal viscera.

The three splanchnic nerves, their ganglia of origin, and the prevertebral ganglion in which they synapse are as follows:

◆ *Greater splanchnic nerve.* This nerve arises from thoracic ganglia five through nine (Figs. 6-7; 6-8, *A*; and 6-9, *A*) and synapses in the celiac ganglion. Some of its fibers do not synapse here but run directly to the medulla of the adrenal gland, which they innervate.

◆ *Lesser splanchnic nerve.* The lesser splanchnic nerve arises from thoracic ganglia 9 and 10 (it may sometimes arise from 10 and 11) (Williams et al., 1989). It synapses in the aorticorenal ganglion.

◆ *Least splanchnic nerve.* This nerve originates from the twelfth thoracic ganglion and synapses within ganglia of the renal plexus.

REFERENCES

Alvarez, O., Roque, C.T., & Pampati, M. (1988). Multilevel thoracic disk herniations: CT and MR studies. *J Comput Assist Tomogr, 12,* 649-652.

Bauduin, E. et al. (1989). Foraminal herniation of a thoracic calcified nucleus pulposus. *Neuroradiology, 31,* 287-288.

Behrsin, J.F. & Briggs, C.A. (1988). Ligaments of the lumbar spine: A review. *Surg Radiol Anat, 10,* 211-219.

Bland, J. (1987). *Disorders of the cervical spine.* Philadelphia: W.B. Saunders.

Cook, S.D. et al. (1986). Upper extremity proprioception in idiopathic scoliosis. *Clin Orthop, 213,* 118-123.

Deacon, P., Archer, J., & Dickson, R.A. (1987). The anatomy of spinal deformity: A biomechanical analysis. *Orthopedics, 10,* 897-903.

Deane, G. & Duthie, R.B. (1973). A new projectional look at articulated scoliotic spines. *Acta Orthop Scand, 44,* 351-365.

Dupuis, P.R. et al. (1985). Radiologic diagnosis of degenerative lumbar spinal instability. *Spine, 10,* 262-276.

Hardy, P.A. (1988). Anatomical variation in the position of the proximal intercostal nerve. *Br J Anaesth, 61,* 338-339.

Hasue, M. et al. (1983). Anatomic study of the interrelation between lumbosacral nerve roots and their surrounding tissues. *Spine, 8,* 50-58.

Humzah, M.D. & Soames, R.W. (1988). Human intervertebral disc: Structure and function. *Anat Rec, 220,* 337-356.

Foreman, S.M. & Crofts, A.C. (1988). *Whiplash injuries: The cervical acceleration/deceleration syndrome.* Baltimore: Williams & Wilkins.

Lipson, S.J. & O'Connell, J.X. (1991). A 47-year-old woman with back pain and a lesion in a vertebral body. *N Engl J Med, 325,* 794-799.

Maigne, J.Y., Maigne, R. & Guerin-Surville, H. (1991). Upper thoracic dorsal rami: Anatomic study of their medial cutaneous branches. *Surg Radiol Anat, 13,* 109-112.

Marchesi, D. et al. (1988). Morphometric analysis of the thoracolumbar and lumbar pedicles, anatomico-radiologic study. *Surg Radiol Anat, 10,* 317-322.

Moore, K.L. (1992). *Clinically oriented anatomy* (3rd ed.). Baltimore: Williams & Wilkins.

Netter, F. (1990). *The Ciba collection of medical illustration. Vol 8: The musculoskeletal system.* Summitt: Ciba Geigy Corp.

Nissinen, M. et al. (1989). Trunk asymmetry and scoliosis. *Acta Paediatr Scand, 78,* 747-753.

Otani, K. et al. (1988). Thoracic disc herniation: Surgical treatment in 23 patients. *Spine, 13,* 1262-1267.

Pal, G.P. et al. (1988). Trajectory architecture of the trabecular bone between the body and the neural arch in human vertebrae. *Anat Rec, 222,* 418-425.

Paris, S. (1983). Anatomy as related to function and pain. From Symposium on Evaluation and Care of Lumbar Spine Problems. *Orthop Clin North Am, 14,* 476-489.

Scapinelli, R. (1989). Morphological and functional changes of the lumbar spinous processes in the elderly. *Surg Radiol Anat, 11,* 129-133.

Singer, K.P. & Giles, L.G.F. (1990). Manual therapy considerations at the thoracolumbar junction: An anatomical and functional perspective. *J Manipulative Physiol Ther, 13,* 83-88.

Singer, K.P., Giles, L.G.F., & Day, R.E. (1990). Intra-articular synovial folds of thoracolumbar junction zygapophyseal joints. *Anat Rec, 226,* 147-152.

Spapen, H.D. et al. (1990). The straight back syndrome. *Neth J Med, 36,* 29-31.

Vernon, L., Dooley, J. & Acusta, A. (1993). Upper lumbar and thoracic disc pathology: A magnetic resonance imaging analysis. *J Neuro musculoskeletal System, 1,* 59-63.

Vital, J. et al. (1989). The neurocentral vertebral cartilage: Anatomy, physiology and physiopathology. *Surg Radiol Anat, 11,* 323-328.

White, A.W. & Panjabi, M.M. (1990). *Clinical biomechanics of the spine.* Philadelphia: J.B. Lippincott.

Williams, P.L. et al. (1989). *Gray's anatomy* (37th ed.). Edinburgh: Churchill Livingstone.

Wyatt, M.P. et al. (1986). Vibratory response in idiopathic scoliosis. *A J Bone Joint Surg, 68,* 714-718.

CHAPTER 7

The Lumbar Region

Gregory D. Cramer

The lumbar portion of the vertebral column is sturdy and is designed to carry the weight of the head, neck, trunk, and upper extremities. Yet, pain in the lumbar region is one of the most common complaints of individuals, experienced by approximately 80% of the population at some time in their lives (Nachemson, 1976). The estimated annual cost for treatment of low back pain and for resulting disability is estimated at more than $13 billion in the United States. Low back pain is the most common complaint of patients who go to clinics that deal primarily with musculoskeletal conditions. Low back pain of mechanical origin is the most frequent subtype found in this group (Cramer et al., 1992a). The most common sources of low back pain are the lumbar zygapophyseal joints (Z joints) and the intervertebral discs (IVDs) (Bogduk, 1985).

> **Eighty Percent of Individuals Will Have Low Back Pain During Their Lifetime**

> **The Annual Cost Related to *Low Back Pain* is $13 Billion in the United States Alone**

Much of the reason for the high incidence of low back pain is probably related to humans being bipedal. Being able to walk on the hind limbs is accompanied by increased freedom of movement and increased ability to interact with the environment, other species, and other members of the same species. Animals that walk on the hind legs (primarily humans) can normally turn their heads to look around on both sides with relative ease. They also have the ability to use their hands for an almost infinite number of tasks without having to be concerned about using their upper extremities to help maintain balance.

However, the ability to walk on the lower extremities (the bipedal stance) has one significant drawback: increased stress is placed on the spine. The weight of the body is concentrated on a smaller region compared with quadrupeds. The weight of the human trunk is completely supported by the lower extremities and lumbar spine during standing, and it is completely absorbed by the lumbar spine and sacroiliac joints during sitting. Therefore the lumbar region, sacrum, and sacroiliac joints are susceptible to more problems than are encountered by four-legged animals. These problems can be divided into three types of lumbar disorders and also sacroiliac joint difficulties:

I. Problems with the lumbar region
    A. The Z joints (facet joints; see Figs. 7-3 through 7-5). Increased weight borne by these joints can be a direct cause of back pain. These joints are also susceptible to arthritic changes (osteoarthritis; arthritis associated with "wear and tear").
    B. The intervertebral disc. The IVDs absorb most of the increased stress received by the low back in bipeds. The discs may bulge or rupture, and by doing so compress the spinal nerves that exit behind them (see Figs. 7-19 and 7-20). This protrusion results in back pain that also has a sharp radiation pattern into the thigh and sometimes into the leg and foot. This type of pain is frequently described as feeling like a "bolt of lightning" or a "hot poker" (see Chapter 11). The IVDs may also undergo degeneration. This narrows the space between the vertebrae, which may result in arthritic changes and additional pressure on the Z joints (see Chapter 2). The discs themselves are supplied by sensory nerves and therefore can be a direct source of back pain (i.e., they do not have to compress neural elements to cause back pain).
    C. The muscles of the low back in bipeds are called on to hold the spine erect (erector spinae muscles; see Chapter 4). Therefore, when they are required to carry increased loads (this sometimes includes the added weight of a protruding abdomen), these muscles can be torn (strained).
       Note: The lumbosacral region, between L5 and the sacrum, receives the brunt of the biomechanical stress of the biped spine. The lumbosacral joints (interbody joint and left and right Z joints between L5 and the sacrum) are a prime source of low back pain. In addition to the stresses previously mentioned, the opening for the mixed spinal nerve at this level is the smallest in the lumbar region, making it particularly vulnerable to IVD protrusions and compression from other sources.
II. The sacroiliac joints are the joints between the sacrum and the left and right ilia. The weight carried in the upright posture can also result in damage to the sacroiliac joint, another source of low back pain (see Chapter 8).

Because of its clinical importance, the lumbar region has been the target of extensive high-quality research. Numerous descriptive and quantitative studies have been completed on this area of the spine. This chapter concentrates on the unique characteristics of the lumbar vertebrae and the ligamentous, neural, and vascular elements of the lumbar region. It also includes the most pertinent results of descriptive and quantitative investigations in an attempt to explain clearly the most important and clinically relevant idiosyncrasies of this intriguing area of the spine.

All the lumbar vertebrae are considered to be typical, although the fifth lumbar vertebra is unique. This chapter presents the typical characteristics of lumbar vertebrae, the lumbar vertebral canal, and the intervertebral foramina (IVFs). A description of the unique characteristics of L5 and the lumbosacral articulation follows. The ranges of motion of the lumbar region are also included. The chapter concludes with a discussion of the nerves, vessels, and related viscera of the lumbar region.

LUMBAR LORDOSIS AND CHARACTERISTICS OF TYPICAL LUMBAR VERTEBRAE
Developmental Considerations and the Lumbar Curve (Lordosis)

The development of lumbar vertebrae is similar to the development of typical vertebrae in other regions of the spine (see Chapter 12). Unique to the lumbar region is the presence of two additional secondary centers of ossification on each lumber vertebra. This brings the total number of secondary centers of ossification per lumbar vertebra to seven. These additional centers are located on the posterior aspect of the superior articular processes and develops into the mamillary processes.

Between 2 and 16 years, the lumbar vertebrae grow twice as fast as the thoracic vertebrae. Because the anteroposterior curves of these two regions face in opposite directions (thoracic kyphosis versus lumbar lordosis), the posterior elements of thoracic vertebrae probably grow faster than their vertebral bodies, and the reverse (lumbar vertebral bodies grow faster than their posterior elements) is true in the lumbar region (Clarke et al., 1985).

Normally the lumbar lordosis is more prominent than the cervical lordosis. The lumbar lordosis extends from T12 to the L5 IVD, and the greatest portion of the curve occurs between L3 and L5. The lumbar lordosis is created by the increased height of the anterior aspect of both the lumbar vertebral bodies and the lumbar IVDs, with the discs contributing more to the lordosis than the increased height of the vertebral bodies.

Either an increase or decrease of the lumbar lordosis may contribute to low back pain (Mosner et al., 1989). This has sparked an interest in measurement of the lumbar curve, and as a result, the lumbar curve has been measured in a variety of ways. One method, developed by Mosner and colleagues (1989), used measurements from lateral x-ray films taken with the patient in the supine position. A line was drawn across the superior vertebral end plate of L2 and another across the superior aspect of the sacral body. These two lines were continued posteriorly until they intersected, and the angle between them was measured. Using this method, an angle of 47° and 43° was found to be normal for women and men, respectively. This is in agreement with the values given by other authors (Williams et al., 1989).

In the past, many clinicians incorrectly assumed that the lumbar lordosis in the black population was greater than that in the white population, but this has been found to be incorrect; the lordosis is approximately the same in both races (Mosner et al., 1989).

The lumbar lordosis is often significantly increased in achondroplasia. This can lead to a marked compensatory thoracic (thoracolumbar) kyphosis, which in some cases can be severe (Giglio et al., 1988).

Vertebral Bodies

When viewed from above, the vertebral bodies of the lumbar spine are large and kidney shaped with the concavity facing posteriorly (Fig. 7-1). The superior surfaces

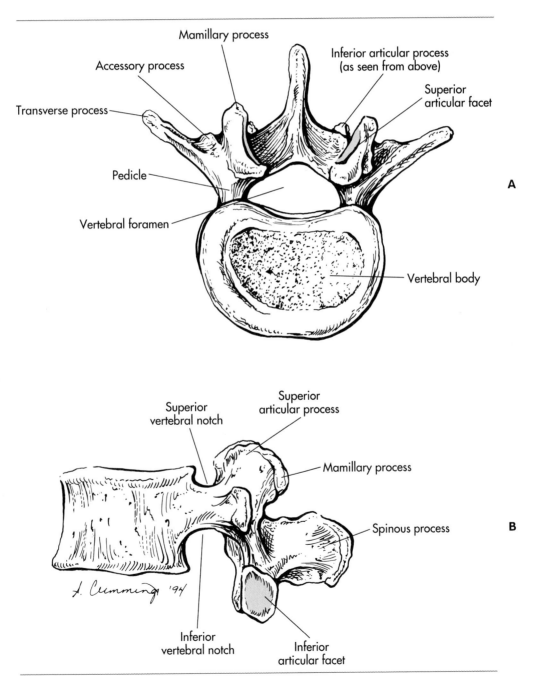

FIG. 7-1 Typical lumbar vertebra. **A,** Superior view. **B,** Lateral view.

of the vertebral bodies possess small elevations along their posterior rim. These represent remnants of the uncinate processes of the cervical region. The inferior surfaces of the vertebral bodies have two small notches along their posterior rim. These notches correspond to the uncinate-like elevations of the vertebra below. These elevations and notches have been used as landmarks on x-ray films as a means for evaluating normal and abnormal movement between adjacent lumbar segments (Dupuis et al., 1985).

The vertebral bodies are wider from side to side (lateral width) than from front to back and are taller in front (anteriorly) than behind. Therefore, as mentioned previously, the vertebral bodies are partially responsible for the creation and maintenance of the lumbar lordosis.

The lateral width of the lumbar vertebrae increases from L1 to L3. L4 and L5 are somewhat variable in width (Williams et al., 1989). Ericksen (1976) found that the L3 and L4 vertebral bodies (the only ones he studied) became wider from side to side with age. Also, he noted a decrease in height of the vertebral body's anterior aspect, corresponding with an increase in its lateral width, in both males and females. Further, Ericksen found that in males the increase in lateral width was accompanied by a corresponding decrease in height of the vertebral body's posterior aspect as well.

The blood supply to the vertebral bodies is extensive and complex (Bogduk & Twomey, 1991). Each lumbar segmental artery gives off up to 20 primary periosteal arteries as it courses across the anterolateral aspect of the vertebral body. The posterior aspect is supplied by many branches of the anterior vertebral canal artery. The anterior vertebral canal artery is the anterior branch of the artery that passes through the IVF. The artery that passes through the IVF is sometimes known as the spinal ramus of the (lumbar) segmental artery.

The end branches of periosteal arteries form a ring around both the superior and the inferior margins of the vertebral body. These rings are known as the metaphyseal anastomoses (superior and inferior). They not only help to supply the metaphyseal region of the vertebral body, but also send penetrating branches (metaphyseal arteries) to the region of the vertebral end plate (Bogduk & Twomey, 1991). A dense capillary network is associated with the superior and inferior vertebral end plates. This network receives contributions from the metaphyseal and nutrient arteries.

Nutrient arteries also arise from the anterior vertebral canal arteries. The nutrient arteries enter the center of the posterior aspect of the vertebral body, pass deep within the substance of the cancellous bone of the vertebral body's center, and then give off superior (ascending) and inferior (descending) branches. In addition to giving off periosteal arteries, the lumbar segmental arteries also send branches that enter the cancellous bone of the anterior and lateral aspects of the vertebral

bodies. These branches enter along the superior-to-inferior midpoint of the vertebral bodies. Known as the equatorial arteries, these vessels are similar to the nutrient arteries in that they also give rise to ascending and descending branches deep within the substance of the vertebral bodies (Bogduk & Twomey, 1991).

Fractures of the secondary centers of ossification associated with the superior and inferior vertebral endplates, the ring apophyses (sometimes known as anular epiphyses, see Chapters 2 and 12), have been reported. These fractures are rather rare but occur most frequently during adolescence. The signs and symptoms of apophyseal ring fractures resemble those of IVD protrusions. Such fractures may go unnoticed on conventional x-ray films. Sagittally reformatted computed tomography (CT) is currently the imaging modality that shows these fractures to best advantage (Thiel, Clements, & Cassidy, 1992).

The lumbar vertebral bodies serve as attachment sites for several structures. Table 7-1 lists those structures that attach to the lumbar vertebral bodies.

Pedicles

The pedicles of the lumbar spine are short but strong (Fig. 7-1). They attach lower on the vertebral bodies than the pedicles of the thoracic region, but higher than those of the cervical region. Therefore each lumbar vertebra has a superior vertebral notch that is less distinct than that of the cervical region. On the other hand, the inferior vertebral notch of lumbar vertebrae is prominent.

Table 7-1	**Attachments to Lumbar Vertebral Bodies**
Region	**Structure(s) attached**
Anterior surface	Anterior longitudinal ligament on superior and inferior borders
Posterior surface	Posterior longitudinal ligament on superior and inferior borders
Lateral surface	Crura of the diaphragm (anterolateral surface of left L1 and L2 and right L1, L2, and L3)
	Origin of the psoas major muscle (posterolateral aspect of superior and inferior surface of all lumbars); a series of tendinous arches between vertebral attachments of the psoas major muscle creates concave openings between arches and vertebral bodies, allowing for passage of segmental arteries, veins, and gray communicating rami of sympathetic chain.

Data from Williams et al. (1989). *Gray's anatomy* (37th ed.). Edinburgh: Churchill Livingstone.

The role of the pedicles in the transfer of loads is discussed in Chapter 2. More study is needed to confirm the role played by the pedicles in the transfer of loads in the upper lumbar region (Pal et al., 1988). However, the trabecular pattern of the L4 and L5 pedicles seems to indicate that most loads placed on these vertebrae may be transferred from the vertebral bodies to the region of the posterior arch, specifically to the pars interarticularis (see Laminae).

Transverse Processes

Each transverse process (TP) (left and right) of a typical lumbar vertebra projects posterolaterally from the junction of the pedicle and the lamina of the same side (Fig. 7-1). It lies in front of (anterior to) the articular process and behind (posterior to) the lumbar IVF.

The lumbar TPs are quite long, the TPs of L3 being the longest. The distance between the apices of the left and right TPs is much greater on L1 than T12. This distance increases on L2 and is the greatest in the entire spine on L3. The intertransverse distance between the left and right L4 TPs is smaller than that of L3 and is even smaller for L5. The lumbar TPs are flat and thin from front to back. They are also narrower from superior to inferior than their thoracic counterparts. They possess neither articular facets (as do thoracic TPs) nor transverse foramina (as do cervical TPs). The anterior aspect of the lumbar TPs are also known as the costal elements, and they may occasionally develop into ribs. This happens most frequently at L1.

The lateral aspect of the anterior surface of the lumbar TPs is creased by a ridge that runs from superior to inferior. This ridge is created by the anterior layer of the thoracolumbar fascia. The middle layer of the thoracolumbar fascia attaches to the apex of the TPs. Table 7-2 lists structures that attach to the lumbar TPs.

Accessory Processes. Unique to the lumbar spine are the accessory processes. Each accessory process projects posteriorly from the junction of the posterior and inferior aspect of the TP with the corresponding lamina. These processes serve as attachment sites for the longissimus thoracis muscles (lumbar fibers) and the medial intertransversarii lumborum muscles (Williams et al., 1989). (See Fig. 4-5, B, for the attachment of the medial intertransversarii lumborum muscles to the accessory processes.)

Articular Processes

Superior Articular Processes. Left and right superior articular processes are formed on every vertebrae of the lumbar spine (Fig. 7-1). Each superior articular process possesses a hyaline cartilage–lined superior articular facet that is oriented in a vertical plane. That is,

these facets are not angled to the vertical plane like the superior articular facets of the cervical and thoracic regions.

All the lumbar superior articular facets face posteriorly and medially. The articular surface of a typical superior articular facet can be gently curved with the concavity facing medially (Figs. 7-2 and 7-3), or the articular surface can be angled abruptly. When the articular surface is angled abruptly, two rather distinct articulating surfaces are formed. One surface faces posteriorly and forms almost a 90° angle with the second surface, which faces medially. As with the curved facet, the concavity faces posteriorly and medially. In either case (curved or angled articular surface), the shape conforms almost perfectly with the inferior articular facet of the vertebra above. The hyaline cartilage of the central region of the superior articular facet (the area of greatest concavity) increases in thickness with age, probably because this region receives much of the load during flexion of the spine (Taylor & Twomey, 1986). Also, the articular processes may fracture as a result of age-related degeneration (Kirkaldy-Willis et al., 1978).

The orientation of the superior articular facets varies from one vertebral level to another (Fig. 7-3). A line passed across each superior articular facet, on transverse CT scans, shows that the L4 superior facets (and therefore the L3-L4 Z joints) are more sagittally oriented than the L5 facets. Also, the S1 superior facets (and therefore the L5-S1 Z joints) are more coronally oriented than the L4 and L5 facets (Van Schaik, Verbiest, & Van Schaik, 1985). (See Zygapophyseal Joints for further detail on the orientation of the superior and inferior articular facets.)

Unique to the lumbar spine are the mamillary processes (Fig. 7-1), which project posteriorly from the superior articular processes of lumbar vertebrae. Each mamillary process is a small rounded mound of

Table 7-2 Attachments to Lumbar Transverse Processes

Region	Structures attached
Anterior surface	Psoas major and quadratus lumborum muscles
	Anterior layer of thoracolumbar fascia (separates psoas major and quadratus lumborum muscles)
	Medial and lateral arcuate ligaments (lumbocostal arches) (L1)
Apex	Middle layer of thoracolumbar fascia
	Iliolumbar ligament (L5, occasionally L4)
Superior border	Lateral intertransversarii muscles
Inferior border	Lateral intertransversarii muscles
Posterior surface	Deep back muscles (longissimus thoracis)

Data from Williams et al. (1989). *Gray's anatomy* (37th ed.). Edinburgh: Churchill Livingstone.

variable size. Some are almost indistinguishable, whereas others are relatively prominent. The mamillary processes serve as attachment sites for the multifidi lumborum muscles.

Mamillo-Accessory Ligament. A mamillo-accessory ligament (Bogduk, 1981; Lippitt, 1984) is found between the mamillary and accessory process on the left and right sides of each lumbar vertebra. Occasionally, one or more of these ligaments may ossify in the lower lumbar levels (L3 to L5). The incidence of ossification increases in frequency from L3 to L5. Ossification of these ligaments at L5 occurs at a 10% (Bogduk, 1981) to 26% (Maigne, Maigne, & Guervin-Surville, 1991) frequency. Maigne and colleagues (1991) studied 203 lumbar spines and found that ossification of this ligament at L5 occurred twice as often on the left. They gave no reason why the ligament ossified more frequently on this side. However, they believed the ossification was the result of osteoarthritis, since they found no evidence of ossification on the spines of children and young adults. These authors also stated that an ossified mamillo-accessory ligament could occasionally be seen on standard lumbar x-ray films.

The mamillo-accessory ligament has been described as a tough, fibrous band that may represent tendinous fibers of origin of the lumbar multifidi muscles or fibers of insertion of the longissimus thoracis pars lumborum muscle (Bogduk, 1981). Regardless of its precise structure, the reported purpose of the mamillo-accessory "ligament" is to hold the medial branch of the dorsal ramus of the above spinal nerve (e.g., L2 medial branch is associated with L3 mamillo-accessory ligament) against (1) the bone between the base of the superior articular process and the base of the transverse process and (2) the Z joint, which is slightly more medial (see Fig. 7-4). As it passes deep to the mamillo-accessory ligament, the medial branch of the dorsal ramus gives off articular branches to the capsule of the Z joint. The medial branch then continues medially across the vertebral lamina to reach the multifidus muscle (Bogduk, 1981). Therefore the medial branch of the dorsal ramus (posterior primary division) is held within a small osteofibrous canal along the posterior arch of a lumbar vertebra. The medial branch could possibly become irritated or even entrapped within this tunnel, which would result in low back pain. However, more investigation is necessary to determine if such irritation or entrapment occurs and, if so, its frequency (Bogduk, 1981; Maigne et al., 1991).

Inferior Articular Processes. The inferior articular processes of lumbar vertebrae are convex anteriorly and laterally. They possess inferior articular facets that cover their anterolateral surface. As with the superior articular facets, the inferior ones vary in shape. Even though articular processes vary from one vertebral level

to another, and even from one side to another, superior and inferior articulating processes of one Z joint conform to one another. This conformation is such that each inferior articular facet usually fits remarkably well into the posterior and medial concavity of the adjoining superior articular facet.

Zygapophyseal Joints

General Considerations. The Z joints have been identified as a source of back pain (Mooney & Robertson, 1976). In addition, Rauschning (1987) states that these joints "display typical degenerative and reparative changes which are known to cause osteoarthritic pain in peripheral synovial joints." Therefore the lumbar Z joints are highly significant clinically. Because these joints are discussed in detail in Chapter 2, this section focuses on the unique and clinically significant aspects of the lumbar Z joints.

The lumbar Z joints are considered to be complex synovial joints oriented in the vertical plane (Williams et al., 1989). They are fashioned according to the shape of the superior and inferior articular facets (see previous discussion). Therefore the lumbar Z joints are concave posteriorly and even have been described as being biplaner in orientation (Taylor & Twomey, 1986). That is, they have a coronally oriented, posterior-facing, anteromedial component and a large, sagitally oriented, medial-facing, posterolateral component. Taylor and Twomey (1986) state that the lumbar Z joints are coronally oriented in children and that the large sagittal component develops as the individual matures. The sagittal component limits rotation, whereas the coronal component limits flexion. More specifically, the shape of the lumbar Z joints allows for a large amount of flexion to occur in the lumbar region, but the size of the lumbar Z joints is what eventually limits flexion at the end of the normal range of motion. Therefore the long contact surfaces between the coronal component of the superior articular processes and the adjacent inferior articular processes finally limit flexion by "restraining the forward translational component of flexion" (Taylor & Twomey, 1986).

Even though the size of the Z joints eventually limits flexion, approximately 60° of flexion is able to occur in the entire lumbar region before the bony restraints of the lumbar articular processes prevent further movement. However, the size and shape of the Z joints greatly limit rotation. During rotation of the lumbar region, distraction (or gapping) occurs between adjacent lumbar articular facets (superior facet of vertebra below and inferior facet of vertebra above) on the side of rotation. For example, right rotation results in gapping of the facets on the right side. Also during rotation, the two opposing facets of the opposite side are pressed together. This causes them to act as a fulcrum for the distracting facets on the side of rotation (Paris, 1983).

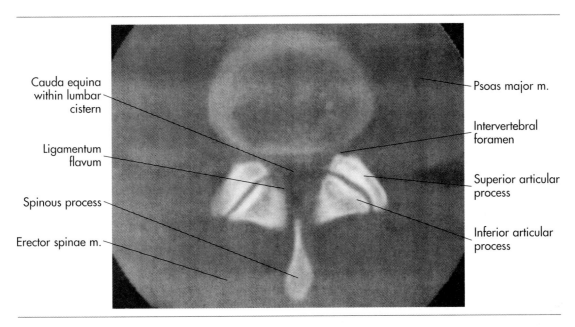

FIG. 7-2 Horizontal computed tomography (CT) scan showing the orientation of the lumbar Z joints. Notice that the left and right superior articular processes face posteriorly and medially.

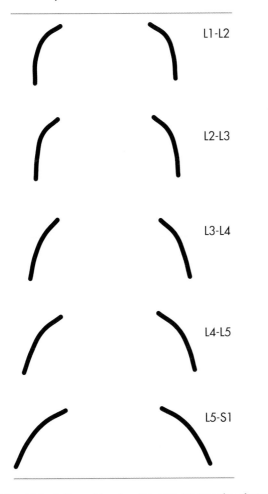

L1-L2

L2-L3

L3-L4

L4-L5

L5-S1

FIG. 7-3 Orientation of lumbar Z joints. Notice the changes from L1-2 to L5-S1. (From Taylor, J.R. & Twomey, L.T. 1986. *Spine, 11,* 739-745.)

Extension of the lumbar region is limited by the inferior articular process on each side of a lumbar vertebra contacting the junction between the lamina and the superior articular process of the vertebra below. This junction between the lamina and the superior articular process is known as the pars interarticularis.

Variation of Zygapophyseal Joint Size and Shape. A considerable degree of variation exists between individual Z joints at different lumbar levels and also between the left and right Z joints at the same vertebral level. The shapes range from a slight and gentle curve, concave posteriorly, to a pronounced, dramatic, posteriorly concave curve, and in some cases to a joint in which the posterior and medial components face one another at an angle of nearly 90°. Generally the Z joints of the upper lumbar levels are more sagittally oriented than those of the lower lumbar levels (Fig. 7-3). This makes the lower lumbar joints more susceptible to recurrent rotational strain (Kirkaldy-Willis et al., 1978).

Biomechanical Considerations. The articular facets do not absorb any of the compressive forces of the spine when humans are sitting erect or standing in a slightly flexed posture. The IVD absorbs almost all the compressive loads under these conditions. However, when standing erect (slight extension), the facets resist approximately 16% of the compressive forces between vertebrae (Dunlop, Adams, & Hutton, 1984). Disc degeneration may lead to increased stress on the Z joints. This results in pain, not from the articular cartilage, but usually either from pressure on the subchondral bone of the articular processes or from soft tissue being caught between the articular facets (Hutton, 1990).

Articular Capsules. An articular capsule covers the posterior aspect of each lumbar Z joint (Fig. 7-4). The ligamentum flavum covers the anteromedial aspect of the Z joint. The articular capsule is tough, possesses a rich sensory innervation, and is well vascularized (Giles & Taylor, 1987). The outer fibers of the articular capsule are horizontally directed, coursing from posterolateral to anteromedial (Paris, 1983). These fibers extend a considerable distance medially and become continuous with the lateral fibers of the interspinous ligament. These characteristics of the capsule help limit forward flexion (Paris, 1983). Laterally, each articular capsule is frequently continuous with the articular cartilage lining the superior articular facet. A gradual transition occurs from the fibrous tissue of the capsule to fibrocartilage and finally to the hyaline cartilage of the superior articular facet (Taylor & Twomey, 1986).

Each capsule has a rather large superior and inferior recess that extends away from the joint. The capsular fibers (or fibers of the ligamentum falvum, anteriorly) surrounding these recesses are very thin and loose, and there may be openings where neurovascular bundles enter the recesses (Taylor & Twomey, 1986). Paris (1983) states that effusion within the Z joint may enter the superior recess, and as little as 0.5 ml of effusion may cause the superior recess to enter the anteriorly located IVF. Once in the IVF, it may compress the exiting spinal nerve. Such a protrusion of the Z joint is known as a synovial cyst (Xu et al., 1991).

Xu and colleagues (1991), in a study of 50 pairs of lumbar Z joints from an elderly population, found that the capsules varied greatly in thickness and regularity. They found that they were "irregularly thickened, amorphous, and calcified in 22 cases." In addition, they found that in most subjects the synovium of the joint space extended 1 to 2 mm outside the boundaries of the joint in one or more locations. These synovial extensions, which could be considered to be small synovial cysts, maintained communication with the joint space. These Z joint extensions were found on both the anterior and posterior aspects of the joint. Anteriorly the spaces most often extended along the posterior border of the ligamentum flavum (64% of Z joints). Sometimes a synovial joint ex-

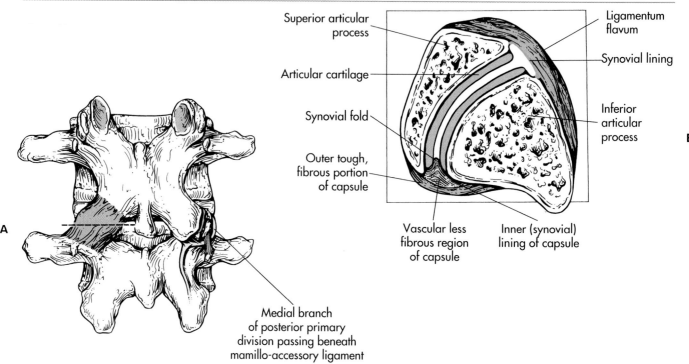

FIG. 7-4   The lumbar Z joints. **A,** Joint capsule *(left)*. Mamillo-accessory ligament and its relationship to the medial branch of the dorsal ramus of the mixed spinal nerve *(right)*. **B,** Cross section through the left Z joint at the level of the dotted line shown in **A.** Notice the ligamentum flavum anteriorly and the Z joint capsule posteriorly. The lateral aspect of the capsule blends with the articular cartilage, and the medial aspect extends for a considerable distance along the posterior aspect of the inferior articular process. Also notice that a synovial fold can be seen extending into the joint space.

tension would extend directly into the ligamentum flavum (8% of cases). Posteriorly the synovial cysts usually extended either laterally along the superior articular process (7% of cases) or medially along the inferior articular process (29%). In 41% of the Z joints, extensions were found on both the inferior and the superior articular processes, and in 23% of the Z joints, no synovial extensions were found (7% of cases). Xu and colleagues believed that the synovial joint extensions (synovial cysts) were probably more common in their older population than in younger age groups. They stated that their findings may explain why Z joint arthrography (visualization of the Z joint after injection with radiopaque dye) could be successful even when the joint space was not entered with the injecting needle.

In another study, Xu, Haughton, & Carrera (1990) visualized the synovial joint extensions (cysts) with magnetic resonance imaging (MRI). Their positive identification of these synovial joint extensions was aided with the injection of paramagnetic contrast medium (gadodiamide, Winthrop Pharmaceuticals). Their imaging was performed on dissected spines using small surface coils, long acquisition times, and thin slice thicknesses. Therefore, clear delineation of these extensions is probably still beyond the resolving capabilities of MRI scans obtained in a typical clinical setting. However, Xu and colleagues thought their results helped to explain the variable appearance of the facet joints on MRI scans. They stated "the inhomogeneity detected at MR imaging and computerized tomography in the ligamentum flavum near the facet joint most likely represents extension of the joint capsule between the ligamentum flavum and the articular processes. . ." (Xu et al., 1990). This is certainly an area of important future investigation.

The superior and inferior recesses are filled with fibrofatty pads. These pads are well vascularized and are lined with a synovial membrane. They also protrude a significant distance into the superior and inferior aspect of the Z joint. Engel and Bogduk (1982) state that adipose tissue pads probably develop from undifferentiated mesenchyme of the embryologic Z joint. Furthermore, they note that in certain instances, mechanical stress to the joint may cause an adipose tissue pad to undergo fibrous metaplasia, which results in the formation of a fibro-adipose meniscoid (an adipose tissue pad with a fibrous tip composed of dense connective tissue). The authors believed that both the adipose tissue pads and the meniscoids "play some form of normal functional role" (Fig. 7-4).

In addition, "fringes" of synovium extend from the capsule to the region between the articular facets. These fringes fill the small region where the facets do not completely approximate one another.

Sometimes a fatty synovial fold develops a rather long fibrous tip that extends a considerable distance between the joint surfaces, where it may become compressed (Taylor & Twomey, 1986). Such protruding synovial folds have been associated with the early stages of degeneration (Rauschning, 1987). Rauschning (1987) typically found hemarthrosis and effusion into the Z joints when the meniscal folds of this type were torn or "nipped" between the joint surfaces.

Occasionally, as humans age, a piece of articular cartilage breaks from the superior or inferior articular facet. The piece usually breaks along the posterior aspect of the Z joint, parallel to the joint space. However, the attachment to the articular capsule is usually maintained. The result is the presence of a large, fibrocartilaginous meniscoid inclusion within the joint. Taylor and Twomey (1986) reported that the formation of this type of meniscoid is partially caused by the regular pulling action on the posterior articular capsule by the multifidi muscles that originate from these capsules. The attachment of the capsule to the periphery of the articular cartilage may then result in the cartilage tears found to run parallel with the joint surface. The torn cartilage fragment is capable of developing into a Z joint meniscoid, which can become interposed between the two surfaces of the joint. The authors also noted that the posterior aspect of the Z joint may open when the multifidi and other deep back muscles relax, allowing the meniscoids and other joint inclusions to become entrapped. The result of this type of entrapment could possibly be (1) loss of motion (locked back), resulting from the cartilage being lodged between two opposing joint surfaces, and (2) pain, because the meniscoids remain attached and therefore might put traction on the very pain-sensitive joint capsule.

Certain Z joint folds possess nociceptive fibers (Giles, 1988; Giles & Taylor, 1987). Entrapment within a Z joint of these innervated folds could be a primary source of back pain and muscle tightness (spasm) even without traction of the capsule. Chapter 2 describes Z joint synovial folds and other Z joint inclusions in further detail.

The pain-sensitive articular capsule and the synovial lining of the ligamentum flavum of each lumbar Z joint are normally held out of the joint by three structures. First, the multifidus lumborum muscles take part of their origin (several originate from each vertebra) from the posterior aspect of each articular capsule (Taylor & Twomey, 1986). These muscles pull the capsule out of the joint's posterior aspect. Second, the ligamentum flavum pulls the synovium out of the joint's anterior aspect. Third, when the joint surfaces are compressed, the Z joint synovial folds push the capsule out of the joint (Paris, 1983). If either of the two mechanisms associated with the articular capsule fails to function properly, the result could be painful pinching of the capsule, with subsequent acute low back pain and muscle tightness (spasm).

Narrowing of the IVD space results in increased pressure on the articulating surfaces of the Z joint. This pressure is further increased with extension of the lumbar region. Disc space narrowing also causes or increases the severity of impingement of synovial folds. Therefore, increased pressure on the subchondral bone of the articular processes and increased impingement of articular tissues (soft tissue "nipped" between the facets) may be two causes of back pain in patients with decreased height of one or more IVDs (Dunlop et al., 1984).

Aging is frequently accompanied by degenerative changes of the Z joints. Kirkaldy-Willis and colleagues (1978) stated that such changes include inflammatory reaction of the synovial lining of the Z joint, changes of the articular cartilage, loose bodies in the Z joint, and laxity of the joint capsule. All these result in joint instability. Changes of the Z joints (left and right) of any given vertebral level are frequently accompanied by degenerative changes in the IVD of the same level. Disc degeneration leads to increased rotational instability of the Z joints, resulting in further degeneration of these structures. Such degenerative changes in the Z joints usually take the form of increased bone formation (arthrosis, spur formation), which can compress the exiting spinal nerve (Rauschning, 1987). Much less frequently, degenerative change takes the form of erosion of the superior articular process (Kirkaldy-Willis et al., 1978). This can lead to

degenerative spondylolisthesis. Fig. 7-5 shows the process of Z joint and disc degeneration and the interrelation between the two.

The articular cartilage lining and the lumbar Z joints usually become irregular with age (Taylor & Twomey, 1986). The cartilage of the posterior aspect of the joint is frequently worn thin or may be completely absent. The articular cartilage of the anterior aspect of the joint usually remains thick but may show many fissures (known as cartilaginous fibrillation) that extend from the articular surface of the cartilage deep to the attachment of the cartilage to the subchondral bone. These types of changes of the articular cartilage are often more pronounced at the most superior and inferior aspects of the joint (Taylor & Twomey, 1986).

As mentioned, osteophytes (or bony spurs) often develop with age on the superior and inferior articular processes. Frequently this occurs along the periphery of the Z joint along the attachment sites of the ligamentum flavum or the articular capsule. The osteophytes most often develop at the attachment site of the ligamentum flavum on the anteromedial aspect of the superior articular process and extend into the posterior aspect of the vertebral canal. Taylor & Twomey (1986) found that fat-filled synovial pads developed in the region of osteophytes associated with the Z joints. These pads formed a cushion between the osteophytes and the inferior artic-

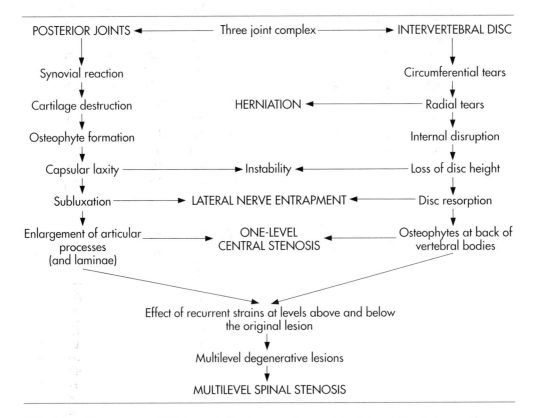

FIG. 7-5. The process of Z joint and disc degeneration and the interrelation between the two. (From Kirkaldy-Willis W.H. et al. *Spine*, 1978, *3*, 319-328.)

ular process. The authors also occasionally found that a prominent pad had developed within the inferior recess of the Z joint. This pad was found to lie between the tip of the inferior articular process and the lamina at the base of the subjacent vertebra's superior articular process. This is where the inferior articular process contacts the lamina during extension of the lumbar spine. This fat pad was often found to become thickened and sclerotic with age, probably in response to the mechanical stimulation of the inferior articular process.

Laminae

The laminae in the lumbar region are broad and thick but do not completely overlap one another. Therefore, in contrast to the thoracic region, a distinct space exists between the laminae of adjacent lumbar vertebrae in a dried preparation. This space allows for relatively easy access to the spinal subarachnoid space and is used in many diagnostic and therapeutic procedures.

Each lumbar lamina can be divided into superior and inferior portions. The superior part is curved and smooth on its inner surface, whereas the inferior part has a rough inner surface for attachment of the ligamentum flavum. Also, the inferior part of the lamina forms a buttress for the inferior articular process (Van Schaik et al., 1985).

The region of the lumbar lamina located between the superior and inferior articular processes is known as the pars interarticularis. This region can be fractured quite easily, a condition known as spondylolysis. As previously mentioned, at the levels of L4 and L5 loads are probably transferred from the vertebral bodies to the pars interarticularis by means of the pedicles. As the trabeculae in the L4 and L5 pedicles pass posteriorly, they are most highly concentrated where they extend into the pars interarticularis. Since trabeculae develop along the greatest lines of stress, the trabecular arrangement leading to the pars interarticularis of the L4 and L5 pedicles has been used to explain the frequency of spondylolysis at these levels.

As a result of spondylolysis, the vertebral body, pedicles, transverse processes, and superior articular processes can displace anteriorly. This anterior displacement is known as spondylolisthesis. Spondylolysis and spondylolisthesis are most common at L5. However, they may occur at any lumbar level. Standard x-ray films and CT remain the imaging modalities of choice for visualizing spondylolysis. However, parasagittal MRI does help to reveal a defect of the pars, which appears as a decrease in signal intensity perpendicular to the plane of the articular facets on these images (Grenier et al., 1989a).

Degenerative spondylolisthesis is a condition in which the superior articular processes undergo erosion with age rather than the usual increase in bone formation that frequently occurs in these processes with age. This erosion results in the vertebrae above (usually L4) moving anteriorly, bringing its posterior arch with it. The consequence is spinal canal stenosis with possible compromise of the cauda equina (Kirkaldy-Willis et al., 1978). Most frequently, L4 moves anteriorly on L5, and the inferior articular processes of L4 entrap the L5 and S1 nerve roots against the posterior aspect of the vertebral body of L5 (Dommisse & Louw, 1990).

Lumbar Vertebral Foramen and Vertebral Canal

General Considerations. The vertebral foramina in the lumbar region are generally triangular in shape, although they are somewhat more rounded in the upper lumbar vertebrae and more triangular, or trefoil, in the lower lumbar vertebrae. The triangular shape of the vertebral foramina of the middle and lower lumbar vertebrae is reminiscent of the shape of these openings in the cervical region; however, the lumbar foramina are smaller than those of the cervical region. On the other hand, the lumbar vertebral foramina are larger and more triangular than the rounded foramina of the thoracic region.

The size of the lumbar vertebral canal ranges from 12 to 20 mm in its anteroposterior dimension at the midsagittal plane and 18 to 27 mm in its transverse diameter. Stenosis has been defined as a narrowing below the lowest value of the range of normal (Dommisse & Louw, 1990). Because of the clinical significance of the vertebral canal, Table 7-3 has been included as a ready source of the dimensions of this region.

The vertebral foramen of L1 contains the conus medullaris, which ends at the level of the L1 IVD. The remainder of the lumbar portion of the vertebral canal (Figs. 7-6 and 7-7) contains the cauda equina. The cauda equina is bathed in the cerebrospinal fluid of the subarachnoid space. The subarachnoid space in the lumbar

Table 7-3 Dimensions of the Lumbar Vertebral Foramina (Vertebral Canal)*

Dimension	Size (range)†
Anteroposterior (in midsagittal plane)	12-20 mm
Transverse (interpedicular distance)	18-27 mm

*Dimensions below the lowest value indicate spinal (vertebral) canal stenosis (Dommisse & Louw, 1990). A typical vertebral foramen is rather triangular (trefoil) in shape. However, the upper lumbar vertebral foramina are more rounded than the lower lumbar foramina. L1 is the most rounded, and each succeeding lumbar vertebra becomes increasingly triangular, with L5 the most dramatically trefoil of all.
†Dimensions of lumbar vertebral foramina are usually smaller than those of the cervical region but larger than those of the thoracic region.

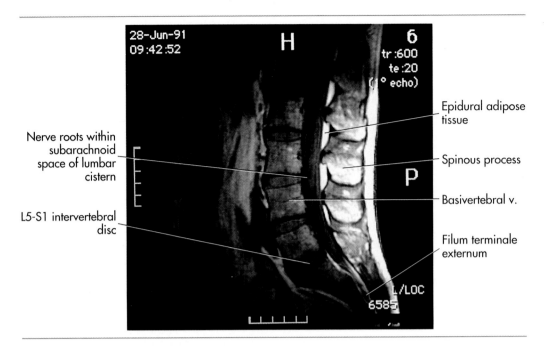

Nerve roots within subarachnoid space of lumbar cistern

L5-S1 intervertebral disc

Epidural adipose tissue

Spinous process

Basivertebral v.

Filum terminale externum

FIG. 7-6   Midsagittal plane MRI scan of the lumbar region.

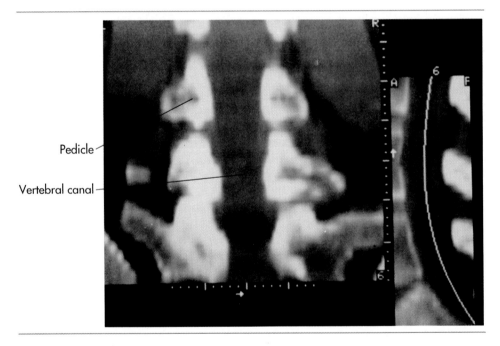

Pedicle

Vertebral canal

FIG. 7-7   Horizontal CT images digitally reformatted by computer to obtain this "curved coronal plane" image of the lumbar vertebral canal.

vertebral canal is quite large compared with that in the cervical and thoracic regions. Because of its size, the subarachnoid space below the level of the L1 vertebral foramen is known as the lumbar cistern. Also within the lumbar vertebral canal are the meninges: pia mater, attached to rootlets; arachnoid; and dura mater, which surrounds the arachnoid and to which the arachnoid is closely applied. In addition, adipose tissue, vessels, and nerves are located within the epidural space of the vertebral canal. Clinicians who specialize in diagnostic imaging frequently use the term *thecal sac* when collectively referring to the dura mater, arachnoid, and subarachnoid space within the vertebral canal. This term is not restricted to the lumbar region of the spine and is used when referring to these structures in the cervical and thoracic regions as well.

Dural Attachments Within the Vertebral Canal. The dura mater of the lumbar spine has a series of attachments to neighboring vertebrae and ligaments. These attachments are found at each segmental level and are usually found in the region of the IVD (Rauschning, 1987). They have been referred to as the dural attachment complex (Dupuis, 1988), or Hoffman ligaments (Dupuis, 1988; Rauschning, 1987). A centrally placed set of connective tissue bands attaches the anterior aspect of the dura mater to the posterior aspect of the lumbar vertebral bodies and the posterior longitudinal ligament. This set of bands has been referred to as midline Hoffman ligaments (Dupuis, 1988). A second set attaches the anterior and lateral aspects of the dura to the lateral, flared extension of the posterior longitudinal ligament, which is attached to the IVD (Fig. 7-8). These bands have been called the lateral Hoffmann ligaments (Dupuis, 1988). A third set of connective tissue bands attaches the exiting dural root sleeves with the inferior pedicles of the IVFs. These are known as the lateral root ligaments (see Lumbar Intervertebral Foramina and the Nerve Root Canals).

Stimulation of the anterior aspect of the lumbar spinal dura mater has been found to result in pain felt in the midline, radiating into the low back and superior aspect of the buttock (Edgar & Ghadially, 1976). This pattern of referral is also seen in irritation of the posterior longitudinal ligament (see Ligaments of the Lumbar Region).

Spinal Canal Stenosis. Narrowing of the vertebral canal (spinal canal) is most often known as spinal canal stenosis. Many variations of this condition exist in the lumbar region, several of which are discussed next. The possible pathologic condition that can result from spinal canal stenosis and that is common to all the variations is compression of one or more of the nerves that run through the vertebral canal. Such compression can lead to pain and dysfunction, probably caused by ischemia of the entrapped nerves (Lancourt et al., 1979). Lumbar spinal canal stenosis affects the nerves of the cauda equina or the dorsal and ventral roots as they leave the vertebral canal and enter IVFs.

Subdivisions of spinal stenosis include lateral recess stenosis and foraminal (intervertebral foraminal) stenosis. The exiting nerve roots travel through the more narrow, lateral aspect of the vertebral canal, known as the lateral recess, before entering the IVF. As the roots pass through this region of the vertebral canal, pressure may be placed on them. This is known as lateral recess stenosis. Another type of stenosis includes narrowing of the IVF. This condition is known as foraminal stenosis.

Causes. Spinal canal stenosis may be **congenital** in nature (Arnoldi et al., 1976). That is, some people are born with a "tight tube," and their vertebral canal remains narrow throughout their lives. Spinal canal stenosis can also be the result of **degenerative** changes.

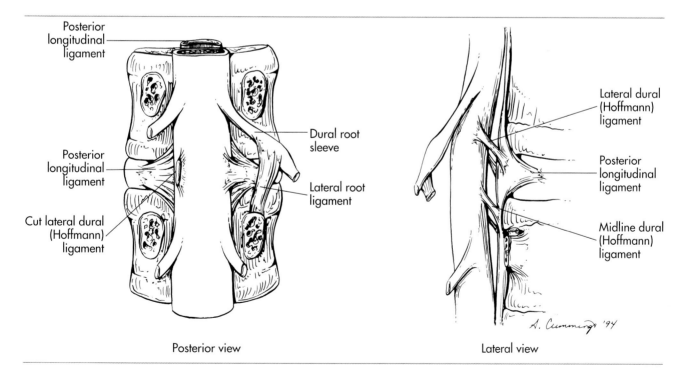

FIG. 7-8 Attachments of the dura mater to surrounding structures. (Modified from Dupuis, P.R. The anatomy of the lumbosacral spine. In W. Kirkadly-Willis (Ed.), *Managing low back pain* (2nd ed.). New York: Churchill Livingstone, 1988.)

Common causes of degenerative spinal canal stenosis include arthrosis (increased bone formation) of the medial aspect of the Z joint, especially of the superior articular process. Also, thickening (hypertrophy) of the ligamentum flavum can be a degenerative cause of spinal canal stenosis (Arnoldi et al., 1976; Liyang et al., 1989).

Other causes of spinal canal stenosis include spondylolisthesis, Paget's disease, fluorosis, degenerative changes following trauma (Kirkaldy-Willis et al., 1978), and iatrogenic (physician-induced) causes. The latter category includes complication after laminectomy, spinal fusion, and chemonucleolysis (Arnoldi et al., 1976). The box below lists possible causes of spinal stenosis.

POSSIBLE CAUSES OF SPINAL (VERTEBRAL) CANAL STENOSIS

Congenital
Degenerative
    Facet arthrosis
    Ligamentum flavum thickening (hypertrophy)
    Following trauma
Spondylolisthesis
Paget's disease
Fluorosis
Iatrogenic
    After laminectomy, spinal fusion, or chemonucleolysis
Any of above causes in conjunction with intervertebral disc protrusion

---

Any combination of congenital and degenerative causes of spinal canal stenosis may be present at one time. In addition, a herniated or bulging IVD can increase the severity of signs and symptoms in a patient who has this condition. Arnoldi and colleagues (1976), who developed a classification system for this condition, have included IVD protrusion in their system of nomenclature for spinal canal stenosis (e.g., congenital stenosis with IVD herniation, degenerative stenosis with IVD herniation). The contents of the lumbar vertebral canal are more frequently affected by disc protrusions than the contents of the cervical and thoracic regions of the vertebral canal (Clarke et al., 1985).

Also important in the development of signs and symptoms of spinal canal stenosis is the ratio between the size of the neural elements within the lumbar vertebral canal (the cauda equina) and the dimensions of the vertebral canal (Liyang et al., 1989). A person with relatively narrow vertebral foramina may be free of symptoms if the size of the roots making up the cauda equina and the surrounding meninges are proportionately small. However, if the vertebral canal is narrow (either congenitally or secondary to pathologic conditions or de-generation) and the roots making up the cauda equina are of normal size, signs and symptoms of spinal stenosis can result. One result of a normal-sized cauda equina within a narrow vertebral canal is a condition known as redundant nerve roots.

Redundant nerve roots. Redundant nerve roots refers to roots of the cauda equina that bend, curve frequently (undulate within the vertebral canal), or buckle during their course through the cauda equina. The buckling can be quite severe, blocking the flow of radiopaque dye on myelography. The roots in some cases appear to form dramatic loops (redundancies) when viewed during spinal surgery (Tsuji et al., 1985). The redundancies usually occur rather high in the lumbar vertebral canal. Degenerative spinal stenosis is thought to be the usual cause of this condition.

Redundant nerve roots once were considered a rare occurrence, but they may occur more frequently than previously expected. Tsuji and colleagues (1985) found this condition in 45% of a series of 117 consecutive cadavers without a recorded history of low back or leg pain. They also found that "22 of 56 patients (39%) had obvious redundant nerve roots, which indicates that this condition is a rather common abnormality in degenerative spinal stenosis."

Tsuji and colleagues (1985) presented a hypothesis of the progression of redundant nerve roots, which is summarized in the box below. Their hypothesis began with the finding that the vertebral column decreases in superior-to-inferior length with age (an average of 14 mm). Shortening of the vertebral canal would force the roots of the cauda equina to become somewhat redundant, causing them to fill the subarachnoid space (thecal space) more completely. Posterior spondylosis (osteophytes) from the vertebral bodies or other constrictions within the vertebral canal, could then more easily rub against the roots during movement. (Their study showed

---

DEVELOPMENT OF REDUNDANT NERVE ROOTS AND THE CONSEQUENCES

Vertebral column decreased in length with age
↓
Redundant nerve roots
↓
Spondylosis results in friction neuritis
↓
Increased root size
↓
Nerve root ischemia
↓
Cauda equina claudication

that considerable movement of the roots probably occurs during flexion-extension excursions of the spine.) The pressure from spondylosis (or other compressive elements) over many years could result in a friction neuritis. The friction neuritis was thought to result in the large redundant roots seen in several specimens. During walking and standing (extension), increased pressure is placed on the nerve roots (Fig. 7-9), which would cause ischemia of the neural elements. Nerve root ischemia would result in the signs and symptoms of intermittent claudication (pain and weakness in the lower extremities during standing and walking), which are frequently associated with spinal stenosis and redundant nerve roots. An average conduction velocity of 50% below normal values was found in cauda equina roots of individuals with redundant nerve roots. Tsuji and colleagues believed such neurologic changes were probably permanent.

Ischemia during stenosis. As mentioned previously, stenosis of the vertebral canal has been implicated as a possible cause of ischemia to the roots of the cauda equina (Dommisse & Louw, 1990; Lancourt, Glenn, & Wiltse, 1979; Tsuji et al., 1985). This ischemia probably occurs in the roots' "vulnerable region" of vascularity. The roots that form the cauda equina receive their blood supply (vasa nervorum) distally from radicular arteries and also proximally from the cruciate anastomosis surrounding the conus medullaris (see Chapter 3). The proximal and distal vessels form an anastomosis at approximately the junction of the proximal and middle thirds of the cauda equina roots. This has been called the "critical zone" of vascularity and represents a region where the roots are vulnerable to compression (Dommisse & Louw, 1990). Compression in this region would result in neural ischemia causing the symptoms and signs usually associated with spinal stenosis (see the following discussion).

Symptoms. The symptoms of spinal canal stenosis usually include pain radiating from the lumbar region into the lower extremities, occasionally inferior to the knee. The symptoms are usually posture dependent and are made worse by standing or walking for variable periods of time. Flexion of the lumbar region usually relieves the pain.

Liyang and colleagues (1989) found that the volume of the dural sac (subarachnoid space), as studied in 10 cadavers, increased by 3.5 to 6.0 ml during excursion from full extension to full flexion. These changes were found to be highly significant ($p < 0.001$). The sagittal diameter of the dural sac (subarachnoid space), as measured from myelograms of the cadaveric spines, was also found to increase significantly during flexion; the greatest increase occurred at the level of L5. Also, the length of the

lumbar vertebral (spinal) canal was found to increase by an average of 19.4 mm during flexion. This helps to explain clinical findings that flexion generally relieves the symptoms of spinal canal stenosis (Fig. 7-9).

Since extension of the lumbar region is accompanied by broadening of the cauda equina, slackening of the ligamenta flava, bulging of the IVDs into the vertebral (spinal) canal, and narrowing of the IVF, one can understand how extension of the lumbar region can increase the symptoms of spinal canal stenosis (Fig. 7-9). Therefore, therapeutic interventions that increase flexion and reduce extension are indicated in patients with this condition (Liyang et al., 1989). Such interventions include exercises that increase tone of abdominal muscles, weight reduction if indicated, and adjustive (manipulative) procedures that promote flexion (Cassidy & Kirkaldy-Willis, 1988; Cox, 1990; Kirk & Lawrence, 1985; Bergmann, Peterson, & Lawrence, 1993). If stenosis is severe, positive effects from manipulation may be more difficult to achieve. "Nevertheless, it can be helpful in some patients and is worth a try in the early management of this syndrome" (Cassidy & Kirkaldy-Willis, 1988). Several authors have reported positive results from wearing a brace to keep the lumbar spine in flexion. Liyang and colleagues (1989) suggested that spinal stenosis be treated by surgical decompression

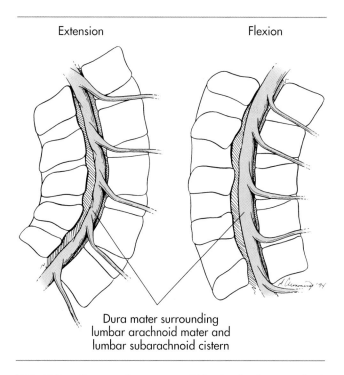

Extension   Flexion

Dura mater surrounding
lumbar arachnoid mater and
lumbar subarachnoid cistern

FIG. 7-9 Changes that occur within the lumbar vertebral canal during flexion and extension. Notice that the lumbar cistern enlarges during flexion and decreases in volume during extension. The lumbar vertebral canal has also been found to increase in length by almost 2 cm during flexion.

(laminectomy) of the spinal (vertebral) canal, followed by fixation of the spine in flexion. Interestingly, Kikuchi and colleagues (1984) found that infiltration of a single nerve root with local anesthetic usually extinguished the symptoms of cauda equina claudication secondary to spinal stenosis. This would seem to be contrary to the widely held belief that neurogenic claudication is the result of compression of the entire cauda equina.

Spinous Process

The spinous processes of lumbar vertebrae are broad from superior to inferior, narrow from side to side, and project directly posteriorly. They are, more or less, flat and rectangular in shape. Their posteroinferior ridge is thickened for the attachment of ligaments and muscles.

The lumbar spinous processes have been found to undergo morphologic changes after age 40, reaching the highest incidence of change in persons over 60 (Scapinelli, 1989). The most common change is the addition of bone along the posterior aspect of the spinous processes, which may increase their anteroposterior length by as much as 1 cm or more. The greatest increase in length is usually at L3. Frequently the added bone presents a sharp, spurlike margin, usually on the posterosuperior aspect of the spinous process. A smaller increase in the superior-to-inferior dimension usually occurs simultaneously with the anteroposterior change. Occasionally the spinous processes touch one another in the neutral position. This is known as "kissing spines," or Bastrup's syndrome.

These changes are created by replacement of ligamentous tissue of the supraspinous and interspinous ligaments and the related fibrous tissue below L3 with fibrocartilage and eventually bone. Scapinelli (1989) believes these changes are associated with decreased movement as one ages, an increased lumbar lordosis, and traction from ligaments and tendons of muscles. The greatest increase in bone is in individuals with degenerative changes of the vertebral bodies and Z joints (degenerative spondyloarthrosis), especially those with diffuse idiopathic skeletal hyperostosis (DISH, or Forestier's disease). With the exception of DISH, the changes are believed to increase the lever arm of the erector spinae muscles, helping with the maintenance of an erect posture (Scapinelli, 1989).

Table 7-4 lists those structures that normally attach to the lumbar spinous processes.

Lumbar Intervertebral Foramina and Nerve Root Canals

General Considerations. The bony and ligamentous canals referred to as the intervertebral foramina (*sing.*, foramen) have been described in Chapter 2. However,

several features of the lumbar IVFs are unique. In addition, these regions have been the subject of extensive descriptive and clinical investigation. The relationship between the lumbosacral nerve roots and their surrounding tissues is important in the proper diagnosis of low back pain and pain radiating into the lower extremity (Hasue et al., 1983). This section therefore focuses on the unique aspects of the anatomy of the lumbar IVFs, the pertinent conclusions of previous and current studies of the IVF, and the clinical relevance of this fascinating area.

Many features of the region of the lumbar IVFs are different from those of the rest of the spine because of the unique characteristics of the lumbar and sacral spinal nerves (Fig. 7-10). Because the spinal cord ends at approximately the IVD of L1, the lumbar and sacral dorsal and ventral roots must descend, sometimes for a considerable distance, within the subarachnoid space of the lumbar vertebral canal. This region of subarachnoid space is known as the lumbar cistern. The exiting nerves (dorsal and ventral rootlets or roots) leave the lumbar cistern by entering a sleeve of dura mater. This usually occurs slightly inferior to the level of the IVD at the level *above* the IVF that the roots will eventually occupy. For example, the L4 roots enter their dural sleeve just beneath the L3-4 disc and then course inferiorly and laterally to exit the L4-5 IVF. More specifically, on leaving the subarachnoid space of the lumbar cistern, the exiting dorsal and ventral roots pass at an oblique inferior and lateral angle while retaining a rather substantial and very distinct covering of dura mater. This covering, known as the dural root sleeve, surrounds the neural elements and their accompanying radicular arteries and veins until they leave the confines of the IVF (see Fig. 2-13). Frequently the dorsal and ventral rootlets that arise from the spinal cord do not all unite to form dorsal and ventral roots until they are well within the dural root sleeve (Dupuis, 1988; Rauschning, 1987). In addition, the dorsal and ventral roots combine to form the mixed spinal nerve while within the distal aspect of the funnel-shaped dural root sleeve. This latter union occurs at the level of the IVF. The exiting mixed spinal nerve has been found to be larger than the combined size of the

Table 7-4 Attachments to Lumbar Spinous Processes

Type	Structures attached
Ligaments	Thoracolumbar fascia (posterior lamella)
	Supraspinous and interspinous
Muscles	Deep back muscles (spinalis thoracis, multifidus, interspinalis)

Data from Williams et al. (1989). *Gray's anatomy* (37th ed.). Edinburgh: Churchill Livingstone.

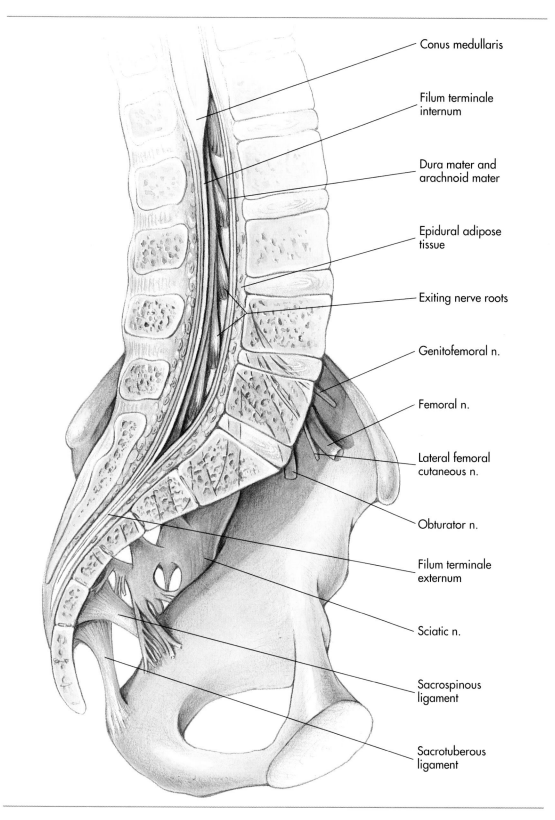

Conus medullaris

Filum terminale
internum

Dura mater and
arachnoid mater

Epidural adipose
tissue

Exiting nerve roots

Genitofemoral n.

Femoral n.

Lateral femoral
cutaneous n.

Obturator n.

Filum terminale
externum

Sciatic n.

Sacrospinous
ligament

Sacrotuberous
ligament

FIG. 7-10 Midsagittal view of the spine showing nerve roots traversing the lumbar vertebral canal, exiting the intervertebral foramina, and forming the lumbar sacral plexuses.

individual dorsal and ventral roots (dePeretti et al., 1989). On reaching the lateral edge of the IVF, the dural root sleeve becomes continuous with the epineurium of the mixed spinal nerve.

Many authors (Bose & Balasubramaniam, 1984; Lee, Rauschning, & Glenn, 1988; Rauschning, 1987; Vital et al., 1983) have described the region beginning at the exit of the neural elements from the lumbar subarachnoid cistern and continuing to the lateral edge of the IVF as having significant clinical importance. Perhaps because of the clinical significance of this region, several terms have been used to describe it, including lumbar radicular canal (Vital et al., 1983), nerve root canal, or simply root canal (Rauschning, 1987) (Fig. 7-11). The term *nerve root canal (NRC)* is used in the following paragraphs when discussing the course of the dural root sleeve and its contents, and the term *IVF* is used to describe the terminal part of the NRC that lies between the pedicles of two adjacent vertebrae.

Within the dural root sleeve an interneural complex of fibrous connections (Dupuis, 1988) anchors the neural elements (rootlets and roots) to the surrounding dura mater of the NRC. More specifically, these connections course from the dura and inner arachnoid of the sleeve to the pia surrounding the rootlets and roots. Recall that farther laterally the root sleeve unites with the mixed spinal nerve to form its epineurium.

Connective Tissue Attachments of the Dura to the Borders of the Intervertebral Foramina. The external surface of the dural root sleeve is usually attached by one or more connective tissue bands to the inferior pedicle of the IVF (see Fig. 7-8). This connective tissue attachment is called the lateral root ligament

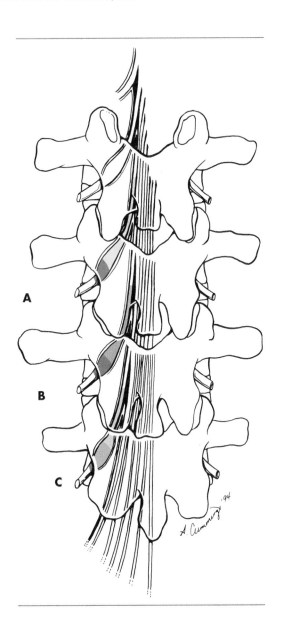

FIG. 7-11　A through C, Regions of the intervertebral foramen (IVF) as described by various authors. A, The nerve root canal (NRC) as the course of the dural root sleeve and its contents (*yellow* and *red* regions combined). Other terms used when referring to this general region are lumbar radicular canal (Vital et al., 1983) and root canal (Rauschning, 1987). The IVF is shown in red as the terminal part of the NRC, located between the pedicles of two adjacent vertebrae. This also represents the classic anatomic description of the IVF. B, Regions of the NRC (lumbar radicular canal) as described by Vital and colleagues (1983). Notice the retrodiscal portion in blue. This is the portion of the NRC that lies posterior to the intervertebral disc (IVD) superior to the level that the spinal nerve eventually exits. The parapedicular portion of the NRC *(green)* is the region medial to the pedicle. Vital and colleagues (1983) refer to the region occupied by the uniting dorsal and ventral roots and the exiting mixed spinal nerve as the IVF proper *(red)*. Table 7-8 describes the borders of the retrodiscal, parapedicular, and IVF proper subdivisions of the NRC. C, Divisions of the NRC (root canal) as described by Rauschning (1987) and by Lee and colleagues (1988). The entrance zone *(pink)* is the region that begins as the dorsal and ventral roots enter the dural root sleeve and extends through the lateral recess. Other authors use lateral recess, lateral canal, subarticular gutter, or lateral nerve canal when referring to the entrance zone. The middle zone, or pedicle zone, *(blue)* is the region of the NRC located between the two adjacent pedicles which make up an IVF. This area was described above (A and B) as the IVF proper (Vital et al., 1983). The term exit zone, or foramen proper, is used by Rauschning (1987), and Lee and colleagues (1988) to refer to the almost two-dimensional opening ("doorway") formed by a parasagittal plane passed along the lateral edge of the two pedicles that help to form an IVF. The exit zone is shown in red in C.

(Dupuis, 1988). It limits the medial and upward mobility of the root sleeve and its contents (Rauschning, 1987). Fibrous connections from the lateral aspect of the IVF to the exiting spinal nerve have also been identified (dePeretti et al., 1989; Hasue et al., 1983). These fibrous attachments have been found to give considerable resistance to traction of the anterior primary divisions. Therefore, they serve to spare the lumbar roots from traction injuries. The dural root sleeve also provides resistance to traction. In fact, the dural root sleeve ruptures before avulsion of the rootlets from the conus medullaris occurs. These resistive forces, when combined with the fact that the rootlets and roots forming the spinal nerves are of excess length within the dura mater, indicates that the IVF seems to provide an almost insurmountable protective barrier to traction forces placed on the exiting spinal nerves (dePeretti et al., 1989).

Entrapment of the Neural Elements. Unfortunately, the exiting neural elements are not as well protected from pressure injuries as they are from traction injuries. Compression, or entrapment, of neural elements as they pass through the NRC or the IVF is of extreme clinical importance (Lancourt et al., 1979). Also, because treatment may differ depending on the cause of entrapment, a detailed understanding of this region is essential. The clinician should attempt to localize a lesion as precisely as possible to determine the structure causing the problem and also to identify the specific neural elements being affected (Rauschning, 1987). These neural elements include the dorsal and ventral roots and their union as the mixed spinal nerve. Causes of such compression include degenerative changes of the superior articular facets and posterior vertebral bodies, IVD protrusion, and pressure from the superior pedicle of the IVF (Hasue et al., 1983; McNab, 1971; Vital et al., 1983) (see Chapter 11).

Occasionally, osteophytes from the Z joints and vertebral bodies can become so large that they can almost completely divide the IVF into two smaller foramina, one on top of the other (Kirkaldy-Willis et al., 1978). Such changes may result in entrapment of the exiting spinal nerve. Because of the clinical importance of the NRCs and the IVFs, a more accurate anatomic description is necessary.

Anatomy of the Nerve Root Canals. The sizes of the NRCs vary considerably from the upper to lower lumbar segments. They are smaller in length at the level of L1 and L2 because, after exiting the lumbar cistern, the L1 and L2 nerves course almost directly laterally to reach the IVF. This led Crock (1981) to state that the concept of a nerve root *canal* at L1 and L2 is useless, since the beginning of the dural root sleeve lies against

the inferior and medial aspect of the IVF's upper pedicle. Therefore, no true dural "canal" exists for these nerve roots.

Table 7-5 gives the obliquities and lengths of the lumbar NRCs. The NRCs become progressively longer from L1 to S1 as the dural root sleeves exit at a more oblique inferior angle. Therefore the NRCs of L5 and S1 are the longest in the lumbar region and the most susceptible to damage from pathologic conditions of surrounding

Table 7-5 Obliquity and Length of the Lumbar Nerve Root Canals

Level	Obliquity*	Length†	Length*
L1	70°	NVG	AN
L2	80°	NVG	AN
L3	60°	NVG	NVG
L4	60°	6.7 mm	25 mm
L5	45°	7.8 mm	30 mm
S1	30°	8.0 mm	35 mm

NVG, No value given; *AN,* almost nonexistent.
*According to Bose and Balasubramaniam (1984); obliquity given in degrees from a sagittal plane (low values, much inferior obliquity).
†According to Vital et al. (1983).

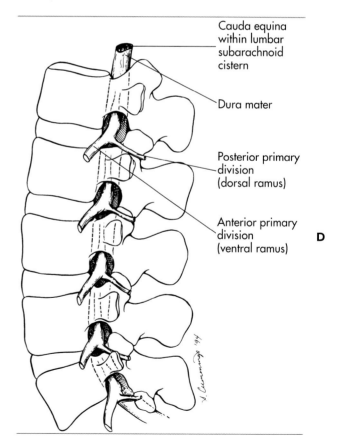

D

Cauda equina within lumbar subarachnoid cistern

Dura mater

Posterior primary division (dorsal ramus)

Anterior primary division (ventral ramus)

FIG. 7-11, cont'd. **D,** Lateral view of the lumbar IVFs. The specific dimensions of the lumbar IVFs are given in Chapter 2 (see Tables 2-3 and 2-4). *Continued.*

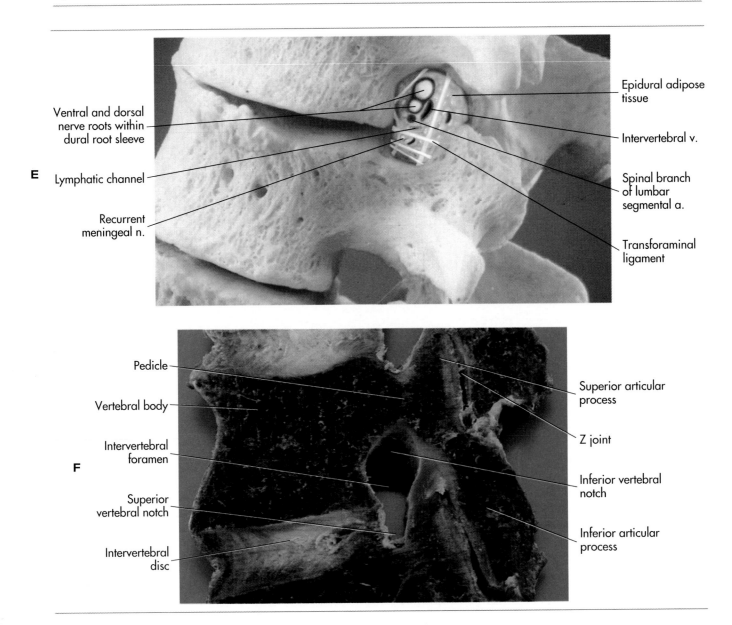

E, Ventral and dorsal nerve roots within dural root sleeve — Lymphatic channel — Recurrent meningeal n. — Epidural adipose tissue — Intervertebral v. — Spinal branch of lumbar segmental a. — Transforaminal ligament

F, Pedicle — Vertebral body — Intervertebral foramen — Superior vertebral notch — Intervertebral disc — Superior articular process — Z joint — Inferior vertebral notch — Inferior articular process

FIG. 7-11, cont'd. **E,** Lateral view of two IVFs. The structures that normally traverse this region have been drawn in the more superior IVF. The most common locations of the transforaminal ligaments are also shown traversing this IVF. **F,** Parasagittal section through the fourth lumbar IVF. A typical lumbar IVF is sometimes described as being shaped like an "inverted teardrop" or an "inverted pear" when viewed from the side. (**E** and **F** courtesy The National College of Chiropractic.)

structures (Crock, 1981). Tables 7-6 and 7-7 describe the relationships of the L5 and S1 NRCs, respectively. Many, if not most, of the types of borders described in Table 7-6 for the L5 NRC also apply to the L3 and L4 NRCs as well.

All the exiting rootlets or roots course over an IVD either just before entering their dural root sleeve (L1 and L2) or, in the case of L3-S1, directly in the region where they enter the dural root sleeve. However, only the S1 dural root sleeve (and contents) passes completely over an IVD (the L5 disc). The S1 NRC passes through a mov-

able, narrow opening between the L5 disc anteriorly and the L5-S1 ligamentum flavum posteriorly. Therefore the S1 nerve is exposed to possible compression both anteriorly (disc protrusion) and posteriorly (ligamentum flavum bulging or buckling, hypertrophy of superior articular process of sacrum) in this region (Rauschning, 1987).

Anomalies of the Neural Elements and the Dural Root Sleeves. Anomalies of the rootlets as they come off of the spinal cord are common. Such anomalies oc-

Table 7-6 Relationships of the L5 Nerve Root Canal

Surface	Relationship
Origin	L4-5 IVD (sometimes does not begin this far superiorly, in which case begins at L5 vertebral body)
Medial surface	Lateral aspect of S1 NRC
Lateral surface	Medial aspect of pedicle of L5, then enters L5 IVF
Anterior surface*	Posterior aspect of L5 vertebral body
Posterior surface†	L5-S1 Z joint and overlying ligamentum flavum
Other relationships	Surrounded by epidural adipose tissue, and small arteries, veins, and lymphatics (very small)

Data partly from Bose, K. & Balasubramaniam, P. (1984). *Spine, 9,* 16-18.
*Just distal to origin.
†Posterior relationships vary considerably depending on length of the nerve roots and orientation of the L5 lamina, which changes with a change in the angle between L5 and the sacrum (Crock, 1981).

Table 7-7 Relationships of the S1 Nerve Root Canal

Surface	Relationship
Origin	Medial aspect of L5 pedicle
Medial surface	Lateral aspect of dural sac
Lateral surface	L5 nerve root, then L5-S1 IVF, then S1 pedicle, then enters S1 IVF
Anterior surface	Posterior aspect of L5 vertebral body, then L5 IVD, then posterior aspect of the S1 vertebral body
Posterior surface*	Bony ridge of anterior aspect of L5 lamina (formed by the attachment of ligamentum flavum), then ligamentum flavum, then anteromedial aspect of S1 superior articular process
Other relationships	Surrounded by epidural adipose tissue, and small arteries, veins, and lymphatics (very small)

Data from Crock, H.V. (1981). *J Bone Joint Surg, 63,* 487-490; and Vital, J.M. et al. (1983). *Anat Clin, 5,* 141-151.
*Posterior relationships vary considerably depending on length of the nerve roots and orientation of the L5 lamina, which changes with a change in the angle between L5 and the sacrum (Crock, 1981).

cur much more often with the dorsal rootlets than the ventral rootlets (Kikuchi et al., 1984). The anomalies take the form of rootlets of one spinal cord segment passing to the root of the nerve below or above. Such anomalies could conceivably result in the perception of radicular symptoms different from the normal dermatomal pattern.

Anomalies of the roots making up the cauda equina while within the lumbar cistern are also quite common.

These usually consist of nerve bundles from one root passing to a neighboring root. The clinical implications of this type of anomaly are the same as those just discussed for anomalous rootlets.

Congenital anomalies associated with the dural root sleeves also occur with some frequency. Hasue and colleagues (1983) found anomalies in 5 of the 59 cadavers (8.5%) in their study. Several types of anomalies have been identified (Bogduk & Twomey, 1991; Hasue et al., 1983; Kikuchi et al., 1984; Neidre & MacNab, 1983) (Fig. 7-12). The first type is known as conjoined nerve roots and is the most common type of dural sleeve anomaly (Fig. 7-12, *C*). With this anomaly, roots of adjacent spinal cord segments share the same dural root sleeve for a short distance. The roots then separate into their own dural root sleeve and exit the appropriate IVF. Conjoined nerve roots cause one of the roots (or both) to take a rather tortuous course, possibly making it more susceptible to traction across a bulging disc or a narrow NRC.

The second type of root sleeve anomaly is the most dramatic. The dorsal and ventral roots of two distinct spinal cord levels, within their appropriate root sleeves, exit the same IVF, leaving the adjacent IVF devoid of exiting roots (Fig. 7-12, *B*). In a variation of this anomaly, an additional dorsal and ventral root and their covering dural root sleeve pass through the same IVF with the neural and dural structures that normally pass through the IVF. In this instance, all of the IVFs have roots within them, and one IVF has two pairs of roots passing through it (Fig. 7-12, *D*). The nerves within an IVF containing more than one set of roots in these types of anomalies are more susceptible to entrapment. Entrapment of two sets of roots within one IVF might lead to radicular symptoms of more than one dermatomes (see Chapters 9 and 11).

In the third type of dural root sleeve anomaly, a communicating branch, surrounded by its own dural sheath, passes from one NRC to its neighbor before either primary root exits its IVF. The result of this anomaly could be similar to that of roots sending connecting branches to neighboring roots, causing dispersion of radicular symptoms to include an adjacent segment (e.g., L5 compression may result in some pain or paresthesia being felt in the L4 dermatome). However, because it runs within its own dural root sleeve, the neural elements within the "bridging sleeve" are more vulnerable to compression either inside a lateral recess or as they pass behind an IVD. This type of anomaly can also occur in conjunction with the variation of the second type of anomaly previously mentioned. In this case a communicating branch is found between two dural root sleeves as they both exit the same IVF (Fig. 7-12, *D*).

Anomalies of the nerve roots and the dural sleeves can be a sole cause of radicular symptoms. They can also

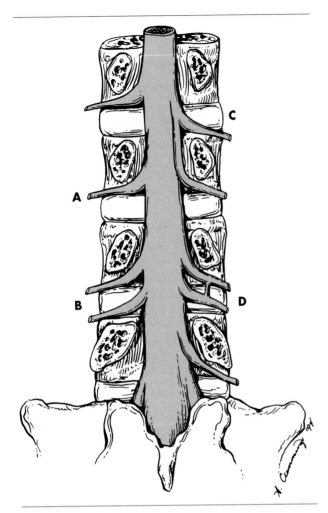

FIG. 7-12 Posterior view of the vertebral canal showing anomalies of dural root sleeves. The dural root sleeve, *A*, is normal. Notice that it is exiting the upper region of the IVF. The anomaly, *B*, shows the roots of two distinct spinal cord levels, within their appropriate root sleeves, exiting the same IVF. This leaves an adjacent IVF devoid of exiting roots. The anomaly, *C*, shows conjoined nerve roots. In this case the roots of adjacent spinal cord segments share the same dural root sleeve for a short distance. The roots then separate into their own dural root sleeve and exit the appropriate IVF. Conjoined nerve roots cause one of the roots (or both) to take a rather tortuous course. The anomaly, *D*, is a variation of *B*. Anomaly *D* shows an additional dorsal and ventral root, and their covering dural root sleeve, passing through the same IVF with the neural and dural structures that normally pass through that IVF. Therefore all the IVFs on the right side of the illustration have roots within them, and one IVF has two pairs of roots passing through it. Also notice another type of anomaly is shown in *D*. A communicating branch, surrounded by its own dural sheath is seen passing from one dural sleeve to its neighbor, before either exits the IVF. All these types of anomalies *(B, C, D)* can have significant clinical implications (see text). (Modified from Bogduk, N. & Twomey, L.T. *Clinical anatomy of the lumbar spine.* London: Churchill Livingstone, 1991.)

augment radicular symptoms from other causes (Hasue et al., 1983). Even though the incidence of symptoms as a result of such NRC anomalies is thought to be rare, they should be kept in mind when patients have unusual distribution patterns of radicular symptoms (Bogduk & Twomey, 1991).

Terminology Associated with the Nerve Root Canals and the Intervertebral Foramina. Terminology with regard to the exiting roots can be rather confusing. Some authors (Vital et al., 1983) describe the beginning of the NRC (that portion posterior to the IVD directly above the level of the IVF of exit) as the retrodiscal portion of the NRC (see Fig. 7-11, *B*). As the nerve continues to descend more laterally in what is described by many as the lateral recess, the nerve lies medial to the pedicle that forms the upper border of the IVF, which the nerve roots eventually exit. This region is sometimes called the parapedicular portion of the NRC (Vital et al., 1983). The portion of the IVF occupied by the uniting dorsal and ventral roots and the exiting mixed spinal nerve is referred to as the IVF proper. Table 7-8 describes the borders of the retrodiscal, parapedicular, and IVF proper subdivisions of the NRC. This table is included to help clarify the regions where the nerve roots and mixed nerve are most vulnerable to various types of pathologic conditions.

Moving from the upper lumbar region to the lower lumbar region, the parapedicular portion (lateral recess) of the NRC widens in the transverse plane (i.e., left to right), becomes shorter from top to bottom, and be-

Table 7-8   Relationships of the Various Regions of the S1 Nerve Root Canal

Region and surface	Relationships
Retrodiscal Region	
Anterior	IVD*
Posterior	Superior articular process*, ligamentum flavum*
Parapedicular region (lateral recess)	
Anterior	Posterior surface of vertebral body
Posterior	Ligamentum flavum*, superior articular process*, pars interarticularis (isthmus)*
Lateral	Medial surface of pedicle
Medial	Dura of lumbar cistern
IVF Proper	
Superior	Lower margin of upper pedicle
Anterior	Upper and lower vertebral bodies, IVD in between them*
Inferior	Upper margin of lower pedicle
Posterior	Z joint and ligamentum flavum*

*Indicates relationships that are of key clinical importance.

comes narrower from anterior to posterior (average of 12 mm at L2 and 8 mm at L5) (Vital et al., 1983). Therefore this part of the NRC becomes more like a true lateral recess, or gutter, as one descends the lumbar spine.

The position of the entire lumbar region affects the NRC and the neural elements (Vital et al., 1983). The anteroposterior dimension of the retrodiscal space narrows in the upright posture. This is because of slight posterior bulging of the IVD and slight anterior buckling of the ligamentum flavum. During flexion of the lumbar region, the neural elements become stretched and pressed against the anterior walls of the retrodiscal and the parapedicular spaces. Also, the IVF proper increases in height and width during flexion. Extension of the lumbar region results in slackening of the neural elements. They also move against the posterior wall of the lateral recess during extension. In addition, the IVF becomes significantly shorter from superior to inferior and anterior to posterior during extension (Mayoux-Benhamou et al., 1989).

A different set of terms was put forth by Rauschning (1987) and by Lee and colleagues (1988) (Fig. 7-11, *C*). These authors used the term *entrance zone* when referring to the region that begins as the roots enter the dural root sleeve and continues through the lateral recess. Other authors use the terms *lateral recess, lateral canal, subarticular gutter,* or *lateral nerve canal* when referring to this region (Rauschning, 1987). This area corresponds to the combination of the retrodiscal and parapedicular regions previously described. The most common cause of stenosis in the entrance zone is hypertrophic osteoarthritis of the Z joint, usually of the superior articular facet. Other causes include congenital variations of the Z joints or a congenitally short pedicle. Also, a bulging anulus fibrosus (e.g., L3 anulus compressing the L4 nerve) or an osteophythic spur from the superior vertebral end plate coursing along the anulus, could compress the neural elements in the entrance zone.

Rauschning (1987) and Lee and colleagues (1988) use the term *mid zone* or *pedicle zone* when referring to the region of the NRC located between the two adjacent pedicles that make up an IVF (Fig. 7-11, *C*). This area was described previously as the IVF proper (Vital et al., 1983) (Fig. 7-11, *A*). The dorsal root (spinal) ganglion and the ventral root are located within this region and can be compressed here. Because of its large size, the dorsal root ganglion is more susceptible to minor compression than the ventral root. Osteophyte formation along the ligamentum flavum (anterior to the pars interarticularis) and hypertrophy of fibrous tissue along a fracture of the pars interarticularis was cited by Lee and colleagues (1988) as being the most common causes of stenosis in the middle zone. Lee and colleagues (1988) also believed that, because the middle zone is difficult to

evaluate with diagnostic imaging procedures, clinicians may overlook stenosis of this region. The authors stated that neural entrapment of the middle zone may result in symptoms of activity-related, intermittent, neurogenic claudication. They also noted that some patients progress until they experience constant pain and diminished sensation even during times of rest. These unprovoked resting symptoms may be caused by spontaneous action potentials arising from compressed or entrapped ganglionic cells (Lee et al., 1988).

The term *exit zone,* or *foramen proper,* was used by Rauschning (1987) and Lee and colleagues (1988) to refer to the almost two-dimensional opening ("doorway") formed by a parasagittal plane passed along the lateral edge of the two pedicles that help to form an IVF (Fig. 7-11, *C*). The most common causes of stenosis in this region are "hypertrophic osteoarthritic changes of the facet joints (Z joints) with subluxation and osteophytic ridge formation along the superior margin of the disc" (Lee et al., 1988).

Clinical Conditions Related to the Nerve Root Canals. Resorption of the IVD (particularly at the L5-S1 level) causes narrowing of the IVF at the same level (L5-S1 IVF in this case) and also narrowing of the NRC of the nerve exiting at the IVF below (the S1 NRC in this case). Crock (1981) stated that the remaining anulus fibrosus of the disc may bulge posteriorly, bringing the posterior longitudinal ligament along with it. The superior articular facet of the segment below (S1) moves superiorly and anteriorly, again compressing the NRC (S1). The combination of posterior anulus bulge along with anterior displacement of the superior articular facet of the vertebra below can result in dramatic narrowing of the NRC that runs between these two structures (Rauschning, 1987). Osteophyte (bony spur) formation is fairly common, both from the vertebral body along the attachment of the anulus fibrosus and from the superior articular process along the attachment of the ligamentum flavum. These spurs can further compress the neural and vascular elements of the NRC (Rauschning, 1987). In addition, a bony ridge may develop along the anterior and inferior surface of the lamina. This can compress the more medial NRC (that of the nerve exiting at the IVF of the level below, S1 in this instance) and also the lateral and distal aspect of the NRC of the nerve exiting at the same level (in this case, L5).

The L5 NRC is related to both the L4-5 (at its origin) and the L5-S1 (at its exit) IVDs. Therefore, with suspected entrapment of the L5 nerve, a differentiation between compression from L4 or L5 disc protrusion (bulge) or from another structure along the L5 NRC must be made (Bose & Balasubramaniam, 1984).

Congenital hypertrophy of the L5-S1 articular facets may cause localized obstruction of the L5-S1 IVF.

Osteoarthritis of the L5-S1 facets may cause the same condition, but usually such arthritis tends to cause obstruction more medially, affecting the descending S1 NRC (Crock, 1981).

Intervertebral Foramina Proper. When viewed from the side, the lumbar IVFs face laterally. A typical lumbar IVF is sometimes described as being shaped like an inverted teardrop or an inverted pear (Fig. 7-13). The specific dimensions of the lumbar IVFs are given in Chapter 2 (see Tables 2-3 and 2-4).

The spinal nerve is located in the upper third of each lumbar IVF. As it enters the IVF, the spinal nerve is very close to the medial and inferior aspect of the superior pedicle that forms the upper boundary of the IVF (Crock, 1981). Here the nerve is accompanied by a branch (or sometimes branches) of the lumbar segmental artery, the superior segmental (pedicle) veins, which connect the external and internal vertebral venous plexuses, and by the sinuvertebral nerve (Rauschning, 1987). The spinal nerve occupies approximately one third of the IVF in the lumbar region. This allows for crowding by the articular facets during extension (Bose & Balasubramaniam, 1984; Rauschning, 1987). The inferior aspect of the IVF is usually narrowed to a slit by the anulus fibrosus, which normally bulges slightly posteriorly. The inferior aspect of the IVF is also narrowed by the posteriorly located ligamentum flavum. The inferior segmental (discal) veins usually lie in this narrow space. As with the superior segmental (pedicle) veins, the inferior veins also unite the internal (epidural) vertebral venous plexus with the external vertebral venous plexus and the ascending lumbar vein.

The lateral borders of the IVFs are covered with an incomplete layer of transforaminal fascia. This fascia condenses in several locations at each IVF to form the accessory ligaments of the IVF (see Chapter 2). An exiting mixed spinal nerve could be affected by these structures at it leaves the IVF (Bachop & Janse, 1983; Bachop & Ro, 1984; Bakkum & Mestan, 1994; Bose & Balasubramaniam, 1984; Rauschning, 1987). In addition to compression by accessory ligaments or transforaminal fascia, Rauschning (1987) states that lateral disc herniations and bony structures such as the TPs (usually of L5, but at higher lumbar levels on rare occasions) "may compress, kink, or constrict the lumbar nerves beyond the foraminal outlet." The author calls this region the extraforaminal region or the postcanal zone.

Also, the lateral borders of the L1 through L4 IVFs are associated with the origin of the psoas major muscle. In fact, because of the posterior origin of the psoas major muscle from the front of the TPs and its anterior origin from the lumbar vertebral bodies and IVDs, the psoas major almost completely surrounds the lateral opening of the first four lumbar IVFs. Therefore the anterior primary divisions (ventral rami), by necessity, run through the substance of the psoas major muscle, frequently uniting with neighboring ventral rami within the muscle to

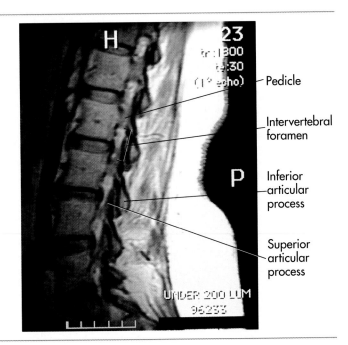

FIG. 7-13 Parasagittal plane MRI scan of the lumbar region. Note the prominent intervertebral foramina.

form the branches of the lumbar plexus. In addition to the protection given by the dural root sleeve and the Hoffman ligaments (see previous discussion), the psoas major muscle may provide some protection for the dorsal and ventral roots during traction of the peripheral nerves of the lumbar plexus (dePeretti et al., 1989). Such traction may occur as a result of hyperflexion or hyperextension of the lower extremity.

The boundaries of the IVF can be imaged well with both MRI and CT (Cramer et al., 1994) (Figs. 7-13 and 7-14). Occasionally, ossification of the superior attachment of the ligamentum flavum results in foraminal spurs, which can be seen on CT. These spurs are considered to be normal variants; may project well into the IVF, posterior to the dorsal root ganglion; are frequently bilateral; and are usually asymptomatic (Helms & Sims, 1986).

Many of the pathologic conditions previously described as affecting the NRC can also diminish the dimensions of the IVF proper. In addition, recall that the IVD forms a part of the anterior border of the IVF. Because of this, a decrease in disc height also results in a decrease of the vertical dimension of the IVF (Crock, 1981). Investigation into the normal size of the lumbar IVFs as they appear on MRI scans is being performed (Cramer et al., 1992b). However, comparisons need to be made between normal IVF size and IVF size in patients with pathologic conditions of this region.

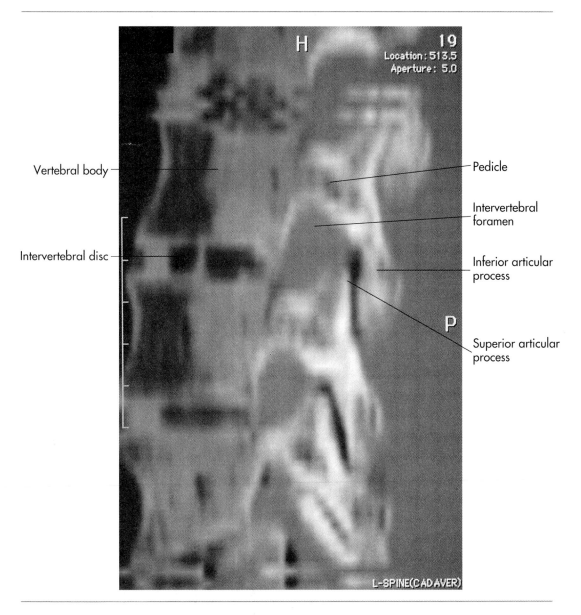

FIG. 7-14 Digitally reformatted parasagittal plane CT image showing the region of the Z joints and IVFs.

L5 Nerve Root Canal and L5 Intervertebral Foramina. The anatomy of the L5 NRC is unique, and because of this the L5 roots and nerve are susceptible to compression in many different locations. This canal is longer and runs at a more oblique anterior angle than the rest of the lumbar NRCs. Also, the lateral recess of the L5 vertebra is the deepest laterally and often the narrowest from anterior to posterior of the entire spine. This narrow lateral recess may lead to compression of the L5 nerve in some instances (Rauschning, 1987). Hasue and colleagues (1983) found histologic evidence of compression (intraneural fibrosis) of the L5 dorsal root. Compression occurred between the superior articular process of S1 and the posterior aspect of the vertebral body of L5 (Hasue et al., 1983).

After leaving the lateral recess, the L5 roots and their dural root sleeve continue along the L5 NRC by wrapping around the posterior and lateral aspect of the L5 vertebral body. The roots continue around the posterolateral aspect of the L5 IVD and unite to form the mixed spinal nerve. The L5 nerve, which is the *largest* of the lumbar nerves, exits the lateral border of the L5 NRC (the IVF proper), which is the *smallest* IVF of the lumbar spine (Cramer et al., 1992b; Olsewski et al., 1991). This makes the L5 nerve particularly susceptible to compression within its IVF.

The anterior primary division (APD) of L5 is given off at the most lateral aspect of the IVF and then passes along a depression on the front of the sacral ala. The APD is frequently bounded anterosuperiorly in this region by the corporotransverse ligament (Bachop & Janse, 1983; Bachop & Ro, 1984; Rauschning, 1987). The corporotransverse ligament runs from the vertebral body and IVD of L5 to the TP of L5. Olsewski and colleagues (1991) and Nathan, Weizenbluth, & Halperin (1982) report that the inferior band of the iliolumbar ligament, known as the lumbosacral ligament (LSL), usually runs from the vertebral body and TP of L5 to the ala of the sacrum (see Fig. 7-19). The descriptions of the corporotransverse ligament by Bachop and Janse (1983) and Bachop and Ro (1984) are consistent with what Nathan and colleagues consider to be the fibers of origin of the LSL. This indicates that the fibers of origin of the LSL are much more substantial than those fibers found more laterally, and that frequently a distinct tough, fibrous band, the corporotransverse ligament, is formed in this region.

After passing beneath the corportranverse ligament and the LSL, the APD of L5 continues inferiorly (Bachop & Janse, 1983; Bachop & Ro, 1984; Nathan et al., 1982; Olsewski et al., 1991). Therefore the corporotransverse ligament of Bachop and the LSL significantly extend the osteoligamentous canal of the L5 NRC, and the most inferior aspect of the LSL forms the anterior and inferior boundary of the L5 osteoligamentous canal. Nathan and colleagues (1982) state that the gray communicating ramus from the sympathetic chain to the APD of L5 pierces the LSL. Previous studies had shown that, throughout the spine, osteophytes from vertebral bodies frequently exert pressure on the sympathetic trunk, rami communicantes, and spinal nerves. This was found to be particularly true with the neural elements of L5 (Nathan et al., 1982). Finally, just inferior to the LSL, a branch of the APD of L4 joins the APD of L5 to form the lumbosacral trunk.

The unique characteristics of the L5-S1 NRC, IVF proper, and the lateral osteoligamentous canal of the L5 APD make the L5 nerve "extremely vulnerable to compression by any of the structures forming the tunnel. A tight LSL, osteophytes on the border of the L5-S1 disc or a combination of the two may impinge on the nerve and compress it against the ala of the sacrum" (Nathan et al., 1982). Olsewski and colleagues (1991) reported that the APD of L5 was observed to be compressed by the LSL in 11% of the 102 cadaveric specimens they studied by gross dissection. Histologic evidence of compression (perineurial and endoneurial fibrosis, peripheral thinning of myelin sheaths, and shift to a smaller fiber diameter) was shown in 3% of specimens studied. Osteophytes extending posterolaterally from both the inferior surface of the L5 body and the upper border of the body of the sacrum were found to narrow the L5 osteoligamentous canal further in 1 of 59 spines (2%) studied by Olsewski and colleagues. This was found to contribute to compression of the APD of L5. Nathan and colleagues (1982) found such osteophytes "frequently" and also noted that the L5 nerve was "very often" entrapped or compressed to some degree by osteophytes or the LSL while passing through the osteoligamentous tunnel.

Compression of the L5 APD by the corporotransverse ligament or the LSL could result in pain along the L5 dermatome (lateral aspect of the leg distally to the great toe [Floman & Mirovsky, 1990]) and possible loss of motor function of the muscles primarily innervated by the L5 APD (extensor hallucis longus muscle). Referred pain may be experienced in the lumbar region (see Chapter 11), although this has not been documented. Myelography, discography, standard CT scans, and transverse plane MRI scans would all be negative (Olsewski et al., 1991). Far lateral parasagittal MRI scans (farther lateral than standard MRI protocols) may show the relationship between the L5 nerve and the corporotransverse ligament and the LSL (Nowicki & Haughton, 1992). Perhaps far lateral parasagittal MRI would be a useful diagnostic procedure for patients exhibiting L5 dermatomal and motor symptoms and signs when other imaging modalities do not reveal a possible cause of entrapment (see Fig. 2-21). Further investigation in this region is warranted. In the meantime, "in the patient presenting with L5 root signs, if the myelogram, discogram, and CT scan do not reveal any defect, then the possibility of extraforaminal compression must be considered as a possible source of the clinical signs" (Olsewski et al., 1991).

Because of the unique anatomy of this region, several distinct conditions, besides those already described, can affect the L5 nerve roots, the L5 mixed spinal nerve, or the APD of L5. For example, because the neural elements of L5 are related to the L5 IVD for a relatively long distance, far lateral L5 IVD protrusion (lateral to the IVF) may affect the L5 mixed spinal nerve or the APD of L5. Another example of the unique vulnerability of the L5 neural elements is spondylolisthesis following spondylolysis (Fig. 7-15). This condition may result in compression of the L5 nerve at any point along its course from behind the L5 disc to the nerve's lateral relation with the corporotransverse ligament and the L5 TP, both of which lie above the nerve (Bachop & Janse, 1983; Bachop & Ro, 1984; Rauschning, 1987).

A 20% or greater anterior shift of a spondylolisthetic L5 vertebra may result in compression of the APD of L5 between the TP of L5 and the sacral ala (Wiltse et al., 1984). Such compression is usually unilateral but may occasionally be bilateral. Also, both asymmetric degeneration of the L5 IVD and degenerative lumbar scoliosis result in lateral tilting and rotation of L5. As with spondylolisthesis, this can also result in compression of the L5 nerve between the TP of L5 and the sacral ala. Such far lateral compressions of the L5 nerve have been called the far-out syndrome (Wiltse et al., 1984) of Wiltse (Dommisse & Louw, 1990). Wiltse and colleagues (1984) stated that the lateral entrapment caused by either degenerative scoliosis or asymmetric disc degeneration was probably most common in elderly patients, whereas lateral entrapment as a result of spondylolisthesis was found most frequently in a somewhat younger group of adult patients. The authors also stated that far lateral entrapment occasionally could occur at levels higher than L5 and may be accompanied by the radiographic findings of marked scoliosis with closely approximated TPs of two adjacent vertebrae. CT was found to be the imaging modality of choice to view the region of entrapment. A "wide window" setting for the CT scan was necessary to view the laterally placed TPs. CT images reformatted in the coronal plane were particularly useful in evaluating the relationship between the L5 TPs and the sacral ala (Wiltse et al., 1984).

Nathan and colleagues (1982) found that branches of the iliolumbar artery and relatively large veins always accompanied the APD of L5 beneath the LSL. Using examples of neuralgias and pareses of cranial nerves caused by compression of these nerves by adjacent arteries, they hypothesized that likewise the APD of L5 could become entrapped within its osteoligamentous tunnel by branches of the iliolumbar artery and accompanying veins. This would be particularly feasible when the APD

of L5 was already partially compressed within a narrow tunnel or by osteophytes extending posterolaterally from the inferior border of the L5 body.

UNIQUE ASPECTS OF THE LUMBAR VERTEBRAE

Fifth Lumbar Vertebra

The L5 vertebra, its relationship with the sacrum, and the soft tissue elements in between are some of the most clinically relevant anatomic structures of the spine. Pain in this region is extremely common (Cramer et al., 1992a), and therefore an accurate working knowledge of the L5-S1 region is essential for those treating patients with low back and leg pain. The anatomy of this region is subject to much variation. Nathan and colleagues (1982) stated that "such skeletal variations are accompanied by changes and adjustments of the related soft tissues, including the nerves and vessels." Therefore, clinically relevant variations frequently accompany the normal anatomy of this region.

The L5 vertebral body is the largest of the entire spine. It is taller anteriorly than posteriorly, which contributes to the increase in the lower lumbar lordosis (the lower lumbar lordosis is frequently called the lumbosacral angle). The spinous process of L5 is the smallest of all those of the lumbar vertebrae. It projects inferiorly, and its posterior aspect is more rounded in appearance than the rest of the lumbar spinous processes. The TPs of L5 are much wider from anterior to posterior and from superior to inferior than those of the rest of the lumbar spine. They originate from the entire lateral aspect of the pedicles, and their origin continues posteriorly to the adjacent lamina. However, the TPs do not extend as far laterally as other lumbar TPs (see Transverse Processes). The lateral aspect of the TPs of L5 also angle slightly superiorly, with the angulation beginning at about the midpoint of each of the two (left and right) processes.

Spondylolysis and Spondylolisthesis. Spondylolysis is a defect of the lamina (Fig. 7-15) between the superior and inferior articular processes. This region is known as the pars interarticularis. Controversy exists as to whether this defect is most frequently caused by trauma or if it is hereditary. Causes of pars (isthmic) defects include lytic or stress fractures of the pars interarticularis (probably the most common cause), elongated but intact pars (not spondylolysis), and acute fracture of the pars (Day, 1991). Bilateral spondylolysis may result in forward slippage of that portion of the vertebra located anterior to the laminar defect (vertebral body, pedicles, TPs, superior articular processes). This leaves the inferior articular processes, a portion of the laminae, and the spinous process behind. Such forward displacement is known as spondylolisthesis and is found in 5% of

FIG. 7-15 **A,** Posterior view of a typical lumbar vertebra. **B,** Bilateral fracture of the pars interarticularis (spondylolysis) and a separation (spondylolisthesis) of the region anterior to the pars interarticularis from the remainder of the posterior arch.

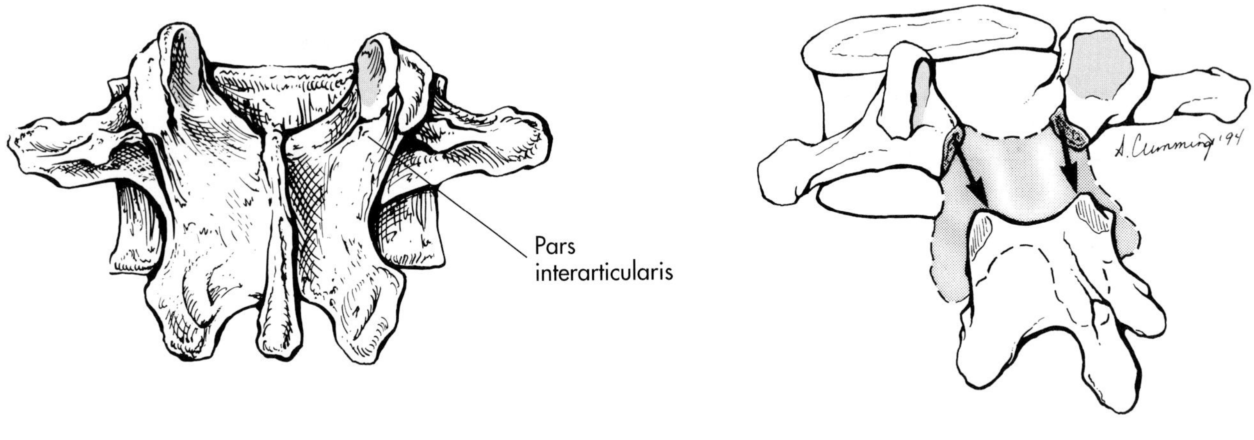

lumbar spines (Williams et al., 1989) (Fig. 7-15). Other causes of spondylolisthesis include (1) improper formation of the posterior vertebral arch, known as the dysplastic type of spondylolisthesis; (2) degeneration and subsequent erosion of the superior articular process; (3) fracture of part of the posterior arch other than the pars interarticularis (e.g., pedicle fracture); and (4) pathologic conditions of the bone forming the posterior arch (e.g., Paget's disease).

Spondylolisthesis is graded by the degree to which the affected vertebral body is anteriorly displaced in relation to the vertebral (or sacral) body located immediately inferior to it. For example, a 25% spondylolisthesis represents forward displacement of a vertebral body (measured at the posterior and inferior border of the vertebral body) by one quarter of the length of the vertebral body (or sacral body) directly inferior to it. Spondylolisthesis can also be graded on a scale of 1 to 4, with each grade representing an additional 25% of anterior slippage. A grade 4 describes a vertebral body that has been displaced completely off of the vertebra (or usually, the sacrum) directly beneath it.

Spondylolisthesis has been implicated as a cause of spinal canal stenosis at the level of the pars interarticularis defect. However, Liyang and colleagues (1989) reported an increase in vertebral canal dimensions at the level of spondylolisthesis in one cadaveric spine, which was included in their study of 10 normal spines. Spondylolisthesis at L5 may also result in entrapment of the L5 nerve as it passes laterally, in front of the pars interarticularis, to exit the L5 IVF. The entrapment is caused by the portion of the pars located above the fracture site. This is the part of the pars that is displaced

anteriorly with the vertebral body and pedicles. By moving anteriorly, it can compress the L5 nerve (Kirkaldy-Willis, 1978).

Although most common at L5, spondylolisthesis is also seen with some frequency at L4 and may be seen at any level of the lumbar spine. Of somewhat related interest, the pars interarticularis can occasionally enlarge as a result of degeneration. This is significant at the level of L5 because it can lead to entrapment of the S1 nerve as it courses along the lateral aspect of the vertebral canal (lateral recess).

Lumbosacral Articulation

The lumbosacral articulation is actually composed of several articulations between L5 and the sacrum. It consists of two components: the joining, by the fifth IVD, of the inferior aspect of the L5 body with the body of the S1 segment; and the joints between the left and right inferior articular processes of L5 and the superior articular processes of the sacrum. These latter joints are not nearly as curved as are the Z joints of the rest of the lumbar spine. The plane of articulation of the lumbosacral Z joints is subject to much variation, ranging 20° to 90° to the sagittal plane (average of 40° to 60°). Frequently, asymmetry, known as tropism, exists between the left and right L5-S1 Z joints. Lippitt (1984) reported that tropism may be a cause of premature degeneration and pain, but the clinical significance of tropism remains a matter of controversy.

The L5-S1 IVD is typically narrower than the IVDs of the rest of the lumbar spine (Nicholson, Roberts, & Williams, 1988). This may contribute to the IVF at this level being smaller than those of the rest of the lumbar spine. Recall that the spinal nerve at this level is the largest lumbar spinal nerve. Therefore, more than one third of the L5-S1 IVF is composed of the mixed spinal nerve. Even though the IVD and IVF are smaller in this region, the L5-S1 articulation is by far the most movable of all the lumbar joints (5° of unilateral rotation, 3° of lateral bending, 10° of flexion, 10° of extension). These factors, along with the others discussed in the previous section devoted to the L5 NRC, make the L5 roots and mixed spinal nerve vulnerable to compression as they traverse the L5 NRC.

The intraarticular space of the left and right lumbosacral Z joints is usually wider than those of the remainder of the lumbar spine. A recess normally exists along the inferomedial edge of the lumbosacral Z joints. This recess has been shown to be filled with a large intraarticular synovial fold. This fold is primarily composed of adipose tissue. Another intraarticular synovial protrusion usually projects into the superomedial aspect of the L5-S1 Z joint (Giles & Taylor, 1987). These synovial folds are susceptible to entrapment between the apposing L5-S1 articular facets and are a likely source of low back pain and subsequent muscle tightness. Gentle, well-controlled spinal manipulation to open the facets, to allow an entrapped synovial fold to be pulled out of the joint by its attachment to the joint capsule, has been suggested as the treatment of choice for this condition (Giles & Taylor, 1987).

A transitional segment between the lumbar spine and the sacrum is found in 5% of the population (Nicholson et al., 1988). This takes the form of either a lumbarization of the S1 segment or, more frequently, a sacralization of the L5 vertebra. Sacralization refers to elongation of the TPs of L5 with varying degrees of fusion or articulation with either the sacral ala or the iliac crest. The union between L5 and the sacrum may be bilateral, but usually it is only unilateral. The L5-S1 IVD in cases of sacralization is normally significantly thinner than that of typical L5-S1 segments (Nicholson et al., 1988). It is also usually devoid of nuclear material, and therefore usually does not undergo pathologic change or degeneration to the degree seen in discs above the sacralized segment (Nicholson et al., 1988).

LIGAMENTS AND INTERVERTEBRAL DISCS OF THE LUMBAR REGION

Most of the ligaments associated with the lumbar region have been discussed in previous chapters. The articular capsules of the Z joints, the ligamenta flava, supraspinous ligament, interspinous ligaments, intertransverse ligaments, and the anterior and posterior longitudinal ligaments are discussed in Chapters 5 and 6, and the IVDs are discussed in Chapter 2. The mamillo-

accessory ligament is discussed previously in this chapter (see Articular Processes). This section is devoted to characteristics of the previously mentioned ligaments that are unique to the lumbar region. The iliolumbar ligaments (left and right), which are found only in the lower lumbar region, are also covered in this section.

Lumbar Anterior Longitudinal Ligament

Unique characteristics of the anterior longitudinal ligament (ALL) in the lumbar region include it being wider from side to side than in the thoracic region. It has also been found to be thicker than the posterior longitudinal ligament (PLL) (Grenier et al., 1989b). The ALL extends across the anterior aspect of the vertebral bodies and IVDs to attach inferiorly to the sacrum. The ALL functions to limit extension, and it may be torn during extension injuries of the spine. It receives sensory (nociceptive and proprioceptive) innervation from branches of the gray communicating rami of the lumbar sympathetic trunk. Therefore, damage to the ALL during extension injuries can be a direct source of pain.

The ALL and PLL have been collectively termed the intercentral ligaments because they connect the anterior and posterior surfaces of adjacent vertebral bodies (centra), respectively (Grenier et al., 1989b). They also help attach the vertebral bodies to the IVDs and are important in stabilizing the spine during flexion (PLL) and extension (ALL). They also function to limit flexion (PLL) and extension (ALL) of the spine.

Lumbar Posterior Longitudinal Ligament

The PLL in the lumbar region is denticulated in appearance (Fig. 7-16). That is, it is narrow over the posterior aspect of the vertebral bodies and flares laterally at each IVD, where it attaches to the posterior aspect of the anulus fibrosus.

The PLL receives sensory innervation from the recurrent meningeal nerve (sinuvertebral nerve). Substance P, a known sensory neurotransmitter that is usually associated with pain sensation, has been found in the terminal fibers of the sinuvertebral nerve innervating the lumbar PLL. Korkala and colleagues (1985) also found enkephalins, a known neuromodulator, in the PLL. Together these findings substantiate previous suppositions that the PLL is pain sensitive and may indicate that the PLL (at least in the lumbar region) is *highly* sensitive to pain. The pain sensitivity of the PLL has been demonstrated by mechanical irritation of the ligament in patients with only local anesthesia of the overlying skin. The pain was felt in the midline and radiated into the low back and superior aspect of the buttock (Edgar & Ghadially, 1976).

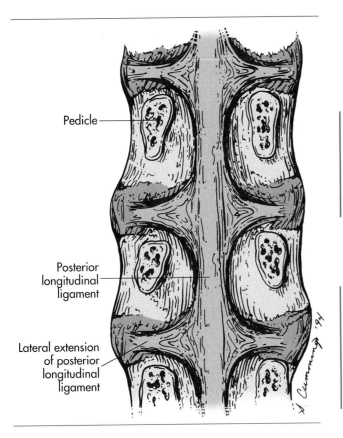

FIG. 7-16 Posterior longitudinal ligament is shown coursing along the anterior aspect of the vertebral canal.

In some instances, posterior and posterolateral IVD protrusions may penetrate the PLL. This is a strong sign that the protrusion is not contained within the anulus fibrosis (see Intervertebral Disc in Chapter 2 and later discussion). This may be an indication for surgical removal of the disc. The penetrated PLL is able to be distinguished from a bulging anulus fibrosus on parasagittal MRI scans. The PLL appears as an area of low signal intensity on these images. Using MRI, Grenier and colleagues (1989b) were able to determine when the PLL was *not* disrupted (not penetrated by the anulus fibrosus or nucleus pulposus) 100% of the time and were able to determine when the PLL *was* disrupted 78% of the time. The authors concluded that MRI was useful in the detection of PLL disruption.

Lumbar Ligamenta Flava

The paired (left and right) ligamenta flava of the lumbar region are the thickest of the entire spine. They extend between the laminae of adjacent vertebrae throughout the lumbar region, including the junction between the laminae of L5 and those of the S1 segment. Each ligamentum flavum is thickest medially. Laterally, the ligament passes more anteriorly to form the anterior joint capsule of the Z joint, attaching to the superior and inferior articular processes that form this joint. The most lateral fibers attach to the pedicle of the vertebra below (Fig. 7-17).

The exiting dorsal and ventral nerve roots of the lumbar region come in direct contact with the anterior aspect of the ligamentum flavum as the ligament forms the anterior capsule of the Z joint within the IVF (Hasue et al., 1983). A recess has been found in the lateral, articular portion of the ligament. Paris (1983) states that this recess may allow the synovium of the facet joint to pass through the ligamentum flavum. Under certain circumstances the synovium could then extend into the IVF, where it could conceivably compress the mixed spinal nerve.

Sensory fibers, probably arising from the medial branch of the posterior primary division (Bogduk, 1983), have been found innervating the most superficial aspect of the posterior surfaces of the ligamenta flava (Edgar & Ghadially, 1976). Therefore, damage to these ligaments may result in back pain. Since the number of nerve endings is small, the significance of the ligamenta flava as a primary source of back pain is uncertain. However, their role as a secondary source of back pain in spinal stenosis is well documented (see Lumbar Vertebral Foramen and the Vertebral Canal; Lumbar Intervertebral Foramina and the Nerve Root Canals).

Lumbar Interspinous Ligaments

The results of descriptive studies of these ligaments in the lumbar region have led to elaboration on their structure in this particular area of the spine. Therefore a brief discussion of the unique aspects of these structures is included here, even though the interspinous ligaments were described with the thoracic region (see Chapter 6).

Several authors have described the structure of a typical lumbar interspinous ligament as being composed of three parts: anterior, middle, and posterior (Behrsin & Briggs, 1988; Bogduk & Twomey, 1991). These three parts run between adjacent spinous processes, filling the gap along the length of these processes.

The anterior portion of the interspinous ligament is paired (left and right) anteriorly, with each part attaching to the ligamentum flavum of the same side. A thin layer of adipose tissue separates the two halves. Posteriorly the two sides of this part of the interspinous ligament unite to form a single ligament. The fibers of this part of the interspinous ligament pass posteriorly and superiorly from their origin (ligamentum flavum) to attach to the anterior half of the inferior aspect of the spinous process of the vertebra above.

The middle portion of the interspinous ligament is the most substantial region. It originates from the anterior half of the upper surface of a spinous process and passes

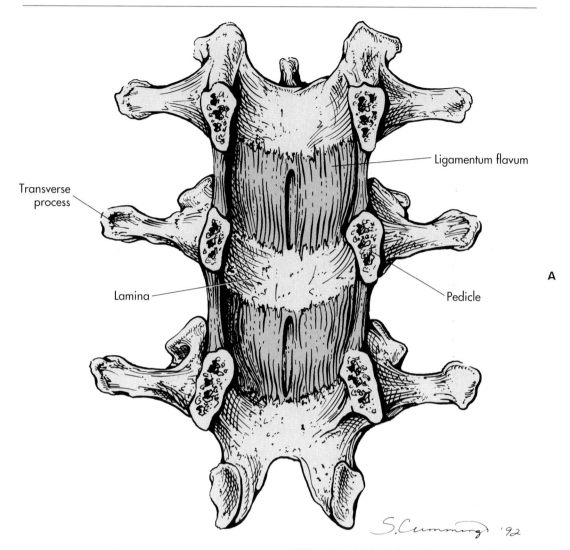

Transverse process

Ligamentum flavum

Lamina

Pedicle

A

S. Cummings '92

FIG. 7-17 Pedicles have been sectioned in a coronal plane to reveal the posterior aspect of the vertebral canal (**A,** Artist's rendering.) **B,** (Cadaveric specimen). Notice the ligamenta flava *(red arrow)* passing between the adjacent laminae. (**B,** Courtesy The National College of Chiropractic.)

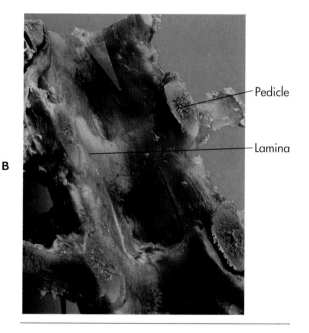

Pedicle

Lamina

B

posteriorly and superiorly to insert onto the posterior half of the lower surface of the vertebra above.

The posterior aspect of the interspinous ligament attaches to the posterior half of the upper surface of a spinous process and continues superiorly to pass behind (posterior to) the vertebra above, becoming continuous with the supraspinous ligament (see following discussion). Bogduk and Twomey (1991) do not consider this posterior portion to be a true part of the interspinous ligament because it does not attach to two adjacent bones.

The interspinous ligament appears to be quite capable of being torn. One investigator found its fibers to be ruptured in 21% of cadavers examined. The middle fibers were found to be torn most frequently (Behrsin & Briggs, 1988).

The interspinous ligaments and supraspinous ligament limit the end stage of lumbar flexion, and they are the first to sprain during hyperflexion of the lumbar region (Hutton, 1990).

Lumbar Supraspinous Ligament

The supraspinous ligament is strongest in the lumbar region. It is classically described as extending to the sacrum (Williams et al., 1989). However, others (Behrsin & Briggs, 1988) believe that the supraspinous ligament ends at L5 and does not extend to the sacrum, and Paris (1983) states that it usually ends at L4 and rarely at L5, never extending to the sacrum. Paris has found that the strong fibers of origin of the lumbar erector spinae muscles and the thoracolumbar fascia take the place of this ligament inferior to the spinous process of L4. This fascia continues inferiorly to the median sacral crest. Bogduk and Twomey (1991) state that the supraspinous ligament is not a true ligament in the lumbar region. They believe it is primarily made up of strong tendinous fibers of the longissimus thoracis and multifidus muscles, and crisscrossing fibers of the thoracolumbar fascia. In addition, a condensation of the membranous (deep) layer of the superficial fascia of the back forms the superficial layer of the supraspinous ligament (Bogduk & Twomey, 1991).

The term supraspinous ligament continues to be used quite frequently by clinicians and researchers alike. In such instances, they are probably referring to the tough combination of midline tendons of the longissimus thoracis muscle, the intersecting fibers of the thoracolumbar fascia, and the membranous layer of superficial fascia. The term *lumbar supraspinous restraints* would seem to reflect more accurately the true nature of the fibrous band of tissue that is found along the posterior aspect of the lumbar spinous processes and interspinous spaces.

Lumbar Intertransverse Ligaments. The general characteristics of the intertransverse ligaments are described in Chapter 5. Some authors describe the lumbar intertransverse ligaments as being thin membranous bands that connect two adjacent TPs (Berhsin & Briggs, 1988). Others consider the intertransverse ligaments to be rather discrete and well-defined bands, although some authors consider them to consist of two lamellae (Berhsin & Briggs, 1988). The latter view appears to be gaining acceptance (Bogduk & Twomey, 1991).

The posterior lamella of the intertransverse ligament passes medially to the posterior aspect of the Z joint. It is pierced by the posterior primary division and continues medially to help reinforce the Z joint capsule from behind. Laterally the membranous intertransverse ligament also has a posterior layer. The posterior layer of the lateral aspect of the intertransverse ligament becomes continuous with the aponeurosis of the transversus abdominis muscle and then becomes continuous with the middle layer of the thoracolumbar fascia (Bogduk & Twomey, 1991).

The anterior lamella of the intertransverse ligament passes medially to form a layer of fascia over the IVF. Here it is pierced by the APD and the spinal branches of lumbar segmental arteries and veins. The anterior lamella then continues anteriorly and medially to become continuous with the ALL. The accessory (transforaminal) ligaments, which span the IVF (see Chapter 2 and previous discussion on corporotransverse ligament under L5 NRC), are probably condensations of the anterior lamella of the intertransverse ligament (Bogduk & Twomey, 1991). Recall that laterally the membranous intertransverse ligament also has anterior and posterior (see preceding paragraph) layers. The anterior layer becomes continuous with the anterior layer of the thoracolumbar fascia and covers the anterior aspect of the quadratus lumborum muscle.

A V-shaped groove (with the apex of the V facing laterally) is formed by the medially located anterior and posterior lamellae of the intertransverse ligament. The region between the two lamellae is filled with a small amount of adipose tissue that is continuous with the adipose tissue within the Z joint. This V-shaped region is known as the superior articular recess (see Zygapophyseal Joints). It aids the Z joint by allowing for its adipose contents to be displaced during extension of the spine (Bogduk & Twomey, 1991).

Iliolumbar Ligaments

The iliolumbar ligament runs from the left and right TPs of L5 (and occasionally L4) to the sacrum and iliac crest of the same side. Each is composed of as many as five parts (Bogduk & Twomey, 1991). The most prominent part consists of an inferior band and a superior band (Olsewski et al., 1991; Williams et al., 1989). The inferior band is present 97% of the time and is also known as the lumbosacral ligament (LSL). The LSL extends from the inferior aspect of the L5 TP and the body of L5 to the anterosuperior aspect of the sacral ala, where it blends with the ventral sacroiliac ligament (Fig. 7-18). The LSL extends from the TP and body of L5 to the sacral promontory at least 3% of the time (Olsewski et al., 1991).

The superior band of the iliolumbar ligament runs farther laterally than the LSL and attaches to the iliac crest in front of the sacroiliac joint. This band is continuous with the attachment of the quadratus lumborum muscle to the TP of L5. Other portions of the iliolumbar ligament include anterior, inferior (not the LSL), and vertical parts. All these originate from the TP of L5 and attach to the ilium.

The iliolumbar ligament was previously thought to develop as a result of metaplasia of epimysium (outer cov-

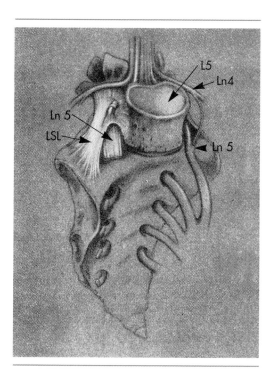

FIG. 7-18   The lumbosacral ligament (**LSL**). Notice the relationship between the LSL and the ventral ramus of L5 (**Ln5**). (From Olsewski, J.M. et al. *Spine*, 1991, *16*, 336-347.)

ering) of the inferior fibers of the quadratus lumborum muscle. However, Uhthoff (1993) found this ligament to be well developed in 12 of 12 fetuses beyond 11.5 weeks of gestational age. Further, he found that the direction of the collagen fibers was 90° to the muscle fibers of the quadratus lumborum muscle. He concluded that the iliolumbar ligament develops in a fashion similar to most of the other ligaments of the body and is not formed by metaplasia of the inferior fibers of the quadratus lumborum muscle.

The iliolumbar ligaments probably function to stabilize the L5-S1 junction, helping to maintain the proper relationship of L5 on S1. This function is enhanced with degeneration of the L5 IVD (Olsewski et al., 1991). In addition, this ligament probably limits axial rotation of L5 on S1. The iliolumbar ligament is innervated by posterior primary divisions of the neighboring spinal nerves and therefore may be a primary source of back pain.

Lumbar Intervertebral Discs

Because of their tremendous clinical significance, much has already been written in this chapter about the lumbar IVDs. In addition, Chapter 2 described the make-up of the IVDs and much of the clinical significance associated with their unique morphology. Chapter 13 discusses the microscopic anatomy of these important structures. This chapter focuses on the unique charac-

teristics of the lumbar IVDs with an emphasis on their clinical significance.

In general, IVDs of the lumbar region are the thickest of the spine. They have the same composition as the discs in the other regions (see Chapter 2), being made up of a central nucleus pulposus, an outer anulus fibrosus composed of 15 to 25 lamellae (Twomey & Taylor, 1990), and the vertebral (cartilaginous) end plates of the two adjacent vertebrae. The thickness of the lamellae of the anulus fibrosus of lumbar IVDs varies considerably from one layer to the next and also varies within the same lamella. Marchand and Ahmed (1990) found that the thickness of the lamellae also increases with age.

The function of the lumbar IVDs is similar to the function of the IVDs throughout the spine. That is, they absorb loads placed on the spine from above (axial loading) and allow for some motion to occur (Hutton, 1990). The lumbar discs become shorter during the day because they carry the load of the torso. They usually regain their shape within 5 hours of sleep. During the active hours the discs require movement to maintain proper hydration. Decreased movement and decreased axial loading have been strongly associated with disc degeneration (Twomey & Taylor, 1990).

Contrary to what was assumed in the past, the IVDs do not normally become narrower from superior to inferior with age (Twomey & Taylor, 1990). Their central region becomes more convex with age and pushes into the central region of the adjacent vertebral bodies. The central aspect of the vertebral bodies lose transverse trabeculae with age and become somewhat shorter from superior to inferior. The peripheral margins of the vertebral bodies lose much less height, causing the end plates to become concave.

The lumbar IVDs are thicker anteriorly than posteriorly. This helps in the formation of the lumbar lordosis. Liyang and colleagues (1989) found that the shapes of the lumbar IVDs change significantly during flexion and extension of the lumbar region. Flexion was found to narrow the anterior aspect of the disc by approximately 1 to 5 mm and to increase the height of the posterior aspect of the disc by between approximately 1.5 to 3 mm.

The IVDs are usually protected from anterior displacement, or shear stress, by the Z joints and the lumbar extensor muscles (Hutton, 1990). However, fracture of the pars interarticularis allows for anterior displacement of the IVDs to occur.

Pain Originating From the Intervertebral Disc. Because each lumbar disc is in direct contact with two or three pairs of dorsal roots (Taylor, 1990), bulging, or protrusion, of the IVD is a major cause of radicular pain (Fig. 7-19). However, clinicians should keep in mind that each IVD is innervated by sensory nerve endings and, as a result, can be a primary source of back pain. The IVD receives both nociceptive and proprioceptive fibers

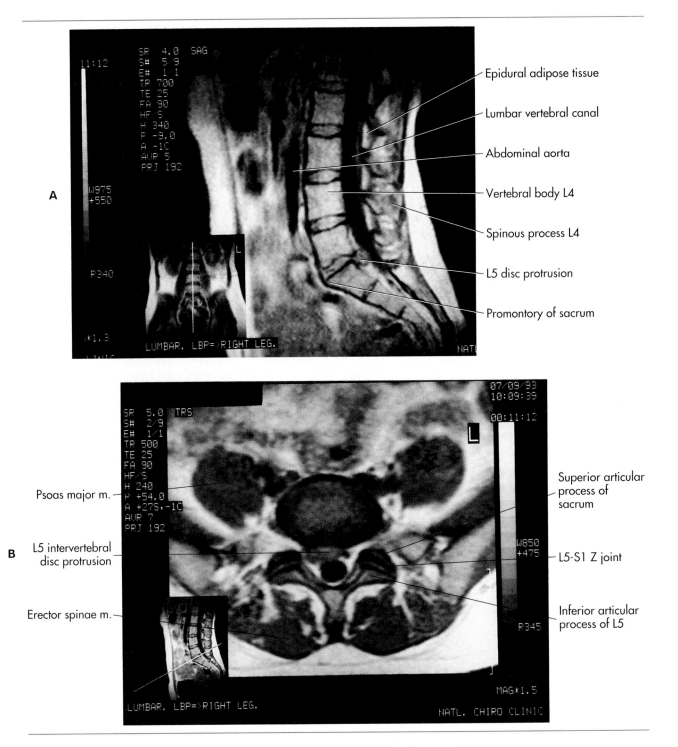

Epidural adipose tissue

Lumbar vertebral canal

Abdominal aorta

Vertebral body L4

Spinous process L4

L5 disc protrusion

Promontory of sacrum

Psoas major m.

L5 intervertebral disc protrusion

Erector spinae m.

Superior articular process of sacrum

L5-S1 Z joint

Inferior articular process of L5

FIG. 7-19 MRI scans demonstrating an intervertebral disc protrusion of the L5-S1 intervertebral disc. **A,** Midsagittal. **B,** Horizontal.

(Chapter 2). The posterior aspect of the disc receives innervation from the recurrent meningeal nerve (sinuvertebral nerve), and the lateral and anterior aspect of the disc is supplied by branches of the gray communicating rami of the lumbar sympathetic trunk (Bogduk, Tynan, & Wilson, 1981; Edgar & Ghadially, 1976).

Nociception from that part of the disc innervated by branches of the gray communicating rami probably courses through the gray rami to the anterior primary division and therefore enters the dorsal horn of the spinal cord in a fashion similar to other nociceptive fibers of the somatic nervous system (Bogduk, 1983).

(Chapters 9 and 11 discuss the central connections of fibers conducting nociception.) Bogduk (1990) has described a series of events that explains the mechanism by which the IVD can be a primary source of pain without IVD herniation. He states that there are primarily two mechanisms by which the disc causes pain without herniation: through torsional injuries to the disc and from compression of the IVD.

Torsional injury to the IVD refers to a sprain of the outer layers of the anulus fibrosus after excessive axial rotation. Normally, tearing of the anulus does not occur because the collagen fibers of the 15 to 25 anular lamellae of a lumbar IVD are able to withstand more than 3° of axial rotation without being stretched beyond their capacity. Rotation of the lumbar spine does not normally cause damage to the IVD (Hutton, 1990), since axial rotation between two adjacent segments is primarily limited by the Z joints and does not usually exceed 3° (see Range of Motion in the Lumbar Spine). However, if flexion is added to axial rotation, the collagen fibers of the anulus fibrosus can be stretched beyond their limits, resulting in circumferential tears of the anulus (Fig. 7-20). Because of the nociceptive innervation of the outer third of the IVD, these tears can result in pain of discal origin. However, even though these injuries have been produced experimentally, have been identified in cadavers, and match the signs and symptoms expressed by many patients who have back pain after injuries involving rotation combined with flexion, no definitive studies irrev-

ocably link isolated circumferential tears of the IVD with low back pain (Bogduk, 1990).

If several episodes of excessive loading of the disc during flexion and axial rotation occur, the result may be circumferential tears of several adjacent lamellae of the anulus fibrosus. If enough anuluar lamellae tear in this way, the anulus fibrosus may be weakened to the point that the nucleus pulposus may be allowed to pass through a path created by the circumferential tears of adjacent lamellae. Such a path courses from the centrally located nucleus pulposus to the periphery through successive layers of the anulus fibrosus. This path, from the nucleus pulposus through several layers of the anulus fibrosus, is known as a radial tear (Fig. 7-20). A radial tear can result in protrusion and herniation of nuclear contents into the vertebral canal. Once in the canal, entrapment or stretching of the neural elements can occur. A protruding or herniated disc can affect the neural elements as they course within the vertebral canal, as they pass through the IVF, or in both regions.

MRI is gaining wide acceptance in the evaluation of disc protrusion. However, a significant number of false-positive findings have been found with MRI. Therefore, close correlation of MRI findings with other clinical findings is essential before a diagnosis of disc protrusion can be made with certainty (Boden et al., 1990).

The second type of injury that can result in pain originating from the IVD itself results from excessive compression of the IVD. Compression injuries can result in

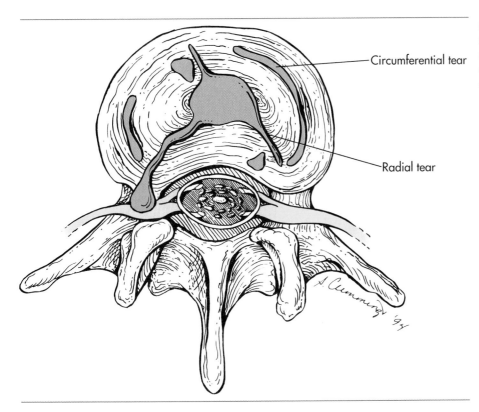

Circumferential tear

Radial tear

FIG. 7-20 Circumferential and radial tears of the IVD. Notice that one of the radial tears is allowing the nucleus pulposus to protrude posterolaterally on the left side.

pain of discal origin by two mechanisms, chemical and mechanical (Bogduk, 1990). Bogduk (1990) has described a series of events that may occur following excessive compression of a lumbar IVD. These events are summarized in the box below. Note that fracture of the vertebral end plate is a key feature in this sequence of events. During compressive loading of the spine (forces being placed on the spine from directly above), the vertebral (cartilaginous) end plates have been shown to fracture before tearing of the anulus fibrosus or herniation of the nucleus pulposus occurs. Such fractures may heal completely and possibly go unnoticed. However, if the fracture extends into the cancellous bone of the vertebral body and the IVD comes in contact with the vascular supply of the vertebral body, a dramatic repair response may occur. This response is characterized by the nucleus pulposus being treated as if it were foreign to the body. The result has been described as an autoimmune type of response (Bogduk, 1990). This response leads to destruction of the proteoglycan aggregates and proteoglycan monomers that make up the disc. The result of this destruction is a condition known as internal disc disruption (Kirkaldy-Willis et al., 1978).

EFFECTS OF COMPRESSIVE LOADING

Fall or excessive compressive load
↓
Fracture of vertebral end plate
↓
Nuclear material exposed to blood supply of vertebral body
↓
Unrestrained inflammatory repair response
↓
Degradation of IVD proteoglycans
↓
Internal disc disruption

Modified from Bogduk, N. (1990). *Manual Med, 5,* 72-79.

Internal disc disruption can result in spinal stenosis (including foraminal stenosis), herniation of the nucleus pulposus, or both. The processes by which these two entities develop are summarized in the boxes Scenario One and Scenario Two.

Internal disc disruption can also result in resorption, or loss, of disc material. The loss of discal material may, over time, make extrusion of the nucleus pulposus less likely. Kirkaldy-Willis and colleagues (1978) state that discography has shown a marked correlation between loss of disc height, the presence of traction spurs (osteophytes), and disruption of the disc. Therefore, even if patients escape nuclear bulge or herniation (presented

---

SCENARIO ONE

Internal disc disruption
↓
Circumferential bulging of the anulus fibrosus
↓
Osteophyte formation
↓
Isolated disc resorption
↓
Foraminal or spinal stenosis

Modified from Bogduk, N. (1990). *Manual Med, 5,* 72-79.

SCENARIO TWO

Rapid internal disc disruption
↓
Centrifugal erosion of the anulus fibrosus
↓
Radial fissures
↓
Fissure track (path)
↓
Nuclear herniation

---

in Scenario Two), they remain vulnerable to lateral recess stenosis (Scenario One).

In addition, as disruption continues toward the outer layers of the anulus fibrosus, pain of purely discal origin can also result. Bogduk (1990) has reviewed two mechanisms by which this can occur. These mechanisms are summarized in the boxes, Pain from Internal Disc Disruption—One and Two. The first mechanism that produces pain of discal origin is chemical in nature. Progression of the inflammatory process of disc disruption results in the direct stimulation of nociceptors in the outer third of the anulus fibrosus. The second process causes pain from the anulus as a result of its decreased ability to handle stress adequately. As the

---

PAIN FROM INTERNAL DISC DISRUPTION—ONE

Degradation of nucleus reaches outer third of anulus fibrosus
↓
Stimulation of nociceptors of outer anulus fibrosus
↓
Chemically induced pain

PAIN FROM INTERNAL DISC DISRUPTION—TWO

Disruption of anular collagen
↓
Decrease in number of collagen fibers
↓
Application of loads results in increased stress
to outer anulus fibrosus
↓
Anular sprain
↓
Mechanically induced pain

process of disruption progresses, the inner lamellae of the anulus break down, causing the outer layers to absorb all the loads placed on the disc. The anulus is rendered more susceptible to circumferential tears, which are pain producing. Therefore this type of pain, secondary to internal disc disruption, is the result of mechanical forces. The two mechanisms just described (pain of chemical and mechanical origin) can occur simultaneously (Bogduk, 1990).

Finally, the box below summarizes the clinical findings in a patient with early internal disc disruption. Note that the neurologic findings are negative. This is because the disc remains contained, especially in the early stages. Pain from internal disc disruption has characteristics similar to those of other somatic causes of low back pain (e.g., Z joint pathology). This makes differentiation from many other causes of back pain very challenging. If the pain is prolonged or becomes severe, injection of radiopaque dye into the disc followed by CT discography usually shows disruption into the anulus fibrosus when internal disc disruption is present. In addition, CT discography reproduces the patient's symptoms. Extrusion of dye into the anulus combined with provocation of the patient's symptoms confirms the condition of internal disc disruption. In addition, a disc affected by internal disc disruption may be identified as an area of reduced signal intensity when viewed on sagittal MRI scans.

CLINICAL FINDINGS WITH INTERNAL DISC DISRUPTION

1. Pain restricted to back or referred to lower limb
2. Pain aggravated by movements or compression of disc
3. Muscle guarding could be present
4. Neurologic examination normal
5. Standard X-ray examination, myelography, and CT scan normal
6. CT discography with pain provocation positive

Other Considerations. The IVD and the two Z joints between two adjacent vertebrae make up a three-joint complex. Pathologic conditions or dysfunction of one component can adversely affect the others (Kirkaldy-Willis et al., 1978). For example, loss of disc height as a result of disc protrusion, internal disc disruption, resorption of the disc, chemonucleolysis, and discectomy may lead to added loads being placed on the Z joint capsules and the articular processes. Disc deterioration at one level can also lead to increased strain and possible degeneration of the discs immediately above or below the level of primary involvement (Kirkaldy-Willis et al., 1978).

Loss of disc height can also result in subluxation of the Z joints and upward and forward displacement of the superior articular processes (Kirkaldy-Willis et al., 1978). This in turn results in narrowing of the lateral recesses of the vertebral canal. Narrowing of the lateral recess may result in entrapment of the exiting nerve roots as they proceed to the medial aspect of the IVF proper. Therefore, loss of disc height from any cause can result in abnormal joint position and abnormal motion. Such abnormal joint position and abnormal motion of both the interbody joint and the Z joints of two adjacent vertebrae has been termed instability (Dupuis et al., 1985). Instability, in turn, can lead to repeated entrapment of the spinal nerve exiting between the two adjacent segments.

RANGES OF MOTION IN THE LUMBAR SPINE

Several factors help to limit specific movements of the lumbar region. These include the unique configuration of the lumbar articular facets and the restraints of the Z joint capsules, ligaments of the lumbar region, deep back muscles, and the lumbar IVDs. For example, flexion of the lumbar region is primarily limited by the Z joint capsules (Hutton, 1990) and the articular processes themselves (Taylor & Twomey, 1986). The ligamenta flava, IVDs, and interspinous and supraspinous ligaments also limit flexion. Hutton (1990) found that the interspinous and supraspinous ligaments (supraspinous restraints) were the first to tear during hyperflexion of the lumbar region.

Extension is limited by the ALL, the Z joint capsular ligaments (Dupuis et al., 1985), and the bony "stop" of the inferior articular processes coming against the pars interarticularis of the subjacent vertebra.

The tightly interlocking facets of this region dramatically limit axial rotation. However, the reciprocal concave and convex surfaces of the respective superior and inferior articular processes do allow for a very small amount of axial rotation to occur. Gapping of the Z joint occurs on the same side of vertebral body rotation (i.e., gapping of right Z joint with right rotation). Axial rotation is finally stopped by the impact of articular processes that make up the Z joint of the side opposite that to which the vertebral body is rotating. This limitation usually occurs at 1° to 2° of axial rotation between adjacent vertebrae from L1 to L4 (Hutton, 1990). The L5-S1 segment is able to attain more axial rotation than the other lumbar segments (see following discussion).

Lateral flexion in the lumbar region is limited primarily by the contralateral intertransverse ligaments. The contralateral capsular ligaments and ligamenta flava are also important in the limitation of lateral flexion. In addition, the configuration of the articular processes help to limit lateral flexion (Dupuis et al., 1985). Lateral flexion in the lumbar region is usually coupled with axial rotation such that left lateral flexion results in right rotation of the vertebral bodies (left rotation of the spinous processes), and vice versa (i.e., right lateral flexion is coupled with left rotation of the vertebral bodies). This is probably caused by the sagittal orientation of the lumbar Z joints, combined with the effect of the relatively strong lumbar interspinous and supraspinous restraints. The latter restraints tend to hold the spinous processes together during lateral flexion. Loose posterior stabilizers (interspinous ligaments, supraspinous restraints, deep back muscles, Z joints) can result in abnormal coupling during lateral flexion so that left lateral flexion is coupled with left rotation of the vertebral body and right rotation of the spinous process (the opposite of the normal coupling pattern). This abnormal coupling pattern, which can be detected on standard x-ray films, is an indication of lumbar instability (Dupuis et al., 1985).

Lumbar instability may result in low back pain if abnormal stress is placed on the unstable segments. A patient with lumbar instability may have centralized low back pain without leg pain or with lateral low back pain combined with radiation into the buttock and thigh. Some patients with lumbar instability have signs of nerve root entrapment. Differentiation between pain caused by lumbar instability and that caused by primary IVD or Z joint pathologic conditions may be challenging. Examination of dynamic x-ray films taken in flexion, extension, and lateral flexion have been found to aid in this differentiation (Dupuis et al., 1985).

Table 7-9 lists the total ranges of motion for the lumbar region as reported by several different authors.

The following is a list of ranges of motion (in degrees) for each lumbar segmental level (White & Panjabi, 1990).

Combined flexion and extension

L1-2	12°
L2-3	14°
L3-4	15°
L4-5	17°

Unilateral lateral flexion

L1-2	6°
L2-3	6°
L3-4	8°
L4-5	6°

Unilateral axial rotation

L1-2	2°
L2-3	2°
L3-4	2°
L4-5	2°

Plamondon and colleagues (1988) used steriometry (method of measurement using sets of x-ray films taken at 90° to one another) to determine the motion of individual lumbar vertebrae. The following list represents the amount of motion they found, *per segment* for the L1 to L4 vertebrae:

Flexion:	10°
Extension:	4°
Axial rotation:	1°
Lateral flexion:	4°

Recall that the L5-S1 articulation is the most movable segment in flexion, extension, and axial rotation in this region. The following is a list of the ranges of motion at this level (White & Panjabi, 1990):

Combined flexion and extension:	20°
Unilateral lateral flexion:	3°
Unilateral axial rotation:	5°

However, some texts present data that show significantly less motion at the L5-S1 region, particularly in axial rotation and lateral flexion (Bogduk & Twomey, 1991).

SOFT TISSUES OF THE LUMBAR REGION: NERVES AND VESSELS

The muscles associated with the lumbar region are discussed in Chapter 4. This includes a discussion of the di-

Table 7-9 Total Ranges of Motion for the Lumbar Region

Direction	Motions and ranges reported in the literature
Flexion	60°
	Range: 39°-55°; average: 45.95° ± 4.28,* 52° ± 18,†
L4-5 segment	Range: 14.5°-19.0°; average: 15.95° ± 1.38*
Extension	20°
	16° ± 10†
Lateral flexion‡	25°-30°
Axial rotation‡	10°-15°
	5°†

*Data from Liyang, D., (1989). *Spine, 14,* 523-525.
†Data from Bogduk, N. & Twomey, L.T. (1991). *Clinical anatomy of the lumbar spine,* London: Churchill Livingstone.
‡Unilateral motion.

aphragm and the muscles of the anterior and posterior abdominal walls, including the abdominal oblique muscles, the transversus abdominis muscle, the rectus abdominis muscle, the quadratus lumborum muscle, and the psoas major and minor muscles. Consequently, this section on soft tissue structures of the lumbar region focuses on vessels and nerves related to the lumbar spine.

Nerves of the Lumbar Region

The innervation of the lumbar portion of the vertebral column and the soft tissue structures of the lumbar region is a topic of supreme clinical importance. Having a knowledge of the innervation of the spine gives the clinician a better understanding of the source of the patient's pain. Perhaps Bogduk (1983) stated it best: "The distribution of the intrinsic nerves of the lumbar vertebral column systematically identifies those structures that are potential sources of primary low back pain." Because the basic neural elements associated with the spine are covered in Chapters 2, 3, 5 and 6, this chapter concentrates on those aspects of innervation unique to the lumbar region. However, many key features of the basic neural elements also are included here to maintain continuity and to minimize the need to refer to previous chapters.

The cauda equina and exiting roots and spinal nerves have been discussed earlier (see Lumbar Vertebral Foramen and Lumbar Intervertebral Foramina and the Nerve Root Canals, respectively). This section briefly covers the dorsal and ventral roots and the mixed spinal nerve. It concentrates on the neural elements once they have left the confines of the IVF. Since the vast majority of spinal structures are innervated by either the recurrent meningeal nerves or the posterior primary divisions (PPDs) these nerves and the structures they innervate are covered in more detail. This is followed by a discussion of the anterior primary divisions (APDs) and the lumbar plexus. Recall that the lateral and anterior aspects of the IVDs and the ALLs are innervated by direct branches of the lumbar sympathetic trunk and also by branches from the lumbar gray rami communicantes. The specific innervation of the IVD has been discussed in greater detail earlier (see Pain Originating from the Intervertebral Disc).

General Considerations. Three types of nerve endings have been found in almost all the structures in the lumbar vertebral column that receive a nerve supply: free nerve endings, other nonencapsulated endings, and encapsulated endings. This would seem to indicate that most innervated structures of the spine are sensitive to pain, pressure, and proprioception (Jackson et al., 1966).

Of particular interest, and sometimes of particular frustration to clinicians and researchers alike, is that innervation overlaps throughout the spine. This has been particularly well documented in the lumbar region. Most spinal structures seem to be innervated by nerves from at least two adjacent vertebral levels. This led Edgar and Ghadially (1976) to state, "The poor localization of much low back pain and its tendency to radiate may be related to this neurological pattern." This can make the task of identifying the cause of low back pain particularly challenging at times.

Dorsal and Ventral Roots and Mixed Spinal Nerves. The dorsal and ventral roots of the lumbar spine travel inferiorly as the cauda equina. They then course through the NRC before exiting the IVF (see previous material). The nerve roots can be irritated by many structures and pathologic processes (see Chapter 11). These include disc protrusion or other space-occupying lesions, structural lesions of the vertebral canal, chemical irritation, and intrinsic radiculitis (Bogduk, 1976). Before exiting the IVF, the dorsal and ventral roots unite to form a mixed spinal nerve. Each lumbar mixed spinal nerve emerges from a lumbar IVF and immediately divides into an APD (ventral ramus) and a PPD (dorsal ramus).

Recurrent Meningeal (Sinuvertebral) Nerves. The recurrent meningeal nerves (RMNs) at each level innervate many structures located within the IVF and the vertebral canal. Because they have been found to carry fibers that conduct nociception (pain), structures innervated by RMNs are considered to be capable of producing back pain. However, in addition to nociceptive input, the RMNs also probably carry thermal sensation and proprioception (Edgar & Ghadially, 1976). Even though the RMNs are discussed in Chapters 5 and 6, they are included here because of their clinical importance.

The RMNs are found at each IVF of the vertebral column. They each originate from the most proximal portion of the APD just distal to the IVF that they eventually reenter. They receive a branch from the closest gray communicating ramus and then enter the anterior aspect of the IVF close to the pedicle that forms the roof of this opening. Usually, more than one RMN enters each IVF, and up to six have been found at one level. Consequently, compression of the RMNs within the confines of the IVF may be a cause of back pain (Edgar & Ghadially, 1976).

On entering the IVF, the RMNs ramify extensively. Great variation is associated with their distribution within the vertebral canal (Groen, 1990). Usually, each gives off a large ascending branch and smaller descending and transverse branches, although the transverse branch is not always present. The ascending branch usually extends superiorly for at least one vertebral level above its level of entrance. The branches of the RMNs anastomose with those of adjacent vertebral segments, including those of the opposite side of the spine (Bogduk, 1976; Edgar & Ghadially, 1976; Groen et al., 1990). They innervate the posterior aspect of the IVD, the PLL, the periosteum of the posterior aspect of the vertebral bodies, the epidural venous plexus, and the anterior aspect of the spinal dura mater (see Chapter 11). Therefore, all these structures have been implicated as a possible source of back pain. In addition, compression of the RMNs in the vertebral canal may be a component of spinal stenosis (Edgar & Ghadially, 1976). However, because of the great variability in the distribution of the RMNs, the pattern of pain referral as a result of nociceptive input received from them may also be quite inconsistent.

Less frequently cited possible causes of back pain that receive innervation by the RMNs include venous congestion within the vertebral bodies (intravertebral venous congestion) and varicosities of the epidural veins (Edgar & Ghadially, 1976) and basivertebral veins (Bogduk, 1976). Edgar and Ghadially (1976) stated that, in addition to relieving pressure on nerve roots, decompression of the vertebral canal via laminectomy may reduce back pain by relieving venous congestion in the epidural and intravertebral veins.

Posterior Primary Divisions. Whereas the recurrent meningeal nerves innervate the structures located on the anterior aspect of the vertebral canal, the posterior primary rami innervate those structures of the posterior aspect of the vertebral canal (vertebral arch structures). This difference of innervation may be of significance; the RMNs may be responsible for information related to potential or real harm to the neural elements of the vertebral canal, and the PPDs may be responsible for relaying information related to the structural integrity of the spine (Edgar & Ghadially, 1976).

Each PPD of the lumbar region leaves the mixed spinal nerve at the lateral border of the IVF and passes over the TP of the lower vertebra participating in the formation of the IVF (e.g., the L3 nerve passes over the L4 TP). The PPD then passes through a small osteoligamentous canal. This canal, which is unique to the lumbar region, lies between the base of the anterior surface of the superior articular process medially and the posterior lamella of the intertransverse ligament laterally. The nerve then sends a twig to the intertransversarius mediales muscle and continues posteriorly, where it divides into a medial and lateral branch. The medial branch passes deep to the mamillo-accessory ligament (see Articular Processes) and supplies sensory innervation to the Z joint and then motor innervation to the multifidi. This innervation to the multifidi has been found to be specific (Bogduk, Wilson, & Tynan, 1982). The medial

branch of a PPD innervates those fibers that insert onto the spinous process "of the same segmental number as the nerve" (Bogduk et al., 1982). For example, the medial branch of the L3 PPD innervates the multifidi that insert onto the L3 spinous process. The medial branch then continues further medially to innervate the rotatores and interspinous muscles and to provide sensory innervation to the interspinous ligament, supraspinous "ligament" (restraints), possibly the ligamentum flavum, and the periosteum of the posterior arch, including the spinous process (see the box below and Fig. 7-21). Along its course the medial branch anastomoses with medial branches of adjacent levels and also sends an inferior branch to the Z joint of the level below (Bogduk, 1976; Edgar & Ghadially, 1976). Therefore, each Z joint is innervated by medial branches of at least two PPDs (Bogduk et al., 1982).

STRUCTURES INNERVATED BY THE MEDIAL BRANCH OF A LUMBAR PPD (STRUCTURES CAPABLE OF PRODUCING PAIN)

Z joint
Interspinous ligament
Supraspinous restraints
Ligamentum flavum (possibly)
Periosteum of posterior arch and posterior aspect of spinous process
Muscles, including intertransversarius mediales, multifidi, rotatores, and interspinous muscles (motor and sensory innervation to these)

The lateral branch of the PPD supplies motor innervation to the erector spinae muscles. Bogduk (1983) found that the lateral branch supplies the iliocostalis lumborum muscle while an intermediate branch stems from the lumbar PPDs to supply the longissimus thoracis muscle. After innervating the longissimus thoracis muscle, the intermediate branches form an anastomosis with the intermediate branches of adjacent levels. The PPD of L5 has only two branches, a medial branch with a typical distribution and a more lateral branch that corresponds with the intermediate branches of higher levels because it innervates the longissimus thoracis muscle. Since the muscle fibers of the iliocostalis lumborum do not extend inferiorly to the level of the L5 nerve, the absence of a nerve corresponding to a typical lateral branch of higher levels is quite understandable (Bogduk, 1983). The L1, L2, and L3 lateral branches are sometimes known as the superior clunial nerves. They supply sensory innervation to the skin over the upper buttocks. Neither the medial branches of the PPDs nor any branches of the L4 and L5 PPDs supply the skin of the back.

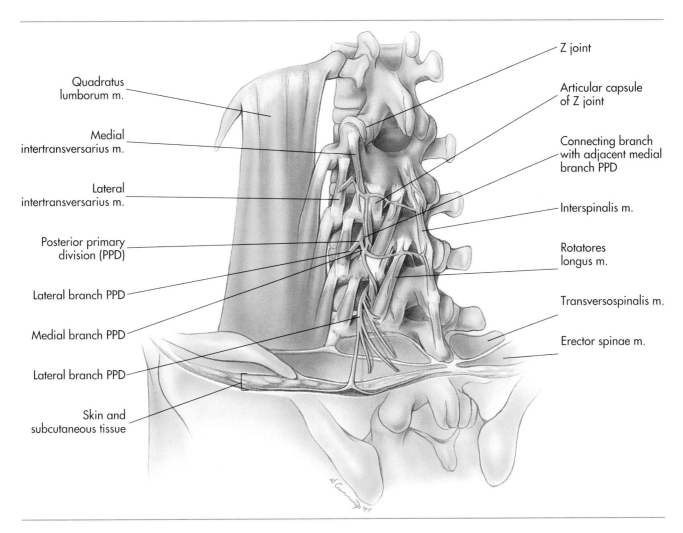

Quadratus
lumborum m.

Medial
intertransversarius m.

Lateral
intertransversarius m.

Posterior primary
division (PPD)

Lateral branch PPD

Medial branch PPD

Lateral branch PPD

Skin and
subcutaneous tissue

Z joint

Articular capsule
of Z joint

Connecting branch
with adjacent medial
branch PPD

Interspinalis m.

Rotatores
longus m.

Transversospinalis m.

Erector spinae m.

FIG. 7-21   Structures innervated by the posterior primary divisions of typical lumbar mixed spinal nerves. The quadratus lumborum muscle, which is innervated by the anterior primary divisions, is also shown.

Anterior Primary Divisions and the Lumbar Plexus. The anterior primary divisions (APDs), or ventral rami, branch from the mixed spinal nerves at the lateral border of the IVF and immediately enter the psoas major muscle. The ventral rami of the first four lumbar nerves then branch within the substance of the psoas major muscle to form the lumbar plexus. As previously mentioned in this chapter, the psoas major muscle may provide some protection for the dorsal and ventral roots from traction forces placed on the peripheral nerves of the lumbar plexus (dePeretti et al., 1989).

The lumbar plexus is derived from the ventral rami of only the first four lumbar nerves. The ventral ramus of L5 unites with a branch of the ventral ramus of L4 to form the lumbosacral trunk. The lumbosacral trunk then enters the pelvis to unite with the APDs of the sacral mixed spinal nerves and in doing so helps to form the sacral

plexus. Frequently the twelfth thoracic (subcostal) nerve also participates in the lumbar plexus.

The branches of the lumbar plexus are listed next, along with the closely related subcostal nerve and lumbosacral trunk.

◆ *Subcostal nerve (T12).* The subcostal nerve is sensory to the region under the umbilicus and is also motor to the pyramidalis and quadratus lumborum muscles.

◆ *Iliohypogastric nerve (L1).* This nerve is sensory to the gluteal, inguinal, and suprapubic regions. It also provides some motor innervation to the muscles of the anterior abdominal wall.

◆ *Ilioinguinal nerve (L1).* This nerve is motor to the muscles of the anterior abdominal wall.

◆ *Genitofemoral nerve (L1 and L2).* The femoral branch is sensory to the region of the femoral triangle, and the genital branch is motor to the dartos and cremaster muscles of the male (no important innervation by this branch in the female).

♦ *Lateral femoral cutaneous nerve (L2 and L3).* This nerve is sensory to the lateral aspect of the thigh.

♦ *Femoral nerve (L2, L3, and L4).* The femoral nerve provides motor innervation to the psoas and iliacus muscles before leaving the abdominopelvic cavity posterior to the inguinal ligament. Distal to the inguinal ligament, this nerve innervates the quadratus femoris and pectineus muscles and supplies sensory innervation to the anterior thigh and medial leg.

♦ *Obturator nerve (L2, L3, and L4).* The obturator nerve is motor to the adductor muscles of the thigh and supplies sensory innervation to the medial aspect of the thigh.

♦ *Lumbosacral trunk (L4 and L5).* The lumbosacral trunk is not officially a part of the lumbar plexus. This nerve passes inferiorly to participate in the sacral plexus. It therefore serves as a connection between the lumbar and sacral plexuses.

Autonomic Nerves of the Lumbar Region. The abdominal and pelvic viscera receive their motor innervation from autonomics derived from both the sympathetic and the parasympathetic nervous systems. Sensory nerves originating from the same visceral structures also travel along the sympathetic and parasympathetic nerve fibers. The diffuse nature of the sympathetic and parasympathetic systems is responsible for the equally diffuse nature of the sensory innervation that travels along with them. This is one reason pain from an abdominal or pelvic viscus may "refer" to a region some distance from the affected organ.

Sympathetic innervation of the abdominal viscera is derived from two sources, the thoracic and lumbar splanchnic nerves. The parasympathetics are supplied by either the left and right vagus nerves or the pelvic splanchnic nerves. The clinical relevance and the specific nerves that comprise both the sympathetic and the parasympathetic divisions of the autonomic nervous system are discussed in detail in Chapter 10.

Vessels of the Abdomen Related to the Spine

This synopsis of the arteries and veins of the abdomen is included because of the close relationship of the abdominal vessels to the anterior and anterolateral aspects of the lumbar vertebral bodies and the lumbar IVDs. This section is by no means complete; it is meant to provide a ready reference for the student and the clinician.

Abdominal Aorta and its Branches. Three large, unpaired branches of the aorta—the celiac trunk, the superior mesenteric artery, and the inferior mesenteric artery—exit the anterior aspect of the abdominal aorta and supply the gastrointestinal tract from the stomach to the superior aspect of the rectum. In addition, the celiac trunk supplies the spleen, liver, gallbladder, and a large part of the pancreas. Paired branches of the abdominal aorta are also present throughout its length and are closely related to the posterior abdominal wall. For this reason, they are more relevant to our current discussion (Fig. 7-22). The paired branches of the abdominal aorta are listed and briefly discussed next.

♦ *Inferior phrenic artery.* The left and right inferior phrenic arteries branch from the aorta as it enters the abdominal cavity through the aortic hiatus. Each courses superiorly to supply the posteroinferior aspect of the diaphragm and, along its way, gives many superior suprarenal (adrenal) arteries.

♦ *Middle suprarenal (adrenal) arteries.* These are several paired branches that run directly to the adrenal gland.

♦ *Renal artery.* The large left and right renal arteries course behind the renal veins to enter the hilus of the left and right kidneys. At the hilus, each divides into five branches (four anterior and one posterior) that supply the five renal arterial segments.

♦ *Gonadal artery* (testicular artery in the male and ovarian artery in the female). The left and right gonadal arteries arise from the anterior aspect of the abdominal aorta in a staggered fashion. That is, one of the arteries (usually the left) originates up to several centimeters superior to the other. The gonadal vessels have a long inferolateral course within the abdomen and pelvis. The testicular artery of each side enters the deep inguinal ring on its way to the testes. The left and right ovarian vessels enter the pelvis by crossing the external iliac artery of the same side before supplying the ovary.

♦ *Lumbar arteries.* These are four paired segmental arteries that arise from the posterolateral aspect of the aorta. They pass laterally along the vertebral bodies, and each artery divides into an anterior and a posterior branch. The anterior branches of the lumbar arteries supply the inferior half of the anterolateral abdominal wall. Each posterior branch provides a spinal branch (ramus), which is an important contribution to the vasculature of the vertebral canal and its contents (see Chapters 2 and 3). The posterior branch of the lumbar segmental artery continues posteriorly to supply the muscles and the skin of the back.

♦ *Median (middle) sacral artery.* This is a small, unpaired artery that arises from the posterior aspect of the abdominal aorta just before its bifurcation into right and left common iliac arteries. The median sacral artery passes inferiorly along the midline of the anterior sacrum.

Veins of the Abdomen. The two large veins of the abdomen are the portal vein and the inferior vena cava

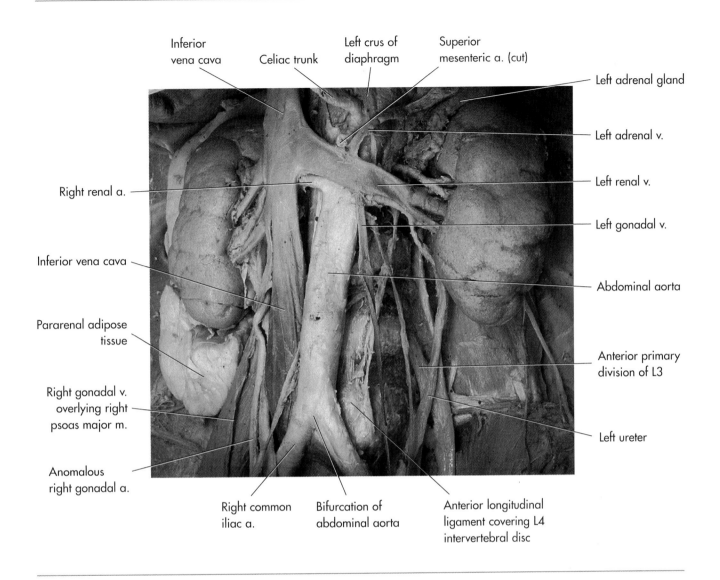

Inferior vena cava · Celiac trunk · Left crus of diaphragm · Superior mesenteric a. (cut) · Left adrenal gland · Left adrenal v. · Left renal v. · Left gonadal v. · Abdominal aorta · Anterior primary division of L3 · Left ureter · Anterior longitudinal ligament covering L4 intervertebral disc · Bifurcation of abdominal aorta · Right common iliac a. · Anomalous right gonadal a. · Right gonadal v. overlying right psoas major m. · Pararenal adipose tissue · Inferior vena cava · Right renal a.

FIG. 7-22 Important vessels of the abdomen related to the lumbar vertebral column.

(IVC). The portal vein receives the blood from the entire gastrointestinal tract and the spleen and pancreas. The IVC receives blood from the remainder of the abdominal and pelvic viscera and the lower extremities. In general the venous return to the IVC follows a similar course to that of the arterial supply. Some unique features of the abdominal venous system are listed next.

♦ *Hepatic veins.* These veins drain the liver and empty into the IVC as it passes through the fossa for the inferior vena cava. This occurs along the posteroinferior surface of the liver.

♦ *Renal veins.* These tributaries of the IVC drain the kidneys. The right renal vein communicates with the azygos vein, whereas the left renal vein communicates with the hemiazygos vein. The azygos and hemiazygos veins course along the right and left sides of the upper lumbar vertebral bodies, respectively.

♦ *Ascending lumbar veins.* The right and left ascending lumbar veins course superiorly along the posterior and lateral aspects of the lumbar vertebral bodies. They receive tributaries from both the internal and the external vertebral venous plexuses. Superiorly, the right and left ascending lumbar veins communicate with the azygos and hemiazygos veins, respectively.

REFERENCES

Arnoldi, C.C., et al. (1976). Lumbar spinal stenosis and nerve root entrapment syndromes. *Clin Orthop, 115,* 4-5.

Bachop, W. & Janse, J. (1983). The corporotransverse ligament at the L5 intervertebral foramen. *Anat Rec, 205,* (abstract).

Bachop, W.E. & Ro, C.S. (1984). A ligament separating the nerve from the blood vessels at the L5 intervertebral foramen. *J Bone Joint Surg, 8,* 437.

Bakkum, B. & Mestan, M. (1994). The effects of transforaminal ligaments on the sizes of T11 to L5 human intervertebral foramina. *J Manipulative Physiol Ther, 17,* 517-522.

Behrsin, J.F. & Briggs, C.A. (1988). Ligaments of the lumbar spine: A review. *Surg Radiol Anat, 10,* 211-219.

Bergmann, T.F., Peterson, D.H. & Lawrence, D.J. (1993). *Chiropractic technique: Principles and procedures.* New York: Churchill Livingstone.

Boden, S.D. et al. (1990). Abnormal magnetic-resonance scans of the lumbar spine in asymptomatic subjects. *J Bone Joint Surg, 72,* 401-408.

Bogduk, N. (1976). The anatomy of the lumbar intervertebral disc syndrome. *Med J Aust, 1,* 878-881.

Bogduk, N. (1981). The lumbar mamillo-accessory ligament: Its anatomical and neurosurgical significance. *Spine, 6,* 162-167.

Bogduk, N (1983). The innervation of the lumbar spine. *Spine, 8,* 286-293.

Bogduk, N. (1985). Low back pain. *Aust Fam Physician, 14,* 1168-1171.

Bogduk, N. (1990). Pathology of lumbar disc pain. *Manual Med, 5,* 72-79.

Bogduk, N. & Twomey, L.T. (1991). *Clinical anatomy of the lumbar spine.* London: Churchill Livingstone.

Bogduk, N., Tynan, W., & Wilson, A. (1981). The nerve supply to the human lumbar intervertebral discs. *J Anat, 132,* 39-56.

Bogduk, N, Wilson, A., & Tynan, W. (1982). The human lumbar dorsal rami. *J Anat, 134,* 383-397.

Bose, K. & Balasubramaniam, P. (1984). Nerve root canals of the lumbar spine. *Spine, 9,* 16-18.

Cassidy, J. & Kirkaldy-Willis, W. (1988). Manipulation. In W. Kirkaldy-Willis (Ed.), *Managing low back pain* (2nd ed.). New York: Churchill Livingstone.

Clarke, G.A. et al. (1985). Can infant malnutrition cause adult vertebral stenosis? *Spine, 10,* 165-170.

Cox, J. (1990). *Low back pain: Mechanism, diagnosis, and treatment* (5th ed.). Baltimore: Williams & Wilkins.

Cramer, G., et al. (1992a). Generalizability of patient profiles from a feasibility study. *J Can Chiropractic Assoc, 36,* 84-90.

Cramer, G. et al. (1992b). Lumbar intervertebral foramen dimensions from thirty-seven human subjects as determined by magnetic resonance imaging. *Proceedings of the 1992 International Conference of Spinal Manipulation, 1,* 3-5.

Cramer, G. et al. (1994). Comparison of computed tomography to magnetic resonance imaging in the evaluation of the lumbar intervertebral foramina. *Clin Anat, 7,* 173-180.

Crock, H.V. (1981). Normal and pathological anatomy of the lumbar spinal nerve root canals. *J Bone Joint Surg, 63,* 487-490.

Day, M.O. (1991). Spondylolytic spondylolisthesis in an elite athlete. *Chiro Sports Med, 5,* 91-97.

dePeretti, F. et al. (1989). Biomechanics of the lumbar spinal nerve roots and the first sacral root within the intervertebral foramina. *Surg Radiol Anat, 11,* 221-225.

Dommisse, G.F. & Louw, J.A. (1990). Anatomy of the lumbar spine. In Y. Floman (Ed.), *Disorders of the lumbar spine.* Rockville, Md, and Tel Aviv, 1990 Aspen and Freund.

Dunlop, R.B., Adams, M.A., & Hutton, W.C. (1984). Disc space narrowing and the lumbar facet joints. *J Bone Joint Surg, 66,* 706-710.

Dupuis, P.R. (1988). The anatomy of the lumbosacral spine. In W. Kirkaldy-Willis (Ed.), *Managing low back pain,* (2nd ed) New York: Churchill Livingstone.

Dupuis, P.R. et al. (1985). Radiologic diagnosis of degenerative lumbar spinal instability. *Spine, 10,* 262-276.

Edgar, M., & Ghadially J. (1976). Innervation of the lumbar spine. *Clin Orthop, 115,* 35-41.

Engel, R. & Bogduk, N. (1982). The menisci of the lumbar zygapophysial joints. *J Anat, 135,* 795-809.

Ericksen, M.F. (1976). Some aspects of aging in the lumbar spine. *Am J Phys Anthropol, 45,* 575-580.

Floman, Y., & Mirovsky, Y. (1990). The physical examination of the lumbosacral spine. In Y. Floman (Ed.) *Disorders of the lumbar spine.* Rockville, Md, and Tel Aviv: Aspen and Freund.

Giglio, G.C. et al. (1988). Anatomy of the lumbar spine in achondroplasia. *Basic Life Sci, 48,* 227-239.

Giles, L.G. (1988). Human zygapophyseal joint inferior recess synovial folds: A light microscopic examination. *Anat Rec, 220,* 117-124.

Giles, L.G. & Taylor, J.R. (1987). Human zygapophyseal joint capsule and synovial fold innervation. *Br J Rheumatol, 26,* 93-98.

Grenier, N. et al. (1989a). Isthmic spondylolisthesis of the lumbar spine: MR imaging at 1.5T. *Radiology, 170,* 489-493.

Grenier, N. et al. (1989b). Normal and disrupted lumbar longitudinal ligaments: Correlative MR and anatomic study. *Radiology, 171,* 197-205.

Groen, G., Baljet B., & Drukker, J. (1990). Nerves and nerve plexuses of the human vertebral column. *Am J Anat, 188,* 282-296.

Hasue, M. et al. (1983). Anatomic study of the interrelation between lumbosacral nerve roots and their surrounding tissues. *Spine, 8,* 50-58.

Helms, C.A. & Sims, R. (1986). Foraminal spurs: A normal variant in the lumbar spine. *Radiology, 160,* 153-154.

Hutton, W.C. (1990). The forces acting on a lumbar intervertebral joint. *J Manual Med, 5,* 66-67.

Jackson, H.C. et al. (1966). Nerve endings in the human lumbar spinal column and related structures. *J Bone Joint Surg, 48,* 1272-1281.

Kikuchi, S. et al. (1984). Anatomic and clinical studies of radicular symptoms. *Spine, 9,* 23-30.

Kirk, C.R. & Lawrence, D.J. (1985). *States manual of spinal, pelvic, and extravertebral technics,* (2nd ed.). Baltimore: Waverly Press.

Kirkaldy-Willis, W.H. et al. (1978). Pathology and pathogenesis of lumbar spondylosis and stenosis. *Spine, 3,* 319-328.

Korkala, O. et al. (1985). Immunohistochemical demonstration of nociceptors in the ligamentous structures of the lumbar spine. *Spine, 10,* 156-157.

Lancourt, J.E., Glenn, W.V., & Wiltse, L.L. (1979). Multiplanar computerized tomography in the normal spine and in the diagnosis of spinal stenosis. A gross anatomic-computerized tomographic correlation. *Spine, 4,* 379-390.

Lee, C.K., Rauschning, W., & Glenn, W. (1988). Lateral lumbar spinal canal stenosis: Classification, pathologic anatomy and surgical decompression. *Spine, 13,* 313-320.

Lippitt, A.B. (1984). The facet joint and its role in spine pain: Management with facet joint injections. *Spine, 9,* 746-50.

Liyang, D. et al. (1989). The effect of flexion-extension motion of the lumbar spine on the capacity of the spinal canal, an experimental study. *Spine, 14,* 523-525.

Maigne, J.Y., Maigne, R., & Guerin-Surville, H. (1991). The lumbar mamillo-accessory foramen: A study of 203 lumbosacral spines. *Surg Radiol Anat, 13,* 29-32.

Marchand, F., & Ahmed, A. (1990). Investigation of the laminate structure of lumbar disc anulus fibrosus. *Spine, 15,* 402-410.

Mayoux-Benhamou, M.A. et al. (1989). A morphometric study of the lumbar spine, influence of flexion-extension movements and of isolated disc collapse. *Surg Radiol Anat, 11,* 97-102.

McNab, I. (1971). Negative disc exploration: An analysis of the causes of nerve-root involvement in sixty-eight patients. *J Bone Joint Surg, 53A,* 891-903.

Mooney, V., & Robertson, J. (1976). The facet syndrome. *Clin Orthop 115,* 149-156.

Mosner, E.A. et al (1989). A comparison of actual and apparent lumbar lordosis in black and white adult females. *Spine, 14,* 310-314.

Nachemson, A.L. (1976). The lumbar spine, and orthopedic challenge. *Spine, 1,* 59-71.

Nathan, H., Weizenbluth, M., & Halperin, N. (1982). The lumbosacral ligament (LSL), with special emphasis on the "lumbosacral tunnel" and the entrapment of the 5th lumbar nerve. *Int Orthop, 6,* 197-202.

Neidre, A. & MacNab, I. (1983). Anomalies of the lumbosacral nerve roots: Review of 16 cases and classification. *Spine, 8,* 294-299.

Nicholson, A.A., Roberts, G.M., & Williams, L.A. (1988). The measured height of the lumbosacral disc in patients with and without transitional vertebrae. *Br J Radiol, 61,* 454-455.

Nowicki, B.H., & Haughton, V.M. (1992). Ligaments of the lumbar neural foramina: A sectional anatomic study. *Clin Anat 5,* 126-135.

Olsewski, J.M. et al. (1991). Evidence from cadavers suggestive of entrapment of fifth lumbar spinal nerves by lumbosacral ligaments. *Spine, 16,* 336-347.

Pal, G.P. et al. (1988). Trajectory architecture of the trabecular bone betwen the body and the neural arch in human vertebrae. *Anat Rec, 222,* 418-425.

Paris, S. (1983). Anatomy as related to function and pain. *Symposium on Evaluation and Care of Lumbar Spine Problems,* 475-489.

Plamondon, A., Gagnon, M. & Maurais, G. (1988). Application of stereoradiographic method for the study of intervertebral motion. *Spine, 13,* 1027-1032.

Rauschning, W. (1987). Normal and pathologic anatomy of the lumbar root canals. *Spine, 12,* 1008-1019.

Scapinelli, R. (1989). Morphological and functional changes of the lumbar spinous processes in the elderly. *Surg Radiol Anat, 11,* 129-133.

Taylor, J.R. (1990). The development and adult structure of lumbar intervertebral discs. *J Manual Med, 5,* 43-47.

Taylor, J.R., & Twomey, L.T. (1986). Age changes in lumbar zygapophyseal joints: Observations on structure and function. *Spine, 11,* 739-745.

Theil, H.W., Clements, D.S., & Cassidy, J.D. (1992). Lumbar apophyseal ring fractures in adolescents. *J Manipulative Physiol Ther, 15,* 250-254.

Tsuji, H. et al. (1985). Redundant nerve roots in patients with degenerative lumbar spinal stenosis. *Spine, 10,* 72-82.

Twomey, L., & Taylor, J.R. (1990). Structural and mechanical disc changes with age. *J Manual Med, 5,* 58-61.

Twomey, L., Taylor, J., & Furniss, B. (1983). Age changes in the bone density and structure of the lumbar vertebral column. *J Anat, 136,* 15-25.

Uhthoff, H. (1993). Prenatal development of the iliolumbar ligament. *J Bone Joint Surg, 75,* 93-95.

Van Schaik, J., Verbiest, H., & Van Schaik, F. (1985). The orientation of laminae and facet joints in the lower lumbar spine, *Spine, 10,* 59-63.

Vital, J.M. et al. (1983). Anatomy of the lumbar radicular canal. *Anat Clin, 5,* 141-151.

White, A.W., & Panjabi, M.M. (1990). *Clinical biomechanics of the spine.* Philadelphia: J.B. Lippincott.

Williams, P.L. et al. (Eds), (1989). *Gray's anatomy* (37th ed.). Edinburgh: Churchill Livingstone.

Wiltse, L.L. et al. (1984). Alar transverse process impingement of the L5 spinal nerve: The far-out syndrome. *Spine, 9,* 31-41.

Xu, G.L., Haughton, V.M., & Carrera, G.F. (1990). Lumbar facet joint capsule: Appearance at MR imaging and CT. *Radiology, 177,* 415-420.

Xu, G.L. et al. (1991). Normal variations of the lumbar facet joint capsules. *Clin Anat, 4,* 117-122.

CHAPTER 8

The Sacrum, Sacroiliac Joint, and Coccyx

Chae-Song Ro
Gregory D. Cramer

This chapter begins with a discussion of the bony sacrum. Then, because of its clinical significance, the sacroiliac joint is covered in detail. This is followed by a discussion of the anatomy of the coccyx.

THE SACRUM

The sacrum is composed of five fused vertebral segments. It is triangular in shape, and therefore the wider superior surface of the sacrum is known as the base, and the smaller inferior surface is known as the apex (Figs. 8-1 and 8-2). The sacrum is concave anteriorly (kyphotic), and, as with the other primary kyphosis (the thoracic region), its curvature helps to increase the size of a bony body cavity, in this case the pelvis. The sacrum is normally positioned so that its base is located anterior to its apex. Therefore the sacral curve faces anteriorly and inferiorly (Williams et al., 1989). The sacral curve is more pronounced in humans than in other mammals, including monkeys and apes. In addition, the human sacral curve is almost nonexistent in infants but becomes more pronounced with age (Abitbol, 1989). The combination of the upright posture, the supine sleeping posture, and humans having a well-developed levator ani muscle are responsible for the increased sacral curve in humans. Abitbol (1989) also found that the frequency of sleeping in the supine posture, and the younger the age when this posture was first assumed for sleeping, were positively associated with the size of the sacral curve.

The sacrum ossifies much like any other vertebra, with one primary center located in the anterior and centrally located primitive vertebral body and one primary center in each posterior arch. Unique to the sacrum is that the costal elements develop separately and then fuse with the remainder of the posterior arch to form the solid mass of bone lateral to the pelvic sacral foramina. Secondary centers of ossification are rather complex, with centers developing on the superior and inferior aspects of each sacral vertebral body, on the lateral and the anterior aspects of each costal element, on the spinous tubercles, and on the lateral (auricular) surface of the sacrum. Most centers fuse by approximately the 25th year of life, but ossification and fusion of individual segments continue until later in life. Early in development, fibrocartilage forms between sacral bodies. These

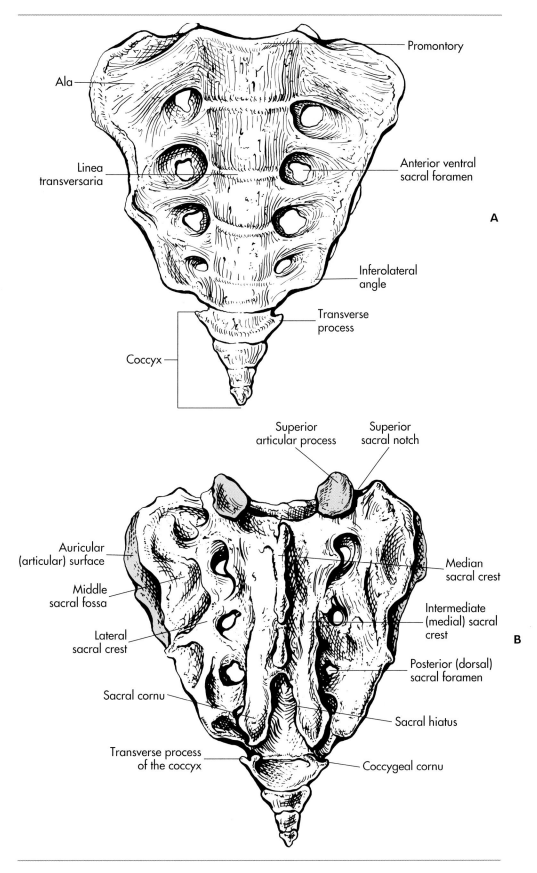

FIG. 8-1 The sacrum. **A,** Anterior view. **B,** Posterior view.

represent rudimentary intervertebral discs (IVDs) and usually become surrounded by bone as the sacral bodies fuse with one another. However, the central region of these "discs" usually remains unossified throughout life.

Sacral Base

The sacral base is composed of the first sacral segment. It has a large body that is the homologue of the vertebral bodies (Figs. 8-1 and 8-2). This body is wider from left to right than from front to back. The anterior lip of the sacral body is known as the promontory. The vertebral foramen of the first sacral segment is triangular in shape and forms the beginning of the sacral canal. This canal extends the length of the sacrum. The pedicles of the first sacral segment are rather small and extend to the left and right laminae. The laminae of the first segment meet posteriorly to form the spinous tubercle. The transverse processes (TPs) extend laterally and fuse with the costal elements to form the large left and right sacral ala, which are also known as the lateral sacral masses. Each lateral sacral mass is concave on its anterior surface, allowing it to accommodate the psoas major muscle. The psoas major passes across the sacrum before inserting onto the lesser trochanter of the femur.

Extending superiorly from the posterior surface of the sacral base are the left and right articular processes. These processes generally face posteriorly and slightly medially. However, the plane in which these processes lie varies considerably (Dommisse & Louw, 1990). Their orientation ranges from nearly a coronal plane to almost a sagittal one. These processes are also frequently asymmetric in orientation, with one process more coronally oriented and the other more sagittally oriented. Such asymmetry is known as tropism and usually can be detected on standard anterior-posterior x-ray films. The superior articular processes possess articular facets on their posterior surfaces that articulate with the inferior articular facets of the L5 vertebra. The zygapophyseal joints (Z joints) formed by these articulations are more planar than those between two adjacent lumbar vertebrae, and they are usually much more coronally oriented than the lumbar Z joints (see Chapter 7). However, because of the wide variation of the plane in which the superior articular processes lie, the orientation of the lumbosacral Z joints also varies in corresponding fashion.

Just lateral to the superior articular facets are the left and right superior sacral notches. These notches allow for passage of the left and right posterior primary divisions of the L5 spinal nerve.

The muscular and ligamentous attachments to the sacral base and the anterior and posterior surfaces of the sacrum are listed in Table 8-1. This table also provides the key anatomic relationships between these regions of the sacrum, and the neural, muscular, and visceral structures that contact them.

Lateral Surface

The lateral surface of the sacrum (Fig. 8-2) is composed of the TPs of the five sacral segments, fused with the

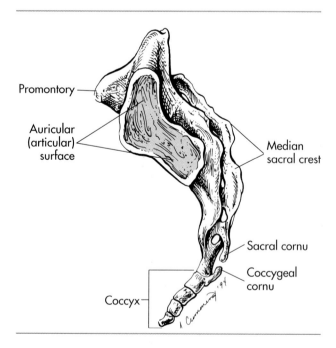

FIG. 8-2   Lateral view of the sacrum.

Table 8-1   Attachments and Relationships to the Sacrum

Surface	Attachments or relationships
Base	
Anterior	Ligaments: anterior longitudinal, iliolumbar, ventral sacroiliac
	Muscles: psoas major and iliacus (cover the base)
	Nerves: lumbosacral trunk (crosses over the base)
Posterior	Ligaments: posterior longitudinal, ligamentum flavum (to lamina of S1), posterior sacroiliac
Ventral	Muscle: piriformis
	Nerves: S1-4 ventral rami (S1-3 are anterior to piriformis), sympathetic trunks (left and right)
	Arteries: median sacral, lateral sacral (left and right), superior rectal
	Viscera: parietal peritoneum (S1-3 bodies), sigmoid mesocolon (S1-3 bodies), rectum (S3-5 bodies)
Dorsal	Muscles: Erector spinae, multifidus (between median and lateral sacral crests)

Data from Williams et al. (1989). Gray's anatomy (37th ed.). Edinburgh: Churchill Livingstone.

costal elements of the same segments. This surface contains the auricular surface. The auricular surface of the sacrum articulates with the auricular surface of the ilium. The sacral auricular surface is concave posteriorly and extends across the lateral aspects of three of the five sacral segments. Within the region formed by the concavity of the auricular surface are several elevations and depressions that serve as attachment sites for the ligaments that support the sacroiliac joint posteriorly. These ligaments and the sacroiliac joint are discussed in detail later in this chapter. Inferior to the auricular surface, the lateral surface of the sacrum curves medially and becomes thinner from anterior to posterior. The inferior and lateral angle of the sacrum is located at approximately the level of the junction of the fourth and fifth sacral segments. Below this angle the sacrum rapidly tapers to the sacral apex. The apex of the sacrum has an oval-shaped facet on its inferior surface for articulation with a small disc between the sacrum and the coccyx.

Sacral Canal and Sacral Foramina

The sacral canal is composed of the vertebral foramina of the five fused sacral segments. The left and right lateral walls of the canal each contain four intervertebral foramina (IVFs). Each IVF is continuous laterally with a ventral (pelvic) and dorsal sacral foramen. The sacral canal ends inferiorly as the sacral hiatus (see following discussion).

The cauda equina extends inferiorly through the beginning of the sacral canal and within the subarachnoid space. The arachnoid mater and dura mater end at approximately the level of the S2 spinous tubercle. The sacral roots exiting below this level must pierce the inferior aspect of the arachnoid and dura to continue inferiorly through the sacral canal. In the process, these roots receive a dural root sleeve. Dorsal and ventral roots unite within their dural sleeve to form a mixed spinal nerve and then exit a sacral IVF.

Structures Exiting the Sacral Hiatus. Both the left and the right S5 nerves and the coccygeal nerve of each side exit the sacral hiatus just medial to the sacral cornua of the same side. They proceed inferiorly and laterally, wrapping around the inferior tip of the sacral cornua (see Dorsal Surface). The posterior primary divisions (PPDs) of these nerves pass posteriorly and inferiorly to supply sensory innervation to the skin over the coccyx. The S5 and coccygeal anterior primary divisions pass anteriorly to pierce the coccygeus muscle and enter the inferior aspect of the pelvis. Here they are joined by the ventral ramus of the S4 nerve to form the coccygeal plexus. This small plexus gives off the anococcygeal nerves that help to supply the skin adjacent to the sacrotuberous ligament.

Also passing through the sacral hiatus is the end of the filum terminale. The filum terminale originates from the most inferior aspect of the spinal cord, where it is known as the filum terminale internum. It passes through the lumbar cistern of cerebrospinal fluid (CSF), pierces the inferior aspect of the arachnoid and dura (at approximately the level of the S2 segment), and then becomes known as the filum terminale externum. After exiting the sacral hiatus, the filum terminale externum attaches to the posterior surface of the first coccygeal vertebral segment.

Ventral Surface

The junctions of the five fused sacral segments form lines that can be seen running across the central aspect of the anterior, or pelvic, surface of the sacrum. These junctions are known as the linea transversaria (also known as transverse lines, or transverse ridges). Remnants of the IVDs are located just deep to the transverse lines. These "discs" frequently remain throughout life and can be seen on standard x-ray films and on magnetic resonance imaging (MRI) scans. The vertebral bodies of the five fused sacral segments lie between the transverse lines and medial to the pelvic sacral foramina (Fig. 8-1).

The ventral surface of the sacrum displays four pairs of ventral (pelvic, or anterior) sacral foramina. These foramina are continuous posteriorly and medially with the sacral IVFs. The sacral IVFs, in turn, are continuous with the more medially located sacral canal. The anterior primary divisions (APDs) of the S1 through S4 sacral nerves exit the pelvic sacral foramina. The APDs are accompanied within these openings by branches of the lateral and median sacral arteries and by segmental veins. Located between the pelvic sacral foramina of the same side are the costal elements. The costal elements fuse posteriorly with the TPs of the sacral segments.

The muscular and ligamentous attachments to the anterior surface of the sacrum are listed in Table 8-1. Also, Figs. 8-18 and 8-19 demonstrate the major arteries and nerves associated with the anterior surface of the sacrum.

Dorsal Surface

The dorsal surface of the sacrum is irregular in shape (Fig. 8-1). The superior articular processes extend from the superior aspect of the sacral base (see Sacral Base).

Four pair of dorsal (posterior) sacral foramina are located among the five fused sacral segments. These openings are continuous anteriorly with the IVFs of the sacral segments. The PPDs of the S1 through S4 mixed spinal nerves exit through these openings. The PPDs are accompanied by small segmental arteries and veins.

The posterior surface of the sacrum contains five longitudinal ridges known as the median, intermediate (left and right), and lateral (left and right) sacral crests

(Fig. 8-1). These crests are homologous to the spinous processes, articular processes, and the TPs of the rest of the spine, respectively.

The median sacral crest is composed of four spinous tubercles that are fused with one another and form the posterior boundary of the sacral canal. Each sacral tubercle is formed by the union of the left and right laminae of the sacral vertebral segments. The median sacral crest ends as the only normally occurring spina bifida of the vertebral column. This is because the left and right laminae of the fifth sacral segment normally do not fuse, forming an opening at the inferior end of the sacral canal known as the sacral hiatus.

The left and right intermediate, or medial, sacral crests are formed by four fused articular tubercles on each side of the sacrum (S2-5 tubercles; the S1 articular process is distinct). The left and right fifth articular tubercles extend inferiorly as the sacral cornua. The sacral cornua come to blunted tips inferiorly. They form the left and right inferior boundaries of the sacral hiatus.

Finally, the left and right lateral sacral crests lie lateral to the dorsal sacral foramina. These crests are formed by the fused transverse tubercles of the five sacral segments.

The muscular and ligamentous attachments to the posterior surface of the sacrum are listed in Table 8-1.

Several differences exist between male and female sacra, although sometimes these changes may be very subtle. Generally the male sacrum is narrower from left to right and longer from superior to inferior than that of the female. The wider sacrum of the female results in a larger pelvic inlet (region bounded by the pecten of the pubis, the arcuate line of the ilium, the sacral ala, and the sacral promontory). A larger pelvic inlet results in more room for the passage of the fetal head during delivery. The sacrum in the female is also oriented slightly more horizontally than that of the male. This results in an increase of the lumbosacral angle. The ventral surface of the female pelvis is more concave than that of the male. This concavity provides more space in the pelvic cavity proper than would otherwise be the case, and it also results in a more prominent S2 spinous tubercle on the posterior surface of the female sacrum.

Fusion of the L5 vertebra with the sacrum (sacralization) was discussed previously (see Chapter 7). The first sacral segment may also separate from the sacrum. This is known as lumbarization. The separation may be complete but is usually unilateral, and a joint may develop between the TP of the lumbarized segment and the remainder of the sacrum. Also, the first coccygeal segment may fuse with the sacrum.

Sacrococcygeal Joint

A fibrocartilaginous disc typically exists between the apex of the sacrum and the coccyx, making this joint a symphysis. However, occasionally a synovial joint develops here. At the other extreme, this region may completely fuse in some older individuals (Williams et al., 1989).

Table 8-2 lists all the ligaments of the sacrococcygeal joint by their coccygeal attachments, as well as the muscles attaching to the coccyx.

CLINICAL IMPLICATIONS

Sacral fractures are present in as many as 45% of pelvic fractures (Gibbons et al., 1990). These fractures may go undetected if caudal, cephalic, and oblique x-ray examinations of the pelvis are not performed. Fractures of the sacrum can damage the APDs of the lumbosacral plexus, and fractures involving the sacral canal may affect the sacral roots before they are able to exit the sacrum.

Gibbons, Soloniuk, & Razack (1990) found neurologic deficits in 34% of patients with sacral fractures. They also noted that the neurologic deficits usually improved with time. The presence and type of nerve injury correlated with the type of sacral fracture. Patients with injuries that involved only the sacral ala had the lowest incidence of neurologic deficit, although L5 or S1 radiculopathy was found in 24%. The mechanism of L5 radiculopathy was thought to be caused by entrapment of the APD of L5 between the fractured, superiorly displaced ala and the TP of L5.

Gibbons and colleagues (1990) also found that fractures involving the pelvic sacral foramina were usually vertical fractures that passed through all four foramina of one side. These injuries were always associated with other pelvic fractures and had a 29% incidence

Table 8-2	Attachments and Relationships to the Coccyx		
Surface	Attachments or Relationships
Anterior	Pubococcygeus, illiococcygeus, and ischiococcygeus (coccygeus) muscles, ventral sacrococcygeal ligament (similar to anterior longitudinal ligament)
Posterior	Gluteus maximus and sphincter ani externus (to tip of apex) muscles, intercornual ligaments, deep and superficial dorsal sacrococcygeal ligament,* filum terminale externum
Lateral	Lateral sacrococcygeal ligament (from transverse process of coccyx to inferolateral angle of sacrum)

Data from Williams et al. (1989). Gray's Anatomy (37th ed.). Edinburgh: Churchill Livingstone.

*The superficial part runs between the sacral cornua (it closes the inferior aspect of the sacral canal at the sacral hiatus). The deep part is similar in location (and function) to the posterior longitudinal ligament. The filum terminale externum passes between the two parts of this ligament before attaching to the coccyx.

(two of seven fractures) of unilateral L5 or S1 nerve root involvement. However, bowel and bladder function was maintained because a bilateral lesion is required to affect these functions.

Fractures involving the sacral canal can be either transverse (horizontal) or vertical and have the greatest chance of causing nerve damage (57% with horizontal and 60% with vertical). Vertical fractures are usually associated with other pelvic fractures and can result in bladder and bowel dysfunction (Gibbons et al., 1990).

Horizontal fractures of the sacrum affecting the sacral canal are not necessarily associated with other pelvic fractures. They could be isolated injuries caused by a direct blow as might occur from a long fall. The inferior fragment is sometimes considerably displaced and severe neurologic deficits, involving bladder and bowel functions, can occur if the fracture is above the S4 segment (Gibbons et al., 1990).

SACROILIAC JOINT

General Considerations

The degree to which low back pain is caused by pathologic conditions or dysfunction of the sacroiliac joint (SIJ) has been discussed for many decades. The SIJ is now gaining added attention as a primary source of low back pain (Cassidy & Mierau, 1992). One reason for this is that herniation of the IVD is now known to be a rather infrequent cause of low back pain, accounting for less than 10% of the pain in this region (Cassidy & Mierau, 1992). On the other hand, pain arising from the SIJ is reported to account for more than 20% of low back pain (Kirkaldy-Willis, 1988) and may be implicated to some extent in more than 50% of patients with low back pain (Cassidy & Mierau, 1992). This makes the SIJ an area of significant clinical importance. An understanding of the unique and interesting anatomy of this joint is essential before a clinician can properly diagnose and treat pain arising from this articulation.

The pelvic ring possesses five distinctly different types of joints: the lumbosacral Z joints, the anterior lumbosacral, coxal (hip), SIJ, and symphysis pubis. The dynamic interactions between these joints are not well understood. Since the pelvic ring is complex and involves a total of eight joints (left and right Z joints, coxals and SIJs; plus the single lumbosacral joint and the pubic symphysis), any change in the trunk or lower extremity is compensated in some way by the complicated dynamic mechanism of the pelvic ring (Drerup & Hierholzer, 1987; Fidler & Plasmans, 1983; Grieve, 1981; LaBan et al., 1978; Lichtblau, 1962; Sandoz, 1978; Wallheim, Olerud, & Ribbe, 1984; Winterstein, 1972). In fact, a survey of the pelvic rings of asymptomatic school children 7 to 8 years of age revealed distortion (asymmetry) in 40% of them. Surgical removal of graft material from the pelvic bone (iliac crest) also causes distortion

of the pelvic ring (Beal, 1982; Diakow, Cassidy, & Dekorompay, 1983; Grieve, 1975).

The SIJ and the symphysis pubis move very little. At first inspection, what little motion they have may seem enigmatic at best. Some authors have stated that the sole function of these two joints simply is to widen the pelvic ring during pregnancy and parturition. The joints aided in this action by the hormone relaxin (Bellamy, Park, & Rodney, 1983; Simkins, 1952). Others believe the SIJs move during many activities. An incomplete list of activities thought to enlist the movement of the SIJ include the following: locomotion, spinal and thigh movement, and changes of position (from lying to standing, standing to sitting, etc.).

The SIJ is thought to move only 2 mm and 2°, but this small amount of movement is complex (Brunner, Kissling, & Jacob, 1991; Colachis et al., 1963; Pitkin & Pheasant, 1936b; Sturesson, 1989; Weisl, 1955; Wood, 1985). Janse (1978) stated that the function of movement in the SIJ is to convert the pelvis into a resilient, accommodating receptacle essential to the ease of locomotion, weight bearing, and shock absorption. This is in agreement with other authors (DonTigny, 1990; King, 1991) who state that the function of SIJ is to buffer, absorb, direct, and compensate for forces generated from above (gravity, carrying the torso, and muscle action) and below (forces received during standing and locomotion).

Unique Characteristics

Differences between humans and quadrupeds. The pelvis tilts anteriorly and inferiorly in the bipedal human, and the SIJ is aligned in parallel fashion with the vertebral column, whereas the pelvis of quadrupedal animals is tilted more posteriorly. The SIJ of the bipedal human has other differences associated with a two-legged stance. These include the articulating surfaces of the SIJ that are shaped like an inverted L, the interosseous ligaments that are more substantial and stronger posteriorly, and the many bony interlockings between the sacrum and the ilium that develop with age (Walker, 1986).

Differences among humans. The weight of the human trunk is transmitted by gravity through the lumbosacral joint and is then divided onto the right and left SIJs. In addition, the ground reaction, or bouncing force, is transmitted through the hip joints and also acts on the SIJs. Adapting to the bipedal requirements of mobility and stability may account for the tremendous amount of variation and asymmetry found in the human SIJ. The joint structure and the surface contours of the SIJ have changes associated with age, sex, and the mechanical loads that are placed on them (Walker, 1986). Therefore the functional requirements of the SIJ, to a great extent, may influence the structural changes found in them (Weisl, 1954a). For example, one may speculate that in younger persons, females around the time of parturition, and in athletes, more mobility is required in the SIJ. On the other hand, more stability is required in older persons, in males (generally larger body weight), and in those who frequently carry heavy weights. This stability may be provided by the development of stronger interosseous ligaments and a more prominent series of bony interlockings (Table 8-3). Also, the osteophytes and ankylosis frequently seen in the SIJs of older individuals may develop to increase stability.

Structure

General Relationships. The SIJ is an articulation between the auricular surface of the lateral aspect of the sacrum and the auricular surface of the medial aspect of the ilium (see Figs. 8-6 and 8-7). Previously this joint was classified as an amphiarthrosis. However, the SIJ is now classified as an atypical synovial joint with a well-defined joint space and two opposing articular surfaces (Cassidy & Mierau, 1992). Each auricular surface is shaped like an inverted L (Williams et al., 1989). Other authors have described it as being C shaped (Cassidy & Mierau, 1992). The superior limb of this surface is oriented posteriorly and superiorly, and the inferior limb is oriented posteriorly and inferiorly (Figs. 8-3 to 8-7). An articular capsule lines the SIJ's anterior aspect, whereas the SIJ's posterior aspect is covered by the interosseous sacroiliac (S-I) ligament. No articular capsule has been found along the posterior joint surface.

The sacral auricular surface has a longitudinal groove, known as the sacral groove, along its center that extends from the upper end to the lower end. The posterior rim of this groove is thick and is known as the sacral tuberosity. The iliac auricular surface has a longitudinal ridge, known as the iliac ridge, which corresponds to the sacral groove. The inferior end of this iliac ridge ends as the posterior inferior iliac spine (PIIS). The sacral groove and the iliac ridge interlock for stability and help to guide movement of the SIJ (Table 8-3 and Figs. 8-8 and 8-9).

The region within the posterior concavity of the SIJ is covered by the interosseous sacroiliac ligament and consists of three fossae (Fig. 8-9). The middle fossa is the approximate location of the axis of SIJ rotation. It is approximately around this fossa that the iliac ridge moves circularly in the sacral groove. Posterior to the auricular surface of the ilium is the iliac tuberosity. The anterior aspect of the iliac tuberosity inserts into the middle sacral fossa, creating a pivot around which the iliac ridge turns within the sacral groove (Bakland & Hanse, 1984) (Table 8-3). Between the iliac tuberosity and the iliac ridge there is a sulcus. The sulcus promotes stability by interlocking with the sacral tuberosity (see following discussion). Finally, anterior and superior to the iliac tuberosity is a depression that interlocks with an additional

elevation on the posterior and superior surface of the sacral ala (alar tuberosity). Therefore, stability of the SIJ is promoted by a series of "tongue and grooves." Figs. 8-8 and 8-9 show this series of interlocking elevations and depressions that aid the stability of the SIJ, and Table 8-3 summarizes the tongue and groove relationships between these "hills and valleys." This series of interlocking prominences and depressions become more enhanced and irregular with age.

Ligaments

Articular capsule. The fibrous articular capsule of the SIJ is only located along the anterior surface of the joint (Fig. 8-10). It is lined internally with a synovial membrane and is innervated with nociceptive and proprioceptive nerve endings. No articular capsule is located along the posterior border of the SIJ.

Interosseous sacroiliac (S-I) ligament. The interosseous ligament of each SIJ connects the three sacral fossae (see previous section) to the area around the iliac tuberosity (Figs. 8-8 to 8-15). The interosseous ligament consists of superficial and deep layers. Further, the deep layer has a cranial band and a caudal band. The cranial band is oriented transversely, and the caudal band is oriented more vertically. The superficial layer is membranous and is covered by the posterior S-I ligaments (long and short). Nerves and blood vessels pass between the posterior sacroiliac ligament and the superficial layer of the interosseous ligament. Since there is no posterior joint capsule of the SIJ, the interosseous S-I ligament is what limits the SIJ posteriorly.

A small band, known as the superior intracapsular ligament, or Illi's ligament (Illi, 1951; Janse, 1976), has been found to extend between the superior aspects of the sacral and iliac auricular surfaces in 75% of 31 cadavers studied (Freeman, Fox, & Richards, 1990). This ligament may be an anterior and superior extension

Table 8-3	"Tongue and Groove" Relationships (Bony Interlockings) Between the Sacrum and the Ilium*
Sacral E or D	**Iliac E or D**
Sacral groove (D)	Iliac ridge (E)
Middle sacral fossa (see text) (D)	Iliac tuberosity (E)
Sacral tuberosity (E)	Sulcus between iliac ridge and iliac tuberosity (iliac sulcus) (D)
Additional elevation on posterior and superior surface of sacral ala (alar tuberosity) (E)	Depression anterior and superior to iliac tuberosity (D)

E, Elevation; *D,* depression.
*Compare with Fig. 8-9.

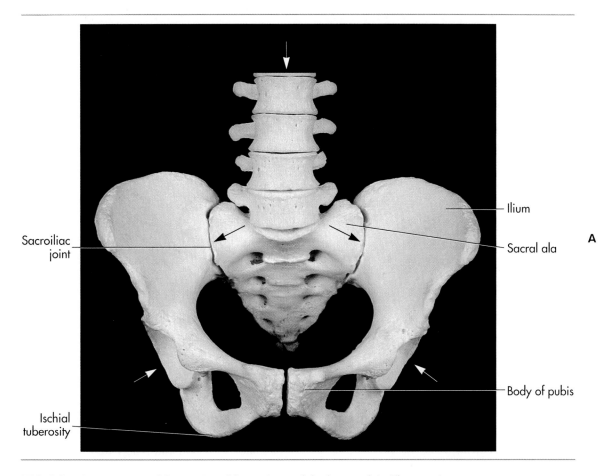

Sacroiliac joint

Ilium

Sacral ala

A

Body of pubis

Ischial tuberosity

FIG. 8-3   **A,** Anterior, and **B,** anterior oblique views of the bony pelvis. The anterior aspect of the left and right sacroiliac joints (SIJs) can be seen. The large arrows in **A** indicate the forces received by the SIJs. Notice that the SIJs receive forces from above and below. Those from above are generated primarily from carrying the weight of the trunk, other weight lifted by the upper extremities, and forces generated during pushing or bending. Forces from below are generated primarily from the lower extremities during walking, running, and so on and are transmitted through the acetabula. Forces from below can also be transmitted through the ischial tuberosities during sitting.   *Continued.*

of the interosseous S-I ligament, but Freeman and colleagues (1990) found that it was quite distinct. The superior intracapsular ligament may have relatively little biomechanical value.

Anterior sacroiliac ligament. The pelvic surface of each SIJ is covered by the anterior, or ventral, S-I ligament (Fig. 8-11). The ventral S-I ligament passes across the anterior aspect of the SIJ in the horizontal plane. It does not support as strongly as either the interosseous or the posterior S-I ligaments. The ventral S-I ligament fuses with the articular capsule of the pelvic side of the SIJ and is thicker inferiorly, near the region of the posterior inferior iliac spine (Freeman et al., 1990; Weisl, 1954b).

Posterior sacroiliac ligament. The posterior (dorsal) sacroiliac (S-I) ligament is made up of two rather distinct parts, which are listed next (Figs. 8-11 and 8-12).

♦ *Long posterior sacroiliac (S-I) ligament.* This ligament originates from the posterior superior iliac spine and the sacral tubercles of S3 and S4. It runs vertically along the posterior aspect of the SIJ and ends by blending inferiorly with the sacrotuberous ligament.

♦ *Short posterior sacroiliac (S-I) ligament.* This ligament originates from the sacral tubercles of S1 and S2. It runs in the horizontal plane covering the SIJ posteriorly, and attaches to the medial aspect of the posterior surface of the iliac crest and the iliac tuberosity.

Accessory sacroiliac ligaments. The stability of the SIJ is enhanced by two accessory S-I ligaments (Fig. 8-11). A third ligament, the iliolumbar ligament (see Chapter 7 and Fig. 8-12), also provides stability to the region.

♦ *Sacrotuberous ligament.* This ligament runs inferiorly and laterally from the posterior and inferior aspect of the sacrum to the ischial tuberosity. The lesser sciatic

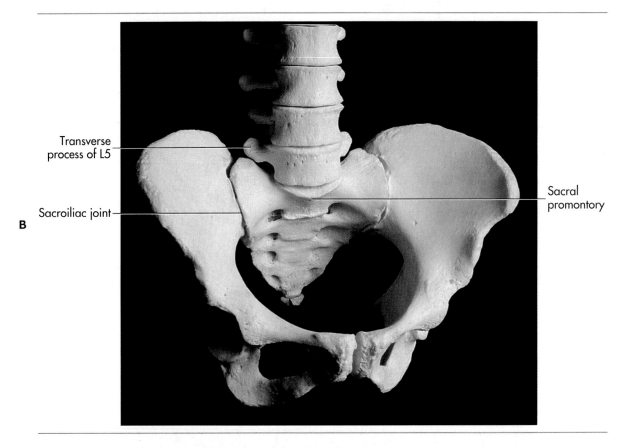

FIG. 8-3, cont'd.   **B,** Anterior oblique view of the bony pelvis.

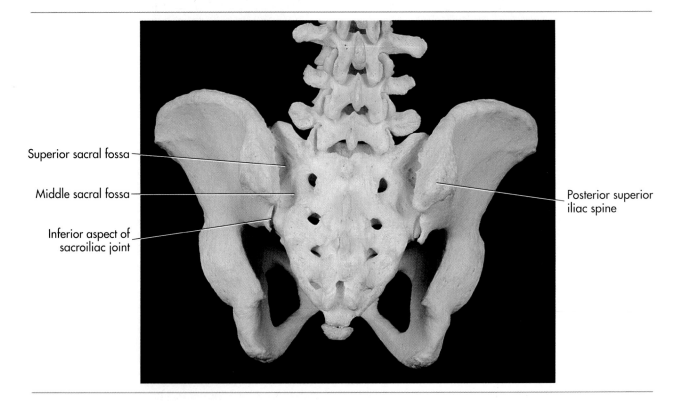

FIG. 8-4   Posterior view of the pelvis. Several sacral fossae associated with the sacroiliac joint are visible from this perspective.

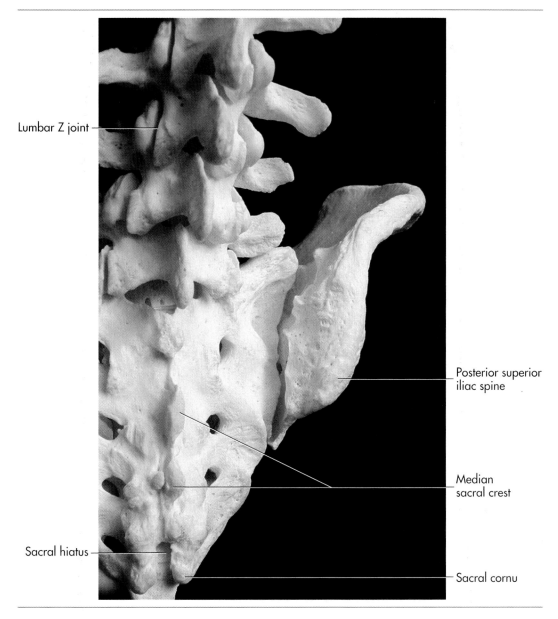

Lumbar Z joint

Posterior superior
iliac spine

Median
sacral crest

Sacral hiatus

Sacral cornu

FIG. 8-5   Close-up of the posterior aspect of the sacroiliac joint, showing the normal anatomic relationships of the sacrum and the ilium.

foramen is formed between this ligament and the sacrospinous ligament.

- *Sacrospinous ligament.* This ligament runs from the anterior surface of the sacrum (fused second, third, and fourth segments) to the spine of the ischium (Fig. 8-11). The greater sciatic foramen is located superior to this ligament.

The sacrotuberous and sacrospinous ligaments help to limit the small amount of anterior and inferior nodding (nutational) motion of the sacrum at the SIJ. This is accomplished by restricting the amount the sacral apex can move posteriorly and superiorly when the promontory of the sacrum moves anteriorly and inferiorly.

- *Iliolumbar ligament.* The iliolumbar ligament connects the iliac crest with the adjacent TP of the L5 vertebra. Part of the iliolumbar ligament (lumbosacral ligament, see Fig. 8-18) attaches to the anterior and superior part of the sacrum (see Chapter 7). The iliolumbar ligament helps to limit lateral tilting of the pelvis and gapping of the SIJ.

Arterial Supply and Venous Drainage

Both the anterior and posterior aspects of the SIJ are served by the superior branch of the lateral sacral artery and vein, which are branches of the internal iliac artery and vein, respectively. These vessels anastomose with

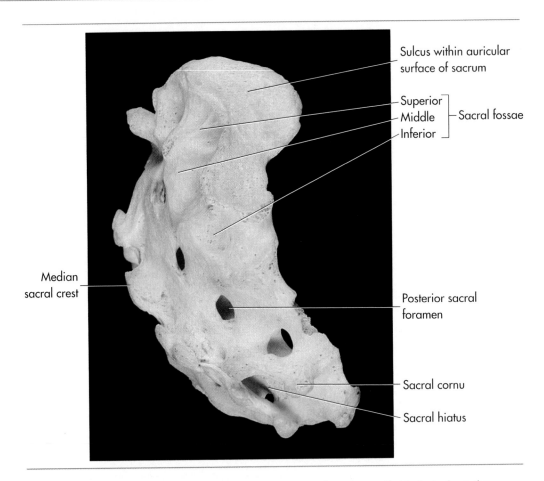

Sulcus within auricular
surface of sacrum

Superior ⎤
Middle ⎬ Sacral fossae
Inferior ⎦

Median
sacral crest

Posterior sacral
foramen

Sacral cornu

Sacral hiatus

FIG. 8-6   Lateral view of the sacrum demonstrating several structures that help to form the sacroiliac joint.

the superficial branch of the superior gluteal artery and vein (Williams et al., 1989). Figs. 8-18 and 8-19 demonstrate the major arteries and nerves associated with the anterior surface of the SIJ.

Innervation

The SIJ is richly innervated, and the joint capsule possesses both nociceptors (pain receptors) and proprioceptors (joint position sensation receptors). This would indicate that the sensory receptors of the SIJ relay information related to movement and joint position and in doing so may help to keep the body upright and balanced. The most pain-sensitive structures in this region are the posterior inferior iliac spine and the superior portion of the sacroiliac fissure (Norman & May, 1956; Pitkin & Pheasant, 1936a). The specific innervation of the SIJ is quite variable, even between the left and right sides of the same individual.

The anterior (pelvic) part of the SIJ is innervated by the APDs of L2 through S2 (Bernard & Cassidy, 1993), with L4 and L5 being the most frequent source of innervation (Cassidy & Mierau, 1992). The posterior part of

the SIJ, according to most authors, is innervated by PPDs of S1 and S2. However, the innervation of this part of the joint is probably more extensive than just the upper sacral segments. Bernard and Cassidy (1993) state that the posterior part of the SIJ is innervated by the lateral branches of the PPDs of L4 to S3. Ro (1990) has demonstrated that the lateral branch of the L5 PPD can extend inferiorly and pass between the superficial layer of the interosseous (S-I) ligament and the posterior S-I ligament.

The variable innervation of the SIJ from person to person and even from the left to the right side of the same person, may be one reason for the wide range of pain referral patterns described by patients experiencing discomfort of SIJ origin (Bernard & Cassidy, 1993). Furthermore, the wide variation of referral patterns may help to explain the difficulty researchers and clinicians have had in identifying the incidence with which SIJ dysfunction occurs.

A portion of the sacral plexus is formed along the anterior surface of the SIJ. Figs. 8-18 and 8-19 demonstrate the relationship of the sacral plexus to the anterior aspect of the SIJ.

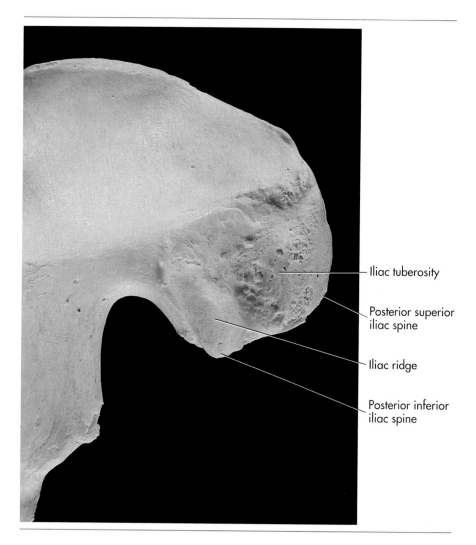

Iliac tuberosity

Posterior superior
iliac spine

Iliac ridge

Posterior inferior
iliac spine

FIG. 8-7 Medial surface of the posterior ilium of a dried skeletal specimen. Several structures that participate in the formation of the sacroiliac joint are demonstrated.

Microscopic Anatomy

The histologic makeup of the cartilage lining the auricular surface of the sacrum differs from that lining the auricular surface of the ilium. The sacral surface is lined by hyaline cartilage, and the iliac surface is lined by what is best described as fibrocartilage. The hyaline cartilage of the adult sacral surface is three times thicker than the cartilage of the iliac surface. Large, round, paired chondrocytes are distributed throughout the hyaline matrix of the sacral auricular surface and are arranged in columns parallel to the articulating surface. The hyaline cartilage is homogeneous with a small amount of fibrous tissue. Its smooth surface aids the gliding motion of the joint.

The iliac cartilage is thin (approximately 1 mm) and contains smaller spindle-shaped chondrocytes clumped in a fibrous matrix. The cell columns are oriented at right angles to the surface. Postpartum the iliac cartilage de-

generates early, and the amount of fibrous tissue increases. The sacral cartilage degenerates throughout life, and in later adult life it may appear fibrous as well (Bowen & Cassidy, 1981; Paquin et al., 1983; Sashin, 1929).

Development

The SIJ begins development during the seventh week of fetal life with the ilia moving superiorly and also posterior to the sacrum. During the eighth week of development, the mesenchyme between the two bones becomes arranged into three layers. At the tenth week, multiple cavities develop in the mesenchyme. These cavities are separated by septa, which disappear by the time the fetus reaches term. The sacral hyaline cartilage develops first, followed by the development of the iliac surface. At birth the sacral hyaline cartilage is thick and

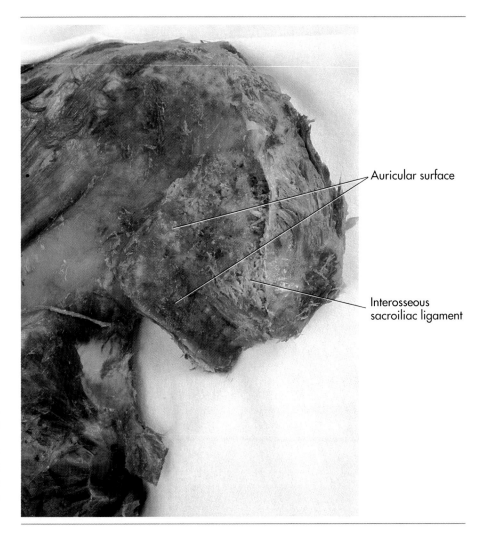

Auricular surface

Interosseous sacroiliac ligament

FIG. 8-8 View similar to that seen in Fig. 8-7, only with more soft tissue visible on this cadaveric specimen. The auricular surface can be readily identified on this medial surface of the posterior ilium. Also notice the cut fibers of the interosseous sacroiliac ligament.

almost fully developed, whereas the iliac cartilage is thin and irregular. The iliac surface has the appearance of fibrocartilage by the time of infancy (Cassidy & Mierau, 1992).

Before puberty, both sacral and iliac auricular surfaces are flat, straight, and vertically oriented (Beal, 1982). The joint can conceivably have a gliding movement in any direction, being restricted only by ligaments. After puberty the auricular surfaces change shape to form a horizontal and vertical limb. The horizontal limb, which can be longer than the vertical limb, is possibly formed to aid stability (Otter, 1985). Also during this time the longitudinal groove is formed in the sacral auricular surface. This groove runs from top to bottom, down the center of this surface. The corresponding iliac ridge develops simultaneously on the iliac auricular surface. The interlocking groove and ridge limit the direction of motion, but increase stability.

During the third decade of life, the interosseous ligaments are strengthened. The many bony tuberosities and corresponding grooves and fossae develop and probably increase the stability of the SIJ by their interlocking relationships (see Table 8-3 and Fig. 8-9). From the fourth decade of life, marginal osteophytes frequently begin to develop, particularly on the anterior and superior portion of the SIJ along the articular capsule. These degenerative changes develop earlier in the male. They probably increase stability of the joint, at the expense of decreased joint mobility. In later life the cartilage undergoes degeneration and further marginal ankylosis develops. Total fibrous ankylosis may eventually occur. After the eighth decade of life, SIJ mobility is usually lost completely, making body movement stiff (Walker, 1986).

Sacroiliac Joint Motion

The SIJ provides substantial, yet resilient, stability to the region between the spine and the lower extremities while also allowing for slight mobility to occur between the sacrum and the ilium. The SIJ has a small amount of movement (Egund et al., 1978; Frigerio, Stowe, & Howe, 1974; Solonen, 1957), but the movement is difficult to evaluate because of its location deep to the origin of the erector spinae muscle group, the posterior S-I ligament, and the interosseous S-I ligament. SIJ movement is three

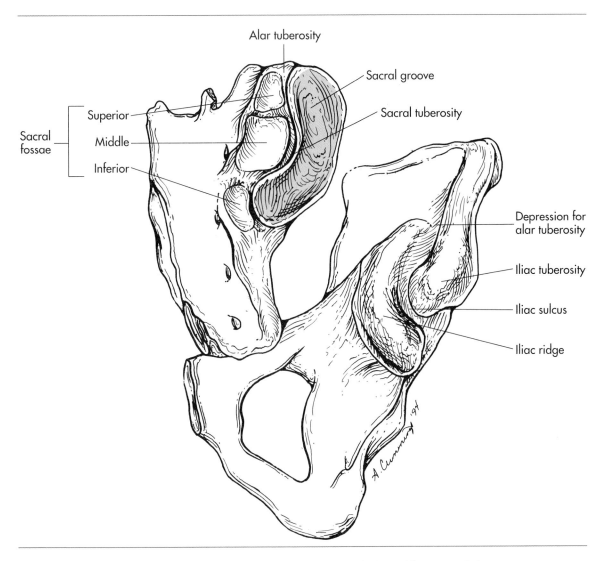

FIG. 8-9   Medial surfaces of the right side of the sacrum and the right ilium. The series of elevations and depressions associated with the sacroiliac joint (SIJ) are accentuated in this illustration. These elevations and depressions are thought to help increase stability of the SIJ. Table 8-3 lists the important elevations and depressions of the SIJ.

dimensional and contains several elements. The primary movements appear to be anteroinferior to posterosuperior nodding (called nutation) of the sacral base in relation to the ilium (Fig. 8-16, *B*). This represents rotation along the sacral groove, with the center of rotation located in the middle sacral fossa of the SIJ.

Another type of movement is rotatory movement along an axis that passes longitudinally through the iliac ridge of the SIJ (Fig. 8-16, *C*). The movement of the posterior aspect of the ilium in this case is superomedial and inferolateral. Although the iliac ridge may move only 2 mm during this type of movement, the distance between the two anterosuperior iliac spines increases or decreases by as much as 10 mm (Ehara, El-Khoury, & Bergman, 1988; Hadley, 1952; Wilder, Pope, & Frymoyer, 1980).

Gapping of the superior and inferior aspects of the SIJ has also been described. This could be interpreted as a third type of SIJ motion (Fig. 8-16, *A*).

Initiation of SIJ movements are made by the vertebral column and the lower extremities. The forces inducing SIJ motion are gravity (trunk weight), ground reaction (bouncing) force, and muscle contraction. Postural changes of the vertebral column (during lying, sitting, standing) and motion of the vertebral column (flexion, extension, rotation) cause the sacrum to move relative to the ilium. Change of thigh position (e.g., during sitting, standing, standing on one leg) and active motion of the thigh during flexion, extension, abduction, adduction, and rotation cause the iliac surface of the SIJ to move relative to the sacral surface of the SIJ. In addition, abduction and adduction of the thigh causes a certain

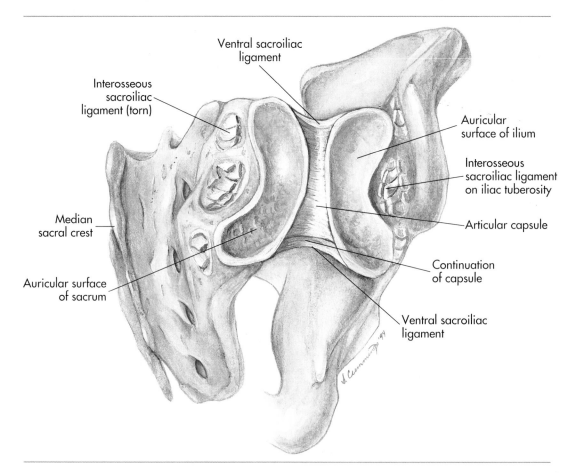

Ventral sacroiliac
ligament

Interosseous
sacroiliac
ligament (torn)

Auricular
surface of ilium

Interosseous
sacroiliac ligament
on iliac tuberosity

Median
sacral crest

Articular capsule

Continuation
of capsule

Auricular surface
of sacrum

Ventral sacroiliac
ligament

FIG. 8-10   Posterior view of an opened right sacroiliac joint demonstrating some of the important bony and soft tissue components. Notice the articular capsule is found only anteriorly. Posteriorly the interosseous sacroiliac ligament supports the joint. This ligament is shown torn to illustrate the deeper structures of the opened joint.

amount of gapping motion. The mechanism of walking is extremely complex, thereby causing movements of the SIJ to be complicated.

Even though there appears to be no muscle specifically designed for movement of the SIJ, approximately 40 muscles can influence this joint. Some of the most important are the erector spinae, quadratus lumborum, multifidus, iliopsoas, rectus abdominis, gluteus maximus, and piriformis muscles (Fligg, 1986).

As mentioned previously, stability is increased and mobility is decreased with age. Until puberty, stability is maintained primarily by ligaments. After puberty, the bony interlockings that enhance stability begin to form (see Table 8-3 and Fig. 8-9). Recall that after the fourth decade of life, osteophytes are formed and ankylosis may begin to occur, increasing stability. Near the eighth decade of life, total fibrous degeneration develops for stability, and consequently, SIJ movement usually completely stops at about this age.

Clinical Considerations

Disorders of the Sacroiliac Joint. Because of its role in weight bearing and perhaps also because of its unique anatomy, the SIJ can become a source of pain. This section briefly highlights some of the most common causes of pain arising from this clinically important articulation. Brief mention also is made of the most important factors involved in the clinical evaluation of the SIJ. Also, some of the most common methods currently used to treat SIJ dysfunction are mentioned in this section. However, a complete consideration of the pathologic conditions, diagnosis, and treatment of SIJ disorders is beyond the scope of this book.

Trauma and repeated minor forces can cause SIJ disorders. Examples of minor forces include those received while driving for long periods over rough terrain or while driving on poorly maintained roads in a vehicle with inadequate suspension (Abel, 1950). The SIJ receives its greatest stresses from below during sitting.

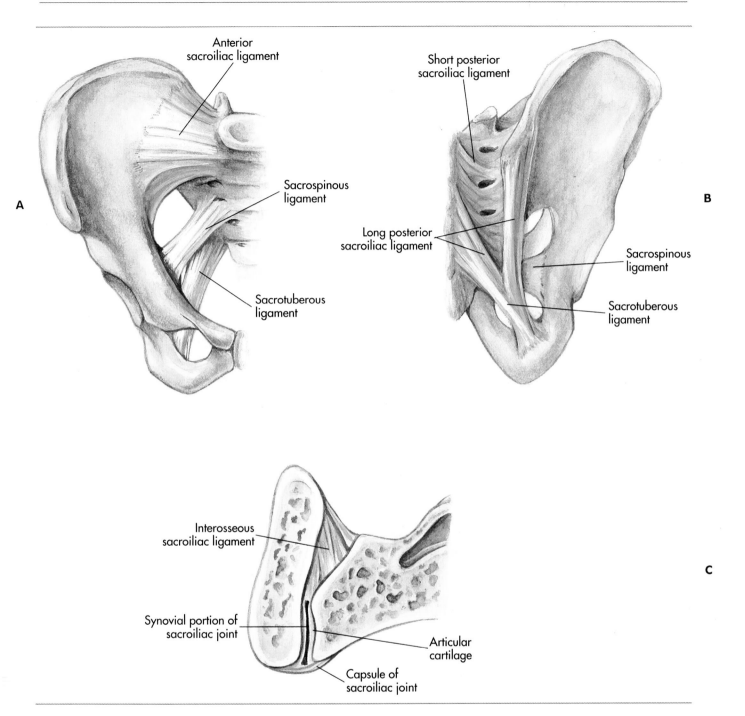

FIG. 8-11   Ligaments of the sacroiliac joint (SIJ.) **A,** Anterior view. **B,** Posterior view. **C,** SIJ in horizontal section. Notice the capsule of the SIJ joint is only present anteriorly.

This is because the ground reaction (bouncing) force reaches the SIJ directly without going through any other joint (Bermis & Daniel, 1987; Johnson, 1964; Schuchman & Cannon, 1986).

Women appear to be more susceptible to SIJ syndrome (pain as a result of mechanical irritation) than men. This is probably caused by the actions of the hormone relaxin during menstruation, pregnancy, and for a short time after childbirth (Cassidy & Mierau, 1992). Re-

laxin decreases the tension of the S-I ligaments, allowing them to become more pliable (or lax). The best known SIJ disease is osteitis condensans ilii, which occurs secondary to pregnancy and parturition (Nykoliation, Cassidy, & Dupuis, 1984; Olivieri et al., 1990).

A partial list of disorders of the SIJ include joint space widening or narrowing, cystic or erosive change, osteosclerosis, osteophytosis, and idiopathic hyperostosis. Some causes of SIJ dysfunction include trauma,

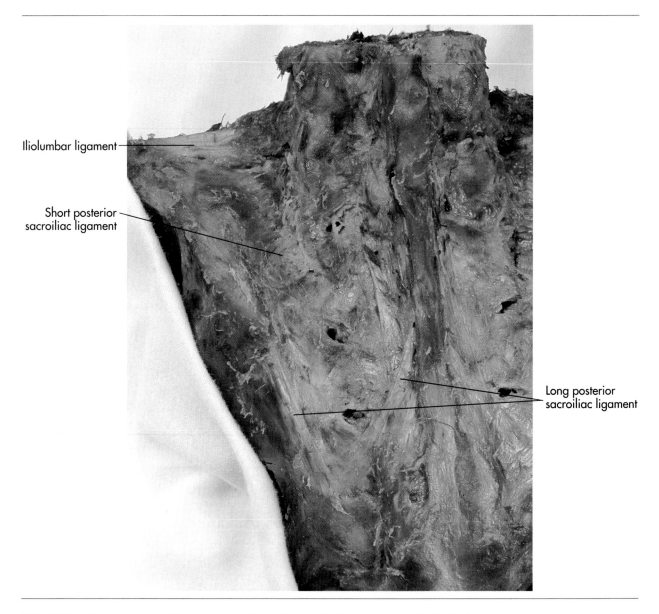

Iliolumbar ligament

Short posterior sacroiliac ligament

Long posterior sacroiliac ligament

FIG. 8-12   Posterior view of the sacrum and the left posterior ilium, showing the iliolumbar ligament and the posterior sacroiliac ligament. The posterior sacroiliac ligament has long fibers, which are vertically oriented, and short fibers, which are horizontally oriented.

disease of bone, infection, and arthropathy (Blower & Griffin, 1984; Blumel, Evans, & Eggers, 1959; Bose, 1982; Cone & Resnick, 1983; Dunn et al., 1976; DeCavalho & Graudal, 1980; Fryette, 1936; Jajic & Jajic, 1987; Resnik, Dwosh, & Niwayama, 1975; Resnik & Resnick, 1985; Romanus, 1955; Vogler et al., 1984). Table 8-4 provides a more complete list of some of the causes of SIJ dysfunction.

Evaluation and Treatment. Examination of the SIJ is challenging for many reasons. First, the SIJ is subject to a wide range of normal anatomic variation. Second, its unusual location and its oblique position make direct palpation almost impossible. Also, evaluation is made more challenging because spinal radiography does not always correspond well with symptoms.

As always, the patient's history can be extremely revealing. The patient may complain of pain over the posterior superior iliac spine (PSIS) that radiates into the buttock and less frequently to the groin and lower extremity (Cassidy & Mierau, 1992). Neurologic signs are negative, and the pain is not of dermatomal distribution.

Useful methods of palpatory examination for the SIJ include the palpation of neighboring prominences (PSIS and the S2 spinous tubercle) during thigh flexion (motion palpation). Potter and Rothstein (1985) investigated the reliability of many physical tests for SIJ dysfunction and found the most reliable test to be a measurable

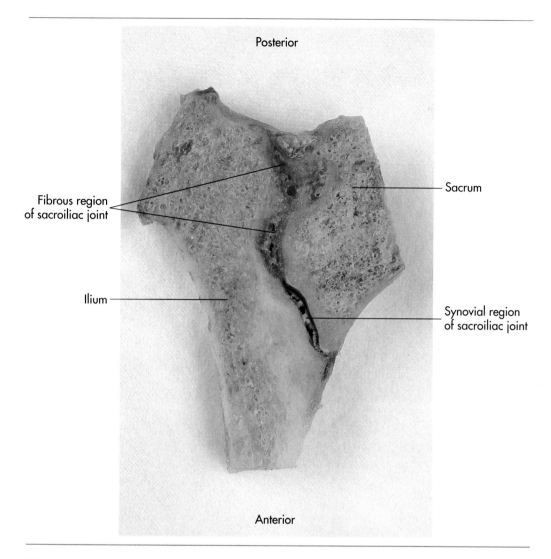

Posterior

Fibrous region
of sacroiliac joint

Sacrum

Ilium

Synovial region
of sacroiliac joint

Anterior

FIG. 8-13   Horizontal section through the right sacroiliac joint. Notice the synovial portion of the joint anteriorly and the fibrous portion posteriorly. The posterior fibrous portion of the joint is filled with the interosseous sacroiliac ligament.

widening of the distance between the left and right anterior superior iliac spines from a standing to a supine position. Using this method, a 94% agreement was found between multiple observers. A measured narrowing of the distance between the left and right anterior superior iliac spines after compression in the side-lying posture was the second most reliable method, with a 76% agreement found among observers. Also, certain orthopedic tests may be helpful in evaluating disorders of the SIJ. Using bone scans, Cassidy and Mierau (1992) found SIJ dysfunction to be particularly correlated with at least two out of three of the following orthopedic tests for SIJ sprain: Patrick-Faber (pathologic conditions of the hip previously ruled out), Gaenslen's test (forced thigh flexion), and Yeoman's test (forced thigh extension). Several other orthopedic tests for SIJ dysfunction also exist (Lawrence, 1990).

Differentiation between enteric disorders, pelvic disorders, and inflammatory arthritides from SIJ dysfunction can be challenging, and two of these disorders may coexist. Such conditions include Crohn's disease, psoriasis, Reiter's syndrome, Behcet's syndrome, and other inflammatory bowel disorders. Differential diagnosis may be aided by anesthetic injection into the SIJ, with relief of pain following anesthetic injection being an indication of SIJ dysfunction (Davis, Thomson, & Lentle, 1978; Dekker-Saeys et al., 1978; McEwen et al., 1971; Olivieri et al., 1990; Russell et al., 1977; Ro, 1990, Yazici, Tuzlaci, & Yurdakul, 1981).

Fortunately, SIJ syndrome is usually self-limiting and responding well to rest. However, in some individuals the condition becomes chronic and disabling. Chiropractic manipulation has been used to treat SIJ disorders. More than 90% of patients presenting to a university

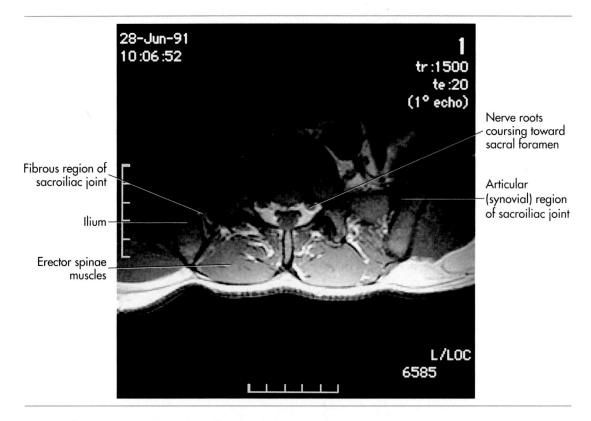

FIG. 8-14 MRI scan performed in a horizontal plane that shows the sacroiliac joint.

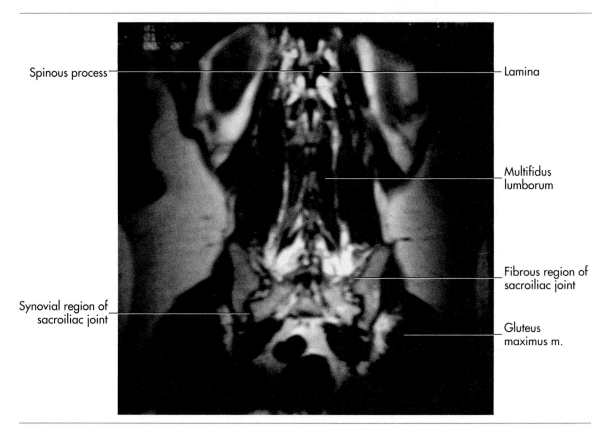

FIG. 8-15 MRI scan taken in a coronal plane that shows the sacroiliac joint.

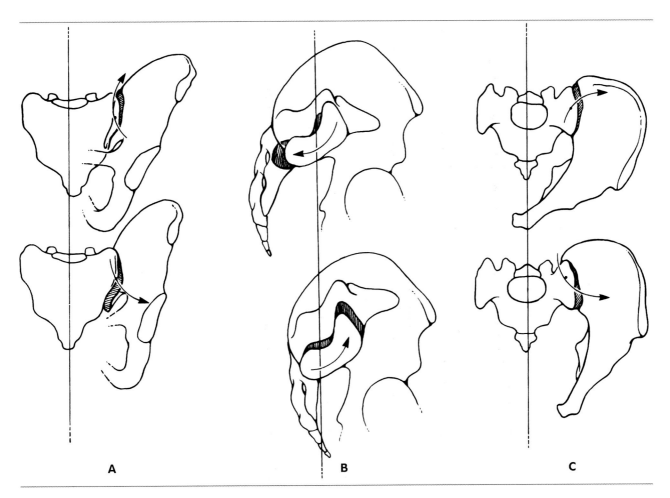

FIG. 8-16   Three types of sacroiliac joint (SIJ) motion. **A,** Superior and inferior aspects of the SIJ are shown gapping. **B,** Anterior and posterior rocking of the sacral base. This is sometimes known as nutation. **C,** Movement of the ilium on the sacrum that takes place in the horizontal plane. The arrows in **A** and **C** show motion of the ilium. The arrows in **B** show sacral motion. These movements are accentuated for demonstrative purposes in this illustration.

Table 8-4   Causes of Sacroiliac Joint Dysfunction

Type	Possible causes
Trauma	Direct trauma, falls, locus minoris resistentiae
Disease of bone	Osteitis condensans ilii, infection
Arthropathies	Ankylosing spondylitis, enteropathic arthropathies, gouty arthritis
Other causes	Hyperparathyroidism, paraplegia, lower extremity disorders, activity related (e.g., athletic activity), after hip surgery, neoplasm.

hospital disabled with chronic SIJ syndrome responded favorably to a regimen of sacroiliac manipulation (Cassidy & Mierau, 1992). Some believe examination and treatment of the soft tissues surrounding the SIJ to be the best way to manage spinal and SIJ problems (Lavignolle et al., 1983; Maltezopoulos & Armitage, 1984). Injection of local anesthetic not only may prove useful in the diagnosis of these disorders, but also may provide long-term relief in some patients who do not respond to other treatments (Cassidy & Mierau, 1992). The use of belts to stabilize the SIJ, injections of proliferants (to decrease mobility), exercises, and fusion have also been used to treat SIJ disorders (Cassidy, 1993).

THE COCCYX

The coccyx (Fig. 8-17) is formed by three to five fused segments (usually four), and each develops from one primary center of ossification. The coccygeal segments develop between ages 1 (first segment) and 20 (fourth segment), although the time when coccygeal ossification centers develop varies. Fusion of the coccygeal segments usually occurs in the late 20s but may be delayed considerably (Williams et al., 1989). Sometimes the first coccygeal segment does not fuse with the remainder of

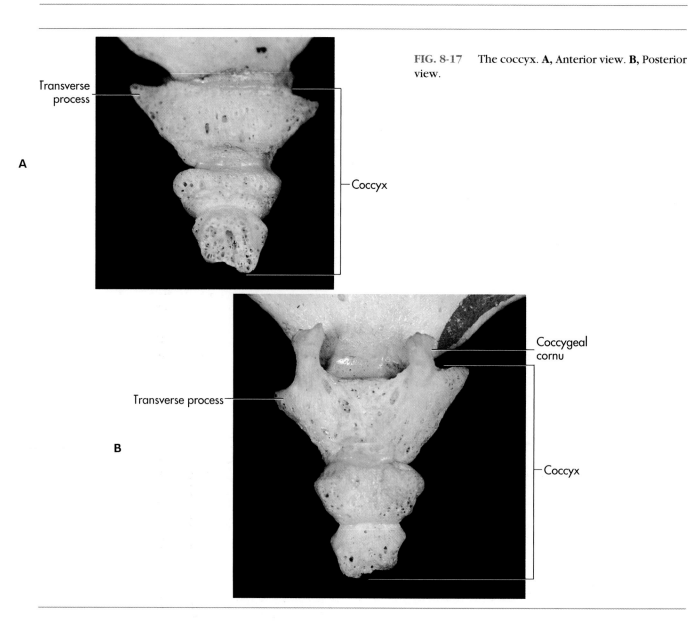

FIG. 8-17   The coccyx. **A,** Anterior view. **B,** Posterior view.

the coccyx at all. The first coccygeal segment has several prominences (see following discussion), whereas the second through the fifth coccygeal segments are rather simple and are homologous to vertebral bodies of typical vertebrae.

As with the sacrum, the coccyx is triangular in shape, with the superior surface the base and the inferior surface the apex (Fig. 8-17). The base of the coccyx is formed by the first coccygeal segment. The top of the base has an articular facet for articulation with a small disc that intervenes between it and the apex of the sacrum. Also, a transverse process extends from the left and right lateral surfaces of the coccygeal base. Posteriorly the coccygeal cornua are in register with the sacral cornua. Intercornual ligaments connect the cornua of the sacrum with those of the coccyx. The S5 and coc-

cygeal nerves of each side exit the sacral hiatus (see The Sacrum) and pass between the apex of the sacrum and the intercornual ligament. They then give off the dorsal rami, which pass posterior to the TP of the coccyx.

A series of fibrocartilaginous discs develop, before and after birth, between the individual coccygeal segments. These discs are eventually replaced by bone as the segments fuse during the second or third decades of life.

Structures That Attach to the Coccyx and the Borders of the Pelvic Outlet

Table 8-2 lists the muscles and ligaments that attach to the coccyx. The apex of the coccyx helps to form the boundaries of the pelvic outlet. The boundaries of this outlet are listed next.

Anterior: pubic symphysis
Posterior: tip of coccyx
Lateral: ischial tuberosities

NERVES AND VESSELS ASSOCIATED WITH THE SACRUM AND COCCYX

Sacral Plexus

The sacral plexus is formed by the anterior primary divisions (ventral rami) of L4 and L5 (lumbosacral trunk), S1-3, and part of S4. The anterior primary division of S4 also contributes to the coccygeal plexus. The plexus is located on the posterior pelvic wall, specifically, anterior to the piriformis muscle (Figs. 8-18 and 8-19). The branches of the sacral plexus are listed next (contributing spinal cord segments appear in parentheses).

- Posterior cutaneous nerve of the thigh (S1-3)
- Pudendal nerve (S2-4)
- Sciatic nerve (L4, L5, S1-3)
- Superior gluteal nerve (L4, L5, S1)
- Inferior gluteal nerve (L5, S1, S2)

- Nerve to the obturator internus (and superior gemellus) (L5, S1, S2)
- Nerve to the quadratus femoris (and inferior gemellus) (L4, L5, S1)

Chapters 9 and 10 provide further information on the nerves of the sacral plexus. Chapter 10 also discusses the relationship between the nerves of the sacral plexus and pelvic autonomic fibers.

Pelvic Autonomic Nerves

The S2 to S4 segments provide parasympathetic innervation to the pelvic viscera via nerves of the sacral plexus. In addition, each sympathetic trunk has five sacral ganglia that are located along the anterior surface of the sacrum. These ganglia supply sympathetic innervation to the pelvic viscera via gray rami. The two sympathetic chains join inferiorly on the anterior surface of the coccyx at a single ganglion, which is called the ganglion impar. The inferior hypogastric autonomic plexus, which receives contributions from the lumbar splanchnic

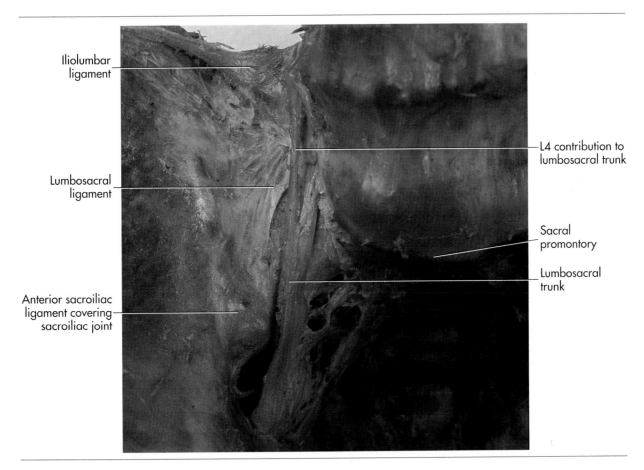

Iliolumbar ligament

Lumbosacral ligament

Anterior sacroiliac ligament covering sacroiliac joint

L4 contribution to lumbosacral trunk

Sacral promontory

Lumbosacral trunk

FIG. 8-18   Anterior and superior view of the region of the sacroiliac joint showing the lumbosacral trunk and its L4 and L5 contributions.

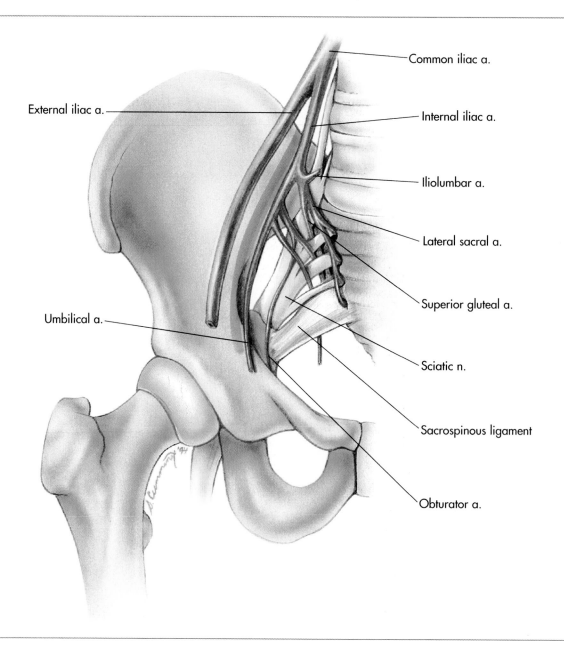

FIG. 8-19   Arteries and nerves associated with the anterior aspect of the sacrum and the sacroiliac joint.

nerves (sympathetic), sacral sympathetics, and pelvic splanchnic nerves (parasympathetic), helps to supply the pelvic viscera with autonomic fibers. Chapter 10 thoroughly discusses the pelvic autonomics.

Arteries Associated with the Sacrum and Coccyx

The aorta bifurcates at approximately the body of L4 into left and right common iliac arteries. Each common iliac artery, in turn, bifurcates into an internal and external iliac artery. The external iliac artery courses toward the inguinal ligament, giving off the inferior epigastric and deep circumflex iliac arteries before crossing under the inguinal ligament to become the femoral artery. The left and right internal iliac arteries supply the pelvic viscera, inferior aspect of the posterior abdominal wall, the pelvic wall, the gluteal region, ischioanal (ischiorectal) fossa, perineum, and adductor region of the thigh. Each internal iliac artery can be described as having an anterior, or visceral, division and a posterior, or somatic, division. The branches of each division of the internal iliac artery are listed in the following section.

Posterior Division of the Internal Iliac Artery

1. *Iliolumbar artery.* This is the first branch of the internal iliac artery. The iliolumbar artery further divides into two branches:
    a. An iliac branch passes along the superior border of the iliac crest to supply the iliacus and quadratus lumborum muscles.
    b. A lumbar branch courses superiorly to help supply the psoas muscle.
2. *Lateral sacral artery.* This artery has been discussed previously and is shown in Figs. 8-18 and 8-19. It courses along the anterior and lateral surface of the sacrum, sending branches into the anterior sacral foramina. It serves as a major source of blood to the sacrum and the sacral nerve roots.
3. *Superior gluteal artery.* This artery usually passes between the lumbosacral trunk and the S1 ventral ramus to exit the pelvis (in some cases it may exit between the S1 and S2 ventral rami). The superior gluteal artery helps to supply the gluteal region.

Anterior Division of the Internal Iliac Artery

1. *Inferior gluteal artery.* This artery usually exits the pelvis by passing between the S1 and S2, or the S2 and S3, ventral rami. As with the superior gluteal artery, this artery also helps to supply the buttock and thigh.
2. *Internal pudendal artery.* This artery usually exits the pelvis between the S2 and S3 ventral rami. It then passes around the posterior surface of the sacrospinous ligament to enter the ischioanal (ischiorectal) fossa, where it continues anteriorly within the pudendal (Alcock's) canal. It terminates near the symphysis pubis by dividing into the deep and dorsal arteries of the penis.
3. *Inferior vesical artery.* This artery is only found in the male. In the female its place is taken by the vaginal artery. The inferior vesical (or a branch of the vaginal artery in the female) supplies the inferior aspect of the bladder.
4. *Middle rectal artery.* This artery is usually small and may arise from the inferior vesical artery or the internal pudendal artery. It helps to supply the rectum.
5. *Obturator artery.* The obturator artery has a rather long intrapelvic course before exiting the pelvis at the obturator foramen. It then supplies the adductor region of the thigh. Before exiting the pelvis, this artery gives a branch that anastomoses with the pubic branch of the inferior epigastric artery. This anasto-

mosis frequently is called the accessory obturator artery. Occasionally the pubic branch of the inferior epigastric artery may replace the obturator artery.
6. *Umbilical artery.* This artery is the direct continuation of the internal iliac artery. It runs from the superior aspect of the bladder to the anterior abdominal wall, where its continuation forms the medial umbilical ligament. The superior vesical arteries are branches of the proximal portion of the umbilical artery. These arteries pass inferiorly from the umbilical artery to supply the superior aspect of the bladder.

Branches Found Only in the Female

1. *Uterine artery.* This artery courses beneath (inferior to) the ureter to reach the lateral aspect of the uterus, which it supplies.
2. *Vaginal artery.* This artery not only supplies the vagina, but also takes the place of the male inferior vesical artery. Therefore it also supplies the inferior aspect of the bladder.

Median Sacral Artery. Another vessel associated with the anterior surface of the sacrum is the median sacral artery. The median (middle) sacral artery (see Chapter 7) is a tiny unpaired artery that arises from the posterior surface of the abdominal aorta just before the aorta bifurcates into right and left common iliac arteries. It then passes inferiorly along the midline of the anterior sacrum, sending branches into the anterior sacral foramina. These foraminal branches are accompanied by branches of the lateral sacral artery.

Veins Associated with the Sacrum and Coccyx

The venous drainage of the sacrum, coccyx, and pelvic viscera generally flows in the opposite direction as the arterial supply and drains into the internal iliac vein. The internal iliac vein drains into the common iliac vein, and the common iliac vein drains into the inferior vena cava. One exception to this is the superior rectal vein, which helps to form the inferior mesenteric vein. The inferior mesenteric vein, in turn, drains into either the splenic or superior mesenteric veins. The latter two veins combine to form the portal vein. Blood from the inferior rectal vein eventually drains into the inferior vena cava. The anastomosis between the superior rectal veins and the inferior and middle rectal veins forms an important portal-caval anastomosis.

The internal and external vertebral venous plexuses also help to drain the sacrum. These venous plexuses are discussed with the vertebral canal in Chapter 2.

REFERENCES

Abel, M.S. (1950). Sacroiliac joint changes in traumatic paraplegics. *Radiology, 55,* 235-239.

Abitbol, M. (1989). Sacral curvature and supine posture. *Am J Phys Anthropol, 80,* 379-389.

Bakland, O. & Hanse, J. (1984). The axial sacroiliac joint. *Anat Clin, 6,* 29-36.

Beal, M.C. (1982). The sacroiliac problem: Review of anatomy, mechanics and diagnosis. *J Am Osteopath Assoc, June,* 667-673.

Bernard, T. & Cassidy, D. (1993). As quoted from: The sacroiliac joints revisited: Report from the San Diego congress on the sacroiliac joint. *Chiro Rep, 7*(2), 1-6.

Bermis, T. & Daniel, M. (1987). Validation of the long sitting test on subjects with sacroiliac dysfunction. *J Orthop Sports Phys Ther, 8,* 336-343.

Bellamy, N., Park, W., & Rodney, P.J. (1983). What do we know about the sacroiliac joint? *Arthritis Rheum, 12*(3), 282-309.

Blower, P.W. & Griffin, A.J. (1984). Clinical sacroiliac joint test in ankylosing spondylitis and other causes of low back pain: 2 studies. *Ann Rheum Dis, 43,* 192-195.

Blumel, J., Evans, E.B., & Eggers, G.W.N. (1959). Partial and complete agenesis or malformation of the sacrum with associated anomalies. *J Bone Joint Surg, 41A,* 497-518.

Bose, R.N. (1982). Ankylosing spondylitis: Treatment. *Am Chiro, June,* 50.

Bowen, V. & Cassidy, J.D. (1981). Macroscopic and microscopic anatomy of sacroiliac joint from embryonic life until the eighth decade. *Spine, 6*(6), 620-628, 1981.

Brunner, C., Kissling, R., & Jacob, H.A.C. (1991). The effects of morphology and histopathologic findings on the mobility of the sacroiliac joint. *Spine, 16*(9), 1111-1117.

Cassidy, D. (1993). As quoted from: The sacroiliac joints revisited: Report from the San Diego congress on the sacroiliac joint. *Chiro Rep, 7*(2), 1-6.

Cassidy, J.D. & Mierau, D.R. (1992). Pathophysiology of the sacroioiac joint. In S. Haldeman (Ed.), *Principles and practice of chiropractic,* (2nd ed.). East Norwalk, Conn: Appleton & Lange.

Colachis, S.C. et al: (1963). Movement of sacroiliac joint in adult male: A preliminary report. *Arch Phys Med Rehabil, 44,* 490-497.

Cone, R.O. & Resnick, D. (1983). Roentgenographic evaluation of the sacroiliac joints. *Orthop Rev, 12*(1), 95-105.

Davis, P., Thomson, A.B.R., & Lentle, B.C. (1978). Quantitative sacroiliac scintigraphy in patients with Crohn's disease. *Arthritis Rheum, 21*(2), 234-237.

DeCavalho, A. & Graudal, H. (1980). Sacroiliac joint involvement in classical or definite rheumatoid arthritis. *Acta Radiol Diagn, 21,* 417-423.

Dekker-Saeys, B.J. et al. (1978). Prevalence of peripheral arthritis, sacroiliitis and ankylosing spondylitis in patients suffering from inflammatory bowel disease. *Ann Rheum Dis, 37,* 33-35.

Diakow, P., Cassidy, J.D., & DeKorompay, V.L. (1983). Post-surgical sacroiliac syndrome: A case study. *J Can Chiro Assoc, 27*(1), 19-21.

Dommisse, G.F. & Louw, J.A. (1990). Anatomy of the lumbar spine. In Y. Floman (Ed.), *Disorders of the lumbar spine.* Rockville, Md, and Tel Aviv: Aspen and Freund.

DonTigny, R.L. (1990). Anterior dysfunction of sacroiliac joint as a major factor in the etiology of idiopathic low back pain syndrome. *Phys Ther, 70*(4), 250-265.

Drerup, B. & Hierholzer, E. (1987). Movement of human pelvis and displacement of related anatomical landmarks on body surface. *J Biomech (Br), 20*(19), 971-977.

Dunn, E.J. et al. (1976). Pyogenic infections of the sacroiliac joint. *Clin Orthop, 118,* 113-117.

Egund, N. et al. (1978). Movement of sacroiliac joint, demonstrated with roentgen stereophotogrammetry. *Acta Radiol Diagn, 19,* 833-846.

Ehara, S., El-Khoury, G.Y., & Bergman, R.A. (1988). The accessory sacroiliac joint, a common anatomic variant. *AJR, 150,* 857-859.

Fidler, M.W. & Plasmans, C.M.T. (1983). The effect of four types of support on segmental mobility of the lumbosacral spine. *J Bone Joint Surg, 65A,* 943-947.

Fligg, D.B. (1986). Piriformis technique. *J Can Chiro Assoc, 30*(2), 87-88.

Freeman, M.D., Fox, D., & Richards, T. (1990). The superior intracapsular ligament of the sacroiliac joint: Confirmation of Illi's ligament. *J Manipulative Physiol Ther, 13*(7), 374-390.

Frigerio, N.A., Stowe, R.R., & Howe, J.W. (1974). Movement of sacroiliac joint. *Acta J Chiro, 8,* 161-166.

Fryette, H.H. (1936). Some reasons why sacroiliac lesions recur. *J Am Osteopath Assoc, 36*(3), 119-122.

Gibbons, K., Soloniuk, D., & Razack, N. (1990). Neurological injury and patterns of sacral fractures. *J Neurosurg, 72,* 889-893.

Grieve, E. (1981). Lumbopelvic rhythm and mechanical dysfunction of the sacroiliac joint. *Physiotherapy, 67*(6), 171-173.

Grieve, G.P. (1975). The sacroiliac joint. *Norfork Norwich Hosp,* pp. 384-401.

Hadley, L.A. (1952). Accessory sacroiliac articulations. *J Bone Joint Surg, 34A*(1), 149-155.

Illi, F.W. (1951). *The vertebral column: Lifeline of the body.* Chicago: National College of Chiropractic.

Jajic, I. & Jajic, Z. (1987). The prevalence of osteoarthrosis. *Clin Rheum, 6,* 39-41.

Janse, J. (1976). *Principles and practice of chiropractic: An anthology.* Lombard, Ill: National College of Chiropractic.

Janse, J. (1978). The clinical biomechanics of sacroiliac mechanism. *ACA J Chiro, 12,* s1-s8.

Johnson, J.W. (1964). Sacroiliac strain. *J Am Osteopath Assoc, 63,* 1132-1148.

King, L. (1991). Incidence of sacroiliac joint dysfunction and low back pain in fit college students. *J Manipulative Physiol Ther, 14*(5), 333-334.

Kirkaldy-Willis, W. (1988). The pathology and pathogenesis of low back pain. In W. Kirkaldy-Willis (Ed.), *Managing low back pain* (2nd ed.), New York: Churchill Livingstone.

LaBan, M.M. et al. (1978). Symphyseal and sacroiliac joint pain associated with pubic symphysis instability. *Arch Phys Med Rehabil, 59,* 470-472.

Lavignolle, B. et al. (1983). An approach to functional anatomy of sacroiliac joint in vivo. *Anat Clin, 5,* 169-176.

Lawrence, D.J. (1990). Sacroiliac joint. Part two. Clinical considerations. In J.M. Cox (Ed.). *Low back pain: Mechanism, diagnosis and treatment* (5th ed.), Baltimore: Williams & Wilkins.

Lichtblau, S. (1962). Dislocation of sacroiliac joint. *J Bone Joint Surg, 44A,* 193-198.

Maltezopoulos, V. & Armitage, N. (1984). A comparison of four chiropractic systems in the diagnosis of sacroiliac malfunction. *Eur J Chiro, 32,* 4-42.

McEwen, C. et al. (1971). Ankylosing spondylitis and spondylitis accompanying ulcerative colitis, regional enteritis, psoriasis and Reiter's disease. *Arthritis Rheum, 14*(3), 291-318.

Norman, G.P., & May, A. (1956). Sacroiliac condition simulating intervertebral disc syndrome. *WJSO & G, (August),* 401-402.

Nykoliation, J.W., Cassidy, J.D., & Dupuis, P. (1984). Osteitis condensans ilii, a stress phenomenon. *J Can Chiro Assoc, 28*(1), 21-24.

Olivieri, I. et al. (1990). Differential diagnosis between osteitis condensans ilii and sacroilitis. *J Rheum, 17*(1), 1504-1512.

Otter, R. (1985). A review study of differing opinions expressed in the literature about the anatomy of the sacroiliac joint. *Eur J Chiro, 33,* 221-242.

Paquin, J.D. et al. (1983). Biomechanical and morphological study of cartilage from adult human sacroiliac joint. *Arthritis Rheum, 26*(6), 887-895.

Pitkin, H.C. & Pheasant, H.C. (1936a). Sacroarthrogenic telalgia. *J Bone Joint Surg, 18A*(1), 111-133.

Pitkin, H.C. & Pheasant, H.C. (1936b). A study of sacral mobility. *J Bone Joint Surg, 18A,* 365-374.

Potter, N.A. & Rothstein, J.M. (1985). Intertester reliability for selected clinical tests of the sacroiliac joint. *Phys Ther, 65*(11), 1671-1675.

Resnik, C.S. & Resnick, D. (1985). Radiology of disorders of sacroiliac joints. *JAMA, 253*(19), 2863-2866.

Resnik, D., Dwosh, I.L., & Niwayama, G. (1975). Sacroiliac joint in renal osteodystrophy: Roentgenographic-pathologic correlation. *J Rheum, 2*(3), 287-295.

Ro, C.S. (1990). Sacroiliac joint. In J.M. Cox (Ed.). *Low back pain: Mechanism, diagnosis and treatment* (5th ed.), Baltimore: Williams & Wilkins.

Romanus, R. (1955). Pelvo-spondylitis ossificans. Chicago: Year Book.

Russell, A.S. et al. (1977). The sacroiliitis of acute Reiter's syndrome. *J Rheum, 4*(3), 293-296.

Sandoz, R.W. (1978). Structural and functional pathologies of the pelvic ring. *Ann Swiss Chiro Assoc,* pp. 101-155.

Sashin, D. (1929). A critical analysis of the anatomy and the pathologic changes of the sacroiliac joints. *Bull Hosp Joint Dis,* pp. 891-910.

Schuchman, J.A. & Cannon, C.L. (1986). Sacroiliac strain syndrome, diagnosis and treatment. *Tex Med, 82,* 33-36.

Simkins, C.S. (1952). Anatomy and significance of the sacroiliac joint. In *AAO Yearbook* 64-69.

Solonen, K.A. (1957). The sacroiliac joint in the light of anatomical, roentgenographical and clinical studies. *Acta Orthop Scand, 27,* 160-162.

Sturesson, B. (1989). Movements of the sacroiliac joint, a roentgen stereopathogrammetric analysis. *Spine, 14*(2), 162-165.

Vogler, J.B. et al. (1984). Normal sacroiliac joint: A CT study of asymptomatic patients. *Radiology, 151*(2), 433-437.

Walker, J.M. (1986). Age-related differences in the human sacroiliac joint: A histological study; implications for therapy. *J Orthop Sports Phys Ther, 7*(6), 325-334.

Wallheim, G.G., Olerud, S., & Ribbe, T. (1984). Motion of symphysis in pelvic instability. *Scand J Rehabil Med, 16,* 163-169.

Weisl, H. (1954a). The articular surface of sacroiliac joint and their relation to the movement of the sacrum. *Acta Anat, 22,* 1-14.

Weisl, H. (1954b). The ligaments of sacroiliac joint examined with particular reference to their function. *Acta Anat, 20*(30), 201-213.

Weisl, H. (1955). The movement of the sacroiliac joint. *Acta Anat, 23,* 80-91.

Wilder, D.G., Pope, M.H., & Frymoyer, J.W. (1980). The functional topography of sacroiliac joint. *Spine, 5*(6), 575-579.

Williams et al. (1989). *Gray's anatomy* (37th ed.). Edinburgh: Churchill Livingstone.

Winterstein, J.F. (1972). *Spinographic evaluation of pelvic and lumbar spine.* Lombard, Ill: National College of Chiropractic.

Wood, J. (1985). Motion of the sacroiliac joint. *Palmer Coll Res Forum, Spring,* 1-16.

Yazici, H., Tuzlaci, M., & Yurdakul, S. (1981). A controlled survey of sacroiliitis in Behçet's disease. *Ann Rheum Dis, 40,* 558-559.

PART II

NEUROANATOMY OF THE SPINAL CORD, AUTONOMIC NERVOUS SYSTEM, AND PAIN PATHWAYS

CHAPTER 9

Neuroanatomy of the Spinal Cord

Susan A. Darby
Darryl L. Daley

The vertebral column and its adjacent musculature have been discussed in detail in the previous chapters. Because of the intimate anatomic and functional relationship between the vertebral column and the spinal cord (which is protected by the vertebral column), knowledge of both is equally important. Chapter 3 describes the meninges, external surface, and vasculature of the spinal cord. In addition, it provides a cursory description of the cord's internal organization. The purpose of this chapter is to elaborate on this internal organization by discussing the neurons, which form the circuitry of the spinal cord, and the ascending and descending tracts, which provide a connection among the spinal cord, the peripheral nerves, and the higher centers of the central nervous system. This information forms the basis of important neuroanatomic concepts that are necessary for an understanding of clinical neuroscience. The knowledge of these concepts is imperative for diagnosing pathologic conditions of the cord, some of which may be caused by vertebral column dysfunction. Examples demonstrating the application of these neuroanatomic principles to pathologic conditions are presented at the end of the chapter.

PERIPHERAL NERVOUS SYSTEM

Peripheral Receptors

Peripheral receptors are sensory endings of peripheral nerves, and they are scattered throughout the body. They are found in great numbers along the vertebral column and within the ligaments, muscles, and skin that surround the spine. These receptors, and the sensory systems that transmit their input, provide information concerning our environment. Each receptor is sensitive to a particular form of physical energy, or stimulus, and transduces the stimulus into electrochemical energy, or action potentials, which is the "language" the central nervous system (CNS) can understand.

Receptors may be divided into two types, rapidly adapting and slowly adapting. A slowly adapting receptor, such as a Merkel's disc, responds continuously to a sustained stimulus, whereas a rapidly adapting receptor does not. A pacinian corpuscle is a rapidly adapting receptor, and it responds at the onset of the stimulus and again at the end of the stimulus. A stimulus furnishes a receptor with four basic characteristics: modality (e.g., pain, temperature, touch), intensity, duration, and location. When a receptor is adequately stimulated, a generator potential occurs across its membrane and may lead to an action potential. The action potential propagates along the sensory neuron into the CNS. The CNS is then able to combine the four characteristics of the stimulus into a perceived sensation.

The sensory neurons of the peripheral nervous system (PNS) are pseudounipolar neurons, and their cell bodies are located in the dorsal root ganglia. The part of the fiber attached to the receptor is the peripheral process, which may be myelinated or unmyelinated, and it is the sensory component of a peripheral nerve. The other part of the fiber enters the CNS and is the central process. A bundle of central processes form a dorsal root. The peripheral processes are classified according to their conduction velocity, and conduction velocity is related to the axon diameter. Fibers with large diameters conduct the fastest. Based on the relationship between velocity and diameter, cutaneous fibers are classified alphabetically as A-beta, A-delta, and C fibers. Similarly, afferents from muscle tissue are usually classified numerically from heavily myelinated to unmyelinated as I, II, III, and IV (Martin & Jessell, 1991b). Type I also has subgroups of Ia and Ib. Afferents from visceral interoceptors are often classified as group B fibers. Motor (efferent) fibers are also classified according to the alphabetic listing. Large somatic motor neurons correspond to the A-alpha and A-gamma group, and autonomic efferent fibers correspond to the B and C groups. Table 9-1 summarizes the classifications of the afferent and efferent fibers.

Peripheral receptors can be classified by their morphology, their location, and the type of stimulus to which they respond. Morphologically, receptors may be encapsulated by connective tissue and nonneural cells, or they may be simple nonencapsulated, bare arborizing endings. Receptors classified by their location of distribution are called exteroceptors, proprioceptors, or interoceptors. Exteroceptors are superficial and located in the skin. Modalities such as nociception (pain), temperature, and touch (and the submodalities of pressure and vibration) are conveyed by these receptors. Proprioceptors are located in the muscles, tendons, and joints of the body and provide information concerning limb position, while the limbs are stationary (static) or moving (dynamic or kinesthetic). Interoceptors are located in the viscera, glands, and vessels and convey poorly localized information from such systems as the digestive and urinary. Examples of the types of information conveyed by interoceptors include distention or fullness and ischemic pain.

Receptors classified by the type of stimulus to which they respond are called mechanoreceptors, thermoreceptors, chemoreceptors, or nociceptors. Mechanoreceptors respond to deformation or displacement of self or of adjacent cells. Thermoreceptors respond to changes in temperature. Chemoreceptors respond to chemical stimuli and are important in the special senses of taste and olfaction. Nociceptors respond to stimuli that damage tissue cells, and their stimulation results in the sensation of pain. The classification of receptors by location overlaps with the classification by stimulus type, such that nociceptors can also be exteroceptors, and mechanoreceptors can also be proprioceptors.

Cutaneous Receptors. Cutaneous receptors (exteroceptors) include mechanoreceptors, thermoreceptors, and nociceptors and subserve such modalities as touch, pressure, vibration, temperature, and nociception (pain). Mechanoreceptors include the nonencapsulated Merkel's discs, nonencapsulated endings surrounding hair follicles (peritrichial), and encapsulated endings such as Ruffini endings, pacinian corpuscles, and Meissner's corpuscles. The fibers supplying these receptors are primarily A-beta. Thermoreceptors are nonencapsulated, free nerve endings that occupy areas approximately 1 mm in diameter. Cold thermoreceptors respond in the range of 1° C (33.8° F) to 20° C (68° F) below the normal skin temperature of 34° C (93.2° F). Warm thermoreceptors are stimulated in the temperature range between 32° C (89.6° F) and 45° C (113° F) (Martin & Jessell, 1991b). Cold receptors are supplied by A-delta or C fibers, but warm receptors are supplied by C fibers alone.

Table 9-1 Summary of the Classification of Peripheral Fibers

Fiber diameter (microns)	Efferent fibers	Afferent fibers (from cutaneous receptors)	Afferent fibers (from skeletal muscle and articular receptors)	Myelination
20	A-alpha (skeletomotor)		Type I (from mechanoreceptors)	Heavily myelinated
		A-beta (from mechanoreceptors)	Type II (from mechanoreceptors)	Myelinated
	A-gamma (fusimotor)			Myelinated
1		A-delta (from nociceptors and thermoreceptors)	Type III (from mechanoreceptors and nociceptors)	Thinly myelinated
1-3	B*† (preganglionic autonomic fibers)			Myelinated
0.2-1.5	C*† (postganglionic autonomic fibers)	C (from nociceptors and thermoreceptors)	Type IV (from nociceptors)	Unmyelinated

*Barr & Kiernan (1988). *The human nervous system* (6th ed.). Philadelphia: JB Lippincott.
†Williams et al. (1989). *Gray's anatomy* (37th ed.). Edinburgh: Churchill Livingstone.

An understanding of nociceptors is helpful in the comprehension of pain of spinal origin. Nociceptors are free nerve endings, and they respond to stimuli that may threaten or actually damage adjacent tissue cells. The damage to cells causes the release of chemical mediators that may sensitize (e.g., prostaglandins) or activate (e.g., histamine, bradykinin, potassium, serotonin) the free nerve endings. In some instances, activated free nerve endings release substance P into the surrounding area, causing vasodilation, extravasation of fluid, and release of histamine from tissue cells (Jessell & Kelly, 1991). Three types of nociceptors appear to exist: mechanical, which are stimulated by mechanical damage such as by a sharp object; thermal, which are stimulated by temperatures higher than 45° C (113° F); and polymodal, which respond to damaging mechanical, thermal, or chemical stimuli. Mechanical and thermal nociceptors send their information via A-delta fibers, whereas polymodal receptors use C fibers.

The cutaneous fibers of these receptors form overlapping horizontal plexuses in the dermis and subcutaneous layers of the skin. The density and variety of receptors vary in different regions. For example, in hairy skin the peritrichial endings are most common, but Merkel's discs and free nerve endings are also present. In glabrous (hairless) skin, free nerve endings are present, as are Merkel's discs and Meissner's corpuscles. The latter two receptors have small receptive fields and help to discriminate the spatial relationship of stimuli. This ability to discriminate is well developed on the fingertips. In fact, Meissner's corpuscles have only been located in primate animals (Barr & Kiernan, 1993). The subcutaneous tissue of both types of skin are provided with pacinian corpuscles and Ruffini endings, both of which have large receptive fields and therefore are less dicriminatory (Martin & Jessell, 1991b).

Cutaneous modalities that may be easily tested during a neurologic examination include vibration, temperature, pain (nociception), and tactile sensation. Tactile sensation can be described as simple touch (which includes light touch, touch pressure, and crude localization) and tactile discrimination (which includes deeper pressure and spatial localization), which is sometimes referred to as two-point discriminatory touch. On the fingertips, for example, tactile discrimination is precise enough to localize two points of stimulation applied simultaneously 2 mm apart. Such tactile discrimination is necessary for further analysis of objects concerning their size, shape, texture, and movement pattern. This analysis is completed in sensory integrative areas of the cerebral cortex. Identifying common objects held in the hand and identifying letters drawn on the back of the hand without visual cues are called stereognosis and graphesthesia, respectively, and are further examples demonstrating tactile discrimination. The clinical relevancy of these cutaneous modalities is discussed at the end of this chapter.

Proprioceptors. The second major class of peripheral receptors consists of the proprioceptors. As defined previously, proprioceptors (excluding the vestibular system of the inner ear) are located in the joints, muscles, and tendons. They function in the coordination and control of movements by monitoring both the stationary position and the movement (kinesthesia) of body parts and relaying that information into the CNS. This information, often referred to as joint position sense, may be perceived consciously. The receptors involved with providing proprioception are the joint receptors, neuromuscular spindles, and Golgi tendon organs (neurotendinous spindles). In addition, it has been shown that for proprioception to be assessed completely, cutaneous mechanoreceptors must also be involved (Martin & Jessell, 1991b).

Joint receptors are located in the superficial and deep layers of the joint capsules and in the ligaments. Four types of receptors exist and are classified as I, II, III, and IV. The first three types are encapsulated mechanoreceptors. The fourth type consists of unmyelinated, free nerve endings. The receptors classified as I, II, or III provide information regarding such activities as the direction, velocity, and initiation of joint movements. They do this by responding to tension applied to the connective tissue surrounding them. The group IV free nerve endings, which mediate nociception and are normally silent, respond to potentially injurious mechanical or inflammatory processes (Wyke, 1985).

Neuromuscular spindles are complex encapsulated proprioceptors that monitor muscle fiber length. They are located within a skeletal muscle close to the tendon and are surrounded by muscle fibers. They provide the sensory arc of the stretch, or myotatic, reflex. Each spindle consists of a connective tissue capsule that is fixed at each end to adjacent muscle fibers. The capsule encloses specialized muscle fibers called intrafusal fibers, which are either nuclear bag fibers or nuclear chain fibers. The total number and individual number of nuclear bag and chain fibers vary among spindles. The innervation of the nuclear bag and chain fibers of the spindle is provided by group Ia and II sensory fibers. In addition, the spindle is a unique peripheral receptor in that it also has a motor innervation furnished by gamma motor neurons. The motor innervation of the intrafusal fibers allows the spindle to remain sensitive to muscle fiber length during muscle contraction. The section Motor Control at the Spinal Level describes the function of the muscle spindle and stretch reflex.

Golgi tendon organs (GTOs), or neurotendinous spindles, respond to tension that is applied to a tendon. They consist of tendon collagen fibers surrounded by connective tissue, with group Ib afferent fibers twisted among the collagen fibers in such a way that they may become "squeezed" under the appropriate amount of tension. On stimulation the group Ib afferent fiber stimulates a Ib interneuron. This interneuron then inhibits the alpha motor neuron that supplies the skeletal muscle associated with that stimulated GTO. This action is opposite to that of a stimulated neuromuscular spindle, which produces excitation of the alpha motor neuron supplying the skeletal muscle associated with that spindle. The GTOs and spindles not only function at the spinal level, but also send input to higher centers (see Ascending Tracts). The section Motor Control at the Spinal Level describes the functional relationship between muscle spindles and GTOs.

Interoceptors. Interoceptors, the third major classification of peripheral receptors, are located in the viscera. They include mechanoreceptors that respond to movement or distention of the viscera. These are found in locations such as the mesentery, connective tissue enclosing the organs, and along blood vessels. Nociceptors are also found in the viscera. These are capable of responding to noxious mechanical, thermal, and chemical stimuli (Willis, Jr., & Coggeshall, 1991). Chapter 10 discusses the relationship of these receptors and their afferent fibers to somatic and autonomic efferents.

Peripheral Nerves

The spinal cord receives impulses from receptors and sends output to effectors via the PNS. Because the PNS transmits this essential information, its components are considered in this section.

Thirty-one pairs of spinal nerves exist, and each is formed by the convergence of a dorsal root and a ventral root usually within the intervertebral foramen (IVF). Just distal to this union, each spinal nerve divides into a dorsal ramus (posterior primary division, PPD) and a ventral ramus (anterior primary division, APD). The dorsal rami of spinal nerves innervate the skin and deepest muscles of the neck and back. The ventral rami innervate the ventrolateral aspect of the trunk and the extremities. Successive thoracic ventral rami retain a clear segmental distribution along the thoracic region. However, the back of the head, the anterior and lateral neck, shoulder, and upper and lower extremities are innervated by plexuses. Each plexus is formed by a regrouping of adjacent ventral rami. The plexuses are called the cervical, brachial, and lumbosacral plexuses, and each is briefly described here.

The cervical plexus is formed by ventral rami of the C1 through C4 cervical nerves. It supplies cutaneous innervation to the dorsolateral part of the head, neck, and shoulder. Motor fibers in this plexus course to the deep cervical muscles, hyoid muscles, diaphragm, and the sternocleidomastoid and trapezius muscles (see Chapter 5).

The brachial plexus is formed by ventral rami of the C5 through T1 spinal nerves (with a possible contribution from C4 and T2). This plexus supplies the upper extremity. Subsequent to the mixing of the ventral rami in the plexus, numerous branches are formed, including five large terminal branches: the axillary, musculocutaneous, radial, ulnar, and median nerves. The axillary nerve (C5 and C6) supplies cutaneous branches to the deltoid region and muscular branches to the deltoid and teres minor muscles. The musculocutaneous nerve (C5 to C7) is sensory to the anterolateral and posterolateral aspect of the forearm. It supplies motor innervation to the flexors of the arm, which include the biceps brachii. The radial nerve (C5 to C8, possibly T1) has an extensive area of distribution in both the arm and the forearm. Its cutaneous branches innervate the posterior aspect of the arm and forearm. The superficial radial nerve supplies the lateral half of the dorsum of the hand and the first three and a half digits, excluding the nails. The radial nerve also innervates the extensor muscles of the upper extremity. The ulnar nerve (C8 and T1, possibly C7) courses through the arm to supply structures in the forearm and hand. Its motor distribution includes one and a half forearm flexors (ulnar side) and intrinsic hand muscles, including the hypothenar and all interossei muscles and the adductor pollicis muscle. Its cutaneous distribution is present only in the hand and encompasses the ulnar half of the hand, including the fifth and one half of the fourth digits. The median nerve (C6 to C8 and T1, possibly C5) supplies motor fibers to the forearm flexors (excluding those with ulnar innervation) and some intrinsic hand muscles, including the thenar muscles. As with the ulnar nerve, its sensory area is only in the hand and includes the lateral palmar surface and first three and a half digits, including the nails (Williams et al., 1989) (Figs. 9-1 and 9-2 and Table 9-2). (See Chapter 5 for a full description of the brachial plexus and its proximal branches.)

The third plexus is the lumbosacral plexus, which is composed of ventral rami L2 through S2 (with contributions from L1 and S3). The major branches of this network are the femoral, obturator, gluteal, sciatic, common peroneal (fibular) (and its branches), and tibial nerves. Cutaneous nerves with large areas of distribution include, but are not limited to, the lateral femoral cutaneous, saphenous, posterior femoral cutaneous, and sural nerves. (Chapters 7 and 8 describe the lumbar plexus and its smaller branches [iliohypogastric and ilioinguinal] and the sacral plexus and its branches.)

The obturator nerve (L2 to L4) supplies motor branches to the adductor muscles of the thigh and gracilis muscle. It also is cutaneous to the inner thigh. The

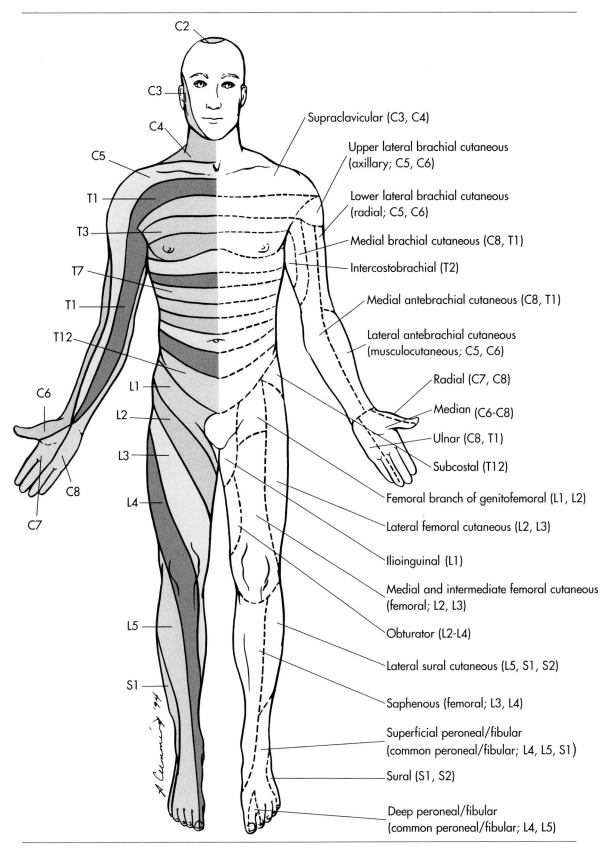

FIG. 9-1 Anterior view of the body showing its cutaneous innervation. *Left,* Dermatomal pattern, which may vary according to different authors. This dermatomal mapping is based on studies by J.G. Keegan and F.V. Garrett (1948). *Right,* Areas of cutaneous peripheral nerve distributions. Note the similarity of cord segment origins between the two sides.

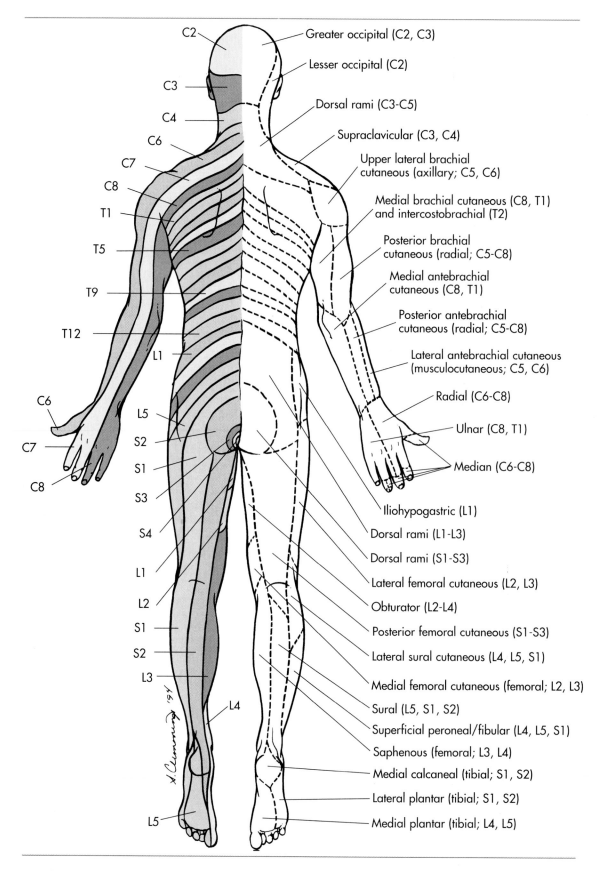

FIG. 9-2   Posterior view of the body showing its cutaneous innervation. *Left,* Dermatomal pattern, which may vary according to different authors. This dermatomal mapping is based on studies by J.G. Keegan and F.V. Garrett (1948). *Right,* Areas of cutaneous peripheral nerve distributions. Note the similarity of cord segment origins between the two sides.

Table 9-2 Muscles Supplied by Terminal Branches of the Brachial Plexus and the Lumbosacral Plexus

Muscle(s) supplied	Peripheral nerve	Cord segments
Deltoid, teres minor	Axillary	C5, C6
Anterior arm	Musculocutaneous	C5-7
Extensors of upper extremity	Radial	C5-8 (T1)*
Flexor carpi ulnaris, flexor digitorum profundus (medial half), hypothenar eminence, interossei, adductor pollicis, lumbricals (3rd and 4th)	Ulnar	(C7), C8-T1
Anterior forearm (except above), thenar eminence (except above), lumbricals (1st and 2nd)	Median	(C5), C6-T1
Medial thigh	Obturator	L2-4
Anterior thigh	Femoral	L2-4 (mostly L4)
Posterior thigh	Sciatic	L4-S3
	Common peroneal (fibular)	L4-S2
Lateral leg	Superficial	(mostly S1)
Anterior leg	Deep	
Posterior leg	Tibial	L4-S3
Gluteus maximus	Inferior gluteal	L5-S2 (mostly S1)
Gluteus medius and minimus	Superior gluteal	L4-S1 (mostly L5)

*Levels in parentheses represent clinically significant contributions in a small portion of the population.

femoral nerve (L2 to L4) sends motor branches to the anterior thigh muscles (e.g., quadriceps), which extend the leg. Cutaneous innervation by the femoral nerve supplies the anterior and anteromedial thigh and, via the saphenous nerve (L3 and L4), the medial leg and foot. The thigh's lateral side is innervated by cutaneous branches of the lateral femoral cutaneous nerve (L2 and L3). The sciatic nerve (L4 to S3) is the body's largest nerve. This nerve is actually composed of two parts (tibial and common peroneal) but is ensheathed to form one nerve in the posterior thigh. Motor branches in the posterior thigh innervate the hamstring muscles (biceps femoris, semitendinosus, semimembranosus), which flex the leg. The cutaneous innervation of the posterior thigh is furnished by the posterior femoral cutaneous nerve (S1 to S3). At varying levels proximal to the knee, the sciatic nerve divides into the common peroneal and tibial nerves.

The common fibular (peroneal) nerve (L4, L5, S1, and S2) courses laterally around the neck of the fibula and divides into two major branches: superficial fibular (peroneal) and deep fibular (peroneal). The superficial fibular (peroneal) nerve supplies muscular branches to the peronei (fibularis) muscles, which are responsible for eversion of the foot, and cutaneous branches to the distal and anterolateral third of the leg and dorsum of the foot (excluding the first interspace). The deep fibular (peroneal) nerve sends motor fibers to the anterior leg muscles, which provide dorsiflexion of the foot and extension of the toes. Cutaneous branches supply the skin between the first two toes. The other branch of the sciatic nerve is the tibial nerve (L4, L5, S1, S2, and S3). This nerve provides motor innervation to posterior leg muscles (including the gastrocnemius muscle), which are responsible for plantar flexion of the foot. A branch of the tibial nerve and contributing fibers from the common fibular (peroneal) nerve form the sural nerve. This supplies sensory innervation to the posterior and lateral surfaces of the leg. At the region of the medial malleolus, the tibial nerve divides into medial and lateral plantar nerves. These nerves supply motor and sensory innervation to the plantar aspect of the foot (Figs. 9-1 and 9-2 and Table 9-2).

Nerves innervating muscles moving the hip joint are the inferior and superior gluteal nerves. The inferior gluteal nerve (L5, S1, and S2) is responsible for the motor innervation of the strongest hip extensor, the gluteus maximus. The superior gluteal nerve (L4, L5, and S1) innervates the gluteus medius and minimus muscles and the tensor fascia latae muscle, which are responsible for hip abduction (Table 9-2).

This has been a cursory description of the innervation of major individual muscles and muscle groups and the cutaneous distribution of the major nerves. Because of developmental events, one muscle is innervated by many cord segments, and one cord segment may be involved with the innervation of more than one muscle. The intermingling of dorsal root fibers in the plexuses produces a peripheral nerve with an area of distribution that is different from a dermatomal pattern. However, the origin (cord segments) of a peripheral nerve innervating a particular cutaneous region includes the same cord segments as those supplying the dermatomes of that same area. For example, the lateral femoral cutaneous nerve is formed from cord segments L2 and L3, and its peripheral nerve pattern includes parts of the L2 and L3 dermatomal regions.

Realizing the differences between peripheral nerve patterns and dermatomal patterns (remembering there is much variation in dermatomal maps) is important (Figs. 9-1 and 9-2). Knowing both the segmental and the peripheral innervation of major skeletal muscles is also important. This knowledge of peripheral innervation of muscles and skin is imperative, since a neurologic examination includes the assessment of a patient's motor functions (reflexes and muscle strength; Table 9-3) and sensory functions. The information gained from this assessment is useful for distinguishing if the lesion is in the CNS or PNS and subsequently for determining the specific location of the lesion along one of those two systems.

INTERNAL ORGANIZATION OF THE SPINAL CORD

Gray Matter

The gray matter of the spinal cord appears in cross section as an H-shaped or butterfly-shaped region. Each of the two symmetric halves consists of a dorsal horn, which includes a head, neck, and base; an intermediate region; and a ventral horn. In cord segments T1 through L2 or L3, an additional lateral horn is present. In general, the dorsal horn is a receptacle for sensory afferent input, and the ventral horn is involved in motor functions, including housing the cell bodies of motor neurons. Microscopically the gray matter is a dense region of neuron cell bodies, cell processes and their synapses, neuroglia cells, and capillaries.

The neurons that compose the gray matter are subdivided into four groups: motor neurons, the axons of which leave the spinal cord and innervate the effector tissues (skeletal, smooth and cardiac muscles, glands); tract neurons, the axons of which ascend in the white matter to higher centers; interneurons, which have short processes; and propriospinal neurons, the axons of which provide communication between cord segments. Kuypers (1981) classified propriospinal neurons as long, intermediate, or short. Long propriospinal neurons extend the length of the cord bilaterally in the ventral funiculus and ventral part of the lateral funiculus (see White Matter). Short propriospinal neurons extend six to eight segments in the ipsilateral lateral funiculus, and intermediate propriospinal neurons course primarily ipsilaterally more than eight segments but less than the cord's entire length.

In the early 1950s, Rexed (1952) studied feline spinal cords and proposed that the organization of the gray matter formed 10 layers, or laminae. He described lamina I as being located at the tip of the dorsal horn, followed sequentially into the ventral horn by laminae II through IX. Lamina X formed the connecting crossbar of the gray matter, that is, the gray commissure. This organization has been accepted for the human spinal cord as well (Fig. 9-3). Each lamina includes at least one of the four general types of neurons: motor, tract, interneuron, or propriospinal. Each lamina may also be the site of the termination of primary afferents, descending tracts, propriospinal neurons, and interneurons of neighboring laminae. The laminae may vary in size throughout regions of the spinal cord and may even by absent in some regions. Also within each lamina, neurons may be organized into smaller groups, called nuclei or cell columns,

Table 9-3   Muscle Testing and Deep Tendon (Muscle Stretch) Reflexes

Muscle action	Cord segments	Peripheral nerve(s)	Reflex
Shoulder abduction (deltoid)	C5	Axillary	
Elbow flexion (biceps brachii, brachialis, brachioradialis)	C5	Musculocutaneous	Biceps
	C6	Radial	Brachioradialis
Elbow extension (triceps brachii)	C7	Radial	Triceps
Wrist extension (posterior forearm muscles)	C6 (C7)*	Radial	
Wrist flexion (anterior forearm muscles)	C7	Median, ulnar	
Finger extension (extensor digitorum)	C7	Radial	
Finger flexion (flexor digitorum)	C8	Median, ulnar	
Finger abduction (interossei)	T1	Ulnar	
Hip flexion (iliopsoas)	T12-L3	Lumbar plexus (L2-4), femoral	
Hip extension (gluteus maximus)	S1	Inferior gluteal	
Hip adduction (adductors)	L2-L4	Obturator	
Hip abduction (gluteus medius and minimus)	L5	Superior gluteal	
Knee extension (quadriceps femoris)	L2-L4	Femoral	Patellar (L4)
Foot inversion and dorsiflexion (tibialis anterior)	L4	Deep peroneal (fibular)	
Foot eversion, with plantar flexion (peronei)	S1	Superficial peroneal (fibular)	
Foot eversion, with dorsiflexion (extensor digitorum longus, peroneus tertius)	L5	Deep peroneal (fibular)	
Foot plantar flexion (gastrocnemius, soleus)	S1 (S2)	Tibial	Achilles
Toe extension (hallux) (extensor hallucis longus)	L5	Deep peroneal (fibular)	
Toe extension, except above (extensor digitorum brevis)	S1, S2	Deep peroneal (fibular)	

*Levels in parentheses represent clinically significant contributions in a small portion of the population.

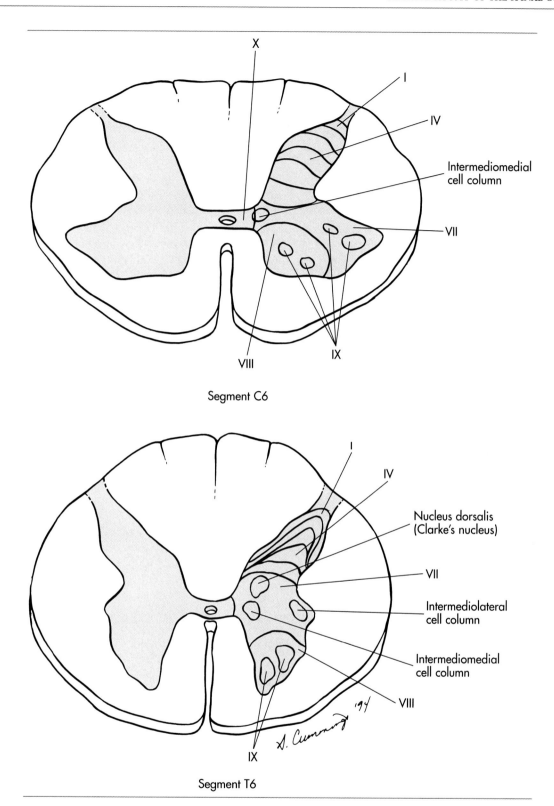

Segment C6

Segment T6

FIG. 9-3   Cross sections of the C6 and T6 spinal cord segments showing the lamination of the gray matter. Examples of nuclei located within the laminae are shown.

based on commonalities such as cell morphology and function. The following is a brief description of each of these laminae.

Laminae I Through VI (Dorsal Horn).

The dorsal horn consists of laminae I through VI. Laminae I through IV form the head, lamina V forms the neck, and lamina VI forms the base of the dorsal horn. Lamina I is also known as the marginal zone of Waldeyer. Most of the primary afferent input into lamina I originates from cutaneous nociceptors and thermoreceptors via A-delta fibers. Additional input is conveyed by C fibers (from nociceptors and thermoreceptors) and by a small group of thinly myelinated muscle, joint, and visceral afferent fibers (Willis & Coggeshall, 1991). Most of the neurons of lamina I are classified as interneurons, although there are some tract neurons as well.

Lamina II is known as the substantia gelatinosa of Rolando. The many processes, the presence of small neurons, and the absence of myelinated axons gives this layer a gelatinous appearance on close inspection. The primary afferent input into lamina II enters by C afferent fibers from cutaneous nociceptors, thermoreceptors, and mechanoreceptors. A few A-delta fibers also terminate here. The neurons of lamina II are interneurons, the dendrites of which arborize within the lamina and also project into other laminae.

Laminae III and IV are similar and are described together. These laminae (and sometimes the upper part of lamina V) are often referred to as the nucleus proprius. The majority of the primary afferent input arrives via A-beta fibers, which transmit input from mechanoreceptors such as pacinian corpuscles, peritrichial endings surrounding hair follicles, and Meissner's corpuscles. Although direct afferent input synapses on the interneurons within laminae III and IV, the dendrites of these interneurons also project dorsally into lamina II. Some lamina II neurons also project axons ventrally into these laminae and thus influence laminae III and IV neurons and their sensory input. Thus, considerable interlaminar communication occurs. The types of neurons present in these laminae include interneurons and some tract neurons.

Lamina V forms the neck of the dorsal horn. Primary afferent input comes via A-delta fibers from cutaneous mechanical nociceptors and from group III and IV muscle, joint, and visceral afferents (Willis & Coggeshall, 1991). Additional input to this lamina is most likely received via the dendritic projections located within more dorsal laminae. Although many interneurons are located in this lamina, there are some tract and propriospinal neuron cell bodies as well.

Lamina VI is the base of the dorsal horn and thus is anatomically close to motor regions in the ventral horn. This lamina exists only in cervical and lumbosacral enlargements. Proprioceptive information enters via large afferent fibers such as the group Ia fibers that form the primary afferent input. In addition, many descending tracts terminate in this area. Numerous interneurons and propriospinal neurons are also present in this lamina.

In summary, the first six laminae of the dorsal horn receive sensory information. Pain and temperature input appears to terminate primarily in superficial layers; mechanical types of stimuli terminate in the middle region; and proprioceptive input ends in the base of the dorsal horn near the motor regions. Many of the laminae communicate with each other via profuse dendritic branching and the axonal projections of their interneurons. This provides a mechanism by which incoming sensory signals may be modified.

Relationship Between the Dorsal Horn and the Trigeminal Nerve.

The dorsal horn of the upper two or three cervical cord segments has an interesting relationship with the trigeminal nerve. The trigeminal nerve (cranial nerve V) provides sensory innervation to the skin of the face and to other structures, including the paranasal sinuses, the cornea, the temporomandibular joint, and the oral and nasal mucosae. Cranial nerve V (CN V) also supplies motor fibers to the muscles of mastication and several other small muscles of the head. The afferent fibers of CN V enter the brain stem at the level of the pons and synapse in a nuclear column that extends from the midbrain through the pons and medulla and into the upper cervical cord segments. The portion of the nuclear column located in the medulla and upper cervical cord segments is known as the spinal trigeminal nucleus (Fig. 9-4). Afferent fibers conveying pain and temperature (and some touch) that enter the brain stem within CN V (and also in the facial and glossopharyngeal nerves) descend as the spinal trigeminal tract and synapse in this nucleus. As the spinal trigeminal nucleus continues from the medulla into the upper two or three cervical cord segments, it blends with laminae I through IV of the dorsal horn of those segments (Carpenter, 1991; Williams et al., 1989). Afferent fibers conveying similar information and traveling in dorsal roots of upper cervical nerves also synapse in these same laminae. In fact, some of these cervical dorsal root afferents may ascend into the rostral medulla and synapse in the spinal trigeminal nucleus (Abrahams, 1989).

The relationship between the dorsal horn and the trigeminal system is clinically significant. The region of convergence between synapsing sensory fibers of CN V and synapsing afferents of upper cervical nerves becomes the anatomic basis for pain referral (cervicogenic head pain or headache) from the neck to regions innervated by CN V (e.g., frontotemporal area), and vice versa (Lance, 1989).

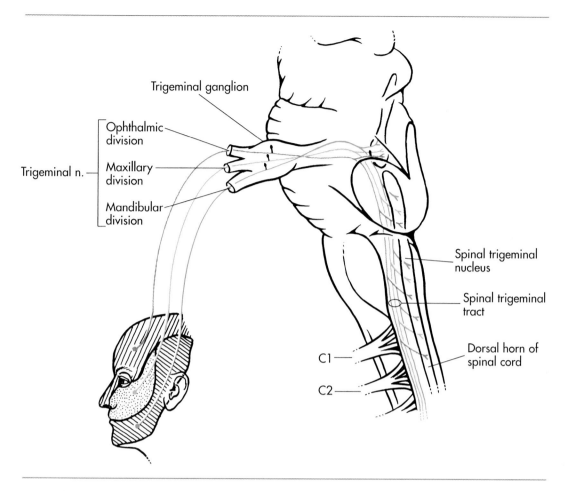

FIG. 9-4   Trigeminal system. The trigeminal nerve fibers conducting pain and temperature enter the pons of the brain stem and descend in the medulla (as the spinal trigeminal tract) and into the upper two or three cervical cord segments. They synapse in the adjacent spinal trigeminal nucleus of the medulla and dorsal horn of the upper cervical cord segments. Note that the descending fibers are arranged within the medulla such that the ophthalmic fibers are ventral, the mandibular fibers are dorsal, and the maxillary fibers are in between.

Laminae VII through X. Lamina VII composes most of the intermediate region of the gray matter and also extends into the ventral horn (see Fig. 9-3). The shape of lamina VII varies in different regions. For example, in the T1 to L2 or L3 segments, lamina VII includes the lateral horn. Most primary afferent input into this lamina and the remaining ventral horn is from proprioceptors. Other input comes from descending tracts and propriospinal neurons. Cell bodies of interneurons and propriospinal neurons are numerous in this region. Clearly defined nuclei and cell columns are also within lamina VII. One of these is the nucleus dorsalis of Clarke (nucleus thoracicus). This oval nucleus consists of tract neurons and is located in the medial part of lamina VII in segments C8 or T1 through L3. It is best defined in the T10 to L2 segments (Carpenter & Sutin, 1983). The axons of these neurons ascend ipsilaterally in the spinal cord

white matter to the cerebellum as the dorsal spinocerebellar tract (see Ascending Tracts). Another cell column in lamina VII is the intermediolateral cell column, which is located in the lateral horn in cord segments T1 to L2 or L3 and consists of autonomic motor neuron cell bodies. The axons of these motor neurons are preganglionic sympathetic fibers that exit in the ventral root and synapse in autonomic sympathetic ganglia. They are involved with the innervation of smooth and cardiac muscles and glands. In cord segments S2 to S4 the sacral autonomic nucleus is found, and although there is no lateral horn at that level, this nucleus is located in a similar position to that of the intermediolateral cell column. The sacral autonomic nucleus contains cell bodies, the axons of which form preganglionic parasympathetic fibers. These fibers exit via the S2 to S4 ventral roots, synapse in autonomic ganglia, and innervate the smooth muscle and glands of the pelvic and lower abdominal regions. An additional group of neurons forms the intermediomedial nucleus of lamina VII. This is found in the medial aspect of this lamina and is considered by some authors to be the termination site of visceral afferent fibers (Carpenter & Sutin, 1983). From this description, it is apparent that lamina VII is composed of all four neuron types: interneurons, tract, propriospinal, and motor neurons.

Lamina VIII is also located in the ventral horn. In spinal cord segments of the cervical and lumbar enlargements, it is found in the medial aspect of the ventral horn. In thoracic segments, lamina VIII is located in the base of the ventral horn. Input to the interneurons and propriospinal neurons of this lamina originates from descending tracts and from some proprioceptive afferents.

Lamina IX is found in the ventral horn and consists of well-defined medial, lateral, and central nuclear groups of motor neurons (anterior horn cells) (see Fig. 9-3) (Williams et al., 1989). The position and presence of the groups vary at different spinal regions. The medial group (subdivided into dorsal and ventral parts) is found in all cord segments and provides the axons that innervate the axial musculature. The lateral group (subdivided into dorsal, ventral, and retrodorsal groups) is responsible for innervating the muscles of the extremities. These clusters of neurons are organized so that the more lateral the motor neurons, the more distal the muscles they innervate. Also, the dorsal motor neuronal groups innervate the flexor muscles, and the ventral motor neuronal groups innervate the extensor muscles. The addition of these lateral motor neuronal groups in cord segments supplying the extremity muscles creates a distinctive lateral enlargement in the ventral horn.

The third nuclear group of lamina IX is the central group. This group has two major nuclei located in specific cord segments. One nuclear column forms the phrenic nucleus, which is found in the C3 to C5 segments. The axons form the phrenic nerve, which provides innervation to the diaphragm. The other nucleus is the accessory nucleus, which is located in the upper five or six cervical segments. Axons from this nucleus form the spinal root of the spinal accessory nerve (CN XI). They ascend in the vertebral canal dorsal to the denticulate ligament and travel through the foramen magnum to enter the cranial cavity and briefly join the cranial root of CN XI. Subsequently, this nerve exits the cranial cavity, and the spinal root fibers branch away to innervate the sternocleidomastoid and trapezius muscles.

Each of these three major groups of lamina IX includes alpha motor neurons, which project to extrafusal skeletal muscle fibers, and gamma motor neurons, which innervate the contractile portion of the neuromuscular spindles located within skeletal muscles. The alpha and gamma motor neurons are tightly packed into pools responsible for the innervation of a particular skeletal muscle. Both types of motor neurons receive input from neighboring interneurons, propriospinal neurons, and some descending tract fibers. Alpha motor neurons also receive the primary afferent fibers from neuromuscular spindles that form the sensory arc of the stretch (myotatic) reflex (see Motor Control at the Spinal Level). The cell bodies of the alpha motor neurons are large and may range from 30 to 70 µm in size. As many as 20,000 to 50,000 neurons may synapse on each motor neuron, indicating the tremendous amount of integration occurring at this cell. Gamma motor neurons are smaller (10 to 30 µm) and have a lower threshold to stimuli than alpha motor neurons (Davidoff & Hackman, 1991; Williams et al., 1989). In addition to the motor neurons, lamina IX includes some interneurons and propriospinal neurons (Barr & Kiernan, 1993; Carpenter & Sutin, 1983; Williams et al., 1989).

The last lamina to be mentioned is lamina X. This region forms the commissural area between the two halves of the gray matter and surrounds the central canal. It consists of interneurons and some decussating axons. Lamina X receives input from A-delta fibers transmitting information from mechanical nociceptors and from group C visceral afferents (Willis & Coggeshall, 1991). Table 9-4 summarizes the types of neuron cell bodies found in each lamina, the primary afferent fiber types terminating in each lamina, and the laminae in which descending (motor) fibers from higher centers synapse.

Dorsal Root Entry Zone

Peripheral receptors and the spinal gray matter are linked together through sensory afferent fibers. Stimulated receptors transmit their information to the CNS via peripheral processes. These processes may be classified according to their velocity of conduction as a group A or group C cutaneous fiber or as a group I, II, III, or IV fiber from muscle or joint receptors. Peripheral processes course with efferent motor fibers in peripheral nerves, dorsal and ventral rami, and spinal nerves. They are processes of pseudounipolar neurons, the cell bodies of which form a dorsal root ganglion. This ganglion is located in the IVF. The pseudounipolar neuron also has a central process, which, with many other central processes, forms a dorsal root. Since each peripheral process and central process are components of one neuron, this sensory or afferent neuron does not synapse until it reaches the CNS. As the dorsal root approaches the spinal cord within the vertebral canal, it branches into numerous rootlets. Each rootlet becomes a myriad of fibers conveying various types of sensory information.

As the rootlet fibers enter the dorsal root entry zone, they become arranged into lateral and medial divisions

Table 9-4 General Summary of Input to and Neurons in the Laminae of Rexed

Lamina	Tract	Types of neurons present			Primary afferent fiber type	Termination of descending motor fibers
		Motor	Interneuron	Propriospinal		
I	X		X		A-delta, (C)	
II			X		C, (A-delta)	
III	(X)*		X		A-beta	
IV	(X)		X		A-beta	(X)
V	X		X	X	A-delta, III, IV	X
VI	(X)		X	X	I, II	X
VII	X	X	X	X	I, II	X
VIII	(X)		X	X	(I, II)	X
IX		X	X	X	I, (II)	(X)
X			X		A-delta	

*All parentheses indicate minor contribution.

(Fig. 9-5). The lateral division contains thinly myelinated and unmyelinated fibers, which include the nociceptive (pain) and temperature, or A-delta and C, fibers. These fibers first enter an area of white matter located at the tip of the dorsal horn called the dorsolateral tract of Lissauer and then continue into the dorsal horn. Within the dorsolateral tract of Lissauer, collateral branches of the entering fibers are given off, some of which ascend and some of which descend a few segments before also synapsing in the dorsal horn. In addition to the ascending and descending branches, the dorsolateral tract of Lissauer also contains fibers from the substantia gelatinosa (lamina II), which interconnect with laminae II of other levels.

The medial division of the dorsal root entry zone contains large-diameter and intermediate-diameter fibers from such receptors as proprioceptors (e.g., neuromuscular spindles) and mechanoreceptors (e.g., Meissner's and pacinian corpuscles). These fibers enter medial to Lissauer's tract. Many ascend in the dorsal white column of the spinal cord to the medulla of the brain stem before synapsing, whereas others enter the dorsal horn from its medial aspect to synapse on neurons in deeper layers, including efferent motor neurons for the stretch reflex and the tract neurons of Clarke's nucleus (located in cord segments C8 or T1 through L3).

When the primary afferents enter the dorsal horn, they synapse in the gray matter and release neurotransmitters. These neurotransmitters include excitatory amino acids and neuropeptides. Many primary afferents appear to release glutamate (and/or aspartate). Glutamate has been localized in peripheral nerves, dorsal root ganglia, dorsal roots, and the dorsal horn. Excitatory neuropeptides found in endings of small-diameter primary afferent fibers include substance P and calcitonin gene-related peptide (CGRP). Substance P, utilized by primary afferents, is synthesized in the dorsal root ganglion and transported to the dorsal horn in small-diameter nociceptive fibers. The fibers' terminals are prevalent in laminae I and II. CGRP has been located in dorsal root ganglion bodies (often localized along with substance P), in group A-delta and C dorsal root fibers, in Lissauer's tract, and in endings of afferent fibers that synapse in dorsal horn laminae. Additional excitatory neuropeptides released by small-diameter afferent fibers are less well known and include somatostatin, cholecystokinin, thyrotropin-releasing hormone, and vasoactive intestinal polypeptide (Willis & Coggeshall, 1991).

In summary, the pathway for sensory information can be generally described as beginning in a peripheral receptor and continuing through peripheral nerves, dorsal or ventral rami, spinal nerves, dorsal roots, and dorsal rootlets. Within each rootlet a fiber travels in either the medial or the lateral division. Once in the spinal cord, the fiber's future course depends on the type of information it is conveying. Most fibers terminate in various laminae of the gray matter. The next section describes the white matter of the spinal cord and the continuation of sensory information to higher centers.

White Matter

The white matter of the spinal cord is seen in cross section to be a distinct region located peripheral to the gray matter. It contains myelinated and unmyelinated axons, glial cells, and capillaries. The white matter consists of three regions: a dorsal funiculus (column) between the dorsal horns, a lateral funiculus (column) between each dorsal horn and ventral horn, and a ventral funiculus (column) between the ventral horns. Tracts, or fasciculi, are present within each of these regions (Fig. 9-6). These may be ascending tracts, which convey sensory information to higher centers, or descending tracts, which originate in higher centers and send descending signals to the cord. These descending signals are involved primarily with some type of motor information. Each tract

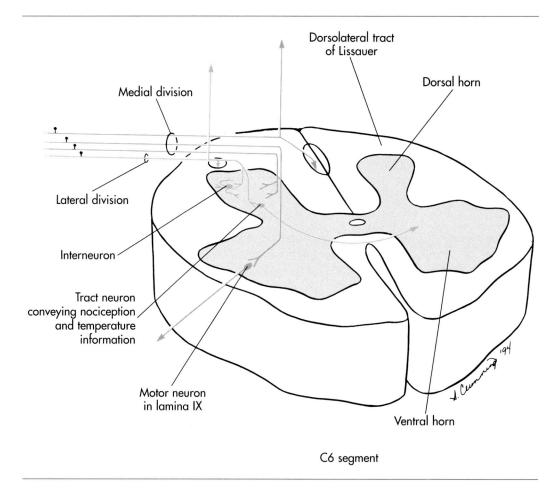

C6 segment

FIG. 9-5 Dorsal root entry zone. The lateral division fibers utilize the dorsolateral tract of Lissauer to enter the laminae associated with nociception (pain) and temperature. Collateral branches of these fibers ascend and descend in Lissauer's tract before they enter the dorsal horn of nearby segments. The medial division fibers, which include large-diameter fibers, enter the cord medial to Lissauer's tract, where many ascend and descend. Others enter the medial aspect of the gray matter to synapse in various laminae, such as lamina IX of the ventral horn, the location of alpha motor neurons.

contains axons that have a common origin, destination, and function. During a neurologic examination, the integrity of certain tracts is tested. Therefore familiarity of the location of these tracts aids the clinician in localizing lesions within the CNS.

Ascending Tracts. Ascending tracts convey information that has originated from a stimulated peripheral receptor located in the skin, muscles, tendons, joints, or viscera. This stimulated receptor transmits an action potential via the peripheral and central processes of sensory (afferent) neurons to the CNS. The sensory fibers that convey the action potential from the peripheral receptors are sometimes referred to as *first-order neurons,* since they are the first neuron in a chain of neurons that proceeds to a higher center (Fig. 9-7). On entering the cord, numerous first-order neurons synapse on neurons

in the gray matter of the spinal cord, while others ascend and synapse in nuclear gray matter in the caudal medulla of the brain stem. The next neuron of the chain that leaves the gray matter of the cord or medulla to ascend to higher centers is known as the *second-order neuron.* Along with many others, this neuron makes up a specific tract. If sensory information is perceived consciously, the second-order neuron decussates and subsequently synapses with a third-order neuron in a nucleus in the thalamus, which is located in the diencephalon of the brain. The *third-order neuron* is necessary to complete the chain to the cerebral cortex. All sensory information traveling to the cerebral cortex (except olfaction) synapses in the thalamus before terminating in the cortex.

When considering the tracts of the CNS, certain important characteristics should be identified. These include the direction of the tract (i.e., ascending or de-

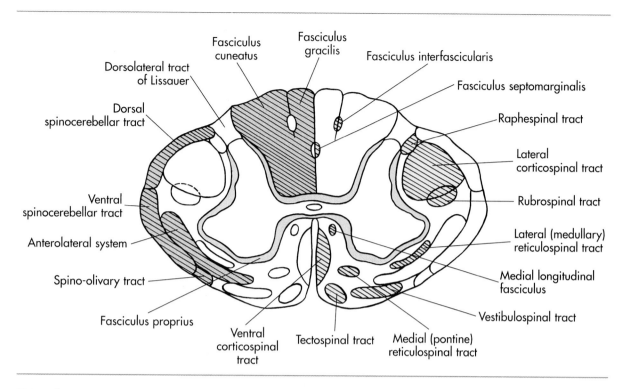

FIG. 9-6 Cross section of the spinal cord illustrating the organization of white matter into fasciculi and tracts. Boundaries usually overlap but are well defined here for illustrative purposes. Ascending tracts are indicated on the left side *(green)*. Descending tracts are indicated on the right side *(yellow)*; the fasciculus proprius is also shown *(blue)*.

scending, which is usually indicated by the name), the specific type of information the tract is conveying, if the tract crosses, and the location of crossing. The ascending tracts are discussed first beginning with the most clinically and anatomically relevant. These major tracts are well defined, and much information has been gathered about them. Secondary tracts are then discussed, about which limited information is available. They appear to supplement the major tracts by conveying similar types of information.

Dorsal column–medial lemniscal system. The first system of ascending fibers to be discussed is the dorsal column–medial lemniscus (DC-ML). Dorsal column refers to the first-order fibers located ipsilaterally (in reference to the side of fiber entry) in the dorsal white column of the spinal cord. Medial lemniscus refers to the second-order fibers located contralaterally in the brain stem. The DC-ML system conveys discriminatory (two-point) touch, some light (crude) touch, pressure, vibration, joint position sense (conscious proprioception), stereognosis, and graphesthesia. This input provides temporal and spatial discriminatory qualities that are perceived subjectively.

The peripheral receptors, which are mechanoreceptors, have been discussed previously in this chapter. The afferent fibers of these mechanoreceptors are large-diameter (group A) fibers; therefore they are located in the medial division of the dorsal root entry zone and subsequently enter the cord just medial to the dorsolateral tract of Lissauer. As these first-order neurons enter, they bifurcate into long ascending and short descending branches. The descending branches descend as the fasciculus interfascicularis in the upper half of the cord and as the fasciculus septomarginalis in the lower cord segments (see Fig. 9-6). These synapse in spinal gray matter and are involved in mediating reflex responses. The longer fibers ascend ipsilaterally in the dorsal (white) column of the cord and continue into the medulla of the brain stem (Fig. 9-8). The first synapse occurs here in the nuclei gracilis and cuneatus, which are deep to the tubercles of the same name (Fig. 9-9, *A*). As the first-order neurons enter the dorsal white column, each neuron comes to lie more lateral to the fibers that entered more inferiorly. For example, information entering via a lumbar nerve ascends in the dorsal column in axons located lateral to the axons conveying information entering via a sacral nerve. In a cross section of the C3 spinal cord,

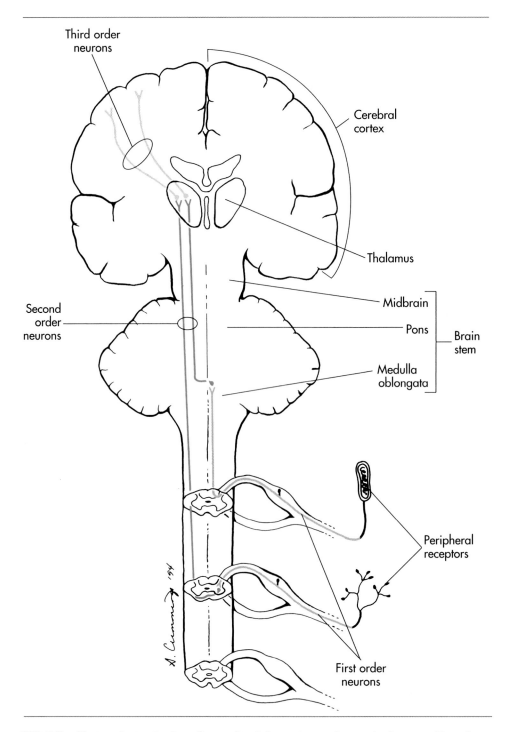

FIG. 9-7 Neuronal organization of ascending information to the cerebral cortex. Note that there are three neurons involved. The first-order neuron *(blue)* cell body is in the dorsal root ganglion. The second-order neuron cell body is located in either the gray matter of the spinal cord or medulla of the brain stem. Its axon *(red)* ascends contralaterally and terminates in the thalamus. The third-order neuron *(green)* courses to the cerebral cortex.

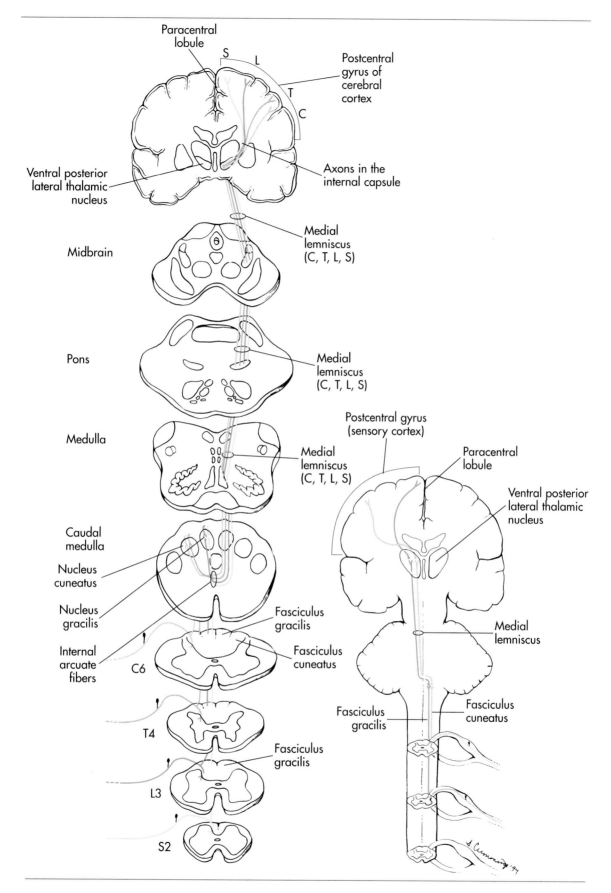

FIG. 9-8 The dorsal column–medial lemniscus (DC-ML) system. The cross sections are through various locations of the CNS and show the location of the ascending fibers. The ascending fibers are color coded (*yellow,* sacral; *red,* lumbar; *blue,* thoracic; *green,* cervical) to correspond to their cord level of entry. Note the organization of these fibers as they ascend to the cerebral cortex.

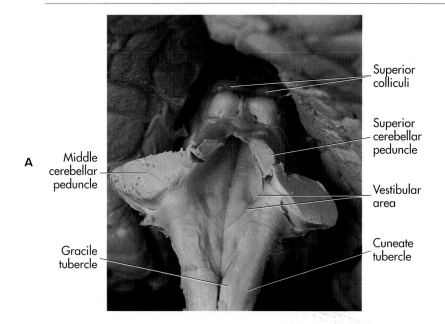

A

Middle
cerebellar
peduncle

Superior
colliculi

Superior
cerebellar
peduncle

Vestibular
area

Gracile
tubercle

Cuneate
tubercle

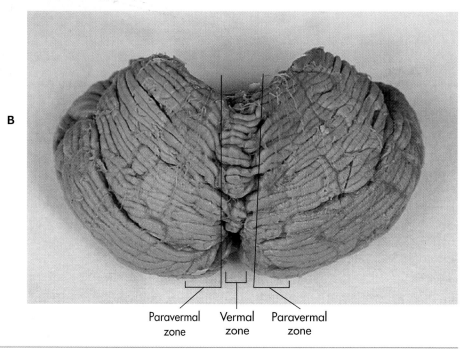

B

Paravermal
zone

Vermal
zone

Paravermal
zone

FIG. 9-9 **A,** Dorsal view of the brain stem. The cerebellum has been removed to expose the floor of the fourth ventricle. **B,** Superior surface of the cerebellum showing the termination sites (vermal and paravermal zones) of the dorsal and ventral spinocerebellar and cuneocerebellar tracts.

first-order neurons conveying information (specific for the DC-ML system) from areas of the body innervated by sacral nerves are found most medial, followed in a lateral sequence by axons conveying information from areas innervated by lumbar, thoracic, and cervical nerves.

At the midthoracic level of the cord and above, the dorsal column is divided by the dorsal intermediate sulcus into a medial fasciculus gracilis and a lateral fasciculus cuneatus. The dorsal intermediate sulcus extends ventrally from the cord's periphery to about one-half the way into the dorsal column. This sulcus acts as a mechanical barrier preventing medial migration of the cuneate fibers (Smith & Deacon, 1984). Thus the fasciculus gracilis, which is found in all cord segments, includes axons of midthoracic, lumbar, and sacral nerves and therefore generally conveys information from the ipsilateral lower extremity. Smith and Deacon (1984) investigated the dorsal columns of human spinal cords and found that the orientation of the fasciculus gracilis fibers varied. In the most caudal part of the fasciculus, the fibers were oriented parallel to the medial side of the dorsal horn, whereas the upper lumbar and lower thoracic fibers were parallel to the dorsal median septum. However, the remaining fibers were oriented obliquely in a ventromedial-to-dorsolateral fashion. The authors also found that some overlapping of fibers occurred within the fasciculus gracilis but little if any between the two fasciculi.

The fasciculus cuneatus includes axons of midthoracic and cervical nerves and, in general, conveys information from the ipsilateral upper extremity (Fig. 9-8). In addition to the mediolateral arrangement of fibers in the dorsal column, the type of modality is organized during the fibers' ascent such that input from hair receptors is superficial, whereas tactile and vibratory information ascends via deeper fibers (Williams et al., 1989). Smith and Deacon (1984) demonstrated that in each of the upper thoracic and cervical segments, the cross-sectional shape of each fasciculus was different and thus characteristic of that particular segment. The authors also believe the fasciculi gracilis and cuneatus should be regarded as separate anatomic entities.

As mentioned, the first-order neurons of the fasciculi gracilis and cuneatus synapse with second-order neurons in the nuclei of the same name in the caudal medulla. The axons of the second-order neurons decussate (cross) in the caudal medulla, and as they do so, they form a bundle of fibers known as the internal arcuate fibers (Fig. 9-8). These second-order neurons then ascend through the brain stem as a fiber bundle known as the medial lemniscus. The lemniscal fibers are organized in the medulla such that information originating from the lower extremity and transmitted to the spinal cord in lumbar and sacral nerves is conveyed by fibers that are ventral to fibers conveying information originating from the upper extremity and transmitted to the cord in (primarily) cervical nerves. In the pons the fibers shift so that the lower extremity information is conveyed by fibers located lateral to the fibers conveying information from the upper extremity. In the midbrain of the brain stem, the lower extremity fibers become located dorsolateral to the upper extremity fibers.

Clinically, it is imperative to recognize that the decussation of fibers occurs in the medulla. A unilateral lesion (trauma, vascular insufficiency, tumor, etc.) in the medial lemniscus of the brain stem produces contralateral deficits (e.g., loss of vibration, loss of joint position sense), whereas a lesion in the dorsal column of the spinal cord produces ipsilateral deficits.

The medial lemniscus ascends to the ventroposterior (lateral part) nucleus of the thalamus and synapses on third-order neurons (Fig. 9-8). The axons of the third-order neurons travel in the internal capsule (a mass of axons going to and coming from the cerebral cortex) and in the corona radiata to the primary sensory area of the cerebral cortex, which is located in the postcentral gyrus and paracentral lobule (posterior part) of the parietal lobe (Figs. 9-8, 9-10, and 9-11). The DC-ML system maintains the spatial relationships of all parts of the body throughout its course in the CNS and allows the surface and underlying body structures to be mapped onto the primary sensory area of the cerebral cortex. This arrangement is referred to as somatotopic organization.

Anterolateral system. The remaining tracts discussed in this chapter follow a basic plan in which first-order neurons synapse in the spinal cord gray matter. One group of tracts conveys nociception (pain) and temperature and some light touch. The tracts of this group ascend in the anterolateral quadrant of the spinal cord white matter and are collectively called the anterolateral system. This system consists of the spinothalamic, spinoreticular, and spinotectal (spinomesencephalic) tracts (Martin & Jessell, 1991a; Nolte, 1993; Willis & Coggeshall, 1991; Young, 1986). The first-order neurons of all these enter the cord via the lateral division of the dorsal root entry zone, pass into the dorsolateral tract of Lissauer, and then synapse in spinal cord laminae (Fig. 9-12).

The spinothalamic fibers are divided into paleospinothalamic and neospinothalamic tracts. Second-order fibers of both originate in laminae I, IV to VI, and even from laminae VII and VIII (Hodge & Apkarian, 1990; Noback, Strominger, & Demarest, 1991; Williams et al., 1989; Willis & Coggeshall, 1991; Young, 1986). Of all of the anterolateral tracts, the neospinothalamic tract is the newest phylogenetically and is best developed in primates. It conveys sharp or A-delta fiber nociception (pain), temperature, light (crude) touch, and pressure. (Sometimes [Carpenter, 1991; Snell, 1992], perhaps unnecessarily [Barr & Kiernan, 1993; Nolte, 1993], this tract is divided into a lateral spinothalamic tract, which is thought to convey nociception and temperature, and a ventral spinothalamic tract conveying light touch and pressure.) The second-order fibers decussate in the cord's ventral white commissure within one or two segments of entry and ascend contralaterally through the brain stem to the ventral posterior (lateral part) nucleus of the thalamus, where they synapse on third-order neurons (Fig. 9-12, *A*). The third-order neu-

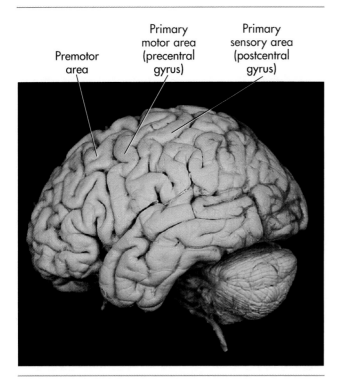

FIG. 9-10   Lateral view of the brain showing the primary motor (precentral gyrus), premotor, and primary sensory (postcentral gyrus) areas of the cerebral cortex.

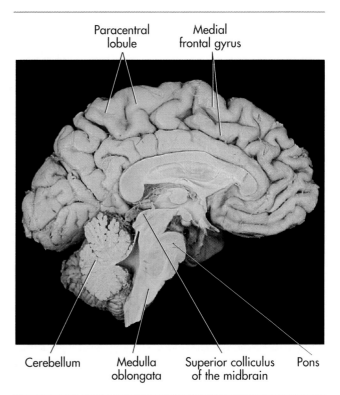

FIG. 9-11   Medial view of the brain. The paracentral lobule, which is the continuation of the primary motor area (precentral gyrus) and primary sensory areas (postcentral gyrus) of the cerebral cortex, is indicated. The medial frontal gyrus (posterior region) is the location of the supplementary motor area.

rons ascend to the sensory part of the cerebral cortex, which is the postcentral gyrus and paracentral lobule (posterior part) of the parietal lobe (Figs. 9-10 and 9-11). The type of pain information ascending in this tract, exemplified by a pinprick, is well localized and discriminatory. The fibers ascend in the spinal cord in a somatotopic fashion such that the axons conveying information from sacral nerves are most superficial and axons conveying information from cervical nerves lie near the ventral horn.

The paleospinothalamic tract conveys dull, achy, or slow C-fiber nociception (pain) and also temperature. The second-order fibers decussate in the ventral white commissure to ascend in the brain stem (Fig. 9-12, *A*). It is generally agreed that the spinothalamic tract sends some collateral branches to the reticular formation of the brain stem on its course to the thalamus (Barr & Kiernan, 1993; Snell, 1992). It is speculated that these collateral branches may originate from the paleospinothalamic tract (Young, 1986). When reaching the thalamus, the second-order neurons of the paleospinothalamic tract synapse in the intralaminar nucleus. From this nucleus, third-order neurons travel to widespread areas of cerebral cortex and even to areas of the limbic system, which is involved with emotions and behaviors necessary for survival.

The spinoreticular tract originates from second-order neurons located primarily in laminae VII and VIII (Jessell & Kelly, 1991; Willis & Coggeshall, 1991; Young, 1986). The second-order fibers ascend bilaterally to the medullary and pontine reticular formation, with a minority of uncrossed fibers reaching the medulla (Fig. 9-12, *B*). From the reticular formation, neurons project to the intralaminar thalamic nucleus and from here to widespread areas of cerebral cortex. It is thought that the spinoreticular tract conveys dull, slow pain and other cutaneous information associated with alertness and consciousness. The brain stem reticular formation is part of the ascending reticular activating system (ARAS), which functions in arousal from sleep and maintenance of alertness and attentiveness.

The third tract found in the anterolateral quadrant consists of a group of fibers that terminates in the midbrain and is called the spinomesencephalic tract (Fig. 9-12, *B*) (Jessell & Kelly, 1991; Martin & Jessell, 1991a; Nolte, 1993; Willis & Coggeshall, 1991; Young, 1986). Others refer to this tract as the spinotectal tract (Barr and Kiernan, 1993; Carpenter, 1991). This crossed

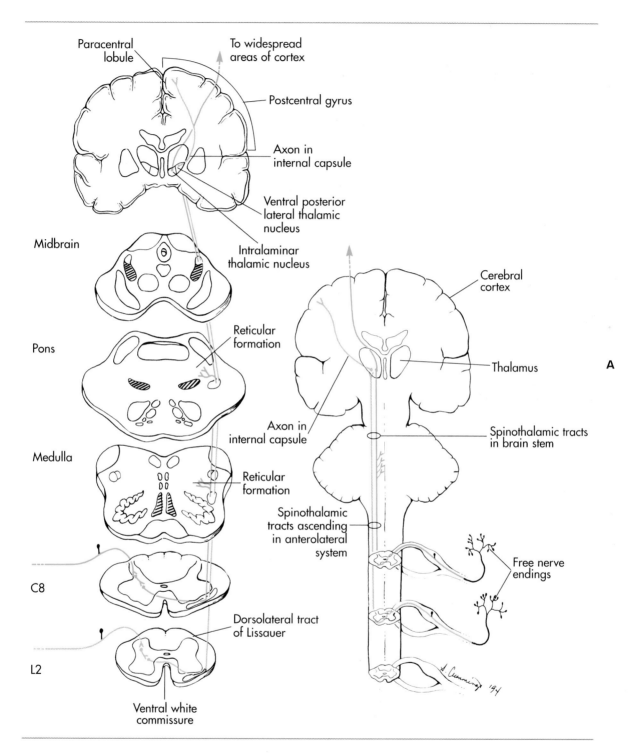

A

FIG. 9-12 Anterolateral system. **A,** Neospinothalamic *(blue)* and paleospinothalamic *(red)* tracts. Note that the second-order neurons cross in the ventral white commissure of the spinal cord. The medial lemniscus is shaded to show its anatomic relationship to the spinothalamic tracts within the brain stem.

Continued.

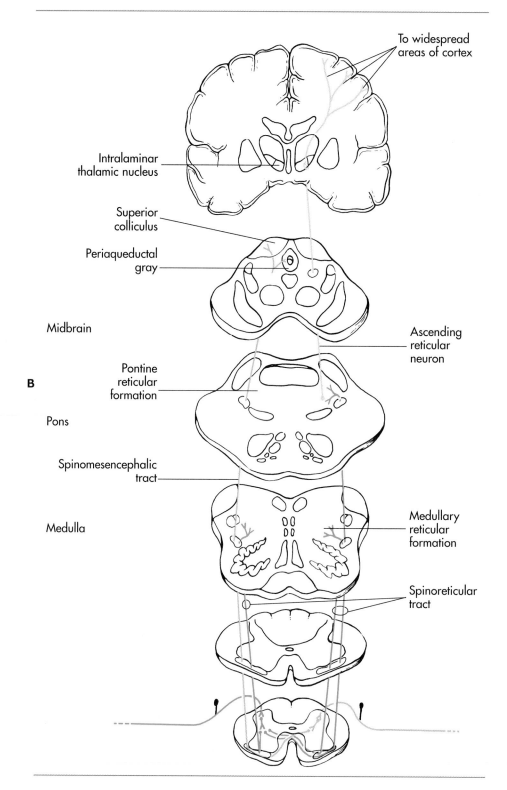

FIG. 9-12, cont'd. **B,** Spinoreticular tract *(red)* terminates in both the pontine and the medullary reticular formations. Information from the reticular formation (represented by the neuron *[green]*) continues to the thalamus and then to the cortex. Spinomesencephalic tract is also shown *(blue)*.

tract originates primarily in laminae I and V and conveys pain and temperature information to midbrain nuclei such as the superior colliculus and to the periaqueductal gray (PAG) of the midbrain (Figs. 9-9, *A*, 9-11, and 9-12, *B*). The superior colliculus is thought to be concerned with spinovisual reflexes, for example, turning the head and eyes toward a stimulus (Williams et al., 1989). The PAG has been implicated as being part of an endogenous pain control system. The PAG is capable of modulating pain circuitry in the dorsal horn of the spinal cord via the descending raphespinal tract (see Other Descending Fibers).

Clinically, it is important to remember that conscious pain and temperature information ascends contralaterally in the anterolateral region and that the decussation of the second-order fibers occurs within the ventral white commissure within one or two segments of entry. Therefore a lesion in the spinal cord or brain stem produces a contralateral loss of pain and temperature.

Spinocervicothalamic tract. Another tract involved with conveying cutaneous sensations such as touch, vibration, and pain is the spinocervicothalamic tract, first recognized in 1955. First-order neurons terminate in the gray matter of the dorsal horn. Axons of tract neurons in laminae III to V (Willis & Coggeshall, 1991) ascend ipsilaterally in the dorsolateral funiculus to synapse in the lateral cervical nucleus. This nucleus is located in the white matter lateral to the tip of the dorsal horn in the first three cervical cord segments and in the lower medulla. Axons of this nucleus decussate and ascend with the medial lemniscus to the thalamus and subsequently to the cerebral cortex. Although the lateral cervical nucleus is prominent in many mammals, especially carnivores, and is likely part of an important somatosensory pathway, its presence and importance in humans are controversial.

Spinocerebellar tracts. The next group of ascending tracts are those that terminate in the cerebellum and convey unconscious proprioception. Numerous spinocerebellar tracts have been implicated, although all their origins are not well known (Ekerot, Larson, & Oscarsson, 1979; Grant & Xu, 1988; Xu & Grant, 1988). The best known of these are the dorsal spinocerebellar tract, the cuneocerebellar tract, and the ventral spinocerebellar tract.

DORSAL SPINOCEREBELLAR TRACT. The dorsal spinocerebellar tract (DSCT) is located on the periphery of the lateral funiculus ventral to the dorsolateral tract of Lissauer and lateral to the lateral corticospinal tract (see Fig. 9-6). It begins in the L2 or L3 segments and ascends (Fig. 9-13). The cell bodies of these tract fibers are located in the nucleus dorsalis (thoracicus) or Clarke's nucleus. This nucleus is located in lamina VII in cord segments C8 or T1 through L3 and is best developed in the T10 to T12 segments (Carpenter & Sutin, 1983). The DSCT is believed to carry information from the trunk and lower extremities. First-order neurons entering at the levels of C8 or T1 to L3 synapse in Clarke's nucleus. However, first-order neurons entering in dorsal roots L4 and inferiorly first ascend in the fasciculus gracilis to reach Clarke's nucleus in the lower thoracic and upper lumbar segments, where they then synapse. Since the second-order neurons originating from Clarke's nucleus ascend in the lateral white column as the DSCT, the tract itself is only present at the levels where Clarke's nucleus is found and superiorly, that is, L3 and above. The DSCT ascends into the medulla of the brain stem and then exits the medulla via the inferior cerebellar peduncle to terminate in the vermal and paravermal region (spinocerebellum) of the cerebellum (Figs. 9-9, *B*, and 9-13).

CUNEOCEREBELLAR TRACT. The upper limb equivalent to the DSCT is the cuneocerebellar tract. Its first-order fibers enter the spinal cord and ascend in the fasciculus cuneatus into the caudal medulla (Fig. 9-13). Here they synapse in the lateral or accessory cuneate nucleus, which is lateral to the nucleus cuneatus of the DC-ML system. Axons from the lateral cuneate nucleus form the cuneocerebellar tract and course with the DSCT, leaving the brain stem via the inferior cerebellar peduncle and terminating in the vermal and paravermal regions of the cerebellum.

VENTRAL SPINOCEREBELLAR TRACT. A third tract that is involved with lower extremity unconscious proprioception is the ventral spinocerebellar tract (VSCT) (Fig. 9-13). This tract does not originate in Clarke's nucleus but instead originates from spinal border cells located in the periphery of the ventral horn (Grant & Xu, 1988; Xu & Grant, 1988) and from other neurons located in laminae V through VII in cord segments L1 and below (Carpenter & Sutin, 1983; Noback et al., 1991). The majority of the tract fibers decussate in the ventral white commissure and are first observed in the lower lumbar cord segments (Carpenter & Sutin, 1983). They ascend in the lateral white column just ventral to the DSCT. The VSCT ascends through the medulla and into the rostral pons and then exits the brain stem via the superior cerebellar peduncle (Fig. 9-9, *A*). Before terminating in the vermal and paravermal regions of the cerebellum (Fig. 9-9, *B*), the majority of the tract fibers decussate again within the cerebellum and thus terminate in the cerebellar hemisphere ipsilateral to the side of the body where the primary afferent fibers originated. The upper

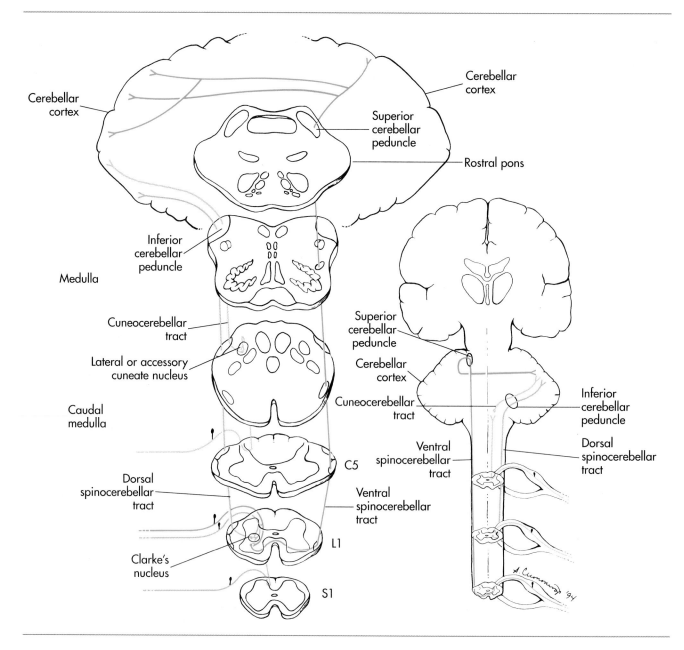

FIG. 9-13   Spinocerebellar tracts as they ascend through the spinal cord, medulla, and rostral pons: the dorsal spinocerebellar tract (and its first-order neuron) *(blue)*, the ventral spinocerebellar tract (and its first-order neuron) *(red)*, and the cuneocerebellar tract (and its first-order neuron) *(green)*. Note that the side of the cerebellum that receives the input is ipsilateral to the side of the body where the input originated.

extremity equivalent to the VSCT, called the rostral spinocerebellar tract, rarely is seen in humans and is not described here.

◆   ◆   ◆

The tracts just discussed are somatotopically organized. The DSCT and VSCT terminate in the region of the cerebellar cortex for the lower limbs, and the cuneocerebellar tract ends in the upper limb area of the

cerebellum. These tracts are involved with muscle coordination during movements and maintenance of posture (Carpenter & Sutin, 1983). The DSCT and cuneocerebellar tract neurons receive input monosynaptically from neuromuscular spindles and GTOs from individual limb muscles, joint receptors, and also from cutaneous (touch and pressure) receptors (Carpenter & Sutin, 1983; Ekerot et al., 1979; Williams et al., 1989). Rather than receiving input from an individual muscle, the

VSCT is thought to convey information from one synergistic muscle group acting on each joint (Carpenter & Sutin, 1983). Based on feline studies, some authors (Ekerot et al., 1979) believe the VSCT neurons are excited or inhibited by segmental motor centers. The motor centers are complex interneuronal pools that receive input from primary afferents and descending tracts and then synapse on local motor neurons. The centers may also be involved with pattern generator areas for automatic movements such as stepping. Therefore, since the VSCT may be relaying information back to the cerebellum in response to some descending input into the segmental motor centers, the VSCT may aid in monitoring the activity of descending paths (Noback et al., 1991).

OTHER PROJECTIONS TO THE CEREBELLUM. In addition to the spinocerebellar and cuneocerebellar tracts, which project to the cerebellum with few synapses, other less direct tracts also convey proprioceptive information to the cerebellum by way of brain stem nuclei. One of these tracts is the *spino-olivary tract.* Second-order neurons from the spinal gray matter decussate in the cord and ascend to the inferior olivary nucleus, which is located deep to the olive of the medulla (see Fig. 9-15). From the inferior olivary nucleus, the axons project through the inferior cerebellar peduncle to the contralateral side of the cerebellum. Another group of nondescript fibers forms the *spinovestibular tract.* The exact location of this tract is unclear, although it does ascend ipsilaterally and terminates in the lateral vestibular nucleus of the vestibular complex, which is located in the floor of the fourth ventricle of the brain stem (Fig. 9-9, *A*). This nucleus, which projects to the ipsilateral side of the cerebellum, also receives a major projection from the receptors for balance located in the inner ear.

◆ ◆ ◆

In summary, unconscious proprioception to the cerebellum is conveyed in the DSCT, cuneocerebellar tract, and VSCT, which use the fewest synapses and are thus the fastest, and also in the spino-olivary and spinovestibular tracts. Pain and temperature sensations are conveyed in the anterolateral quadrant in the spinothalamic, spinoreticular, and spinomesencephalic tracts, which cross in the spinal cord. Discriminative qualities of sensation (e.g., two-point touch) ascend in the DC-ML system, which decussates in the lower medulla. Light (crude) touch ascends in both the spinothalamic tract and the DC-ML system.

Clinically, the most important ascending tracts are the DC-ML and spinothalamic. These tracts convey information that can be tested during a neurologic examination, such as vibration, joint position sense, stereognosis, light touch, pain, and temperature. Since lesions may disrupt these tracts, it is crucial that their functions, locations

within the CNS, and points of decussation be remembered in order to localize the lesion site.

Descending Tracts. As discussed in the previous section, ascending tracts convey sensory information to higher centers. Some of this processed information is integrated to enable the human brain to form a conscious perception of the environment. Sensory input also is used by autonomic centers to help maintain homeostasis and by motor centers to allow for efficient control of somatic movement. Continuous sensory input such as visual, auditory, cutaneous, and proprioceptive input keeps higher centers informed about such facts as an object's location in space relative to body position and body position (stationary or moving) in space. This information is integrated and assessed and used for programming and adjusting movements (Ghez, 1991a).

Three major motor areas receive this input and are involved with controlling movements. They are arranged in a hierarchy, and the first is the spinal cord. Neurons in the spinal cord form local circuits that are involved with reflex and automatic movements. The second motor area is the brain stem, which includes nuclear regions that receive input from ascending tracts and also information from the eyes, inner ear, and even higher centers. The brain stem in turn sends information back to spinal cord neurons to modulate circuitry and thus to influence the alpha and gamma motor neurons involved with postural adjustments and with the control of coordinated head and eye movements. The third motor area is the cerebral cortex. The frontal lobe of the cerebral cortex includes three specific motor areas: primary, located in the precentral gyrus and anterior part of the paracentral lobule; premotor, located in the region anterior to the precentral gyrus; and supplementary, located in the medial frontal gyrus anterior to the paracentral lobule (see Figs. 9-10 and 9-11). These areas project directly to the spinal cord and to brain stem nuclei, which in turn project to the spinal cord. The premotor and supplementary areas also project to the adjacent primary area and, in general, are involved with coordinating and planning complex motor activities (Ghez, 1991a). Two additional higher centers, the basal ganglia and cerebellum, through their projections to the cortex and brain stem nuclei, are also involved with planning, coordinating, and correcting motor activities.

All these motor areas provide control over such activities as maintaining balance and posture and performing skilled movements. In general, three classes of movements can be described. These classes, which may function separately or be combined, are reflex movements, which are the simplest and involuntary; automatic movements such as locomotion, which are rhythmic and voluntary at their initiation and cessation; and voluntary movements, which are performed for a purpose and may be learned and subsequently improved. Voluntary movements vary in complexity from turning a doorknob to playing the piano (Ghez, 1991a).

All three types of movements are influenced by the brain stem and cerebral cortex. These areas produce two sets of parallel descending pathways, through which they can control somatic motor activity by indirectly (via interneurons) and directly influencing the alpha and gamma motor neurons that innervate the muscles that produce movements. Although most descending tracts are involved with somatic motor control, some influence primary sensory afferents and autonomic functions. The location of the tracts within the spinal cord are described in general terms because their boundaries often overlap.

Corticospinal tract. The largest descending tract is the corticospinal tract (CST), which is often referred to as the pyramidal tract (Fig. 9-14). This tract transmits information concerning voluntary (especially skillful) motor activity. The vast majority of the fibers (80%) originate in the motor cortex of the frontal lobe (Schoenen, 1991), although some cell bodies are located in the primary sensory cortex. The CST courses through the internal capsule and continues to descend within the ventral (basal) portion of the brain stem (Fig. 9-14). In the medulla the fibers become very compact and form two elevations called the medullary pyramids (Fig. 9-15). At the caudal level of the medulla, 80% to 90% of the fibers cross as the pyramidal decussation. The crossed fibers become the lateral CST and descend in the lateral white column (funiculus) of the spinal cord between the fasciculus proprius and the DSCT. When the DSCT is not present, the lateral CST may extend to the periphery of the cord.

The CST is relatively new phylogenetically and found only in mammals. It is best developed in humans and becomes fully myelinated by the end of the second year of life. In each human medullary pyramid, there are approximately 1 million axons, and approximately 94% are myelinated (DeMyer, 1959). Axons with a diameter of 1 to 4 μm make up about 90% of the tract fibers (Carpenter & Sutin, 1983; Williams et al., 1989). As the tract descends in the white matter, the size of the tract becomes progressively smaller. In the cervical cord segments, 55% of the fibers leave the tract and synapse on neurons in the gray matter. (It is understandable that such a large percentage of fibers terminates in these segments, since this is the location of the neurons that supply the muscles of the upper extremity, including the hand, which can perform highly skilled movements.) The gray matter in the thoracic cord segments receives 20% of the descending fibers, and the gray matter of the lumbar and sacral segments receives the remaining 25% of the tract axons. The lateral CST, as with the spinothalamic and

DC-ML tracts, is somatotopically organized. The fibers that synapse in the cervical segments are located most medial, followed laterally by the fibers that synapse in the thoracic, lumbar, and sacral segments, respectively. The lateral CST fibers terminate in laminae IV to VII. Some also synapse directly on motor neurons in lamina IX. Rat studies have shown that at least some of these fibers release the neurotransmitters glutamate and aspartate, which are thought to be excitatory (Carpenter, 1991).

A small number (about 2%) of the fibers that do not decussate descend ipsilaterally just ventral to the lateral CST. These thin fibers synapse in lamina VII and in the base of the dorsal horn (Carpenter, 1991). The larger remaining group of uncrossed fibers forms the ventral CST (Fig. 9-14). This tract descends in the ventral white funiculus and is best seen in cervical segments. Before terminating in the intermediate gray and ventral horn (primarily lamina VII), most fibers cross in the ventral white commissure. Therefore approximately 98% of all corticospinal fibers terminate contralaterally.

Studies by Nathan, Smith, and Deacon (1990) have resulted in more information concerning adult human spinal cord CSTs. They found that the extent of the area occupied by the lateral CST varied as a result of the size of the dorsal and ventral horns, the width of the fasciculus proprius that surrounds the gray matter, and the shape of the cord. In some cases the CST extended throughout a wide area of the dorsolateral white column, reaching the cord's periphery, and even extended ventral to a coronal plane through the central canal. In cervical regions the lateral CST varied from segment to segment, whereas in thoracic segments it became more constant.

This variability is important clinically because surgical procedures, such as percutaneous cordotomy and dorsal root entry zone coagulation, may damage these fibers because of the tract's proximity (although the denticulate ligament provides a landmark) to the anterolateral system and to entering dorsal roots, respectively. The ventral CST also was described by Nathan and colleagues (1990) as being located in the ventral white funiculus adjacent to the ventral median fissure. Although some authors believe it is found primarily in cervical and upper thoracic levels (Carpenter, 1991; Nolte, 1993; Snell, 1992; Williams et al., 1989), Nathan and his colleagues (1990) found that it was a distinct tract, and in some cases it extended into sacral segments. Curiously, but of related interest, they also found that cord asymmetry was a common characteristic. In the 50 normal spinal cords studied, 74% were asymmetric, and in spinal cords of 22 patients with amyotrophic lateral sclerosis, 73% were unequal. Of the total asymmetric cords, 75% were found to be larger on the right side. This asymmetry appears to be caused by the size of the CSTs. In cases in

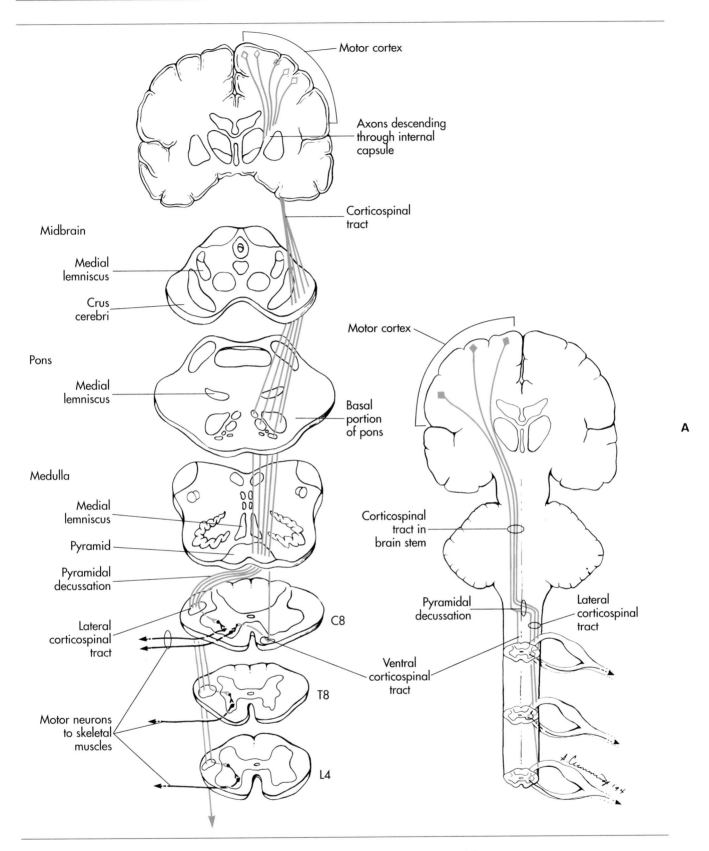

FIG. 9-14   Corticospinal tract (CST). **A,** CST descends within the basal (ventral) region of the brain stem. Most fibers cross in the caudal medulla and descend in the lateral funiculus of the cord as the lateral CST. The uncrossed fibers descend in the ventral funiculus as the ventral CST. These fibers cross before terminating in the gray matter.   *Continued.*

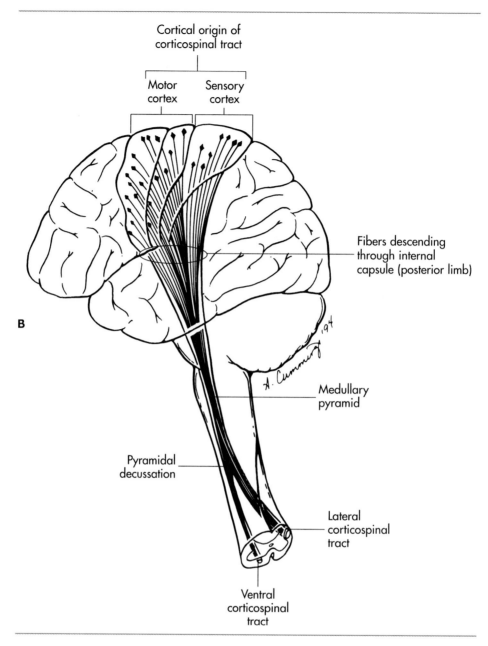

FIG. 9-14, cont'd. **B,** Origin of the CST, its course through the internal capsule, and its continuation into the brain stem and spinal cord.

which the right side was larger than the left, it was observed that a larger number of CST fibers were located in the right side. This was because more CST fibers crossed from the left pyramid into the cord's right side than CST fibers crossing from the right pyramid into the left side. Also, more ventral CST fibers were found on the right side of the cord, since a reciprocal relationship exists between the number of ventral CST fibers and the number of contralateral lateral CST fibers. Therefore the larger (right) half included the larger lateral CST and also the larger ventral CST. A disproportionately large number of uncrossed fibers in spinal cords may explain why lesions

in the internal capsule may produce ipsilateral hemiplegia. Although this asymmetry is quite interesting, it does not appear to be related to handedness, and handedness does not appear to be related to the fact that fibers decussating from left to right do so at a higher level than those that decussate right to left (Nathan et al., 1990).

The CST functions to augment the brain stem's control of motor activity and also to provide voluntary skilled movements. The CST allows movements of manual dexterity and manipulative movements to be performed, primarily by control of the distal musculature of the extremities, through the independent use of indi-

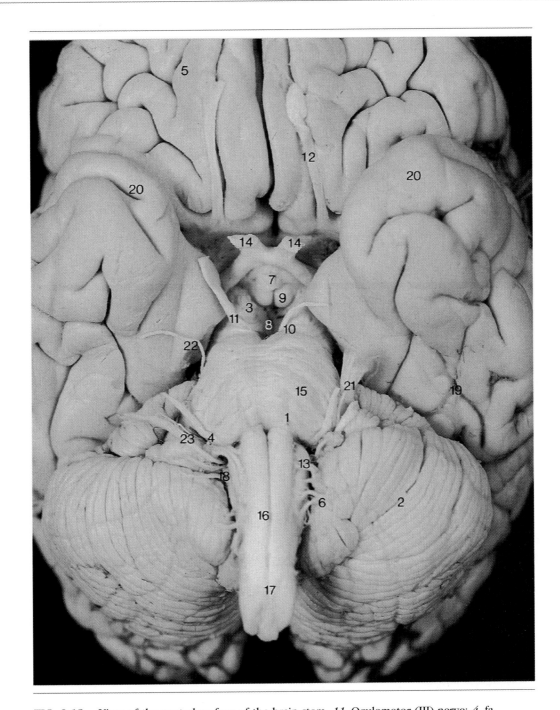

FIG. 9-15   View of the ventral surface of the brain stem. *11,* Oculomotor (III) nerve; *4,* facial (VII) nerve; *18,* glossopharyngeal (IX) nerve and vagus (X) nerve; *16,* pyramid; and *13,* olive, located behind, *6,* hypoglossal (XII) nerve rootlets. (From England, M.A. & Wakely, J. [1991]. *Color atlas of the brain & spinal cord.* St. Louis: Mosby.)

vidual muscles of the hand and fingers. This type of fine motor activity is called fractionation, and the integrity of the motor cortex is essential for it to occur. In addition, the CST adds precision and speed to fractionation and other basic voluntary movements (Wise & Evarts, 1981). As stated previously, the CST takes its origin in part from the sensory cortex. These CST fibers descend and provide feedback to sensory relay areas such as the dorsal horn and gracile and cuneate nuclei (of the DC-ML sys-

tem). The corticocuneate fibers have been implicated in the primate to function as a means for regulating and adjusting (modulating) spatial and temporal input to this nucleus before and during hand movements (Bentivoglio & Rustioni, 1986). The descending fibers also are likely to modulate sensory input to motor areas. The variability of the CST in mammalian species may indicate its functional importance to that species. In the rat the CST synapses in the dorsal horn and intermediate zone, indicating it may be part of that animal's sensory system (Miyabayashi & Shirai, 1988). In species in which manual dexterity is nonexistent, such as the pig, the CST is not evident in the spinal cord (Palmieri et al., 1986). It is best developed in humans, providing feedback to sensory systems and controlling voluntary skilled movements.

Other descending tracts—general considerations. The remaining descending tracts that influence motor activity originate in the brain stem and can be divided into two groups based on their location in the cord's white matter, their termination in the gray matter, and their general functions. The ventral funiculus or ventral white column includes the vestibulospinal tract, medial (pontine) reticulospinal tract, and tectospinal tract (Fig. 9-6). The lateral funiculus or lateral white column includes the rubrospinal tract and lateral (medullary) reticulospinal tract (Barr & Kiernan, 1993; Carpenter & Sutin, 1983; Kuypers, 1981; Williams et al., 1989).

The tracts of the ventral group, in addition to their location, also have the following functional characteristics in common: they give off many collateral fibers (collaterization), which become involved with maintaining posture; they integrate axial and limb movements and provide input associated with movements of an entire limb; and they govern head and body position in response to visual and proprioceptive stimuli. Also, they terminate in the ventromedial gray (e.g., laminae VII and VIII) on long and intermediate propriospinal neurons (which in turn project bilaterally in the fasciculus proprius) and on interneurons associated with the motor neurons supplying the axial muscles and proximal muscles of the extremities.

The tracts located in the lateral funiculus are located near the lateral corticospinal tract. They have little collateralization and enhance the functions of the ventral group by providing independent flexion-based movements of the extremities, especially through their influence on the neurons that innervate the distal muscles of the upper extremity. These tracts terminate in laminae V, VI, and VII (dorsal part) on short propriospinal neurons (which in turn project ipsilaterally in the fasciculus proprius), numerous interneurons, and on some motor neurons (Carpenter & Sutin, 1983; Kuypers, 1981; Schoenen, 1991). Each of the tracts in these two groups are discussed in detail in the following paragraphs.

Reticulospinal tracts. The reticulospinal tracts (ReST) consist of the lateral (medullary) and medial (pontine) tracts (Fig. 9-16, *A*). These tracts originate in the medullary and pontine reticular formation, respectively, and show little if any somatotopic organization. The lateral ReST arises from neurons in the medial two thirds of the medullary reticular formation and descends

bilaterally in the ventral part of the cord's lateral white column. The medial ReST originates in the reticular formation of the medial pontine tegmentum (core of the pons) and descends ipsilaterally in the ventral white column. These tracts are difficult to evaluate in humans, and most data have been compiled from feline studies. During movements these tracts adjust and regulate reflex actions. Depending on the area of stimulation in the reticular formation, either facilitation or inhibition can be produced.

The medial (pontine) ReST facilitates motor neurons supplying axial muscles and limb extensors. The lateral (medullary) ReST monosynaptically inhibits neurons innervating the neck and back muscles. The lateral ReST also polysynaptically inhibits extensor motor neurons and excites flexor motor neurons, although there appear to be some fibers that excite extensor and inhibit flexor motor neurons (Ghez, 1991b). The reticular formation integrates large amounts of information from the motor areas of the cerebral cortex and from other systems involved with motor control (e.g., cerebellum), and it functions to control and coordinate automatic movements such as locomotion and posture. For example, when a standing cat lifts its front paw off the ground (corticospinal input), its body weight shifts to other paws to ensure balance while the movement is occurring. However, if the medullary reticular formation is inoperative, the postural correction does not occur although the limb movement is attempted (Ghez, 1991b). In addition to its influence on somatic motor activity, the ReSTs transmit information that effects autonomic function. Stimulation of reticular formation neurons in the caudal pons and the medulla produces changes in cardiovascular and respiratory functions (Carpenter, 1991).

Vestibulospinal tract. The vestibulospinal tract originates in the lateral vestibular (Deiter's) nucleus located in the vestibular area in the floor of the brain stem's fourth ventricle (see Fig. 9-9, *A*). This nucleus receives proprioceptive input from the body (spinovestibular tract) and the inner ear and information from the cerebellum. The tract fibers descend ipsilaterally in the ventral white column of the cord and synapse in the medial gray of the ventral horn (Fig. 9-16, *B*). This tract facilitates the antigravity muscles of the extremities (lower extremity extensors and upper extremity flexors).

Rubrospinal tract. The rubrospinal tract originates in the red nucleus of the midbrain. It crosses in the midbrain as the ventral tegmental decussation and descends somatotopically in the lateral white column just ventral to the lateral CST (Fig. 9-16, *B*). Although the rubrospinal tract is well established in the cat and monkey and extends the length of the spinal cord, its extent in the human cord is still unclear. Some authors assert its

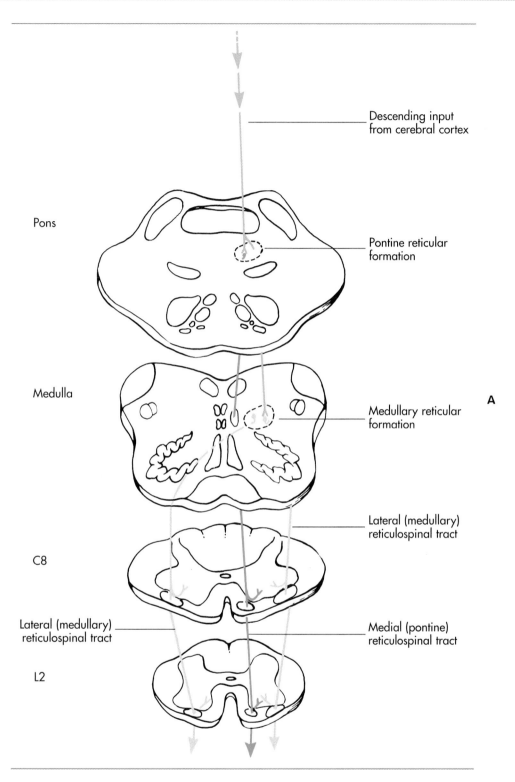

Pons

Medulla

C8

Lateral (medullary) reticulospinal tract

L2

Descending input from cerebral cortex

Pontine reticular formation

Medullary reticular formation

Lateral (medullary) reticulospinal tract

Medial (pontine) reticulospinal tract

A

FIG. 9-16 Descending tracts that originate in the brain stem. **A,** Reticulospinal tracts: lateral (medullary) *(green)* and medial (pontine) *(red)*. Descending input from the cerebral cortex is represented by arrows and the neuron *(blue)*. *Continued.*

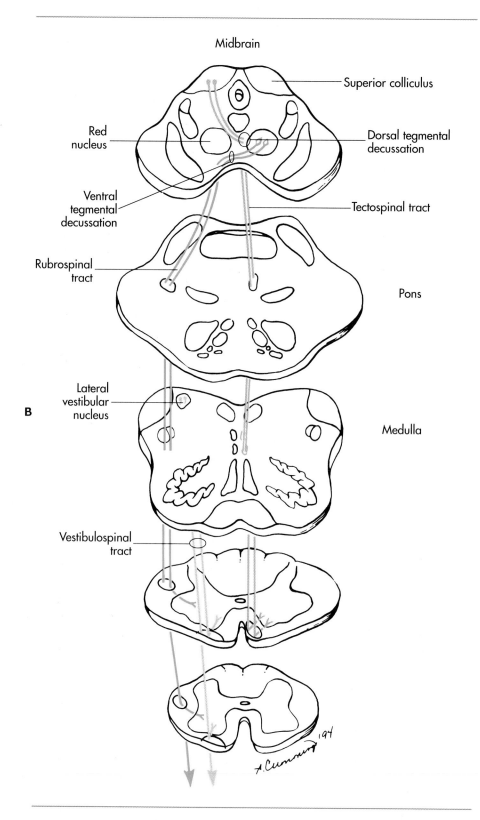

FIG. 9-16, cont'd. **B,** Vestibulospinal tract *(green)*, rubrospinal tract *(red)*, and tectospinal tract *(blue)*.

presence throughout the length of the spinal cord (Carpenter, 1991; Williams et al., 1989). However, Nathan and Smith (1982) studied the human rubrospinal tract from the brains of nine patients and found that the tract was small, and when it could be traced into the cord, it extended only into the upper cervical segments. Stimulation of the red nucleus produces excitation of the contralateral motor neurons supplying flexor muscles and inhibits contralateral motor neurons supplying extensors. Although it is well developed in lower mammals, its importance probably diminished phylogenetically as the CST became more developed.

Tectospinal tract and medial longitudinal fasciculus. The tract fibers that have just been discussed are located throughout the spinal cord and most likely influence somatic motor activity in the trunk in all four extremities. Two additional descending tracts located in the ventral funiculus also influence skeletal muscle activity but are not found in all cord segments. These are the tectospinal tract and the medial longitudinal fasciculus (MLF).

The tectospinal tract originates in the superior colliculus of the midbrain (see Fig. 9-9, *A*). The fibers cross in the midbrain as the dorsal tegmental decussation and descend through the brain stem (Fig. 9-16, *B*). The majority terminate in the upper four cervical cord segments (Carpenter, 1991), although in lower mammals (rat, cat, monkey), fibers also terminate in the segments of the cervical enlargement (Coulter et al., 1979). This tract is involved with orienting an animal toward stimuli in the environment (visual, auditory, cutaneous) by reflex turning of the head (and eyes via tectal fibers to cranial nerve nuclei) toward the stimulus. It is also involved with the head and eye movements used in tracking a moving visual stimulus.

The MLF (descending component) originates primarily in the medial vestibular nucleus of the vestibular area of the brain stem and is sometimes referred to as the medial vestibulospinal tract (Barr & Kiernan, 1993; Nolte, 1993). The tract is located in the cord's ventral white column, descends partly crossed (Kelly, 1991; Nolte, 1993; Williams et al., 1989), and terminates in the cervical cord segments. (Ascending fibers of the MLF are involved with eye movements and course to brain stem motor nuclei of the oculomotor, trochlear, and abducens nerves.) Some authors also include the tectospinal, pontine reticulospinal, and medial vestibulospinal tracts as part of the descending MLF. The tract is responsible for accurately maintaining head position relative to eye movements in response to vestibular stimuli.

Other descending fibers. Two other groups of descending fibers are located in the spinal cord white matter, although they are not well defined. One of these is a group of fibers that originates in the hypothalamus. These fibers descend in the lateral funiculus to synapse on preganglionic autonomic neurons located in cord segments T1 to L2 (L3) and S2 to S4 (see Chapter 10). The other group of fibers are aminergic (Ghez, 1991a) and include the raphespinal tract and the ceruleospinal system. These fibers descend in the lateral white column and synapse in the dorsal horn. They are involved with the endogenous analgesic system (see Chapter 11).

◆ ◆ ◆

In summary (Tables 9-5 and 9-6), ascending fibers conveying input from peripheral receptors and descending axons from higher centers (e.g., motor areas of cerebral cortex, brain stem nuclei) are organized into fairly well-defined, although often overlapping, bundles in the spinal cord white matter. Ascending sensory input is ultimately integrated within the cerebral cortex, and along with visual, auditory, and olfactory information, it allows the human brain to form an overall perception of the environment.

The descending tracts can be classified as medial or lateral depending on their spinal cord location, function, and site of termination; or they may be classified as those that terminate in cervical cord segments (tectospinal and MLF) and those that terminate in all cord segments (corticospinal or pyramidal tract, vestibulospinal tract, rubrospinal tract, ReSTs). Most descending tracts are involved with motor control of posture and equilibrium, automatic movements, and voluntary purposeful movements. These tracts act primarily through interactions with interneurons that, in turn, synapse with the motor neurons that innervate the musculature. Although these tracts obviously are of major importance in providing normal motor activity, neuronal interactions at the segmental level form connections essential for normal motor activity. These segmental connections are influenced by descending tracts that allow for an increase in the complexity of movements. The next section briefly discusses spinal cord segmental control of skeletal muscle.

MOTOR CONTROL AT THE SPINAL LEVEL
Spinal Motor Neurons and the Control of Skeletal Muscle

Human movement results because the nervous system generates a properly timed sequence of contractions of skeletal muscles. The contraction of skeletal muscle is controlled by the motor neurons of the spinal cord. Three types of motor neurons can be found in the cord's ventral horn. The largest motor neurons are the alpha motor neurons (skeletomotor efferents), which exclusively innervate skeletal muscle. The smallest motor neurons are the gamma motor neurons (fusimotor efferents), which exclusively innervate the more polar

Table 9-5   Ascending Tracts

Tract	Information conveyed	First-order cell bodies	Second-order cell bodies	Crossed	Third-order cell bodies	Termination
Dorsal column–medial lemniscus	Two-point touch, light touch, joint position sense, vibration, pressure, stereognosis, graphesthesia	Dorsal root ganglia (DRG)	Gracilis and cuneate nuclei	Yes; internal arcuate fibers	Ventral posterior (lateral) nucleus of thalamus (VPL)	Postcentral gyrus
Spinothalamic: neo and paleo	Pain, temperature, light touch	DRG	Dorsal horn laminae	Yes; in ventral white commissure	VPL (neo) and intralaminar (paleo) thalamic nuclei	Postcentral gyrus (neo) and widespread cortex/limbic system (paleo)
Spinoreticular	Pain and temperature	DRG	Intermediate gray laminae	Majority; in ventral white commissure	—	Pontine and medullary reticular formation
Spinomesencephalic (spinotectal)	Pain (and temperature)	DRG	Dorsal horn laminae	Yes; in ventral white commissure	—	Midbrain: superior colliculus and periaqueductal gray
Dorsal spinocerebellar	Lower limb and joint position	DRG	Clarke's nucleus (nucleus dorsalis)	No	—	Cerebellum via inferior cerebellar peduncle
Cuneocerebellar	Upper limb and joint position	DRG	Lateral cuneate nucleus	No	—	Cerebellum via inferior cerebellar peduncle
Ventral spinocerebellar	Lower limb and joint position	DRG	Lamina VII	Yes; in cord and recrosses in cerebellum	—	Cerebellum via superior cerebellar peduncle
Spino-olivary	Limb and joint position	DRG	Spinal gray	Yes	—	Inferior olivary nucleus
Spinovestibular	Limb and joint position	DRG	Spinal gray	No	—	Lateral vestibular nucleus

regions of muscle spindles (stretch receptors) (Leksell, 1945) and control their sensitivity (see Receptors in the Motor System). Some motor neurons have been found to innervate both skeletal muscle and muscle spindles. This group of motor neurons is known as the beta motor neurons (skeletofusimotor efferents) (Bessou, Emonet-Demand, & Laporte, 1965).

These three types of motor neurons are not segregated within the spinal cord but rather are mixed together into groupings called pools. A given motor neuron pool innervates one particular muscle. The various motor neuron pools, however, are segregated into longitudinal columns extending for two to four spinal segments.

Each mature human skeletal muscle fiber is innervated by one alpha motor neuron. However, a given alpha motor neuron generally innervates more than one muscle fiber. An alpha motor neuron, together with all the skeletal muscle fibers it supplies, is termed a *motor unit.* Motor unit sizes vary dramatically. In a small motor unit a given alpha motor neuron innervates only a few muscle fibers. In contrast, in a large motor unit a given motor neuron may innervate as many as 1000 to 2000 muscle fibers. Muscles of the fingers and the extrinsic eye muscles tend to have small motor units, whereas limb muscles such as the gastrocnemius tend to have large motor units. This size difference is significant because the smaller the motor unit size, the greater the resolu-

Table 9-6 Descending Tracts

Tract	Function	Origin	Crossed	Termination
Corticospinal	Voluntary (skilled) movement	Motor (some sensory) cerebral cortex	Majority cross (lateral corticospinal tract) as pyramidal decussation	Intermediate gray and ventral horn
Rubrospinal	Facilitates flexor and inhibits extensor muscle groups	Red nucleus	Yes; ventral tegmental decussation	Intermediate gray and ventral horn
Lateral reticulospinal	Facilitates/inhibits muscle groups	Medullary reticular formation	Bilateral	Intermediate gray and ventral horn
Medial reticulospinal	Facilitates/inhibits muscle groups	Pontine reticular formation	No	Ventral horn
Vestibulospinal	Facilitates antigravity muscles	Lateral vestibular nucleus	No	Ventral horn
Tectospinal	Reflex postural movements in response to visual, auditory; and somatic sensory stimuli	Superior colliculus	Yes; dorsal tegmental decussation	Ventral horn of cervical segments
Medial longitudinal fasciculus	Coordinates head and eye movements	Vestibular nuclei	Bilateral	Ventral horn of cervical segments
Raphespinal	Pain inhibition	Raphe nuclei	No	Dorsal horn
Descending autonomic fibers	Modulates autonomic nervous system functions	Hypothalamus and brain stem nuclei	No	Spinal gray matter

tion of the movement. That is, small motor units provide a means of achieving fine motor control.

The force of contraction of skeletal muscle fibers is controlled by two separate mechanisms. First, muscle force can be increased by increasing the frequency of motor neuron firing. As a motor neuron increases its firing rate, individual muscle contractions summate, and if the motor neuron firing frequency is high enough, a partial or complete tetanus can occur. This summation process in skeletal muscle results because there is insufficient time between successive action potentials to pump all the calcium ions (Ca^{++}) back into the sarcoplasmic reticulum before the next action potential occurs. Thus, successive Ca^{++} pulses summate to maintain saturation Ca^{++} levels in the cytoplasm of the muscle cells (myoplasm). Many naturally occurring steady muscle contractions are produced by motor neurons firing at relatively moderate rates (8 Hz) far below rates that would produce smooth tetanic contractions. These movements are not jerky but rather are smooth because the motor neurons and the muscle fibers they innervate are activated asynchronously, so these individual motor units do not peak at the same time but average out. Also, during sustained contractions the involved motor units are rotated so as to minimize muscular fatigue.

The second way to increase muscle force is by the orderly recruitment of alpha motor neurons according to size. This is accomplished by increasing synaptic input to the motor neuron pool. Motor neurons with the smallest-diameter axons also have the smallest cell bodies and the lowest threshold to synaptic activation. Thus, weak afferent input to spinal motor neurons recruits only the smallest motor neurons of a pool. As the strength of afferent input increases, larger and larger motor neurons are recruited. This recruitment of motor neurons according to size is called the size principle (Henneman, Somjen, & Carpenter, 1965). This recruitment also applies to voluntary movement. An important consequence of the size principle is that as motor neurons are recruited, progressively greater and greater increments of contractile force are added. This progression of force development results because a good correlation exists between the size of the motor neuron and the number of muscle fibers it innervates. Thus large motor neurons usually innervate large numbers of muscle fibers, whereas small motor neurons tend to innervate only small numbers of muscle fibers.

Receptors in the Motor System

Golgi tendon organs (GTOs) and muscle spindles are the two most important mechanoreceptors involved in the control of skeletal muscle. GTOs are present in virtually all skeletal muscle and are located at the junction between the muscle fibers and tendon and not in the tendon proper (Jami, 1992). The GTO is a capsule of connective tissue that is in series with a discrete number of muscle fibers. The capsule is about 0.5 mm long and about 0.1 mm in diameter (Jami, 1992). The number of GTOs per muscle varies widely; however, there are usually more muscle spindles than GTOs in a given muscle. Within the capsule a single large afferent fiber (group Ib) entwines the fascicles of collagen that compose the GTO (Fig. 9-17, *A*). Not all the collagen bundles are

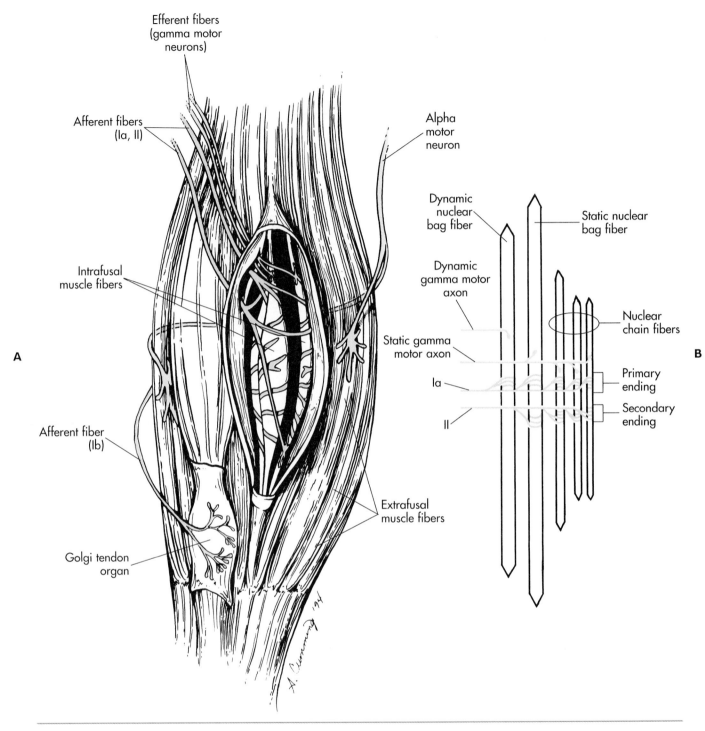

FIG. 9-17 **A,** Golgi tendon organs (GTOs) and muscle spindles are two types of specialized receptors associated with skeletal muscle. Extrafusal muscle fibers make up most of the muscle and are innervated by alpha motor neurons. Located in the fleshy part of skeletal muscle are the muscle spindles composed of intrafusal muscle fibers. These intrafusal fibers are innervated by both afferent and efferent fibers. The GTOs are positioned at the junction between extrafusal muscle fibers and the tendon and are innervated by only one afferent fiber. **B,** Each muscle spindle is composed of three types of intrafusal muscle fibers. The average muscle spindle contains one dynamic nuclear bag fiber, one static nuclear bag fiber, and three or more nuclear chain fibers. Two types of afferents are found to innervate the equatorial regions of the spindle. A group Ia fiber innervates every intrafusal fiber regardless of the number. A group II afferent fiber innervates the static nuclear bag fibers and all nuclear chain fibers. The motor innervation to the spindle is also demonstrated. The dynamic nuclear bag fiber is innervated by dynamic gamma motor axons. The static nuclear bag fiber and the nuclear chain fibers are innervated by static gamma motor axons. (Modified from Gordon, J. & Ghez, C. [1991]. Muscle receptors and spinal reflexes: The stretch reflex. In E.R. Kandel, J.H. Schwartz, & T.M. Jessell [Eds.], *Principles of neural science* [3rd ed.]. New York: Elsevier.)

innervated. The entire GTO is surrounded by a thick lamellar sheath, which is continuous with the perineural sheath of the group Ib afferent. Group Ib afferents are sensitive to changes in muscle tension, particularly when caused by contraction (Houk & Henneman, 1967). Thus, GTO afferents function as monitors of muscle tension. In this role they can monitor the muscle tension produced during ongoing activities and provide the information crucial to maintain muscle output in the face of fatigue.

Muscle spindles are stretch receptors located in the fleshy parts of skeletal muscle (Fig. 9-17, *A*). The density of spindles seems to be correlated with the degree of control required by muscle function. Postural muscles have a much lower density of spindles than muscles of the digits. Muscle spindles are fusiform or spindle-shaped capsules containing 2 to 12 specialized muscle fibers called *intrafusal* fibers (Fig. 9-17, *A* and *B*). All other ordinary muscle fibers are termed *extrafusal* fibers. Spindles range from 6 to 10 mm in length and are surrounded by a connective tissue sheath (Hunt, 1990). Within the capsule the intrafusal fibers are innervated by both sensory and motor fibers.

Three types of intrafusal fibers have been identified (Fig. 9-17, *B*). The nuclear chain fibers compose one group. These fibers are smaller than the other two types, and the nuclei of these fibers line up in a row. The other two types of intrafusal fibers appear similar because their nuclei are clumped together and are jointly known as nuclear bag fibers. Two distinct types of nuclear bag fibers (static and dynamic) can be identified based on physiologic properties. An average muscle spindle contains two nuclear bag fibers, one of each physiologic subtype, and four or more nuclear chain fibers (Hunt, 1990).

Muscle spindles contain two types of sensory endings. Primary, or annulospiral, endings (group Ia) terminate on each nuclear bag and each nuclear chain fiber. Spindles also contain one secondary, or "flower spray," ending (group II) that terminates on the static nuclear bag and all the nuclear chain fibers. The motor innervation of intrafusal fibers by gamma efferents is well documented. In addition to the gamma innervation, beta (skeletofusimotor) motor neurons (Bessou et al., 1965), as well as sympathetic efferents (Hubbard & Berkoff, 1993), have been shown to innervate intrafusal fibers. However, the extent, nature, and clinical relevance of beta and sympathetic innervation of the muscle spindles are not yet well understood.

Muscle spindle afferents are sensitive to muscle stretch. However, the response of group Ia and II afferents is different. Primary endings (group Ia) are most sensitive to the velocity of muscle stretch. Therefore a group Ia afferent can provide the CNS with information about muscle length and thus the position of a joint, as well as how fast the muscle length changed. In contrast, group II afferents do not change their firing as a function of contraction velocity and thus monitor the constant stretch (muscle length) applied to the muscle.

A comparison of muscle spindle afferent discharge with GTO afferent discharge during passive stretch and active muscle contraction highlights the difference in the information these receptors can relay to the CNS. A passive stretch applied to a muscle evokes an increase in firing of both spindle (called loading the muscle spindle) and tendon afferents (Fig. 9-18, *A* and *B*). However, the frequency of firing of the tendon afferents is not as great as the frequency of firing of the spindle afferents. In contrast, if skeletal muscle is stimulated to shorten, the spindle is unloaded (intrafusal fibers go slack) and stops firing while the GTO afferent increases its rate of discharge (Fig. 9-18, *C* and *D*). This difference in response is caused by differences in the physical arrangement of the receptor relative to the skeletal muscle fibers. GTOs are functionally in series with extrafusal muscle, whereas spindles are in parallel with extrafusal muscle. A passive stretch of extrafusal muscle elongates intrafusal fibers and stimulates the innervating afferents to increase their firing rate. In GTOs the same passive stretch is partially absorbed by the compliant extrafusal muscle fibers and only transmits a small stretch to the Ib afferents, and they fire at a moderate rate. When extrafusal muscle fibers shorten during contraction, Ib afferents further increase their firing because the extrafusal muscle fibers directly pull on the collagen fibers of the GTOs and more effectively activate the afferents. In contrast, when extrafusal muscle fibers shorten during contraction, the intrafusal fibers of the muscle spindle do not shorten but slacken, and the innervating afferents stop firing.

The in-series location of GTOs means that Ib afferents are subject to any increase in tension, active or passive, and thus generate action potentials in response to both active and passive stretch. Therefore, GTOs are tension monitors. Muscle spindles are in parallel with extrafusal muscle, and the innervating afferents respond when the muscle is stretched but stop responding when the length of the muscle is shorter (i.e., contracted) than the spindle's length. This is because the spindle does not "see" the load. Spindle afferents are therefore sensitive to increases in muscle length.

The gamma motor neuron system functions to regulate the sensitivity of muscle spindles. As discussed earlier, when extrafusal muscle contracts, the spindle afferents are unloaded and stop firing. Thus, during contraction of skeletal muscle, spindle afferents cannot signal information about changes in muscle length. However, if a gamma motor neuron is stimulated just before contraction of the skeletal muscle, the spindle does not stop responding and can signal any changes in muscle length that might occur. Therefore the gamma motor neuron is reloading the spindle.

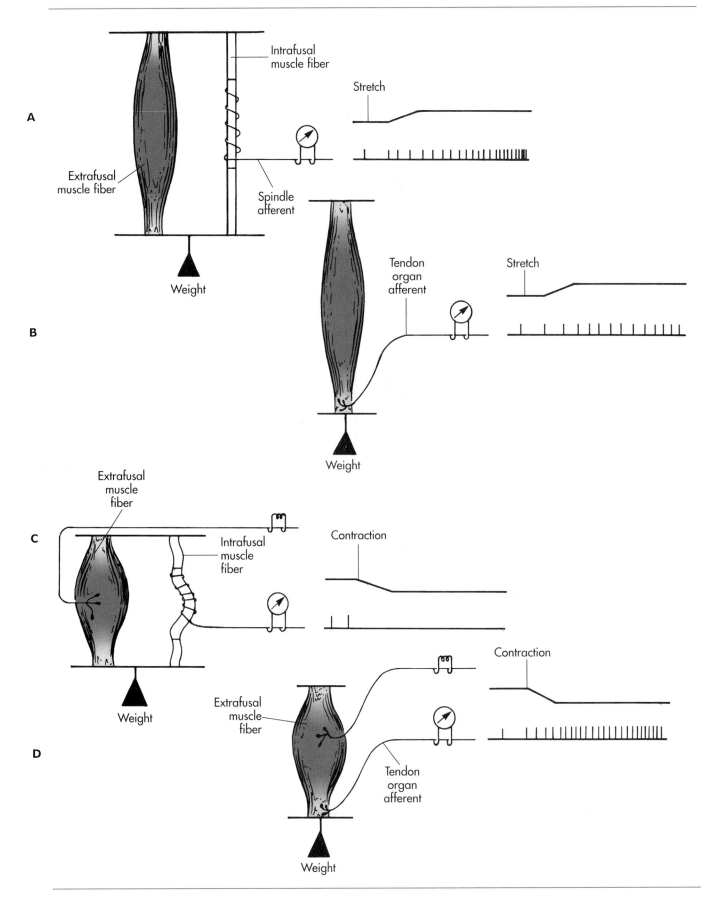

FIG. 9-18 Responses of the two types of muscle receptors to muscle stretch and contraction of skeletal muscle. **A,** Response of a spindle afferent to muscle stretch. **B,** Response of a GTO afferent to muscle stretch. **C,** Spindle afferent response stops when the extrafusal muscle contracts. **D,** GTO afferent response increases when the extrafusal muscle contracts. (Modified from Gordon J. & Ghez, C. [1991]. Muscle receptors and spinal reflexes: The stretch reflex. In E.R. Kandel, J.H. Schwartz, & T.M. Jessell [Eds.], *Principles of neural science* [3rd ed.]. New York: Elsevier.)

Two types of gamma motor neurons exist. Gamma dynamic motor neurons innervate the dynamic type of nuclear bag fiber. Gamma static motor neurons innervate nuclear chain and static nuclear bag fibers. This difference in innervation functions to alter spindle sensitivity selectively during the various phases of a stretch. The gamma dynamic fibers regulate spindle sensitivity during the dynamic phase of stretch (while the muscle length is changing), and the gamma static fibers regulate spindle sensitivity during the static phase of a stretch when the muscle has lengthened but is not undergoing any further change in length. If a gamma dynamic fiber is stimulated before and during the stretch of skeletal muscle fibers, group Ia afferents show a great increase in discharge frequency during the dynamic phase of stretch and also a slight elevation of response during the static phase of stretch. In contrast, stimulation of a gamma static fiber causes the greatest response elevation during the static phase of stretch.

The functional role of gamma efferents is to preserve muscle spindle sensitivity over the wide range of muscle lengths that occurs when a muscle is shortening during a voluntary contraction. This function was first demonstrated in preparations where single afferents and efferents were dissected apart. Recordings from Ia afferents show that during active contractions of extrafusal muscle, the spindles were unloaded, and Ia discharge dropped off. However, if gamma motor neurons were stimulated at the same time the muscle was made to contract, the Ia response did not decline and the spindle was reloaded. Thus the spindle is capable of continually signaling changes in muscle length. Gamma motor neurons for spindles of a particular muscle lie within the alpha motor neuron pool for that muscle. Most descending motor commands for voluntary and postural movements activate not only appropriate alpha motor neurons, but also gamma motor neurons. Thus, both groups of motor neurons are activated simultaneously, and this pattern of activation is called alpha-gamma co-activation.

Spinal Reflexes

Spinal reflexes are among the simplest motor actions and have relatively simple neural circuits. These reflexes are typically used by descending influences to generate more complex motor actions. Spinal reflexes are also a valuable clinical tool, since they serve as a means for assessing the integrity of sensory and motor pathways and the general level of spinal cord excitability. Group Ia afferents from muscle spindles are involved in the stretch reflex, or myotatic reflex. The stretch reflex is composed of two components. A *phasic component* is identified as short and intense and is clinically referred to as a tendon jerk. The *static component* of a reflex is less intense, is

longer lasting, and is involved in maintaining posture and controlling muscle tone.

The central connections responsible for a stretch reflex are relatively simple. Group Ia afferents make direct monosynaptic connection with alpha motor neurons that innervate the same muscle from which the Ia afferent originated (Fig. 9-19, *A*). The Ia afferents also make direct monosynaptic connection with alpha motor neurons, which innervate muscles that are synergistic. Direct excitatory connections of Ia afferents are also made on local inhibitory interneurons (Ia inhibitory interneurons) that inhibit alpha motor neurons controlling muscles that are antagonistic to those from which the Ia fiber originated (Fig. 9-19, *A*). Inhibition of antagonistic motor neurons at the same time the homonymous (agonist) and synergists are excited is called reciprocal inhibition.

The Renshaw cell is a second type of inhibitory interneuron in the ventral horn (Fig. 9-19, *B*). Renshaw cells receive excitatory input from collateral branches of spinal motor neurons and inhibit all neighboring motor neurons of the pool, including the one that activated the Renshaw cell. This inhibition is termed *recurrent,* or *feedback,* inhibition and tends to shorten the motor output from a pool of motor neurons. Renshaw cells also connect with and inhibit Ia inhibitory interneurons and gamma motor neurons. The resulting decrease in inhibition (disinhibition) of the antagonist motor neurons probably functions to shorten the duration of Ia afferent mediated reflex responses. Descending pathways from supraspinal centers and also from segmental afferents provide both excitation and inhibition directly onto Renshaw cells (Davidhoff & Hackman, 1991). These complex inputs suggest that Renshaw cells are controlling the excitability of motor neurons and are probably important in ongoing postural adjustments and minor changes in muscle length (Brooks, 1986).

Group Ib afferents from GTOs also mediate a reflex. All connections in this reflex are made by Ib interneurons that inhibit alpha motor neurons to the same muscle and to the synergists and excite the motor neurons to the antagonists (Fig. 9-19, *C*). This inverse myotatic reflex cannot be demonstrated clinically. However, a crossed-cord component of the reflex called Phillipson's reflex is excitatory and can be observed. Note the myotatic reflex discussed previously does not have a crossed-cord component. The Ib inhibitory interneurons also receive convergent excitatory input from many sources (Fig. 9-19, *C*) including low-threshold cutaneous afferents, group Ia afferents and joint receptors, as well as several higher centers (Jami, 1992). Thus, Ib afferents share these central interneurons, and the Ib inhibition of motor neurons is aided by all these other inputs. This co-processing of sensory input and descending motor commands represents a spinal mechanism that helps to

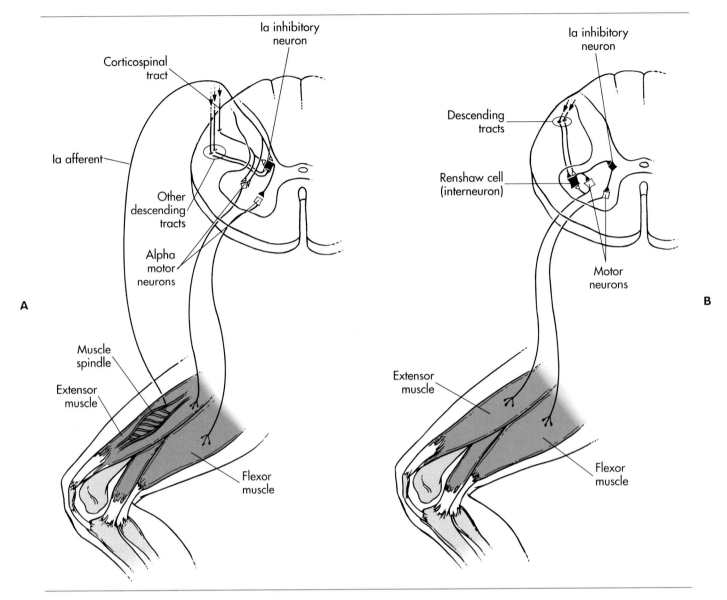

FIG. 9-19 Myotatic and inverse myotatic reflex circuitry. **A,** Ia afferent fiber from the spindle enters the dorsal horn and makes direct synaptic connection with an alpha motor neuron that goes back to the muscle. The Ia afferent also makes synaptic contact with a Ia inhibitory interneuron that inhibits the alpha motor neuron that innervates the antagonist. This inhibition is called reciprocal inhibition. **B,** Renshaw cell is another type of inhibitory interneuron that is part of the myotatic reflex circuitry. A collateral branch of an alpha motor neuron makes excitatory synaptic contact with the Renshaw cell, which then inhibits the motor neuron from which it gained its activation. This negative feedback shortens the motor neuron's response. Other motor neurons of the same pool are also inhibited. The Renshaw cell also inhibits the Ia inhibitory interneuron. Thus the motor neurons of the antagonist are disinhibited. (Δ, Excitatory; ▲, inhibitory.)

guide limb and hand movements during exploration, allowing for precise adjustments of muscle tension once physical contact is made with an object.

A diverse group of somatosensory receptors, including A-beta afferents mediating nonnoxious stimuli and A-delta and C afferents mediating noxious stimuli, elicits a withdrawal reflex consisting of ipsilateral flexion and contralateral extension (Fig. 9-20) (Gordon, 1991). This flexion reflex is protective and involves the coordinated activity of many muscles at multiple joints. All central connections involve polysynaptic pathways, and reciprocal inhibition is the rule. Thus a group A-delta afferent activates an excitatory interneuron that causes excitation of motor neurons to ipsilateral flexors. This same afferent also activates an inhibitory interneuron, which inhibits motor neurons to ipsilateral extensors. The crossed extensor reflex also is polysynaptic, and the interneurons involved excite contralateral extensor motor neurons and reciprocally inhibit flexor motor neurons. Thus a flexor reflex acts to remove the stimulated

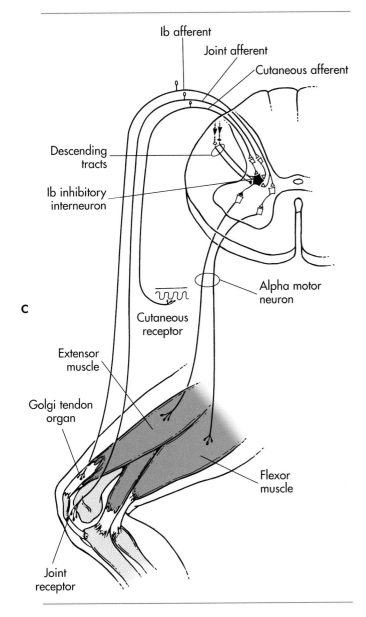

FIG. 9-19, cont'd. **C,** Ib afferent fiber from a GTO activates a Ib inhibitory interneuron that inhibits the motor neuron to the homonymous muscle. The motor neuron to the antagonist is simultaneously excited. The Ib inhibitory interneuron receives both descending input and input from other peripheral receptors. (△, Excitatory; ▲, inhibitory.)

surface from the noxious stimuli, whereas the contralateral component helps to stabilize posture.

Muscle Tone and the Role of Stretch Reflexes

Muscle tone is the resistance of a muscle to active or passive stretch. Skeletal muscle has its own inherent resistance to stretch because skeletal muscle fibers have intrinsic elasticity, as do tendons and muscle connective tissue. The myotatic reflex also functions to resist the

active or passive stretch of extrafusal muscle and works together with the elastic elements of muscle to resist stretch. In a deeply relaxed individual, resistance to passive movement of a limb is moderate and uniform at all speeds of movement and thus solely caused by the elastic properties of the muscle itself (Brooks, 1986). When an individual becomes more active or is agitated, stretch reflexes are activated and thus are under supraspinal control. Automatic adjustments in muscle tone are accomplished by the stretch reflex. Low levels of muscle tone are generated by nonsynchronous activation of small motor units. Increased stretch of extrafusal muscle results in increased motor recruitment. Here the stretch reflex is acting as a feedback system that is attempting to maintain a set muscle length.

Postural maintenance is accomplished largely through reflex adjustments of antigravity muscles. Important examples of these muscles are extensors of the lower extremities. If the floor or platform on which an individual is standing is suddenly moved, appropriate compensatory movements are made to stabilize the individual upright posture. These stabilizing movements are accomplished by stretch reflexes under descending control (Nashner, 1976).

Lesions at various levels of the neural axis can dramatically alter muscle tone. In such cases a limb tested with relatively slow joint rotation may show normal tone. However, with more rapid rotation, increased tone may occur. This hypertonia usually results because of disturbances in the gamma motor system. If a lesion removes major descending inhibition onto the gamma system, the sensitivity of muscle spindles increases and myotatic reflex responses may become quite exaggerated. The resulting hypertonia or spasticity is observed in both phasic and static components of stretch reflexes. Clonus, a series of alternating contractions and relaxations, is often associated with hypertonia. These alternating contractions are caused by exaggerated fusimotor activity that increases the excitability of the stretch reflex. Thus a stimulus elicits a stretch reflex that repeats because the stretch imposed by the muscle returning to the resting position elicits a second response, and so forth.

Hypotonia is abnormally low muscle tone. Spinal transection results in spinal shock, or atonia, as a result of the loss of all spinal reflexes. The acute phase lasts for several weeks before reflexes return. This loss of reflex activity is probably caused by the drastic reduction of descending input to the gamma motor system. However, when reflex activity returns, it may show signs of spasticity and clonus because of the loss of normal descending corticospinal inhibition of the gamma system. Hypotonia may also develop with cerebellar disease. This effect may also be a result of decreased gamma motor neuron output. This explanation of cerebellar

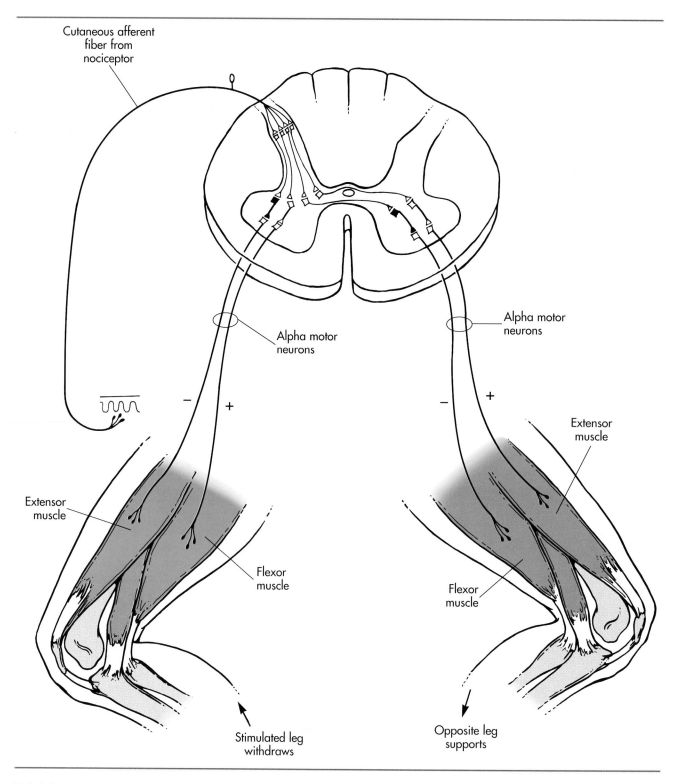

FIG. 9-20   Flexion withdrawal reflex circuitry. Input from a cutaneous nociceptor activates polysynaptic inputs that produce flexion of the stimulated limb and extension of the contralateral limb helping maintain stability. (△, Excitatory; ▲, inhibitory.)

hypotonia has been based on data from lower-primate experiments (Gilman, 1969) but has yet to be assessed in humans.

Spinal Control of Locomotion

Locomotion is a rhythmic behavior that functions to move an animal (human or otherwise) from one location to another. For locomotion to occur, a tonic (nonpatterned) descending message from supraspinal centers must be translated into a patterned alternating stepping of the legs. The step cycle of an individual limb, in its simplest form, can be divided into two phases. During the swing phase of stepping, the foot is off the ground and moving forward. The stance phase represents the part of the stepping cycle when the foot is on the ground and the leg is moving backward with respect to the body. The repetitive swing and stance phases of the two limbs tend to overlap slightly, and forward progression occurs in what appears to be a totally automatic fashion.

The repetitive motor pattern observed in a walking animal is produced by a neural oscillator, or central pattern generator, which resides in the spinal cord. This was first demonstrated in spinal cats. In these animals all dorsal roots were severed, and they were treated with L-dopa or clonidine to stimulate descending noradrenergic pathways involved in turning on locomotion at the spinal level. Cats so treated were made to walk on a treadmill and showed a near-normal walking pattern (Grillner & Zangger, 1975). These same studies showed that each limb had a separate control center, since a right limb held in midcycle would stop stepping although other limbs would continue stepping normally (Grillner, 1975).

The control center, or central pattern generator, represents a collection of interconnected neurons that are capable of producing a patterned motor output without the need of sensory feedback for its pattern or maintenance. Also, alpha and gamma motor neurons have been found to be coactivated during locomotion, and thus spindle afferents increase their discharge during stepping (Severin, Orlovsky, & Shik, 1967). Thus, spindle afferents continually can signal information about muscle length and limb loading throughout the stepping cycle.

Sensory feedback during locomotion may not be necessary for the basic rhythmic motor output, but it is essential for normal stepping movements. This is because afferent input about stepping is used to make corrective adjustments to the central pattern generator so that the motor output is adapted to the particular demands of an individual's environment. Afferent input arising from muscle spindles is capable of modulating the step cycle. The swing phase of stepping can be inhibited in cats if a leg is held during the stance phase (Grillner, 1975).

However, if the leg is slowly moved backward, a swing occurs when the held leg is in the position where swing would occur during normal walking.

Two conditions must be fulfilled for swing to occur: the hip joint must be extended, and the leg extensor muscles and spindles must be unloaded. Both of these conditions are fulfilled at the end of the stance phase when the other limb has touched down. The muscle spindles signal the unloading of the limb by decreasing their output, which allows the central pattern generator to switch from stance to swing. This type of sensory feedback is important to normal walking. It prevents a premature swing by the central pattern generator if, at the end of stance, there is still a significant load on the extensors. Therefore this feedback system preserves an individual's balance. Stretch receptors can also reinforce motor output; this would be necessary when carrying a heavy load or walking uphill. Thus, stretch reflexes are important in normal everyday activities such as walking.

The central pattern generator for locomotion is not only acted on by afferent input, but it can also alter the way sensory feedback is channeled through the spinal cord. An illustration of this is seen during locomotion in the response of a limb to touch. During stepping, it is possible that a particular reflex is useful during one phase of the step cycle and not useful during another phase. In such cases the central pattern generator should make adjustment in the excitability of the reflex to make certain the motor output produces the most appropriate behavior. Phase-dependent reflex reversal to cutaneous stimulation of a cat hind limb is an example of this type of interaction (Forssberg, Grillner, & Sjöström, 1975). If a chronic spinal cat is walking on a treadmill and the dorsum of the foot is touched during the swing phase of stepping, a short latency activation of flexor muscles for all joints of that limb is observed. Thus the animal lifts its leg over an encountered obstacle. However, the same stimulus applied during the stance phase of stepping results in a dramatic increase in extensor activity. This functions to thrust the limb backward, and then the limb is lifted over the obstacle by subsequent flexor activity. This latter response is called the *stumbling corrective reaction* and illustrates that the same stimulus has been channeled through the CNS circuitry differently during different phases of the stepping cycle.

CLINICAL APPLICATIONS

Neuroanatomy is the foundation on which clinical neurology is based. A clinician makes a neurologic assessment of a patient with back and extremity pain based on his or her knowledge of spinal cord anatomy and on the results of the neurologic examination performed. The examination typically includes testing motor functions influenced by the descending tracts and sensory functions conveyed primarily by the spinothalamic tract and DC-ML system. The derivation of an anatomic diagnosis of a disorder affecting the nervous system is essential to the development of an accurate pathologic or etiologic diagnosis (Adams & Victor, 1989). The purpose of this section is to highlight the application of neuroanatomy to the localization of pathologic conditions causing signs and symptoms in a particular patient. Clinical neurology is a subject unto itself, and therefore the following paragraphs are intended to exemplify briefly the clinical application of only portions of the material discussed in this chapter.

Damage to areas of the body resulting in loss or alteration of function is referred to as a *lesion*. Lesions of the spinal cord can occur in many ways. One means is by trauma. Spinal cord trauma occurs in approximately 8000 to 10,000 individuals per year in the United States. The most common cause is automobile accidents (32%), followed by falls (26%), gunshot wounds (9%), and recreational activities such as diving accidents (8%). Direct injury to the cord (knife, bullet), compression by vertebral fragments, compression secondary to hemorrhage and coagulation, damage to vessels, or stretching of the cord can be caused by trauma. Regions most often affected are the cervical and thoracolumbar junction, followed by the thoracic and lumbar segments (Meyer et al., 1991).

Other nontraumatic examples that can cause lesions are vascular insufficiency, tumor, infections, demyelinating diseases (e.g., multiple sclerosis), or degenerative diseases (e.g., amyotrophic lateral sclerosis, Friedreich's ataxia). Patients with lesions of the spinal cord or related nerves may have strictly motor deficits, strictly sensory deficits, or a combination of the two. Disorders may also be either acute or chronic. In the following section the examples are presented in a fairly "cut and dried" manner. However, in a clinician's office a lesion may not always present as a "textbook" case.

Motor Assessment

Lower Motor Neurons. This section discusses the motor aspect of lesions, that is, lesions affecting descending tracts and the somatic motor neurons of the CNS. Two types of motor neurons are referred to clinically. One type is called the lower motor neuron (LMN) and includes the alpha and gamma motor neurons. As noted in the section on gray matter, the cell bodies of LMNs reside in lamina IX of the cord's ventral horn. Because of their location, LMNs are also referred to as anterior horn cells. Their axons leave the cord in the ventral root, enter a spinal nerve, and continue in peripheral nerves to skeletal muscles. In general, LMNs can be de-

fined as the only neurons that innervate skeletal muscle and are thus the final common pathway to the muscle. Without intact LMNs, the skeletal muscle cannot work properly, or even at all. These neurons are found in spinal nerves originating from the spinal cord and also in those cranial nerves emerging from the brain stem that innervate skeletal muscles located in the head region. It is important to realize that LMNs are found in the CNS (i.e., cell bodies in the ventral horn of the cord or motor nuclei of the brain stem) and in the PNS (i.e., axons in peripheral nerves). Therefore a lesion of an LMN can occur anywhere along the entire neuron: at the level of the CNS and its cell body and more distally in the PNS, affecting the axon. Lesions of LMNs produce various signs and symptoms based on the LMN being responsible for the contraction of muscle. Because of its developmental origin, a skeletal muscle becomes innervated by more than one cord segment, and any one cord segment can innervate more than one muscle. Therefore, to eliminate completely a muscle's innervation at the CNS level, a lesion must encompass all cord segments involved. However, a lesion of only one peripheral nerve distal to the brachial or lumbosacral plexuses may be all that is necessary to eliminate the innervation of a muscle of the extremities.

A lesion of LMNs produces characteristic signs, including the following:

◆ Muscle weakness
◆ Absent or diminished muscle tone. Tone is the amount of a muscle's resistance to stretch and is tested by passively flexing or extending a patient's joint. In LMN lesions there is a decreased resistance to passive movement referred to as flaccid paralysis.
◆ Spontaneous contraction of muscle fascicles (fasciculations). This is caused by spontaneous discharging of the dying motor neurons and is visible as muscle twitching under the skin (spontaneous contractions of muscle fibers also occur but are evident only through electromyographic [EMG] recordings). The contractions peak approximately 2 or 3 weeks after denervation (Noback et al., 1991).
◆ Severe neurogenic atrophy caused by denervation of the muscle
◆ Absent or decreased myotatic/stretch/deep tendon reflexes (areflexia or hyporeflexia, respectively). This depends on the number of LMNs that remain intact to an individual muscle. One means of testing the health of a skeletal muscle, its sensory and motor fibers, and the general excitability of the CNS at a segmental level is through the muscle stretch reflex. Tapping a tendon elicits a stretch reflex that may be nonexistent, diminished, normal, or exaggerated. If an LMN lesion involves the nerve fibers innervating the muscle being tested, the reflex response of that particular muscle is

nonexistent (areflexic) or diminished, depending on how much of the muscle's innervation (by LMNs) is affected. For example, a lesion of an entire peripheral nerve or all the cord segments and roots forming that peripheral nerve results in areflexia, while a lesion of just some of the cord segments and roots results in hyporeflexia.

Upper Motor Neurons. The other type of motor neuron is the upper motor neuron (UMN). UMNs are clinically referred to as neurons that influence LMNs. Often UMNs are considered to be the descending corticospinal fibers. In the context of this chapter, UMNs also include the vestibulospinal, rubrospinal, and reticulospinal tracts. Since UMNs are descending tracts, it is apparent that UMNs, unlike LMNs, remain in the CNS and that UMNs extend from the location of their cell bodies to the termination of their axons. Therefore they are located in the cerebral cortex, internal capsule, brain stem, and white matter of the spinal cord.

Lesions of the spinal cord probably interrupt a number of descending tracts (UMNs) and produce characteristic signs that are evident after the acute effects are gone. These include the following:

- Muscle weakness
- Slow disuse atrophy
- Diminished or absent superficial (cutaneous) reflexes. An example of this type of reflex is the abdominal reflex. Stroking lateral to medial in a diamond-shaped pattern around the umbilicus normally causes the umbilicus to move toward the stimulus. This is mediated by the T8 to T12 nerves to the abdominal musculature. Another superficial reflex is the cremasteric reflex, which is tested by stroking the inner thigh. This results in elevation of the ipsilateral testicle and is mediated by the L1 and L2 nerves. This reflex is elicited best in infants. A third reflex is the plantar reflex. Stroking the lateral sole of the foot and under the toes produces a curling under of the toes and is mediated by the S1 and S2 nerves. These reflexes are under the influence of UMNs.
- Pathologic reflex. The most common pathologic reflex is the Babinski sign (extensor toe sign). Providing an uncomfortable stimulus to the lateral sole of the foot and continuing under the toes produces dorsiflexion of the big toe and fanning of the other digits. This is a withdrawal response normally suppressed by the CST (Daube et al., 1986; deGroot & Chusid, 1988).
- Spastic paralysis. This type of paralysis is characterized by hypertonia (increased resistance to passive movement especially evident in the antigravity muscles, i.e., upper extremity flexors and lower extremity extensors). During passive movement of an extremity, the resistance suddenly disappears. This action is similar

to the opening of a pocket knife and is referred to as the "clasp-knife" phenomenon.

It is speculated that afferents from the GTOs (proprioceptors located in muscle tendons) are stimulated, causing inhibition and release the muscle. In addition to hypertonia, myotatic (stretch) reflexes are exaggerated (hyperreflexia). Lesioning UMNs eliminates descending inhibitory input to LMNs. However, the components of the stretch reflex (Ia afferents and alpha motor neurons) and gamma motor neurons are still intact. This allows the gamma motor neurons to discharge at a higher rate. The spasticity produced by UMN lesions is caused by lesions in descending tracts, such as the reticulospinal tract (Bucy, Keplinger, & Siqueira, 1964; deGroot and Chusid, 1988; Nolte, 1993) rather than the corticospinal fibers. In addition, lesions of the cortical fibers projecting to the reticular formation (e.g., within the internal capsule) can cause dysfunction of the reticulospinal tract (deGroot & Chusid, 1988; Lance, 1980; Nolte, 1993).

The lack of involvement of the CST in producing spasticity is supported by experimental evidence. Selective lesions placed in the medullary pyramids of monkeys resulted in weakness of distal musculature and impairment of skilled movements of the hands but did not result in spasticity (Barr & Kiernan, 1993; Ghez, 1991a; Kuypers, 1981; Nolte, 1993). However, isolated case studies report that lesions in the pyramidal tract of humans cause increased tone. This may be because the lesions included reticulospinal fibers that lie close to the pyramidal fibers (Lance, 1980; Paulson, Yates, & Paltan-Ortiz, 1986).

- Clonus. This is another abnormal muscle activity sometimes seen with UMN lesions. Clonus is the rapid alternating contraction and relaxation of antagonistic muscles. For example, forceful and maintained dorsiflexion of the ankle joint results in continued rapid flexion and extension of the foot (see Muscle Tone and the Role of Stretch Reflexes).

Certain aspects should be evaluated when assessing the motor system. These include reflexes, muscle strength, muscle tone, muscle bulk, movements, and posture. Whenever possible, sides of the body should be compared, and proximal muscle groups should be compared with distal muscle groups. LMN lesions may be restricted to individual muscle groups, whereas UMN lesions may affect entire limbs. Both result in voluntary paralysis for different reasons. Paralysis of all four extremities is known as quadriplegia, paralysis in both lower extremities is paraplegia, one-sided paralysis is hemiplegia, and paralysis of one extremity is monoplegia. The presence of UMN lesion signs localizes the lesion to the CNS. However, LMN lesion signs may result from a lesion in the PNS or CNS. In determining the location of the lesion, knowledge of the peripheral nerve and cord segment innervation of muscles is imperative (see Table 9-3 and Peripheral Nerves).

Sensory Assessment

Evaluating the sensory systems involves testing the integrity of the DC-ML system and the spinothalamic tract. Sensory modalities that may be tested include pain, temperature, touch, vibration, and conscious proprioception. Pain (nociception), which ascends contralaterally in the spinothalamic tract, is tested by pinpricking the skin in a dermatomal pattern. Light (crude) touch, which can be evaluated by brushing a wisp of cotton across the skin, ascends in both the spinothalamic tract and the DC-ML system. Testing for its presence gives general information about CNS integrity. Vibration is tested by placing a vibrating tuning fork over various bony prominences, such as the malleoli or olecranon process. This information ascends ipsilaterally in the cord's dorsal column. Conscious proprioception is evaluated by the clinician flexing or extending the patient's big toe or finger and asking the patient to identify if the digit is up or down. During each part of the examination, the patient's eyes are closed. More discriminative sensations, including two-point touch, stereognosis, and graphesthesia, also ascend in the DC-ML system. These are complexly integrated in the parietal lobe of the cerebral cortex. The analysis by the cortex produces discriminatory capabilities that are important in the daily activities of human existence.

Two-point touch is tested on the patient's fingertips by stimulating two points on the skin simultaneously. The two points should be recognized within 2 to 3 mm of each other. Graphesthesia is tested by tracing numbers or letters on the skin of the back of the patient's hand and having the patient identify them. Stereognosis is tested by placing a common object in the hand and asking for its identification. The patient's eyes should be closed during these tests. Whenever possible, symmetry must be considered while evaluating these systems. As with motor assessment, knowledge of the innervation of the area tested, as well as knowledge of the ascending tracts involved, is imperative. Peripheral nerve and dermatomal patterns of innervation (see Figs. 9-1 and 9-2) differ and must be distinguished.

Lesions

Discussing the pathologic conditions of the CNS is beyond the scope of this chapter. Therefore the following discussion generally describes specific lesions with the sole intent of emphasizing the key concepts in this chapter.

Lesions of the Dorsal and Ventral Roots. Depending on the extent of injury to a dorsal root, various symptoms are present. Cutaneous afferents in the dorsal root are destined to innervate a specific strip of skin (dermatome). Therefore a lesion at this site produces symptoms that are localized in a dermatomal distribution rather than a peripheral nerve distribution (see Figs. 9-1 and 9-2). Because dermatomes overlap each other, sectioning (rhizotomy) one dorsal root produces different symptoms than sectioning many dorsal roots. For example, sectioning one dorsal root produces hypesthesia (slightly diminished sensation) or paresthesia (abnormal spontaneous sensation such as "tingling" or "pins and needles" typically experienced as when the foot "falls asleep"). Cutting several consecutive dorsal roots produces anesthesia except in the outermost dermatomes; that is, lesioning the L2 to L4 dorsal roots causes loss of all sensation only in the L3 dermatome. Some injuries may not be as severe, and lesions instead may cause pressure or irritation to the root (radix). Pressure may produce paresthesia and hypesthesia in a dermatomal pattern whereas irritation and subsequent inflammation (or pressure resulting in ischemia) may result in radicular (root) pain located in a dermatomal area (see Chapters 7 and 11).

In addition to the cutaneous effects seen, lesioning dorsal roots also disturbs motor function, producing observable motor deficits. The destruction of all dorsal roots involved with the innervation of an extremity, for example, results in hypotonia and areflexia, even though the LMNs are intact. This occurs because the afferents of the stretch reflex are destroyed. Sensory afferents, such as from touch receptors and proprioceptors, also provide feedback regarding motor activity, which is essential for movements to occur properly. In fact, the extremity is frequently regarded by the individual as useless without this input, although it can be voluntarily moved. Experimental lesions of this nature on primates show that the animal does not use the extremity for climbing, walking, or grasping (Carpenter, 1991).

Tabes dorsalis, a form of neurosyphilis, affects the dorsal roots and also causes degeneration of the dorsal white columns. Initially, radicular pain and paresthesias are present, followed later by impairment of sensation and reflexes, hypotonia, and loss of proprioception. Loss of proprioception results in sensory ataxia and an ataxic gait, described as being broad based with the feet slapping the ground. Visual cues become important in maintaining balance. This loss of proprioception is evidenced by the patient's inability to stand with the feet together and eyes closed without swaying or falling. This is referred to as a Romberg sign and is indicative of damage to the dorsal column.

Ventral root lesion signs reflect the loss or disruption of the innervation to effectors. Destroying LMN fibers produces LMN lesion signs whereas destroying autonomic efferents in the T1 to L2 (L3) and S2 to S4 roots affects visceral function (see Chapter 10). Pressure applied to the roots results in diminished reflexes and muscle weakness.

Cord Transection. A complete transection through the spinal cord isolates the spinal cord from higher centers and other cord segments. It may produce a paraplegic or quadriplegic patient depending on the lesion's location. Initially, and lasting for approximately 1 to 6 weeks, a phenomenon called spinal shock ensues in which all neural functions below the lesion level cease. This includes loss of somatic motor and sensory functions, such as reflexes and tone, and loss of autonomic functions, including autonomic reflexes and thermoregulation.

After the period of spinal shock, UMN lesion signs appear, such as the Babinski sign and muscle spasms. At first, bilateral flexor muscle spasms predominate. In the lower extremity the flexors of the hip, knee, and foot may contract, producing the "triple-flexor response of Sherrington." In some severe cases the neurons become so hyperexcitable that the flexor response may occur in response to minimal cutaneous stimuli (e.g., pulling the bedsheet across over the lower extremities of a patient) or even without any obvious stimulus. After several months of flexor spasms, extensor tone gradually returns, and in most patients, extensor muscle spasms prevail (Carpenter, 1991; Noback et al., 1991) and are observed in conjunction with other UMN lesion signs. Permanent loss of voluntary autonomic control produces profound effects on the sexual activity and the bladder and bowel activities of these patients (see Chapter 10).

A hemisection of the left or right side of the spinal cord destroys several clinically important areas and produces a Brown-Séquard syndrome. Although most often a lesion is partial or incomplete, this syndrome is very instructive for applying concepts of neuroanatomy. In destroying a left or right half of the cord, numerous structures that are tested during a neurologic examination are involved. These are UMNs (located in the white matter), LMNs (located in the ventral horn), the clinically important ascending tracts (the dorsal column of the DC-ML and the spinothalamic tract), and the entry zone of afferent fibers and the dorsal horn (Fig. 9-21). Thus the following signs and symptoms (some of which are ipsilateral to and some contralateral to the side of the lesion) are seen at and below the level of the lesion (Fig. 9-22).

Motor assessment of cord hemisection

◆ Lower motor neuron lesion signs (e.g., fasciculations and flaccidity) are seen in the ipsilateral muscles in-nervated by the nerves originating in the lesioned cord segments.
◆ Upper motor neuron lesion signs (e.g., hyperreflexia, Babinski sign) are seen in the ipsilateral muscles innervated by the nerves originating from cord segments below the level of the lesion. Note that for UMN lesion signs to occur, the LMNs must be functioning.

Sensory assessment of cord hemisection

◆ Signs resulting from the loss of DC-ML functions are present ipsilaterally and below the level of the lesion. This includes loss of discriminating abilities (two-point touch, stereognosis, graphesthesia) and impaired joint position sense and vibratory sense. (Some patients with dorsal column lesions also experience increased sensitivity to pain, temperature, and even tickling [Nathan, Smith, & Cook, 1986].)
◆ Because of the interruption of the spinothalamic tract in the anterolateral quadrant, pain and temperature sense is lost on the contralateral side from approximately one or two segments below the level of the lesion.
◆ On the ipsilateral side and at the level of the lesion, anesthesia is present in a dermatomal pattern. In addition, because of the overlapping of adjacent dermatomes, hypesthesia and paresthesia are present ipsilaterally in dermatomal areas adjacent to the lesioned segments. Also, at the level of the lesion and depending on the number of cord segments involved, there is usually some contralateral impairment of pain and temperature because of the interruption of the decussating fibers that originate from the contralateral side.
◆ Little or no impairment of light (crude) touch exists, since this modality ascends in both the spinothalamic and the DC-ML tracts.

In localizing the site of the pathologic conditions, the UMN lesion signs are indicative of a CNS lesion, and the characteristic features of ipsilateral loss of discriminatory touch, vibration, and joint position sense and contralateral loss of pain and temperature suggest a hemisection of the spinal cord.

Syringomyelia. Syringomyelia is the progressive destruction of the central parts of the spinal cord as a result of the formation of a cavity (syrinx) in the region of the central canal (Figs. 9-23 and 9-24). As the cavity enlarges ventrally (into the ventral white commissure), it disrupts the decussating spinothalamic fibers (Fig. 9-24). This results in bilateral segmental loss of pain and temperature, with other sensory modalities spared. This condition is called sensory dissociation. The lesion may extend into the ventral horn, at which time it affects LMNs, producing atrophy, impaired reflexes, and weakness. The syrinx may even extend into adjacent white matter, affecting descending tracts. The lesion may not be

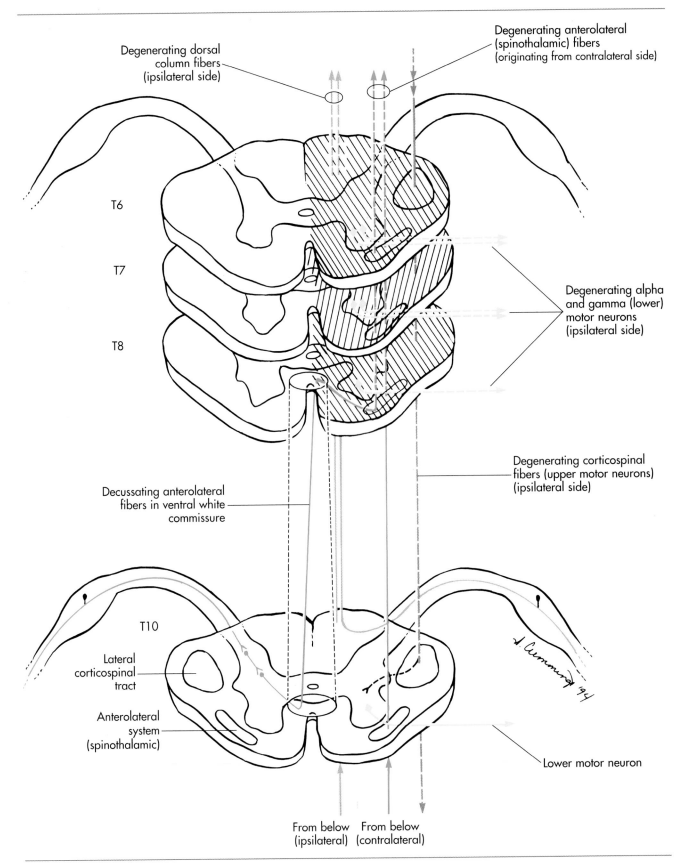

FIG. 9-21 Brown-Séquard syndrome. Hemisection of the spinal cord *(diagonal lines)* located in cord segments T6 through T8. The corticospinal tract *(green),* spinothalamic tract *(red),* dorsal column fibers *(blue),* and lower motor neurons *(yellow)* have been lesioned in those cord segments. The degenerating fibers are shown *(dashed lines).*

symmetric and may vary in size from one segment to the next. Syringomyelia occurring in cervical segments and affecting the upper extremities is most common, and half of patients affected also have associated Arnold-Chiari malformation (inferior displacement of the cerebellar tonsils) (Adams & Salam-Adams, 1991).

Amyotrophic Lateral Sclerosis. Amyotrophic lateral sclerosis (ALS, or Lou Gehrig's disease) is a progressive and degenerative motor neuron disease. It affects LMNs in the ventral horn, producing LMN signs in the affected muscles (atrophy, fasciculations, weakness, etc.). It also causes degeneration of upper motor neurons, and a Babinski sign may be present, as well as hyperreflexia and paralysis. Both types of motor neurons may be affected bilaterally. In addition to affecting skeletal muscles of the extremities and trunk, ALS causes degeneration of LMNs of the cranial nerves that innervate muscles of the face, pharynx, larynx, and tongue and may lead to serious problems of swallowing and breathing. A distinctive characteristic of this disease is that sensory functions are not impaired.

Combined Systems Disease. Combined systems disease is the combined bilateral degeneration of the dorsal white columns and the lateral white columns of the spinal cord. It is relatively rare and is usually associated with pernicious anemia (subacute combined degeneration). Pernicious anemia is caused by the inability to absorb vitamin B_{12} because of a lack of intrinsic factor. Combined systems disease begins with paresthesias in the hands and arms, followed by sensory ataxia as the dorsal columns of the lumbosacral cord become involved. As the disease progresses, UMN lesion signs appear, such as the Babinski sign and hyperreflexia. Peripheral nerves also may be involved; however, the symptoms are masked by those produced by the CNS lesions. Combined systems disease is treatable by the administration of weekly doses of vitamin B_{12} (cobalamin) (Adams & Salam-Adams, 1991).

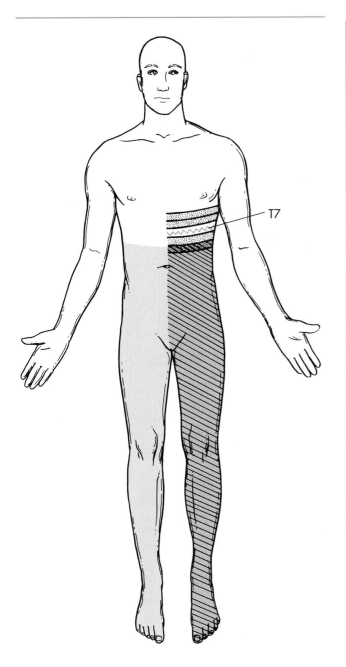

FIG. 9-22 Regions of the body affected by a hemisection (Brown-Séquard syndrome) of cord segments T6 through T8 as illustrated in Fig. 9-21. The T7 dermatome *(red)* is a zone of anesthesia. Because of the overlapping between adjacent dermatomes, an area of hypesthesia and paresthesia exists *(stippled area)* on both sides of the T7 dermatome. Loss of pain and temperature sense *(blue)* occurs contralaterally below the level of the lesion. Impaired joint position sense and vibratory sense and loss of discriminatory abilities occur ipsilaterally below the level of the lesion *(light green)*. Upper motor neuron lesions signs *(diagonal lines)* are present in muscles innervated by neurons originating in cord segments ipsilateral to and below the level of the lesion. Lower motor neuron signs are present in muscles innervated by neurons originating in the lesioned cord segments.

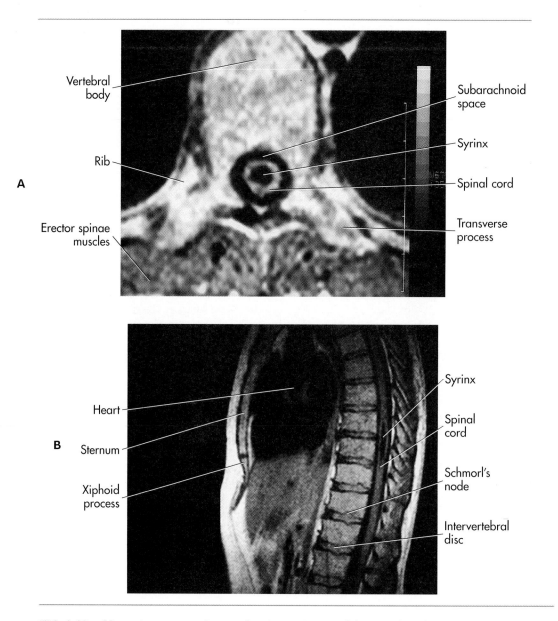

FIG. 9-23   Magnetic resonance images showing cavitation of the spinal cord resulting in syringomyelia. **A,** Horizontal section. **B,** Midsagittal section.

Acquired Immunodeficiency Syndrome. Acquired immunodeficiency syndrome (AIDS) is caused by the human immunodeficiency virus type I (HIV-I). In addition to systemic disorders, AIDS patients may also have neurologic components. In fact, HIV-I has been located in the brains, cerebrospinal fluid (Sharer, 1992), and spinal cords (Eilbott et al., 1989; Weiser et al., 1990) of AIDS patients. Researchers have reached general agreement at this time that the monocyte/macrophage cell line is infected. The pathologic condition seen in the spinal cord is referred to as vacuolar myelopathy and is characterized by vacuoles infiltrated by macrophages in the dorsal and lateral white columns. When first described by

Goldstick, Mandybur, & Bode (1985), the histopathologic resemblance to combined systems disease was noticed. However, Petito and colleagues (1985) found that the 20 patients they studied had no deficiency in cobalamin (vitamin B_{12}). Although variable, patients with vacuolar myelopathy have spasticity and leg weakness (often paraplegia), ataxia, incontinence, and sensory deficits (Adams & Salam-Adams, 1991; Sharer, 1992). Postmortem studies have shown that the average incidence of vacuolar myelopathy in HIV-I patients is 20% to 30%. Children with the HIV-I infection rarely exhibit this condition (Sharer, 1992).

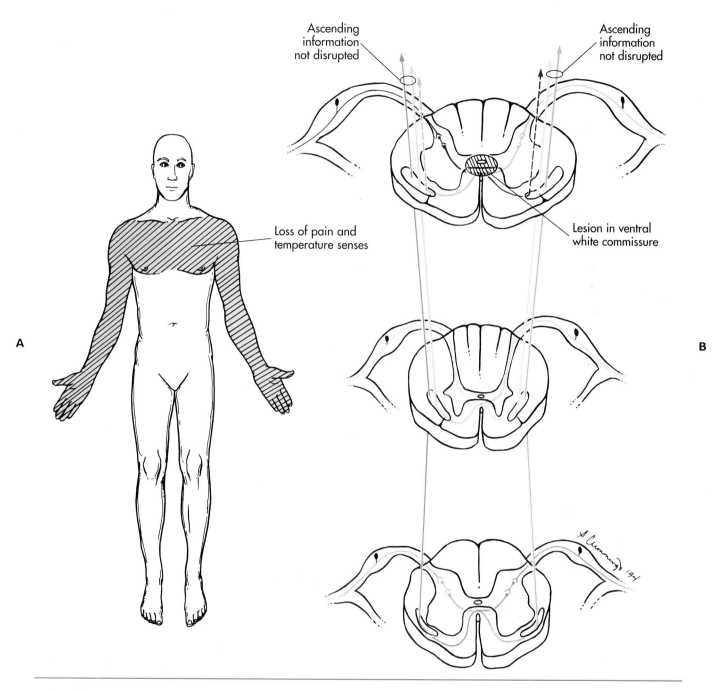

FIG. 9-24 Pain and temperature deficit seen in a "shawl-like" distribution that is characteristic of syringomyelia. The purple and orange areas correspond to the lesioned fibers illustrated in **B**. **B**, Three spinal cord cross sections. The top cross section represents spinal cord segments where cavitation has resulted in syringomyelia. The diagonal lines indicate the lesioned area, which includes the ventral white commissure, where pain and temperature fibers from both sides of the body decussate. These lesioned fibers *(dashed lines)* are colored purple and orange. Ascending information entering the spinal cord below the lesion ascends in axons *(red, green, yellow, blue)* that are not disrupted.

REFERENCES

Abrahams, V.C. (1989). The distribution of muscle and cutaneous projections to the dorsal horn of the upper cervical cord of the cat. In F. Cervero, G.J. Bennett, & P.M. Headley (Eds.), *Processing of sensory information in the superficial dorsal horn of the spinal cord.* New York: Plenum Press.

Adams, R.D. & Salam-Adams, M. (1991). Chronic nontraumatic diseases of the spinal cord. *Neurol Clin, 9* (3), 605-623.

Adams, R.D. & Victor, M. (1989). *Principles of neurology* (4th ed.). St Louis: McGraw-Hill.

Barr, M.L. & Kiernan, J.A. (1993). *The human nervous system* (6th ed.). Philadelphia: JB Lippincott.

Bentivoglio, M. & Rustioni, A. (1986). Corticospinal neurons with branching axons to the dorsal column nuclei in the monkey. *J Comp Neurol, 253,* 260-276.

Bessou, P., Emonet-Demand, F., & Laporte, Y. (1965). Motor fibers innervating extrafusal and intrafusal muscle fibers in the cat. *J Physiol Lond, 180,* 649-672.

Brooks, V.B. (1986). *The neural basis of motor control.* New York: Oxford University Press.

Bucy, P.C., Keplinger, J.E., & Siqueira, E.B. (1964). Destruction of the "pyramidal tract" in man. *J Neurol, 21,* 385-398.

Carpenter, M.B. (1991). *Core text of neuroanatomy* (4th ed.). Baltimore: Williams & Wilkins.

Carpenter, M.B. & Sutin, J. (1983). *Human neuroanatomy* (8th ed.). Baltimore: Williams & Wilkins.

Coulter, J.D. et al. (1979). Cortical, tectal and medullary descending pathways to the cervical spinal cord. *Prog Brain Res, 50,* 263-279.

Daube, J.R. et al. (1986). *Medical neurosciences* (2nd ed.). Boston: Little, Brown.

Davidoff, R.A. & Hackman, J.C. (1991). Aspects of spinal cord structure and reflex function. *Neurol Clin, 9* (3), 533-550.

deGroot, J. & Chusid, J.G. (1988). *Correlative neuroanatomy* (20th ed.). Norwalk, Conn: Appleton & Lange.

DeMyer, W. (1959). Number of axons and myelin sheaths in adult human medullary pyramids. *Neurology, 9,* 42-47.

Eilbott, D.J. et al. (1989). Human immunodeficiency virus type I in spinal cords of acquired immunodeficiency syndrome patients with myelopathy: Expression and replication in macrophages. *Proc Natl Acad Sci, 86,* 3337-3341.

Ekerot, C.F., Larson, B., & Oscarsson, O. (1979). Information carried by the spinocerebellar paths. *Prog Brain Res, 50,* 79-90.

Forssberg, H., Grillner, S., & Sjöström, A. (1975). Phase dependent reflex reversal during walking in chronic spinal cats. *Brain Res, 85,* 103-107.

Ghez, C. (1991a). The control of movement. In E.R. Kandel, J.H. Schwartz, & T.M. Jessell (Eds.), *Principles of neural science* (3rd ed.). New York: Elsevier.

Ghez, C. (1991b). Posture. In E.R. Kandel, J.H. Schwartz, & T.M. Jessell (Eds.), *Principles of neural science* (3rd ed.). New York: Elsevier.

Gilman, S. (1969). The mechanism of cerebellar hypotonia: An experimental study in the monkey. *Brain, 92,* 621-638.

Goldstick, L., Mandybur, T.I., & Bode, R. (1985). Spinal cord degeneration in AIDS. *Neurology, 35,* 103-106.

Gordon, J. (1991). Spinal mechanisms of motor coordination. In E.R. Kandel, J.H. Schwartz, & T.M. Jessell (Eds.), *Principles of neural science* (3rd ed.). New York: Elsevier.

Grant, G. & Xu, Q. (1988). Routes of entry into the cerebellum of spinocerebellar axons from the lower part of the spinal cord. *Exp Brain Res, 72,* 543-561.

Grillner, S. (1975). Locomotion in vertebrates: Central mechanisms and reflex interaction. *Physiol Rev, 55,* 247-306.

Grillner, S. & Zangger, P. (1975). How detailed is the central pattern generator for locomotion? *Brain Res, 88,* 367-371.

Henneman, E., Somjen, G., & Carpenter, D.O. (1965). Functional significance of cell size in spinal motoneurons. *J Neurophysiol, 28,* 560-580.

Hodge, Jr., C.J. & Apkarian, A.V. (1990). The spinothalamic tract. *Crit Rev Neurobiol, 5*(4), 363-397.

Houk, J. & Henneman, E. (1967). Responses of Golgi tendon organs to active contraction of the soleus muscle of the cat. *J Neurophysiol, 30,* 466-481.

Hubbard, D.R. & Berkoff, G.M. (1993). Myofascial trigger points show spontaneous needle EMG activity. *Spine, 18*(13), 1803-1807.

Hunt, C.C. (1990). Mammalian muscle spindles: Peripheral mechanism. *Physiol Rev, 70,* 643-663.

Jami, L. (1992). Golgi tendon organs in mammalian skeletal muscle: Functional properties and central actions. *Physiol Rev, 72,* 623-666.

Jessell, T.M. & Kelly, D.D. (1991). Pain and analgesia. In E.R. Kandel, J.H. Schwartz, & T.M. Jessell (Eds.), *Principles of neural science* (3rd ed.). New York: Elsevier.

Keegan, J.G. & Garrett, F.V. (1948). The segmental distribution of the cutaneous nerves in the limbs of man. *Anat Rec, 102,* 409-437.

Kelly, J.P. (1991). The sense of balance. In E.R. Kandel, J.H. Schwartz, & T.M. Jessell (Eds.), *Principles of neural science* (3rd ed.). New York: Elsevier.

Kuypers, H.G. (1981). Anatomy of the descending pathways. In V.B. Brooks (Ed.), *Handbook of physiology, section 1, vol II, part 1.* Bethesda, Md: American Physiological Society.

Lance, J.W. (1980). The control of muscle tone, reflexes, and movement: Robert Wartenberg Lecture. *Neurology, 30,* 1303-1313.

Lance, J.W. (1989). Headache: Classification, mechanism and principles of therapy, with particular reference to migraine. *Rec Prog Med, 80*(12), 673-680.

Leksell, L. (1945). The action potential and excitatory effects of the small ventral root fibers to skeletal muscle. *Acta Physiol Scand, 10*(suppl 31), 1-84.

Martin, J.H. & Jessell, T.M. (1991a). Anatomy of the somatic sensory system. In E.R. Kandel, J.H. Schwartz, & T.M. Jessell (Eds.), *Principles of neural science* (3rd ed.). New York: Elsevier.

Martin, J.H. & Jessell, T.M. (1991b). Modality coding in the somatic sensory system. In E.R. Kandel, J.H. Schwartz, & T.M. Jessell (Eds.), *Principles of neural science* (3rd ed.). New York: Elsevier.

Meyer, Jr., P.R. et al. (1991). Spinal cord injury. *Neurol Clin, 9*(3), 625-661.

Miyabayashi, T. & Shirai, T. (1988). Synaptic formation of the corticospinal tract in the rat spinal cord. *Okajimas Folia Anat Jpn, 65*(2-3), 117-140.

Nashner, L.M. (1976). Adapting reflexes controlling the human posture. *Exp Brain Res, 26,* 59-72.

Nathan, P.W. & Smith, M.C. (1982). The rubrospinal and central tegmental tracts in man. *Brain, 105,* 223-269.

Nathan, P.W., Smith, M.C., & Cook, A.W. (1986). Sensory effects in man of lesions of the posterior columns and of some other afferent pathways. *Brain, 109,* 1003-1041.

Nathan, P.W., Smith, M.C., & Deacon, P. (1990). The corticospinal tracts in man. *Brain, 113,* 303-324.

Noback, C.R., Strominger, N.L., & Demarest, R.J. (1991). *The human nervous system* (4th ed.). Philadelphia: Lea & Febiger.

Nolte, J. (1993). *The human brain* (3rd ed.). St. Louis: Mosby.

Palmieri, G. et al. (1986-1987). Course and termination of the pyramidal tract in the pig. *Arch d'Anat Micro, 75,* 167-176.

Paulson, G.W., Yates, A.J., & Paltan-Ortiz, J.D. (1986). Does infarction of the medullary pyramid lead to spasticity? *Arch Neurol, 43,* 93-95.

Petito, C.K. et al. (1985). Vacuolar myelopathy pathologically resembling subacute combined degeneration in patients with the acquired immunodeficiency syndrome. *N Engl J Med, 312,* 874-879.

Rexed, B. (1952). The cytoarchitectonic organization of the spinal cord in the cat. *J Comp Neurol, 96,* 415-495.

Schoenen, J. (1991). Clinical anatomy of the spinal cord. *Neurol Clin, 9*(3), 503-532.

Severin, F.V., Orlovsky, G.N., & Shik, M.L. (1967). Work of the muscle receptors during controlled locomotion. *Biofizika, 12,* 575-586.

Sharer, L.R. (1992). Pathology of HIV-I infection of the central nervous system: A review. *J Neuropathol Exp Neurol, 51*(1), 3-11.

Smith, M.C. & Deacon, P. (1984). Topographical anatomy of the posterior columns of the spinal cord in man. *Brain, 107,* 671-698.

Snell, R.S. (1992). *Clinical neuroanatomy for medical students* (3rd ed.). Boston: Little, Brown.

Weiser, B. et al. (1990). Human immunodeficiency virus type I expression in the central nervous system correlates directly with extent of disease. *Proc Natl Acad Sci, 87,* 3997-4001.

Williams, P.L. et al. (1989). *Gray's anatomy* (37th ed.). Edinburgh: Churchill Livingstone.

Willis, Jr., W.D. & Coggeshall, R.E. (1991). *Sensory mechanisms of the spinal cord* (2nd ed.). New York: Plenum Press.

Wise, S.P. & Evarts, E.V. (1981). The role of the cerebral cortex in movement, *TINS, Dec,* 297-300.

Wyke, B.D. (1985). Articular neurology and manipulative therapy. In E.F. Glasgow et al. (Eds.), *Aspects of manipulative therapy* (2nd ed.). New York: Churchill Livingstone.

Xu, Q. & Grant, G. (1988). Collateral projections of neurons from the lower part of the spinal cord to anterior and posterior cerebellar termination areas. *Exp Brain Res, 72,* 562-576.

Young, P.A. (1986). The anatomy of the spinal cord pain paths: A review. *J Am Paraplegia Soc, 9,* 28-38.

CHAPTER 10

Neuroanatomy of the Autonomic Nervous System

Susan A. Darby

The autonomic nervous system (ANS) functions to maintain homeostasis by providing the optimal internal environment for the cellular components of the organism during normal and stressful periods. The ANS accomplishes this task through its control of visceral function, and it is generally considered to be a motor system consisting of fibers that innervate the smooth muscle, cardiac muscle, and glands of the body. However, sophisticated neuroanatomic techniques, such as immunocytochemistry and axonal tracing methods, have produced data indicating that visceral control involves much more than the efferents of the sympathetic and parasympathetic divisions of the ANS. Recent information suggests that other structures and regions are intimately associated with these efferents. These include visceral afferent fibers and the reflexes they may initiate, the widespread influence and variety of chemical mediators, and the central autonomic circuitry, which is involved with the integration and dissemination of visceral input. Therefore, each of these topics is generally described along with the origin and course of the sympathetic and parasympathetic efferent fibers to present a composite picture of the ANS. The chapter concludes with examples of pathologies that affect the ANS.

AUTONOMIC EFFERENTS—SYMPATHETIC, PARASYMPATHETIC, AND ENTERIC DIVISIONS

The ANS is composed of a sympathetic division and a parasympathetic division. These two divisions are discussed here, followed by a description of a third division of the ANS. This third division is the enteric nervous system, which is a complex network of neurons located within the wall of the gut.

The ANS can best be described after certain characteristics common to both the sympathetic and the parasympathetic divisions have been reviewed. The parasympathetic and sympathetic innervation of autonomic effectors (organs, vessels, glands) is organized differently than the innervation of skeletal muscle (Fig. 10-1). Although the axons of alpha and gamma motor neurons course directly to skeletal muscles, the innervation of ANS effectors requires a chain of two neurons (Fig. 10-1). These two neurons are called the preganglionic and postganglionic neurons. The cell body of the preganglionic neuron is always located in the central nervous system (CNS); either in the spinal cord or in the brain stem (Fig. 10-2). The axon is thinly myelinated and immediately leaves the CNS within a specific ventral root of the spinal cord or within certain cranial nerves exiting the brain stem. The cell body of the postganglionic neuron is located in an autonomic ganglion that may be found in numerous places outside the CNS (Fig. 10-2). The preganglionic neuron synapses with the postganglionic neuron within this ganglion. The axon of the postganglionic neuron is unmyelinated and innervates the effector. Both the preganglionic and the postganglionic neurons frequently travel in components of the peripheral nervous system (PNS) (spinal nerves, cranial nerves) and are intermingled with afferents and somatic motor neurons of peripheral nerves. Most effectors are

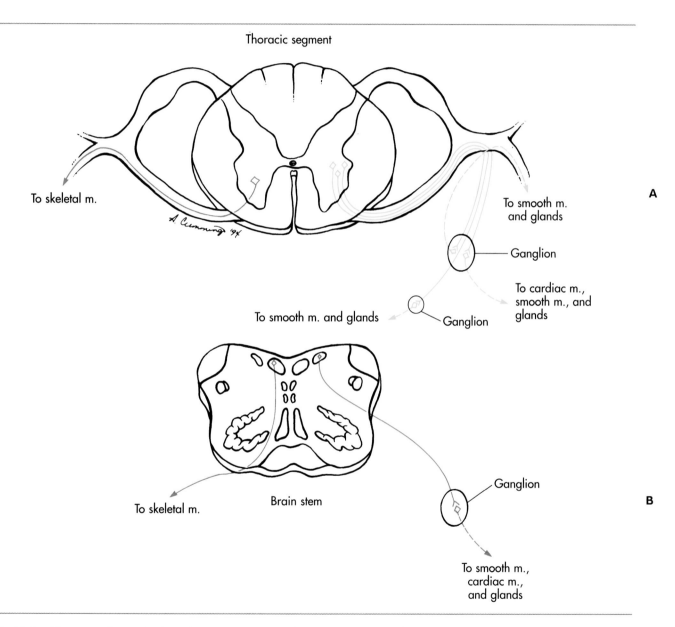

FIG. 10-1 The general organization of autonomic preganglionic *(solid line)* and postganglionic *(dashed line)* neurons *(right)* compared to somatic efferent neurons *(left).* **A,** Sympathetic output and somatic output from the spinal cord. **B,** Parasympathetic output and somatic output from the brain stem.

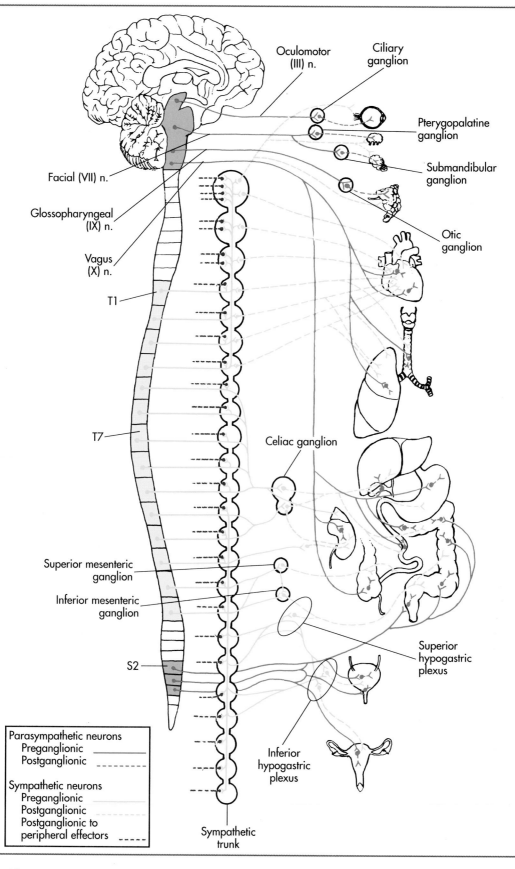

FIG. 10-2 The parasympathetic and sympathetic divisions of the autonomic nervous system. Preganglionic neuron cell bodies are located in the brain stem and sacral cord segments (parasympathetic or "cranio-sacral" division) and thoracic and upper lumbar cord segments (sympathetic or "thoraco-lumbar" division). The axons of these neurons synapse with postganglionic neurons, which course to the smooth muscle, cardiac muscle, and glands of the body. The postganglionic neuron cell bodies may be located in distinct autonomic ganglia, or in or very near the wall of the innervated visceral organ.

innervated by both sympathetic and parasympathetic fibers (Fig. 10-2 and Table 10-1). These fibers produce antagonistic but coordinated responses in the effectors. Descending input from higher integrative centers such as the hypothalamus and areas of the brain stem reaches the cell bodies of preganglionic fibers to regulate and adjust their activity. This descending input is a part of several specific visceral reflex pathways and is also used by higher centers to institute widespread bodily changes.

Sympathetic Division

The general function of the sympathetic nervous system (SNS) is to help the body cope with stressful situations. The response is usually the rapid release, and subsequent use, of energy. This is best exemplified by the reaction of the body to a dangerous situation. In this instance, sympathetic involuntary responses occur, including increased heart and respiratory rates, cold and clammy hands, wide-eyed stare, and dilated pupils. Blood is redistributed by means of vasoconstriction and vasodilation from such areas as the abdominal and pelvic organs and skin, to more important tissues such as the brain, heart, and skeletal muscles. The level of blood glucose increases, as does blood pressure. Activity of the gastrointestinal (GI) and urinary systems is less important during this stressful situation, and therefore the smooth muscle of these organs is inhibited. Because of this overall response, the sympathetic division is often referred to as the fight-or-flight division of the ANS.

Preganglionic Sympathetic Neurons. The cell bodies of the preganglionic sympathetic neurons are located in the spinal cord in all thoracic segments and in the upper two or three lumbar segments (Fig. 10-2). Because of the distribution of these preganglionic cell bodies, the sympathetic division of the ANS is often referred to as the thoracolumbar division. These preganglionic neurons comprise a heterogeneous population within the spinal cord. The dendritic arrangement of these neurons ranges from simple to complex arborizations. The cell bodies are of different shapes, and their size falls in a range between the size of smaller dorsal horn neurons and larger somatic motor neurons. Of the total membranous surface area of these neurons, the cell body of each composes a maximum of 15%, which likely indicates the importance of the dendritic surface area of that neuron (Cabot, 1990).

The cell bodies of the preganglionic neurons are found in four nuclei within the intermediate gray matter of the spinal cord (Cabot, 1990). The largest group of these cell bodies is the intermediolateral (IML) cell column that forms the lateral horn. Throughout this column are clusters of 20 to 100 neurons that are separated by distances ranging from 200 to 500 μm in the thoracic

Table 10-1 Functions of the Sympathetic and Parasympathetic Divisions

Structure	Sympathetic function	Parasympathetic function
Eye		
Pupil	Dilates	Constricts
Ciliary muscle	Relaxes (slightly; far vision)	Contracts (near vision)
Heart		
Rate	Increases	Decreases
Force of ventricular contraction	Increases	Decreases
Lungs		
Bronchi	Dilates	Constricts
Glands		Stimulates secretion
Skin		
Sweat glands	Increases secretion (cholinergic)	—
Arrector pili muscle	Contracts	
Glands of head		
Lacrimal	Reduces secretion	Increases secretion
Salivary	Secretion reduced and viscid	Secretion increased and watery
Arteries		
Skin	Constricts	—
Coronary	Constricts (alpha receptors) and dilates (beta receptors)	Dilates
Bronchial	Constricts	—
Abdominal	Constricts	—
Skeletal muscle	Constricts (alpha receptors) and dilates (beta receptors)	—
Gastrointestinal tract		
Motility/tone	Inhibits	Stimulates
Sphincters	Constricts	Relaxes
Secretion	Inhibits	Stimulates
Liver	Breaks down glycogen (glycogenolysis)	—
Gallbladder	Relaxes	Contracts
Urinary bladder		
Detrusor muscle	Little or no role in micturition	Contracts
Sphincter (nonstriated)		Relaxes
Sex organs	Contracts smooth muscle (ejaculation)	Erection
	Vasoconstriction	Vasodilation
Adrenal medulla	Stimulates secretion	—

region and 100 to 300 μm in the lumbar region. The cell bodies are approximately 12 to 13 μm in diameter and histologically are similar to motor neurons (Harati, 1993). The diameters of the axons range from 2 to 5 μm, and their speed of conduction is about 3 to 15 m per second. These fibers are often classified in the B group (see Chapter 9). At the T6 and T7 levels, the mean number of these cells is about 5000, but it has been shown that the number decreases with age at the rate of about 8% per decade (Harati, 1993).

The other three nuclear groups of preganglionic neurons have been described by Cabot (1990) and are the lateral funicular area (located lateral and dorsal to the intermediolateral group), the intercalated cell group (located medial to the IML column and possibly the same cluster of neurons typically referred to as the intermediomedial group), and the central autonomic nucleus (located lateral and dorsal to the central canal). In longitudinal sections the combination of these groups forms a ladderlike structure in which the paired IML cell columns form the sides of the ladder and the interconnected central autonomic nucleus and intercalated cell group form the rungs (Fig. 10-3). Although the anatomic characteristics of these four nuclei have been described, the functions still remain unclear.

Postganglionic Sympathetic Neurons. According to the general rule of organization of the ANS, two neurons are necessary for the impulse to reach the effector. One is the preganglionic neuron, which has just been briefly discussed. The second neuron in the pathway to an autonomic effector is the postganglionic neuron. This neuron's axon is classified as a group C fiber (see Chapter 9). It is generally described as unmyelinated, with a diameter ranging from 0.3 to 1.3 μm and a slow conduction speed ranging from 0.7 to 2.3 m per second (Carpenter & Sutin, 1983). The cell body is located outside the CNS in an autonomic ganglion. Unlike a sensory ganglion of cranial nerves and a dorsal root ganglion of spinal nerves where no synapses occur, an autonomic

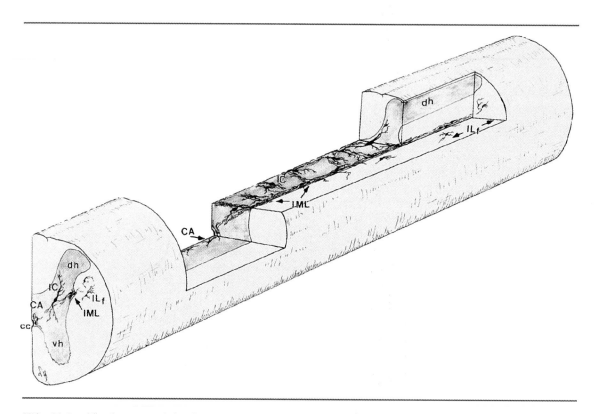

FIG. 10-3   The location of the four groups of sympathetic preganglionic neurons within the spinal cord gray matter. In the middle of the spinal cord, the horizontal plane shows the "ladderlike" arrangement of these neurons (*IL_f,* lateral funicular nucleus; *IML,* intermediolateral nucleus; *IC,* intercalated nucleus; *CA,* central autonomic nucleus; *dh,* dorsal horn; *vh,* ventral horn; *cc,* central canal.) (From Cabot, J.B. [1990]. Sympathetic preganglionic neurons: Cytoarchitecture, ultrastructure, and biophysical properties. In A.D. Loewy and K.M. Spyer [Eds.], *Central regulation of autonomic functions.* New York: Oxford University Press.)

ganglion is the location of the synapse between the preganglionic neuron and the postganglionic neuron. Preganglionic fibers disseminate their information by diverging and synapsing on numerous postganglionic fibers. This principle of divergence is based on studies of the superior cervical ganglion of mammals. Results of different studies show preganglionic to postganglionic ratios of 1:4 (Loewy, 1990a), 1:15 to 1:20, and 1:176 (Williams et al., 1989). (The parasympathetic division has also been found to exhibit divergence, but to a lesser degree.) This divergence may allow the effects of sympathetic stimulation to be more widespread throughout the body and to be of greater magnitude.

The autonomic ganglion in which the synapse occurs may be one of a chain of ganglia (referred to as the sympathetic chain, sympathetic trunk, or paravertebral ganglia) located near the vertebral bodies of the spinal column, or it may be a prevertebral ganglion (see Fig. 10-2) found within one of the autonomic nerve plexuses. These plexuses surround the large arteries in the abdominal and pelvic cavities. Regardless of location, the ganglion is encapsulated by connective tissue. The connective tissue capsule is continuous with the epineurium of the bundle of entering preganglionic neurons and the bundle of exiting postganglionic neurons. Within the capsule are multipolar postganglionic neurons. These neurons consist of cell bodies that have diameters ranging from 20 to 60 μm and dendrites that branch in a complex pattern. Surrounding the cell bodies and dendrites are satellite cells that are similar to those found in the dorsal root ganglia. Other cells, referred to as small intensely fluorescent cells (SIFs), are present singly or in clusters. These latter cells release the neurotransmitter dopamine and may function as interneurons connecting the preganglionic and postganglionic cells (Carpenter & Sutin, 1983; Harati, 1993; Williams et al., 1989).

Sympathetic Trunk. Two sympathetic trunks are located in the body, each of which lies on the anterolateral side of the vertebral column (Fig. 10-4). They both extend from the base of the skull to the coccyx. Because they lie next to the vertebral column, the ganglia of the sympathetic trunks are also called the paravertebral ganglia. Inferiorly the two trunks join in the midline and terminate on the anterior surface of the coccyx as the ganglion impar.

Each sympathetic trunk shares important anatomic relationships with surrounding structures. In the neck it lies between the carotid sheath and the prevertebral muscles, which cover the transverse processes (TPs) of the cervical vertebrae. It is found anterior to the heads of the ribs in the thorax, anterolateral to the bodies of the lumbar vertebrae in the abdomen, and medial to the anterior sacral foramina in the pelvis (Williams et al., 1989). As the name sympathetic chain ganglia implies,

this structure consists of 22 ganglia that are linked together by connective tissue surrounding ascending and descending fibers. The total number of ganglia does not correspond exactly to the number of spinal nerves because some of the ganglia have fused with one another. This fusion is most evident in the cervical region, where there are only three cervical ganglia. The thoracic portion of the sympathetic trunk includes 10 to 12 ganglia (70% of the time there are 11), the lumbar region exhibits 4 ganglia, and 4 or 5 ganglia appear in the sacral region of the trunk. The union of the two sympathetic trunks forms the one coccygeal ganglion.

The preganglionic fibers exit the spinal cord in the ventral roots of cord segments T1 to L2 or L3 to reach the postganglionic neurons. Therefore, at these particular levels, the ventral roots include both preganglionic sympathetic fibers and fibers to skeletal muscle, that is, alpha and gamma motor neurons. The preganglionic fibers continue into the spinal nerve, and at the division of the spinal nerve into its dorsal and ventral rami (posterior and anterior primary divisions, respectively), the myelinated preganglionic fibers exit, forming the white (myelin is a white substance) ramus communicans, and then continue into the sympathetic trunk. (There are only 14 or 15 white rami because there are only 14 or 15 spinal cord segments [T1 to L2-3] that provide preganglionic sympathetic fibers.)

The sympathetic system innervates autonomic effectors throughout the entire body. In general, cord segments T1 through T6 are involved with sympathetic innervation of autonomic effectors in the head, neck, upper extremities, and thorax. The cord segments from approximately T7 through L2 or L3 innervate the effectors in the lower extremities, abdominal cavity, and pelvic cavity. Recall that the sympathetic trunk is the location where synapses occur between preganglionic and postganglionic sympathetic fibers. Since the sympathetic trunk extends rostrally, adjacent to cervical vertebrae to reach the base of the skull, and caudally, adjacent to the sacrum to reach the coccyx, this trunk provides the means by which preganglionic fibers may ascend or descend to reach spinal nerves formed above or below the levels of T1 through L2 or L3. Once the preganglionic fibers pass through the white rami communicantes and enter the sympathetic trunk, they may proceed in different directions.

Autonomic fibers innervating peripheral blood vessels (including those in the skeletal muscles and in the skin), sweat glands, and arrector pili muscles of hair follicles travel in spinal nerves and subsequently peripheral nerves, to innervate the appropriate effectors. These effectors are located in the area of distribution of each of the peripheral nerves. After entering the sympathetic trunk, preganglionic fibers associated with these effectors do one of three things (Fig. 10-5): ascend to synapse

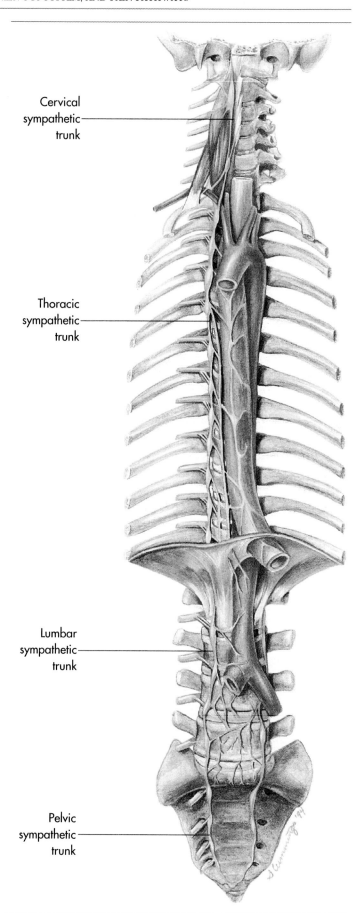

Cervical sympathetic trunk

Thoracic sympathetic trunk

Lumbar sympathetic trunk

Pelvic sympathetic trunk

FIG. 10-4 The sympathetic chain ganglia (trunk) and its anatomic location in the cervical region and in the thoracic, abdominal, and pelvic cavities. (For the sake of clarity, the left sympathetic trunk in the cervical and thoracic regions has been omitted.)

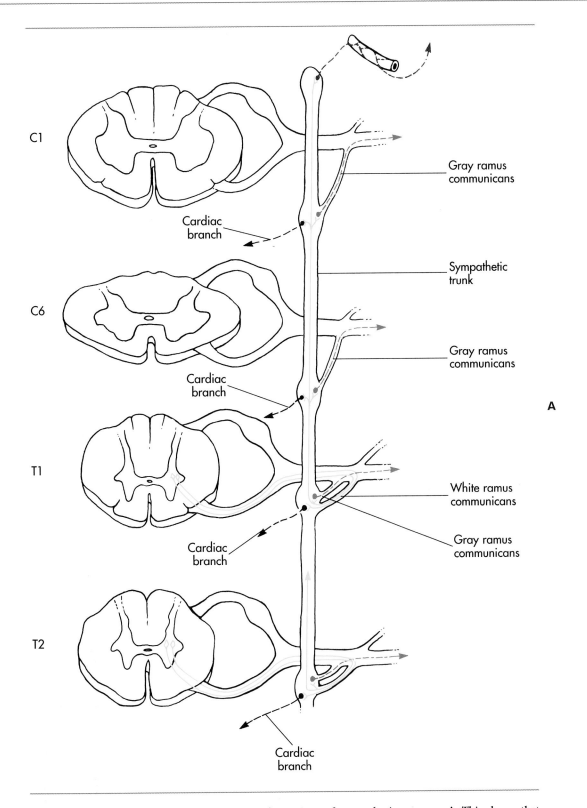

C1

Gray ramus
communicans

Cardiac
branch

Sympathetic
trunk

C6

Gray ramus
communicans

Cardiac
branch

A

T1

White ramus
communicans

Gray ramus
communicans

Cardiac
branch

T2

Cardiac
branch

FIG. 10-5 A diagrammatic scheme showing the options of sympathetic neurons. **A,** This shows that once preganglionic fibers *(yellow)* have entered the chain, they may: *ascend* to higher levels and synapse with postganglionic fibers that may enter gray rami *(blue)* or travel on blood vessels *(green)*; synapse in numerous ganglia with postganglionic neurons that leave the chain as cardiac branches *(black)*; synapse *at the level of entry* with postganglionic neurons that enter gray rami *(blue).*

Continued.

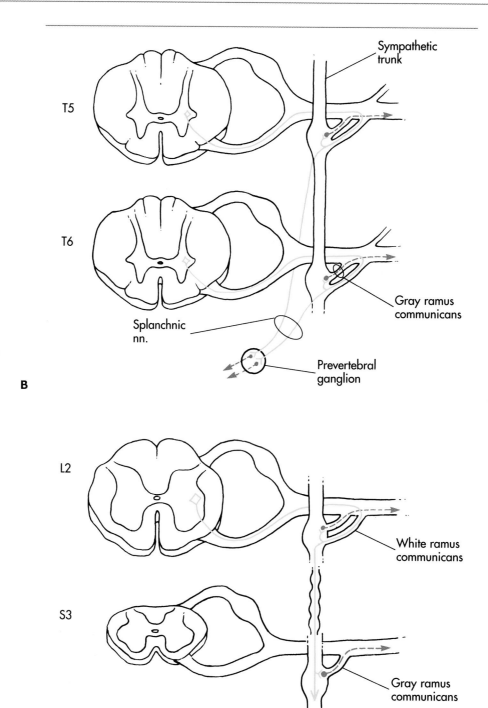

FIG. 10-5, cont'd. **B,** This shows that once preganglionic fibers *(yellow)* have entered the chain they may: synapse *at the level of entry* with postganglionic neurons that enter gray rami *(blue)*; *descend* to lower ganglia and synapse on postganglionic neurons that enter gray rami *(blue)*; pass through the chain *(purple)* without synapsing and travel to prevertebral ganglia, where they synapse with postganglionic neurons, the axons of which course to effectors in the abdominal and pelvic cavities.

with postganglionic neurons in ganglia above T1 (for cervical nerves); synapse with postganglionic neurons at the level of entry into the trunk, that is, T1 to L2 or L3 for those corresponding nerves; or descend to synapse with postganglionic neurons in ganglia below L2-3 (for lumbar and sacral nerves). From the sympathetic trunk the postganglionic fibers course through gray (these are unmyelinated fibers) rami communicantes (usually located proximal to the white rami), enter the spinal nerve at the location of its division into dorsal and ventral rami, and continue to the ANS effectors. Therefore the dorsal and ventral rami and subsequently formed peripheral nerves include sensory afferent fibers, motor neurons to skeletal muscle, and postganglionic sympathetic fibers. The ventral roots of T1 to L2-3 cord segments are unique in that they contain motor neurons to skeletal muscle and also preganglionic sympathetic fibers.

Sympathetic Preganglionic and Postganglionic Fibers. Sympathetic preganglionic fibers sending nerve impulses to effectors in the head enter the sympathetic trunk, ascend to the superior cervical ganglion, and synapse with postganglionic neurons. The postganglionic fibers course with large blood vessels to reach effectors located in the head region (Fig. 10-5, *A*). Such effectors include glands, the smooth muscle of blood vessels, and the smooth muscle of the eye. Some preganglionic fibers sending impulses to smooth muscle, cardiac muscle, and glands of the thorax ascend on entering the trunk and synapse at rostral levels, whereas others synapse with postganglionic fibers at the level of entry. These postganglionic fibers leave the chain as branches that merge with other nerve fibers, including parasympathetic vagal fibers, to form plexuses innervating the heart and lungs. Abdominal and pelvic effectors are innervated in a different manner than the effectors of the head, thorax, and cutaneous regions. Preganglionic fibers enter the sympathetic trunk via white rami communicantes but do not synapse in the chain ganglia. Instead, they pass through the chain ganglia and emerge as a collection of fibers called sympathetic splanchnic (referring to the viscera) nerves. These nerves course inferiorly in an anteromedial direction, pass through the diaphragm, and end in various prevertebral ganglia. Here they synapse on postganglionic neurons that then continue to the effectors of the abdominal and pelvic cavities (Fig. 10-5, *B*). The sympathetic prevertebral ganglia are enmeshed in plexuses of sympathetic and parasympathetic fibers and are located near large arteries found in the abdominal cavity. Examples are the celiac, superior mesenteric, aorticorenal, and inferior mesenteric ganglia.

On entering the sympathetic trunk, a preganglionic neuron may either ascend or descend and, in each case, subsequently synapse in more than one ganglion. A preganglionic neuron may also synapse at the entry level

and send collateral branches up or down to other ganglia. However, less than 2% of the neurons send a branch both up and down (Cabot, 1990). In all cases described thus far, a preganglionic neuron has synapsed with a postganglionic neuron. However, a notable exception is the innervation of the medulla of the adrenal gland. The adrenal medulla develops from the same embryonic neural crest as postganglionic neurons. Although the medullary chromaffin cells do not resemble postganglionic neurons in appearance, they do function in a similar manner. Preganglionic neurons innervate the medulla directly, which in turn releases epinephrine and some norepinephrine into the bloodstream. These neurotransmitters circulate throughout the body, stimulating effectors and assisting in the overall sympathetic response. A summary of the various sympathetic nerve pathways is provided in Fig. 10-6.

Specific Regions of the Sympathetic Trunk

Cervical sympathetic trunk. The fusion of the eight cervical ganglia results in three distinct ganglia in the region of the neck (Figs. 10-4, 10-7, *A,* and 10-8). These are known as the superior, middle, and cervicothoracic (stellate) ganglia. (Twenty percent of the time the T1 ganglion is separate, and then the cervicothoracic ganglion is referred to as the inferior cervical ganglion [Harati, 1993].) The superior ganglion (Figs. 10-7, *A*, 10-8, and 10-9, *A*) is the largest of the three and lies high in the neck adjacent to vertebrae C2 and C3, anterior to the longus capitis muscle and posterior to the cervical part of the internal carotid artery. It is also in the vicinity of the internal jugular vein and the glossopharyngeal, vagus, spinal accessory, and hypoglossal cranial nerves (Williams et al., 1989). The proximity of the ganglion to these nerves may account for the autonomic effects seen when these nerves are lesioned in this location (Cross, 1993b). The ganglion is formed by the fusion of the first four cervical ganglia, is 2.5 to 3.0 cm long, and includes more than 1 million neurons (Carpenter & Sutin, 1983; Harati, 1993; Williams et al., 1989). Postganglionic fibers leaving this ganglion course to various regions. Some ascend as perivascular plexuses on the internal and external carotid arteries. A large branch (internal carotid nerve) from the superior cervical ganglion ascends with the internal carotid artery and divides into branches that form the internal carotid plexus (Fig. 10-7, *A*) (Williams et al., 1989). This plexus continues to travel with that artery, and within the cranial cavity the fibers innervate the autonomic effectors. In addition, some are sympathetic vasoconstrictor fibers and innervate cerebral branches of the internal carotid artery. Other postganglionic fibers leave the ganglion as medial, lateral, and anterior branches and course directly to effectors. The lateral branches include gray rami that join the first four cervical spinal nerves. They travel with those

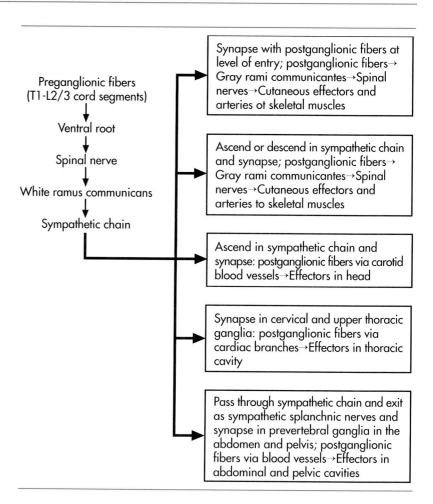

FIG. 10-6   Flow chart of pathways of the preganglionic and postganglionic sympathetic neurons.

spinal nerves to effectors in the areas of distribution of the nerves. The medial branches include laryngopharyngeal and cardiac branches. The anterior branches travel with the common and external carotid arteries. Fibers continue with branches of the external carotid artery to innervate such structures as the facial sweat glands by traveling with terminal branches of the trigeminal nerve (cranial nerve [CN] V) (Williams et al., 1989).

The middle cervical ganglion (Figs. 10-7, *A*, and 10-8), formed by the fusion of the C5 and C6 ganglia, is the smallest (0.7 to 0.8 cm), and sometimes may be absent. It lies adjacent to the C6 vertebra and near the inferior thyroid artery, which is a branch of the thyrocervical trunk. Postganglionic fibers include gray rami that enter the C5 and C6 spinal nerves (sometimes the fourth and seventh), thyroid branches, and the largest sympathetic cardiac branch. The ganglion is continuous with the cervicothoracic ganglion by anterior and posterior branches. Although there is variation to this connection, typically the posterior branch splits around the vertebral artery as it descends to the cervicothoracic ganglion; the anterior component descends and loops around the first part of the subclavian artery before connecting with the

cervicothoracic ganglion. This loop is called the ansa subclavius (Fig. 10-9, *B*).

The cervicothoracic (stellate) ganglion (Figs. 10-7, *A*, and 10-9, *B*) is formed by the fusion of the seventh, eighth, and first thoracic ganglia. It is approximately 2.8 cm long and is located between the base of the TP of C7 and the neck of the first rib. Some postganglionic fibers travel in gray rami communicantes to enter the C7, C8, and T1 spinal nerves, whereas others form a cardiac branch. Some other fibers form branches that course on the subclavian artery and its branches. One of these is large, and because it ascends with the vertebral artery (Fig. 10-7, *A*, and 10-9, *B*), it is frequently called the vertebral nerve (see Chapter 5 and Fig. 5-19). This nerve is joined by other branches and forms the vertebral plexus. This plexus travels into the cranial cavity on the artery and continues on the basilar artery, where it joins the internal carotid artery plexus. Some consider the vertebral plexus to be the major continuation of the sympathetic system into the cranium (Williams et al., 1989).

Although the cervical sympathetic chain has no white rami communicantes associated with it, numerous gray rami are present. As many as three gray rami may connect with each of the C5 to C8 spinal nerves (Carpenter

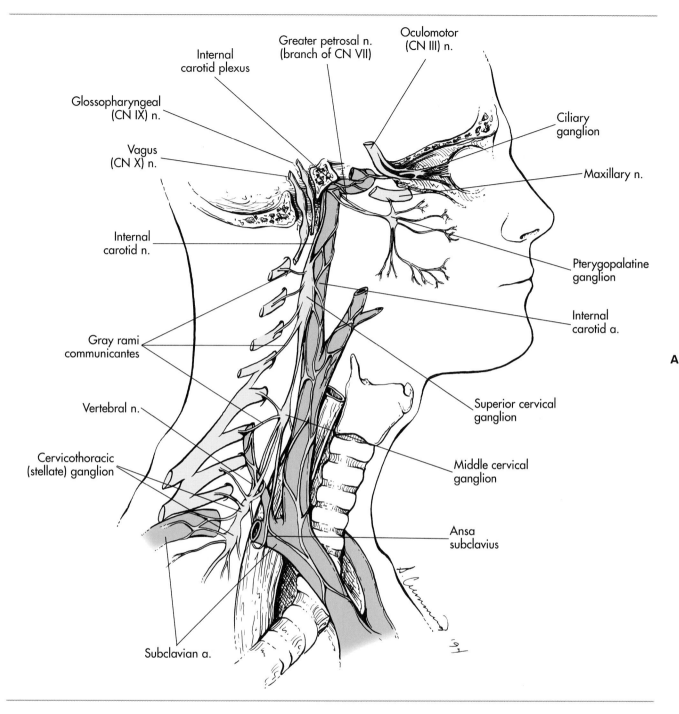

Internal
carotid plexus

Glossopharyngeal
(CN IX) n.

Greater petrosal n.
(branch of CN VII)

Oculomotor
(CN III) n.

Ciliary
ganglion

Maxillary n.

Vagus
(CN X) n.

Internal
carotid n.

Pterygopalatine
ganglion

Internal
carotid a.

Gray rami
communicantes

Vertebral n.

Superior cervical
ganglion

Cervicothoracic
(stellate) ganglion

Middle cervical
ganglion

Ansa
subclavius

Subclavian a.

A

FIG. 10-7   **A,** The cervical sympathetic trunk and the continuation of autonomic fibers to effectors in the head. Note the relationship of the superior cervical ganglion to the vagus and glossopharyngeal cranial nerves and the internal carotid artery. Gray (not white) rami communicantes course from the cervical chain to the cervical spinal nerves. Leaving the cervicothoracic ganglion is the vertebral nerve and plexus that travel with the vertebral artery. Fibers of some postganglionic neuron cell bodies located in the superior cervical ganglion initially form the internal carotid nerve, which travels with the internal carotid artery, and subsequently branches to form the internal carotid plexus. Fibers of other postganglionic neuron cell bodies located in the superior cervical ganglion course with branches of the external carotid artery. Note that postganglionic fibers leave the blood vessels and travel with branches of cranial nerves. On the way to their destination, the sympathetic fibers may pass through, but do not synapse in, parasympathetic ganglia (e.g., ciliary and pterygopalatine).

Continued.

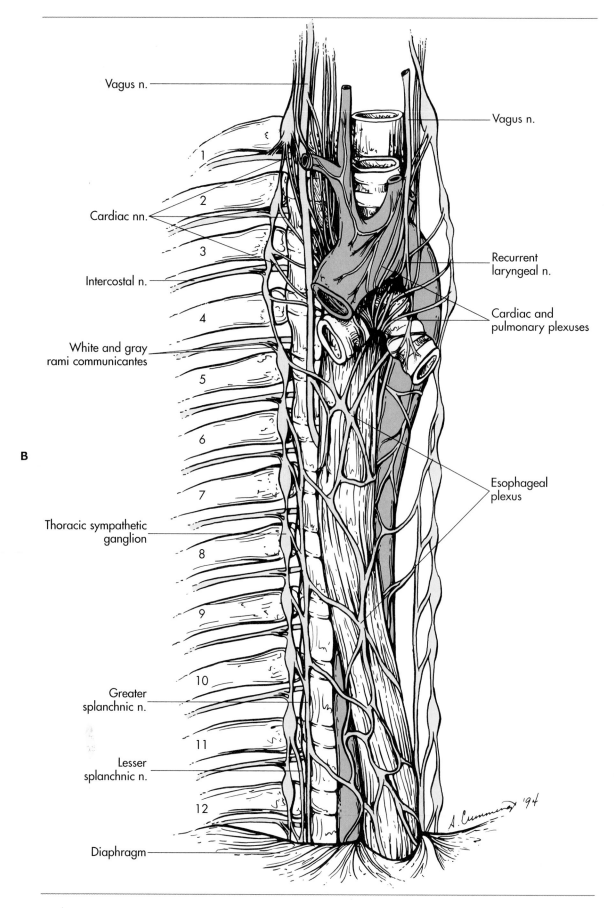

FIG. 10-7, cont'd.   B, The thoracic sympathetic trunk shows that gray (medial) and white (lateral) rami communicantes are present. Thoracic autonomic plexuses (e.g., cardiac, pulmonary, and esophageal), which are formed by postganglionic sympathetic fibers and vagal preganglionic fibers, are shown. Cardiac nerves and greater and lesser splanchnic nerves are also illustrated.

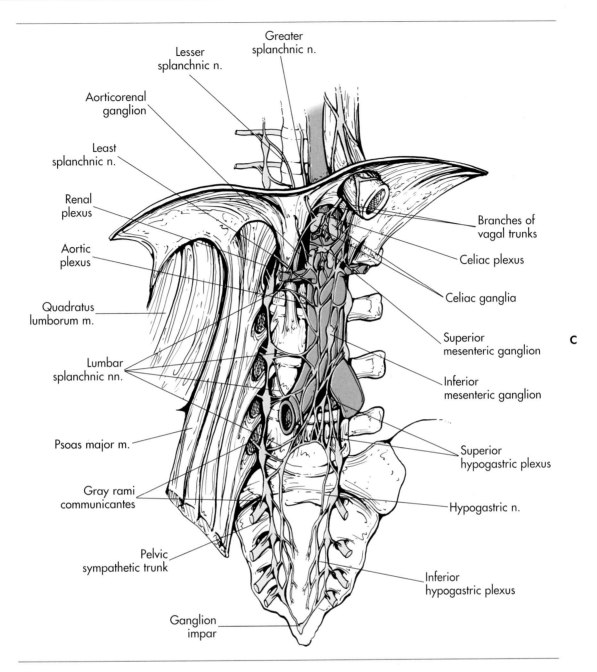

Greater
splanchnic n.

Lesser
splanchnic n.

Aorticorenal
ganglion

Least
splanchnic n.

Renal
plexus

Aortic
plexus

Quadratus
lumborum m.

Lumbar
splanchnic nn.

Psoas major m.

Gray rami
communicantes

Pelvic
sympathetic trunk

Ganglion
impar

Branches of
vagal trunks

Celiac plexus

Celiac ganglia

Superior
mesenteric ganglion

Inferior
mesenteric ganglion

Superior
hypogastric plexus

Hypogastric n.

Inferior
hypogastric plexus

C

FIG. 10-7, cont'd.   C, The lumbar and pelvic sympathetic trunks and autonomic plexuses. The psoas major muscle has been reflected laterally to show the lumbar chain more clearly. The left and right pelvic sympathetic trunks can be seen uniting on the anterior surface of the coccyx to form the ganglion impar. Gray rami communicantes connecting the sympathetic trunk with spinal nerves are present at all levels. Also notice the major autonomic plexuses found in the abdominal and pelvic cavities. Sympathetic prevertebral ganglia located in the abdominal cavity (such as the celiac, superior mesenteric, and inferior mesenteric) are also shown. In the pelvic cavity the superior hypogastric plexus continues as the left and right hypogastric nerves that, with parasympathetic fibers, form the left and right inferior hypogastric (pelvic) plexuses.

& Sutin, 1983). Also, cervical gray rami may pierce the longus capitis and scalenus anterior muscles as they course to the cervical spinal nerves (Williams et al., 1989).

Thoracic sympathetic trunk. Eleven small ganglia are usually (70% of the time) found in the thoracic sym- pathetic chain (Figs. 10-7, *B,* and 10-10). Each ganglion includes 90,000 to 100,000 neurons (Harati, 1993). The thoracic chain lies adjacent to the heads of the ribs. In this region of the chain, white rami communicantes, as well as the gray rami communicantes, are clearly evident (Fig. 10-10, *B*). The white rami lie more distal (lateral) than the gray rami, and two or more rami may be

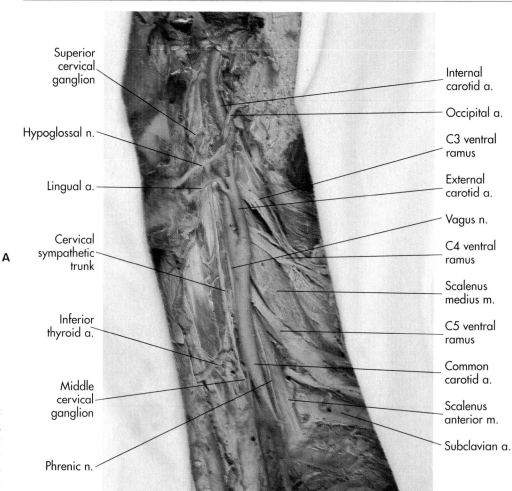

Superior cervical ganglion

Hypoglossal n.

Lingual a.

A

Cervical sympathetic trunk

Inferior thyroid a.

Middle cervical ganglion

Phrenic n.

Internal carotid a.

Occipital a.

C3 ventral ramus

External carotid a.

Vagus n.

C4 ventral ramus

Scalenus medius m.

C5 ventral ramus

Common carotid a.

Scalenus anterior m.

Subclavian a.

FIG. 10-8 A, The left side of the neck showing the cervical sympathetic trunk. The veins and the superior portion of the external carotid artery have been resected.

connected to one spinal nerve. Postganglionic fibers originating from all thoracic ganglia enter the thoracic spinal nerves and travel with them to effectors. Some postganglionic fibers from the T1 to T5 ganglia form direct branches to the aortic, cardiac, and pulmonary plexuses of the thorax. Other branches of the T5 to T12 ganglia are associated with the three splanchnic nerves involved with the sympathetic innervation of the abdominal and pelvic viscera. These splanchnic nerves consist of preganglionic fibers.

The greater splanchnic nerve (Figs. 10-7, *B,* and 10-10, *A*) is formed from preganglionic fibers exiting from the T5 to T9 or T10 ganglia. It courses to the medulla of the adrenal gland, to the celiac ganglion, and sometimes to the aorticorenal ganglion. In the ganglia, the preganglionic fibers of the greater splanchnic nerve synapse on postganglionic neurons. The lesser splanchnic nerve consists of preganglionic fibers from the T9 and T10 or T10 and T11 ganglia and is present 94% of the time. It courses into the abdominal cavity to synapse in the aorticorenal ganglion (which is the detached

lower part of the celiac ganglion). The third splanchnic nerve is the lowest or least splanchnic nerve and is present 56% of the time. This nerve is sometimes called the renal nerve and emerges from the T12 ganglion to terminate in many small ganglia located in the renal plexus (Harati, 1993; Williams et al., 1989). From these prevertebral ganglia, postganglionic fibers participate in the formation of the various perivascular plexuses as they travel to abdominal effectors.

Lumbar sympathetic trunk. The thoracic sympathetic trunk passes posterior to the medial arcuate ligament (or sometimes through the crura of the diaphragm) to become continuous with the lumbar sympathetic trunk found within the abdominal cavity. The trunk consists of four interconnected lumbar ganglia (each of which contains 60,000 to 85,000 neurons [Harati, 1993]) and lies adjacent to the anterolateral aspect of the lumbar vertebrae and the medial margin of the psoas major muscle (Figs. 10-7, *C,* and 10-11). The inferior vena cava, right ureter, and lumbar lymph nodes

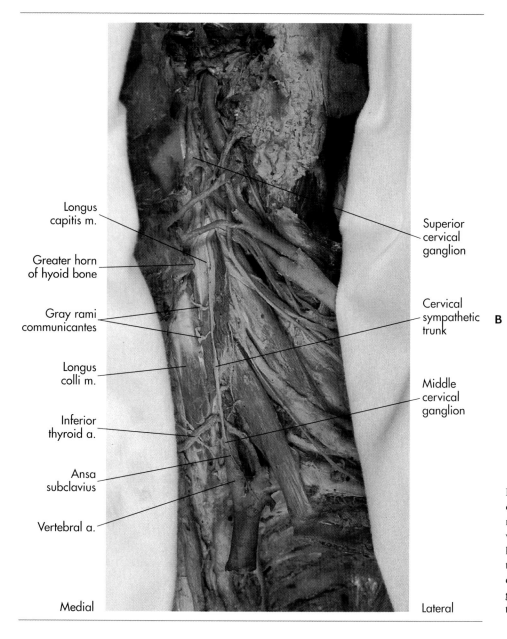

Longus
capitis m.

Greater horn
of hyoid bone

Gray rami
communicantes

Longus
colli m.

Inferior
thyroid a.

Ansa
subclavius

Vertebral a.

Medial

Superior
cervical
ganglion

Cervical
sympathetic
trunk

B

Middle
cervical
ganglion

Lateral

FIG. 10-8, cont'd. B, The common carotid artery has been reflected laterally to expose the vertebral artery. Notice the relationship of the sympathetic trunk to the longus colli and capitis muscles and note the gray rami coursing between the two muscles.

lie anterior to the right sympathetic trunk. The left sympathetic trunk lies posterior to the aortic lymph nodes and lateral to the aorta. These relationships are of importance surgically because lumbar ganglia may need to be removed (lumbar sympathectomy) to treat certain arterial diseases of the lower extremities (Moore, 1980).

White rami communicantes are associated with the upper two or three ganglia. The gray rami are long as they course along the sides of the vertebral bodies to join each lumbar spinal nerve (Fig. 10-11). The majority of these postganglionic fibers are thought to use the femoral nerve, the obturator nerve, and their branches to reach the adjoining blood vessels and cutaneous effectors. In a manner similar to the lower thoracic ganglia, some preganglionic fibers pass through the lumbar

ganglia to form lumbar splanchnic nerves. In general, each lumbar splanchnic nerve corresponds to its ganglion of the same number, although the second lumbar splanchnic nerve receives additional fibers from the third ganglion, and the third lumbar splanchnic nerve also receives a contribution from the fourth ganglion. The four splanchnic nerves course into the abdomen and become part of the abdominal plexuses: the first splanchnic nerve courses within the celiac, aortic, and renal plexuses; the second splanchnic nerve contributes to the inferior part of the aortic plexus; the third splanchnic nerve travels within the superior hypogastric plexus (Figs. 10-7, *C,* and 10-11); the fourth splanchnic nerve contributes to the lowest portion of the superior hypogastric plexus (Williams et al., 1989). The lumbar

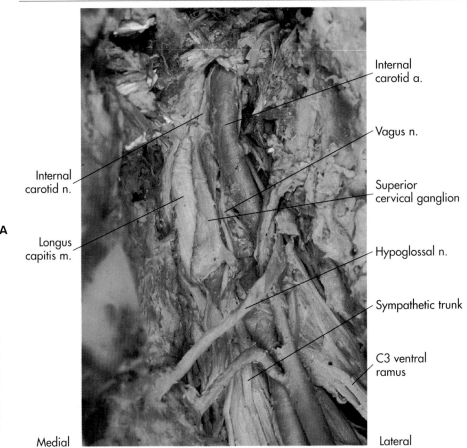

Internal carotid a.

Vagus n.

Superior cervical ganglion

Hypoglossal n.

Sympathetic trunk

C3 ventral ramus

Internal carotid n.

Longus capitis m.

A

Medial

Lateral

FIG. 10-9   **A,** Lateral view of the superior aspect of the deep region of the neck near the base of the skull showing the superior cervical ganglion. The internal carotid nerve (postganglionic fibers) is coursing with the internal carotid artery into the carotid canal.

portion of the sympathetic trunk passes inferiorly, posterior to the common iliac vessels, and becomes continuous with the pelvic portion of the trunk.

Pelvic sympathetic trunk. The pelvic chain consists of four or five ganglia that lie on the anterior aspect of the sacrum. Each side unites to form the ganglion impar on the anterior aspect of the coccyx (Figs. 10-7, *C,* and 10-12). Postganglionic fibers leave the chain in gray rami to enter the sacral spinal nerves and the coccygeal nerve. Fibers destined for blood vessels in the leg and foot course primarily with the tibial nerve to connect subsequently with (and supply) the popliteal artery and its branches. Other fibers travel with the pudendal and gluteal nerves to the internal pudendal artery and gluteal arteries. In addition, some fibers from the first two ganglia send postganglionic branches into the inferior hypogastric plexus.

Plexuses of the Autonomic Nervous System. The autonomic plexuses that have been previously mentioned are a network of autonomic fibers (both sympathetic and parasympathetic) and ganglia found in the thoracic, abdominal, and pelvic cavities. They surround, and are usually named after, the large blood vessels with

which they travel. The plexuses supply the autonomic effectors within the thorax, abdomen, and pelvis. The effectors and their specific innervation are discussed later in this chapter.

The cardiac, pulmonary, celiac, and hypogastric plexuses are the major plexuses (Williams et al., 1989), although secondary plexuses may emanate from each one. The cardiac plexus consists of cardiac branches from cervical and upper thoracic ganglia mixed with cardiac branches of the vagus nerve (Fig. 10-7, *B*). A continuation of the cardiac plexus forms secondary coronary and atrial plexuses. The pulmonary plexus is an extension of fibers of the cardiac plexus that course with the pulmonary arteries to the lungs. Therefore the cardiac and pulmonary plexuses consist of the same sympathetic and vagal branches.

The celiac plexus is the largest autonomic plexus (Fig. 10-7, *C*). It is located at the level of the T12 and L1 vertebrae and surrounds the celiac artery and the base of the superior mesenteric artery. This plexus is a dense fibrous network that interconnects the paired celiac ganglia. Mingling with the celiac plexus and ganglia are the greater and lesser splanchnic nerves and also branches of the vagus and phrenic nerves (Williams et al., 1989). Numerous subsidiary ganglia and fibers extend from the

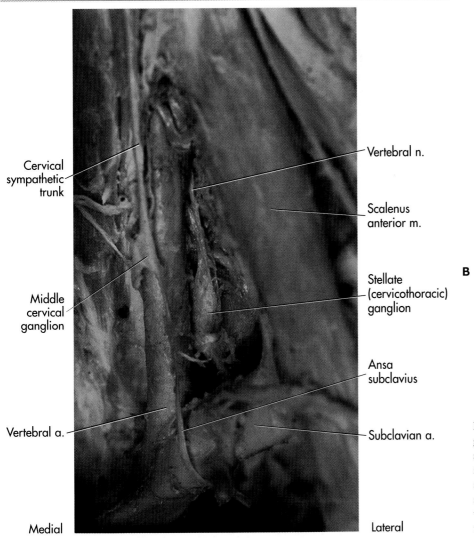

Cervical sympathetic trunk

Middle cervical ganglion

Vertebral a.

Medial

Vertebral n.

Scalenus anterior m.

B

Stellate (cervicothoracic) ganglion

Ansa subclavius

Subclavian a.

Lateral

FIG. 10-9, cont'd. **B,** The stellate ganglion, middle cervical ganglion, and the ansa subclavius. The inferior thyroid artery has been resected. Coursing from the superior aspect of the stellate ganglion is the vertebral nerve, which travels with the vertebral artery.

celiac plexus and course along abdominal blood vessels to autonomic effectors. Examples of these plexuses include the hepatic, splenic, superior mesenteric (to small and large intestines), renal, inferior mesenteric (to lower GI tract), and aortic (intermesenteric). The latter three plexuses also include lumbar splanchnic nerves. Anterior to the bifurcation of the aorta, the superior hypogastric plexus (Fig. 10-7, *C*) is formed by the third and fourth lumbar splanchnic nerves and fibers of the aortic plexus. As the superior hypogastric plexus descends into the pelvic cavity, it divides into left and right hypogastric nerves that continue caudally to form the inferior hypogastric (pelvic) plexuses (Fig. 10-7, *C*). Within the pelvis, pelvic splanchnic parasympathetic fibers join each inferior hypogastric plexus. Extensions of the inferior hypogastric plexus, which include the middle rectal and vesical plexuses, continue along the branches of the internal iliac artery to innervate autonomic effectors of the pelvis. The ANS innervation of

the most clinically important effectors of the pelvis is discussed later in this chapter.

Parasympathetic Division

The parasympathetic division is generally concerned with conserving and restoring energy. It is coordinated with the sympathetic division in the dual and antagonistic innervation of autonomic effectors (see Table 10-1). However, there is no parasympathetic innervation of autonomic effectors located in the extremities and body wall (sweat glands, arrector pili muscles, peripheral blood vessels). Since the sympathetic division has been nicknamed the flight-or-fight division, the parasympathetic division could appropriately be named the rest-and-digest division. In contrast to the widespread control by the sympathetic system, the parasympathetic division controls effectors at a more local level. This relates to the overall pattern of organization of the

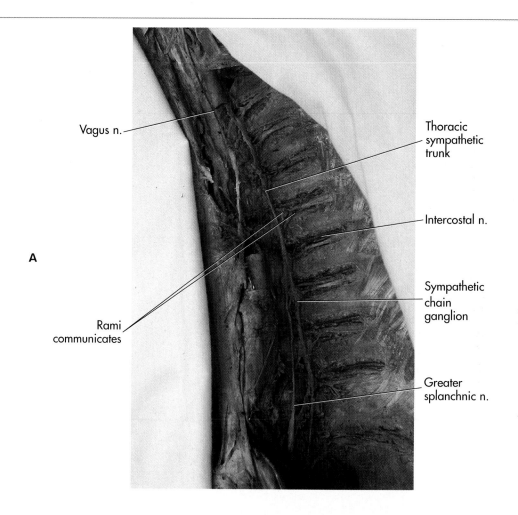

A

Vagus n.

Thoracic
sympathetic
trunk

Intercostal n.

Sympathetic
chain
ganglion

Greater
splanchnic n.

Rami
communicates

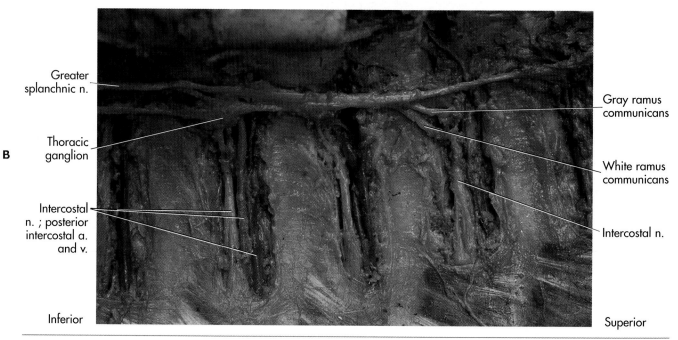

B

Greater
splanchnic n.

Thoracic
ganglion

Intercostal
n. ; posterior
intercostal a.
and v.

Gray ramus
communicans

White ramus
communicans

Intercostal n.

Inferior

Superior

FIG. 10-10   A, The thoracic sympathetic trunk. **B,** A closer view of the left thoracic sympathetic trunk. Both white and gray rami communicantes are shown in relationship to the in-tercostal nerve, artery, and vein. The greater splanchnic nerve (preganglionic fibers) is coursing inferiorly and medially from the sympathetic trunk into the abdominal cavity.

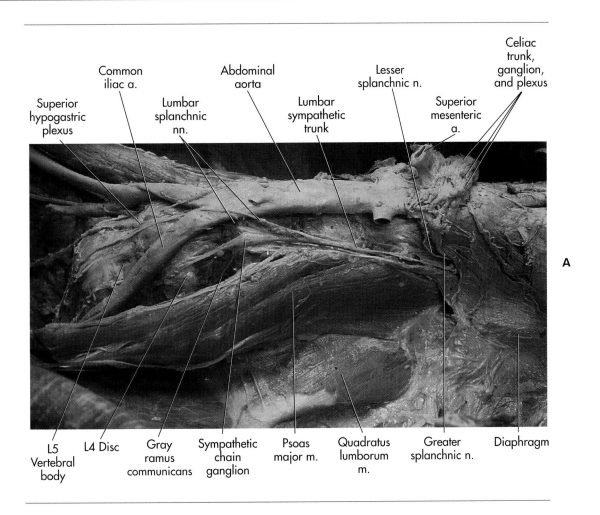

FIG. 10-11 The left lumbar sympathetic trunk. **A,** Notice the relationship of the sympathetic trunk with the psoas major muscle and the vertebral bodies and discs. Lumbar splanchnic nerves are coursing from the sympathetic trunk to the superior hypogastric plexus. The greater and lesser splanchnic nerves pass through the diaphragm to synapse in the celiac ganglion and aorticorenal ganglion. The celiac trunk, superior and inferior mesenteric, and renal arteries have been resected. The inferior vena cava has also been resected.

Continued.

parasympathetic division of the ANS. Compared with the sympathetic division, the parasympathetic division has a lower ratio of preganglionic to postganglionic neurons, and the location of the parasympathetic ganglia is near, or frequently within, the wall of the effector organ.

The parasympathetic division is also referred to as the craniosacral division. As with the thoracolumbar (sympathetic) division, this name refers to the location of the cell bodies of preganglionic neurons (see Fig. 10-2). These cell bodies are located in autonomic nuclei of the brain stem (cranio) and in the second, third, and fourth sacral cord segments (sacral). The parasympathetic efferents of the sacral cord course within the ventral roots and subsequently form pelvic splanchnic nerves. These nerves do not use the sympathetic trunk. Axons of the cell bodies located in the brain stem leave the brain stem in the oculomotor, facial, glossopharyngeal, and vagus cranial nerves. Although numerous branches of various

cranial nerves include these parasympathetic efferents, only the major branches are described. Since this chapter is devoted to autonomic effectors, the somatic functions of the four cranial nerves are not discussed.

Cranial Portion of the Parasympathetic Division

Oculomotor nerve. The oculomotor nerve (CN III) emerges from the ventral surface of the midbrain of the brain stem (see Chapter 9, Fig. 9-15). The origin of the autonomic efferents is in the Edinger-Westphal nucleus, which is located in the midbrain ventral to the cerebral aqueduct of Sylvius. These preganglionic fibers course within the oculomotor nerve to the ciliary ganglion, where they synapse with postganglionic neurons (Fig. 10-13). This ganglion is less than 2 mm long and contains 3000 multipolar neurons (Harati, 1993). It is located in the orbit just anterior to the superior orbital fissure. Postganglionic fibers course in the short ciliary nerves to

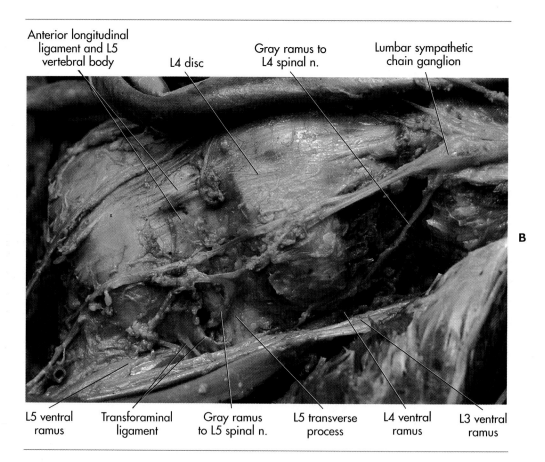

Anterior longitudinal ligament and L5 vertebral body

L4 disc

Gray ramus to L4 spinal n.

Lumbar sympathetic chain ganglion

B

L5 ventral ramus

Transforaminal ligament

Gray ramus to L5 spinal n.

L5 transverse process

L4 ventral ramus

L3 ventral ramus

FIG. 10-11, cont'd. **B,** The lumbar sympathetic trunk at the level of the L4 and L5 vertebrae. The left common iliac artery has been reflected. The psoas major muscle has also been reflected. Notice the long gray rami communicantes. In this specimen, a transforaminal ligament spanning the IVF is present. Note the relationship of the L5 ventral ramus and gray ramus communicans to this ligament.

the eye and travel between the choroid and sclera of the eye wall. Here the fibers innervate the smooth muscle of the iris (sphincter pupillae) and ciliary body (ciliary muscle). The sphincter muscle of the iris functions to constrict the pupil during the pupillary light reflex and during the accommodation-convergence reflex. Contraction of the ciliary muscle occurs during the accommodation-convergence reflex. The result of this contraction is a thickening of the lens, which improves near vision.

Facial nerve. The facial nerve (CN VII) also contains preganglionic fibers. The cell bodies of these fibers are located in the superior salivatory nucleus. This nucleus is located in the caudal part of the pons near the facial motor nucleus. The fibers emerge from the pontomedullary junction in the nervus intermedius portion of CN VII (see Chapter 9, Fig. 9-15). Some of the fibers travel in the chorda tympani nerve, which in turn joins the lingual branch of the mandibular division of the trigeminal nerve (CN V). These preganglionic fibers continue to the submandibular (sublingual) ganglion, where they synapse with postganglionic neurons (Fig. 10-13).

The postganglionic fibers are secretomotor and course to minor salivary glands, as well as to the larger submandibular and sublingual salivary glands. (It has also been reported that stimulation of the chorda tympani nerve results in vasodilation in the salivary glands [Williams et al., 1989].) In addition to the preganglionic fibers en route to the submandibular ganglion, other secretomotor preganglionic fibers from the lacrimal portion of the superior salivatory nucleus course in the greater petrosal nerve to the pterygopalatine ganglion (Fig. 10-13). This ganglion is about 3 mm long and contains 56,500 compactly arranged neurons (Harati, 1993). It is located in the pterygopalatine fossa behind and below the orbit. Postganglionic fibers exit from here and travel in the zygomatic nerve (a branch of the maxillary division of the trigeminal nerve) and terminate in the lacrimal gland. Other secretomotor branches of the pterygopalatine ganglion course to the glands and mucous membranes of the palate and nasal mucosa.

Glossopharyngeal nerve. The glossopharyngeal nerve is CN IX. Preganglionic neurons that course in this

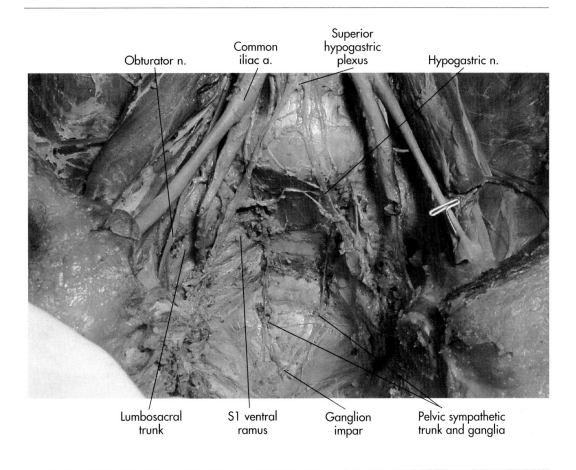

FIG. 10-12   The pelvic sympathetic trunk and ganglia. The left and right trunks join at the level of the coccyx to form the ganglion impar. The superior hypogastric plexus and hypogastric nerves are also present.

nerve originate in the inferior salivary nucleus, which is located caudal to the superior salivary nucleus. CN IX emerges as three to five rootlets from the dorso-olivary sulcus on the lateral side of the medulla of the brain stem (see Chapter 9, Fig. 9-15). The preganglionic fibers travel in the lesser petrosal nerve to the otic ganglion, where they synapse with postganglionic neurons (Fig. 10-14, *A*). The postganglionic fibers are secretomotor, and the axons of these neurons travel in the auriculotemporal nerve (a branch of the mandibular division of the trigeminal nerve) to reach the parotid gland that they innervate. Evidence shows that stimulation of the lesser petrosal nerve results in vasodilation in the parotid gland, as well as serous secretion (Williams et al., 1989).

◆   ◆   ◆

Regarding these three cranial nerves and their ganglia, it is of interest to note that sympathetic postganglionic fibers coursing to their effectors may pass through (but not synapse in) the parasympathetic ganglia. They may also travel along with branches of various cranial nerves. Parasympathetic fibers may also "hitch a ride" with cranial nerves other than III, VII, and IX.

Vagus nerve. The vagus nerve (CN X) also conveys parasympathetic fibers. In fact 75% of the total parasympathetic efferents are carried by the vagus nerve. This nerve is closely related to the glossopharyngeal nerve both anatomically and functionally. Just caudal to the glossopharyngeal nerve the vagus nerve emerges as 8 to 10 rootlets from the dorso-olivary sulcus of the medulla (see Chapter 9, Fig. 9-15). Most preganglionic fibers (some of which are extremely long) arise from the dorsal motor nucleus, which is a column of cell bodies located in the medulla of the brain stem. (It is also speculated that some preganglionic fibers destined for cardiac muscle originate in [or very near] the nucleus ambiguus [Barr & Kiernan, 1993; Loewy and Spyer, 1990; Noback et al., 1991; Nolte, 1993; Williams et al., 1989], which is located in the medulla ventral to the dorsal motor nucleus. However, the nucleus ambiguus is involved primarily with supplying skeletal muscles via CNs IX, X, and XI.) All the preganglionic fibers travel in the vagus nerve and its numerous branches (Fig. 10-14, *B*). Some mingle with sympathetic fibers to form the extensive autonomic plexuses of the thoracic and abdominal cavities. The long preganglionic fibers are destined to synapse in

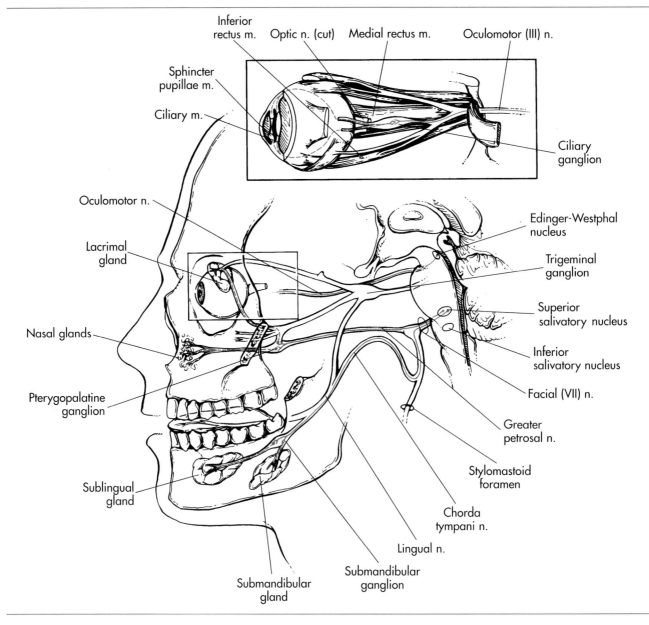

FIG. 10-13 The course of parasympathetic fibers in the oculomotor nerve *(red)* (cranial nerve III) and the facial nerve *(green)* (cranial nerve VII). Oculomotor preganglionic neuron cell bodies are found in the midbrain in the Edinger-Westphal nucleus. Their axons *(solid line)* synapse with postganglionic neurons in the ciliary ganglion located in the orbit. Postganglionic axons *(dashed line)* travel to the smooth muscles of the eye (sphincter pupillae and ciliary). Facial nerve pre-ganglionic neuron cell bodies are found in the caudal pons in the superior salivatory nucleus. Their axons *(solid line)* synapse with postganglionic neurons in the pterygopalatine ganglion and submandibular ganglion. From these ganglia, postganglionic axons *(dashed line)* travel to the lacrimal gland, nasal mucosal, and sublingual and submandibular salivary glands.

small ganglia located within plexuses near the effector organ or in ganglia within the wall of the organ itself. Some of the specific branches that conduct preganglionic parasympathetic fibers are the following: in the thorax—cardiac, pulmonary, and esophageal branches that join the plexuses of the same name; and in the abdomen—gastric and intestinal branches that join in the celiac plexus (and its subsidiary plexuses) en route to the stomach, small intestine, ascending colon and most of the transverse colon, accessory glands, and kidneys.

As can be seen, the vagus nerve has an extensive area of distribution. However, note that the vagus nerve does not supply autonomic effectors of the head. These are innervated by CNs III, VII, and IX. Although vagal effer-

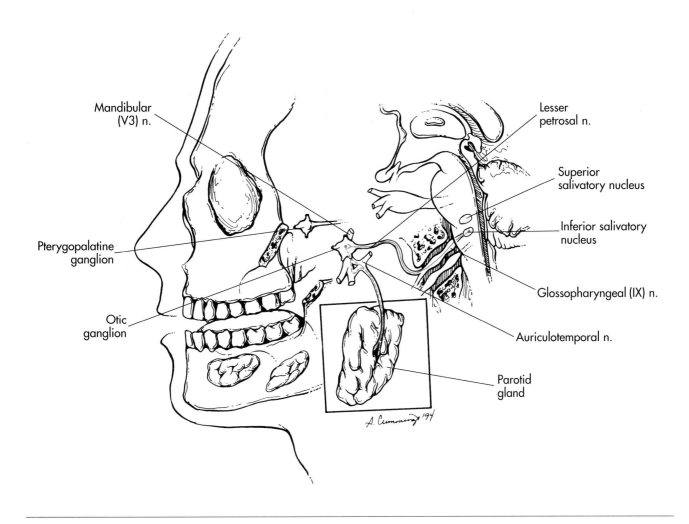

Mandibular
(V3) n.

Lesser
petrosal n.

Superior
salivatory nucleus

Inferior salivatory
nucleus

Pterygopalatine
ganglion

Glossopharyngeal (IX) n.

Otic
ganglion

Auriculotemporal n.

Parotid
gland

FIG. 10-14   **A,** The course of parasympathetic fibers within the glossopharyngeal nerve (cranial nerve IX) to the parotid gland. Preganglionic neuron cell bodies are found in the inferior salivatory nucleus in the rostral medulla. Their axons *(solid line)* synapse with postganglionic neurons *(dashed line)* in the otic ganglion.   *Continued.*

ents are important, the afferent fibers conveying sensory information in the vagus nerve outnumber the efferent fibers (Williams et al., 1989).

Sacral Portion of the Parasympathetic Division. As can be noted from the previous discussion, most effectors innervated by parasympathetic fibers are served by cranial nerves. The remaining effectors, for example, the smooth muscle and glands of the pelvis, not innervated by the vagus nerve are innervated by the sacral portion of the craniosacral parasympathetic division. The origin of these preganglionic fibers is in the sacral autonomic nucleus of lamina VII of sacral cord segments two, three, and four (Fig. 10-15). The preganglionic fibers exit the cord in the ventral roots of these cord segments and leave the ventral rami as pelvic splanchnic

nerves. These fibers course through the hypogastric plexuses, which are formed by both parasympathetic and sympathetic fibers. They synapse in ganglia within those plexuses or in ganglia within the wall of the effector organ. In general, these fibers innervate part of the transverse colon, descending colon, sigmoid colon, rectum, bladder, and reproductive organs. In addition, these parasympathetic fibers convey important sensory information (Barr & Kiernan, 1993; Williams et al., 1989) that provides reflex control of normal bladder, colon, and sexual organ function.

Enteric Nervous System

Extensive research on the enteric nervous system has finally led most authors to recently consider it to be a

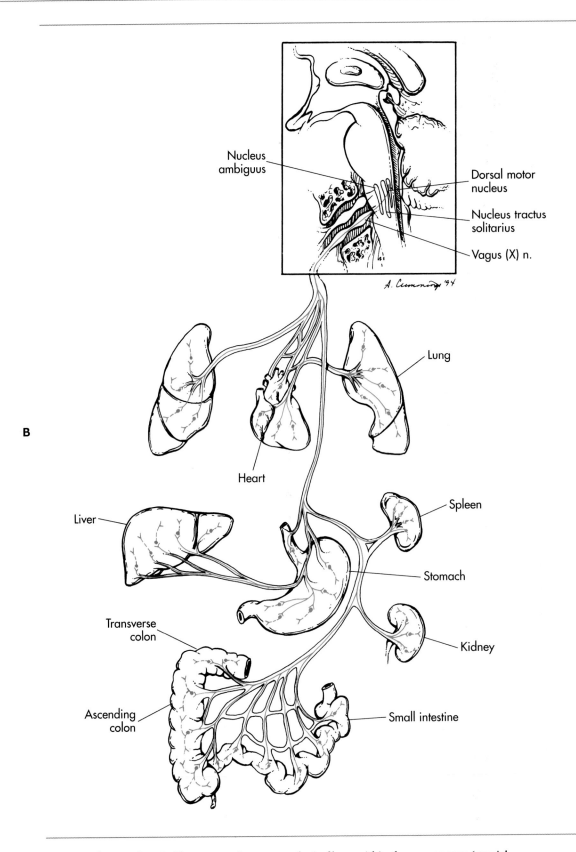

FIG. 10-14, cont'd. **B,** The course of parasympathetic fibers within the vagus nerve (cranial nerve X) to smooth muscle, cardiac muscle, and glands. Preganglionic neuron cell bodies are found in the dorsal motor nucleus located in the medulla. Their axons *(solid line)* synapse with postganglionic neurons *(dashed line)* that are in or very near the wall of innervated thoracic and abdominal visceral organs.

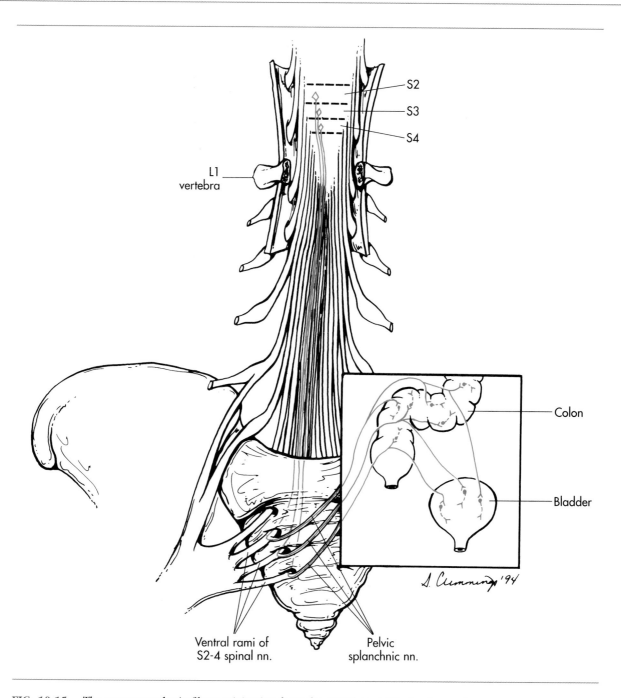

S2

S3

S4

L1
vertebra

Colon

Bladder

S. Cummings '94

Ventral rami of
S2-4 spinal nn.

Pelvic
splanchnic nn.

FIG. 10-15 The parasympathetic fibers originating from the spinal cord. The lumbar vertebral bodies have been removed to expose the sacral cord segments and cauda equina. The preganglionic neurons originate in the S2-S4 cord segments, course within ventral roots of the cauda equina, and exit through their corresponding IVFs. They branch from ventral rami of S2-4 spinal nerves, form pelvic splanchnic nerves, and travel to ganglia (where they synapse) near or within the walls of the pelvic viscera. From the ganglia, postganglionic neurons travel to the smooth muscle and glands of the pelvic viscera.

third division of the ANS, although it was first recognized as such by Langley in 1921 (Gershon, 1981). In 1899 it was first acknowledged that motility of the GI system was under autonomous control by an intrinsic nervous system, when well-coordinated and purposeful motility still occurred independently after severing nerves to the GI system (Gershon, 1981). Since that time the concept that an intrinsic group of neurons exists in the wall of the gut has been fully accepted. This group of neurons extends from the esophagus to the rectum, and it regulates GI vasomotor tone and motility and helps to regulate secretion and reabsorption. All of these activities are necessary for maintaining homeostasis. However, extrinsic postganglionic sympathetic fibers from prevertebral ganglia and preganglionic parasympathetic fibers via the vagus and pelvic splanchnic nerves provide input into these enteric neurons. This input can adjust and regulate and in some emergency situations override this intrinsic system (Dodd & Role, 1991; Loewy, 1990a).

The enteric nervous system is found within the four layers of the wall of the GI tract and is considered to contain as many neurons as the spinal cord itself, about 100 million (Barr & Kiernan, 1993; Camilleri, 1993; Noback, Strominger, & Demarest, 1991). The enteric system consists of two plexuses of neuron cell bodies and their processes (Fig. 10-16). One of these is the myenteric plexus of Auerbach, which is located between the inner circular and outer longitudinal smooth muscle layers of the muscularis externa. This plexus regulates the motility of the GI tract. The second plexus is the submucosal plexus of Meissner, which is found in the submucosa of the GI tract. The submucosal plexus mediates the epithelial functions of secretion and absorption (Jänig, 1988; Loewy, 1990a; Taylor & Bywater, 1988).

Recently it has become apparent that these plexuses are more than just large, extensive parasympathetic ganglia as previously thought. A closer look at these areas reveals that they also receive input from sympathetic postganglionic fibers, as well as preganglionic parasympathetic fibers (Fig. 10-17). In addition, they consist of cell populations different from, and more complex than, other autonomic ganglia. Each plexus contains clusters of neurons that are interconnected, and each cluster is made up of a heterogeneous population of neurons (Barr & Kiernan, 1993; Camilleri, 1993; Loewy, 1990a). Generally, three types of neurons, which form complex circuits, have been classified. These are motor neurons, interneurons, and sensory neurons (Fig. 10-17). The motor neurons provide the innervation to the smooth muscle, vasculature, and secretory cells and receive input from sensory neurons and interneurons. The interneurons aid in forming the circuitry necessary for processing sensory input. They then project to the motor neurons. The sensory neurons have dendrites that project

into the mucosal layer (near the lumen). This allows them to act as mechanoreceptors (in response to stretch), thermoreceptors, and chemoreceptors (e.g., detecting pH and glucose concentration) (Camilleri, 1993; Dodd & Role, 1991; Jänig, 1988). The axonal process of the sensory neuron synapses with interneurons and motor neurons.

The sensory neurons also appear to have a broader function that involves the sympathetic system. These neurons are involved with reflexes mediated by postganglionic sympathetic fibers. Postganglionic sympathetic neurons project to numerous effectors in the GI system, including blood vessels, the smooth muscle of the sphincters, the myenteric plexus (concerning motility), the submucosal plexus (regulating secretion and absorption), and even the organized lymphatic tissue of the GI wall (Jänig, 1988). The axons of the sensory (enteric) afferent neurons project from the myenteric plexus to sympathetic prevertebral ganglia (Fig. 10-17). From here, postganglionic sympathetic fibers course back to the myenteric plexus, resulting in reflex sympathetic inhibition on regions of the GI wall. Numerous data support this intestino-intestinal reflex, and it is likely that similar reflexes exist to control other areas of the gut, including the stomach and colon (Jänig, 1988).

The functional relationship between the sensory afferent fibers and the sympathetic system becomes somewhat more complex when it is noted that sympathetic prevertebral ganglia receive additional input from the CNS via preganglionic sympathetic fibers (splanchnic nerves) and from collateral branches of visceral afferent fibers that are conveying information to the spinal cord (Fig. 10-17). Therefore the sympathetic ganglia may serve a variety of functions related to GI activity. Sympathetic fibers controlling the vasculature may use these ganglia simply as a relay station where preganglionic fibers cause the firing of postganglionic vasomotor fibers. However, the ganglia may also serve as an integrative center for collecting CNS input from preganglionic fibers, as well as peripheral input from sensory neurons in the GI wall. Neither of these alone is capable of causing the postganglionic neurons to reach their firing threshold. Therefore the continual activity of sensory neurons from the gut, in essence, determines the firing threshold of the postganglionic neurons. As long as this activity is at a high enough level, the spatial summation of these afferent fibers, together with the input from preganglionic sympathetic fibers, allows CNS information to reach the effectors. The necessity of summation to allow for proper GI function demonstrates the importance of sensory input to the prevertebral sympathetic ganglia. This input provides a means by which the prevertebral ganglia can regulate and adjust (modulate) incoming information from the CNS that is destined for the GI tract (Jänig, 1988).

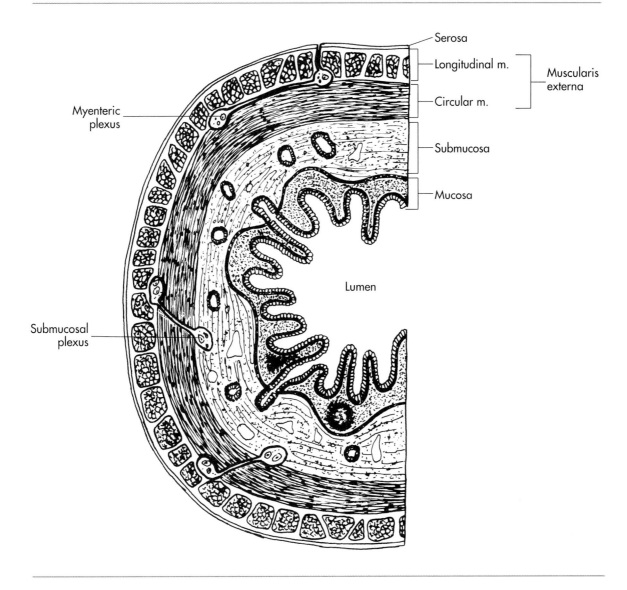

FIG. 10-16 A cross-section through the wall of the gut showing the myenteric plexus (located between the two layers of smooth muscle) and the submucosal plexus (located within the submucosa layer) of the enteric nervous system. Each plexus consists of small ganglia that are interconnected.

Perhaps of equal importance is the speculation that the prevertebral ganglia are involved in the circuitry that protects the GI tract from potential or real injury. GI visceral afferents, the cell bodies of which are located in dorsal root ganglia, have been shown to transmit information from mechanoreceptors and receptors sensitive to molecules such as bradykinin and hydrogen chloride. As they course to the spinal cord, these afferent fibers send collateral branches into the prevertebral ganglia. This input to the prevertebral ganglia and to the spinal cord provides the sensory limb for viscerovisceral, viscerosympathetic, and viscerosomatic reflexes (discussed later in this chapter), as well as for visceral sensation.

The collateral branches synapsing in the ganglia are thought to cause a lowering of the firing threshold of the postganglionic fibers. This would allow spatial summation of the sensory afferent fibers and preganglionic fibers to occur more readily, thereby facilitating, for example, the motor limb of the intestino-intestinal reflex (Jänig, 1988).

In summary, the enteric nervous system not only independently controls the GI tract, but also has an important functional relationship with extrinsic autonomic fibers. By modulating the enteric nervous system, parasympathetic preganglionic fibers stimulate gut motility and secretion and also relax the GI sphincters. The

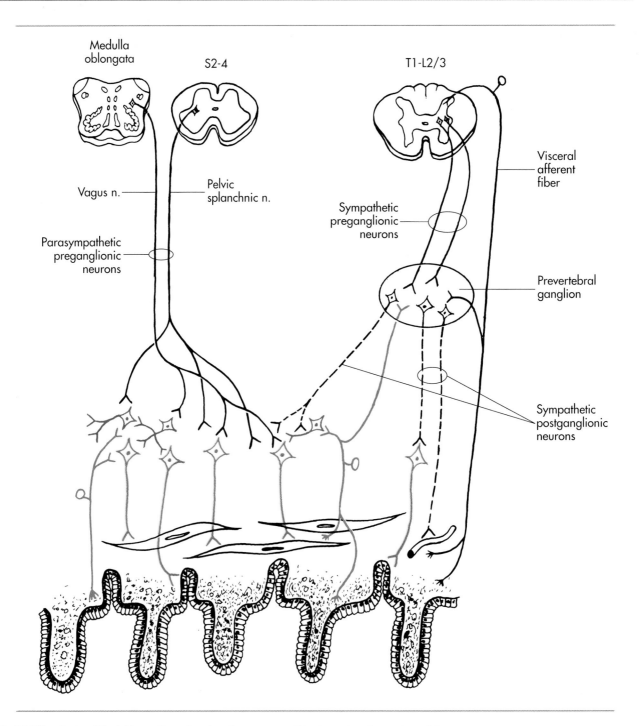

FIG. 10-17 A simplified illustration showing the sensory *(blue)*, motor *(green)*, and interneurons *(purple)* that compose a plexus of the enteric nervous system. Input into this group of neurons is from preganglionic parasympathetic neurons and postganglionic sympathetic neurons, both of which may modulate the function of the enteric neurons. Notice that the prevertebral sympathetic ganglion integrates input from collateral branches of primary visceral afferent fibers destined for the spinal cord, and sensory enteric neurons, thus establishing a reflex arc with postganglionic sympathetic neurons.

sympathetic postganglionic fibers not only synapse on cells of the enteric plexus, but also presynaptically inhibit preganglionic parasympathetic fibers (Barr & Kiernan, 1993; Gershon, 1981) and thus function to inhibit GI motility and secretion and also constrict the sphincters.

INNERVATION OF AUTONOMIC EFFECTORS
Innervation of Peripheral Effectors

Cutaneous Effectors. Cutaneous autonomic effectors include blood vessels, sweat glands, and arrector pili muscles. Unlike most autonomic effectors, these are innervated by only the sympathetic division. Preganglionic fibers originate from cell bodies located in the intermediolateral cell column of the T1 to L2 or L3 cord segments, leave via ventral roots, and after traversing the white rami communicantes, synapse in the sympathetic chain ganglia. Postganglionic fibers, which include vasoconstrictor fibers, sudomotor fibers (to sweat glands), and pilomotor fibers, travel in gray rami to join the spinal nerve on its course to its dermatomal area of supply. (However, the area of skin innervated by sympathetic fibers has been found to be wider than the dermatomal distribution of the somatic fibers [Ogawa & Low, 1993].) More specifically, superior and middle cervical ganglia send postganglionic fibers to the head and neck; the stellate (cervicothoracic) ganglion (in conjunction with a small contribution from the middle ganglion) supplies the upper extremities; thoracic ganglia supply the trunk; and lower lumbar and upper sacral ganglia furnish postganglionic fibers for the skin of the lower extremities (Jänig, 1990; Williams et al., 1989). Because sympathetic efferents innervate cutaneous effectors covering the entire body, nearly all spinal nerves are likely to contain postganglionic sympathetic fibers. The sympathetic innervation of these cutaneous effectors is controlled primarily by the hypothalamus, and stimulation of these effectors is important for thermoregulation.

Blood Vessels Supplying Skeletal Muscles. During muscle activity, vasodilation (and subsequent increased blood flow) is primarily a result of local muscle tissue effects, for example, decreased oxygen in the contracting muscle and release of vasodilator substances. However, sympathetic fibers also innervate these blood vessels and cause vasoconstriction (in some lower animals, sympathetic vasodilator fibers also exist) (Guyton, 1991). The adrenal medulla (innervated by preganglionic sympathetic fibers) is also involved in the regulation of blood flow to skeletal muscles by causing vasoconstriction (via the neurotransmitter norepinephrine, which binds to vasoconstrictor alpha receptors) and some vasodilation

(via the neurotransmitter epinephrine, which binds to vasodilator beta receptors) (Guyton, 1991).

The origin of preganglionic neurons for the upper extremity blood vessels is the intermediolateral cell column of the T2 to T6 or T7 (primarily T2 and T3) cord segments. The axons enter the sympathetic chain ganglia through white rami communicantes and synapse predominantly in the stellate (cervicothoracic) ganglion (Williams et al., 1989). Postganglionic fibers leave the ganglion within gray rami to join spinal nerves and, subsequently, ventral rami destined to form the brachial plexus. The C8 and T1 ventral rami receive the greatest contribution of fibers, and therefore the lower trunk of the brachial plexus conveys most of the peripheral sympathetic efferents. The lower trunk provides fibers to numerous terminal branches of the brachial plexus, including the median, ulnar, and radial nerves. As the postganglionic neurons travel with these nerves, they supply branches to the accompanying brachial, ulnar, and radial arteries, respectively (Williams et al., 1989). The lower extremity muscular arteries are supplied by sympathetic fibers originating in the T10 to L2 or L3 cord segments. These preganglionic fibers enter the sympathetic chain and synapse in the lumbar and sacral ganglia. Postganglionic neurons traverse the gray rami, join spinal nerves, and then enter ventral rami of the lumbosacral plexus. Some postganglionic efferents course with the femoral nerve to supply muscular branches of the femoral artery, whereas others travel with the tibial nerve to innervate the tibial vascular tree (Williams et al., 1989).

Surgical denervation of the peripheral vasculature can be accomplished by cutting the sympathetic chain or removing sympathetic ganglia (sympathectomy) or by cutting preganglionic fibers at the appropriate location (Williams et al., 1989). This provides a treatment for relief of vasomotor spasms that occur in such disorders as Raynaud's disease and intermittent claudication. Sympathectomy has also been performed to influence vasomotor tone in hypertensive patients.

Innervation of the Heart and Lungs

Sympathetic Innervation. As with most autonomic effectors, the heart and lungs are innervated by both the sympathetic and parasympathetic divisions of the ANS. Sympathetic preganglionic neurons to both the heart and the lungs originate in the T1 to T4 or T5 cord segments, enter the sympathetic chain, and synapse. The preganglionic sympathetic fibers associated with the innervation of the heart synapse in the thoracic ganglia that correspond to the spinal cord segments of origin. Many also ascend to synapse in all three cervical ganglia. Postganglionic fibers leave the ganglia as cardiac branches (nerves), which form part of the cardiac plexus (Fig. 10-7, *B*). Sympathetic innervation of the heart results in cardiac acceleration and increased force of ventricular contraction. Coronary blood flow is primarily controlled by autoregulation of the coronary arteries in response to increased and decreased cardiac activity and subsequent metabolic needs of the muscle tissue. However, the coronary arteries are well innervated by sympathetic fibers and, although of minor importance functionally, these fibers on stimulation cause either vasoconstriction or vasodilation depending on which receptor (alpha or beta, respectively) is activated (Guyton, 1991). Afferent information from the heart travels in all cardiac branches except the branch associated with the superior cervical ganglion (Williams et al., 1989).

Postganglionic sympathetic fibers to the lungs originate from the T2 to T5 sympathetic chain ganglia and pass through the cardiac plexus. However, they continue into this plexus and course along the pulmonary arteries to form the pulmonary plexus. These postganglionic efferents provide bronchodilation and vasoconstriction to the lungs.

Parasympathetic Innervation. Parasympathetic innervation to the heart and lungs is provided by the vagus nerve (CN X). Cardiac preganglionic fibers originate in the brain stem medulla. Although most parasympathetic visceral efferents originate in the dorsal motor nucleus, there is controversy as to whether efferents to the heart originate solely in the dorsal motor nucleus or "in" (Barr & Kiernan, 1993; Nolte, 1993; Williams et al., 1989) or "in the region of" (Loewy & Spyer, 1990; Noback et al., 1991) the nucleus ambiguus. Regardless of origin, the preganglionic fibers descend within the vagus nerve into the thoracic cavity as cardiac branches and become part of the cardiac plexus (Fig. 10-7, *B*). They synapse in small cardiac ganglia located in the cardiac plexus and in the walls of the atria. Postganglionic parasympathetic fibers cause a decrease in ventricular contraction and cardiac deceleration. Although autoregulation of coronary arteries is the primary mechanism of controlling coronary blood flow, a few parasympathetic fibers innervate these arteries and, on stimulation, result in a slight vasodilation (Guyton, 1991).

Vagal preganglionic fibers that innervate the lung aid the sympathetics in forming the pulmonary plexus. The preganglionic parasympathetic fibers synapse in small ganglia adjacent to the lung hilum. Postganglionic fibers continue into the lung to stimulate bronchoconstriction, vasodilation, and glandular secretion (Williams et al., 1989). These actions help to maintain the integrity of the epithelial lining of the bronchial tree.

Innervation to the Head

In general preganglionic sympathetic cell bodies for the head (and neck) are located in the T1 to T3 (and some in T4 and T5) spinal cord segments. These fibers enter the sympathetic chain and ascend to the superior cervical ganglion, where they synapse. Postganglionic fibers leave the ganglion and travel with branches of the carotid arteries to gain access to autonomic effectors in the head (Fig. 10-7, *A*). These fibers are vasomotor and secretomotor to sweat glands of the face. One large branch (the internal carotid nerve) leaving the ganglion branches to form the internal carotid plexus, which travels on the internal carotid artery into the cranial cavity. Some fibers (vasoconstrictors) of the plexus continue to the cerebral arteries, where they meet additional sympathetic fibers of the vertebral plexus. Other fibers leave the artery and travel to their destination by "hitching a ride" on cranial nerves in the region. While sympathetic efferents employ arterial transportation, parasympathetic fibers to the head emerge from the brain stem as a part of the oculomotor, facial, and glossopharyngeal nerves. These nerves innervate glandular tissue and smooth muscle.

Although there is dual innervation to the lacrimal, mucosal, and salivary glands, the secretomotor fibers are parasympathetic (sympathetic fibers produce vasoconstriction). Parasympathetic fibers that innervate the lacrimal gland, nasal and palate mucosal glands, and major salivary glands (sublingual and submandibular) travel with the facial nerve. Preganglionic neurons originate in the superior salivatory nucleus located in the brain stem. Those en route to the lacrimal and mucosal glands synapse in the pterygopalatine ganglion, and those destined for the salivary glands synapse in the submandibular ganglion. Parasympathetic efferents innervating the parotid salivary gland course in the glossopharyngeal cranial nerve. These preganglionic fibers originate in the inferior salivatory nucleus of the brain stem and course to the otic ganglion. After synapsing, the postganglionic secretomotor fibers travel to the parotid gland (Figs. 10-13 and 10-14, *A*).

The ANS is also intimately involved with the innervation of effectors located in the region of the orbit. These include the smooth muscle (Müller's) of the eyelids, blood vessels of the eye, and the smooth muscle of the iris and ciliary body. This innervation is responsible for some of the functions that can be assessed during a neurologic examination. Regulation of blood flow to the eye is extremely important in maintaining an adequate nutrient supply to the retina. Retinal arterioles are autoregulated, but choroidal arterioles are autonomically innervated. Sympathetic activation causes vasoconstriction, whereas parasympathetic stimulation, via the facial nerve, is vasodilatory (Loewy, 1990b).

The upper eyelid contains skeletal muscle (levator palpebrae superioris), which is innervated by somatic efferents of the oculomotor nerve. It (and the lower eyelid to a lesser extent) also contains smooth muscle fibers (Müller's) (Williams et al., 1989). The smooth muscle is innervated by sympathetic fibers. Since ptosis (drooping) of the upper eyelid is an important indicator of damage to the sympathetic nervous system, knowledge of the two innervations is necessary for differentiating a lesion involving the oculomotor nerve from a lesion of the sympathetic system.

Other smooth muscle fibers in this region are the intrinsic muscles of the eye, that is, the sphincter and dilator pupillae muscles of the iris and the ciliary muscle of the ciliary body. The iris acts as a diaphragm and regulates the amount of light entering the eye. The dilator muscle is innervated by sympathetic postganglionic efferents that have left the internal carotid plexus to travel with the ophthalmic fibers of the trigeminal nerve. The parasympathetic innervation supplies the sphincter muscle fibers and is the motor arc of the pupillary light reflex. The origin of the parasympathetic preganglionic fibers is the Edinger-Westphal nucleus of the midbrain. The fibers emerge from the brain stem in the superficial aspect of the oculomotor nerve and travel to the ciliary ganglion located in the orbit (Fig. 10-13). After synapsing, postganglionic fibers innervate the sphincter muscle fibers of the iris. When these fibers are activated to cause pupillary constriction, there is an accompanying inhibition of the innervation to the dilator muscle (Loewy, 1990b). During alert but resting periods, a constant sympathetic tone is sustained through hypothalamic input, and at the same time, parasympathetic fibers are inhibited (Cross, 1993b).

An additional smooth muscle, the ciliary muscle, is also involved in the normal function of the eye. This muscle controls the tension of the suspensory ligaments attached to the lens. Parasympathetic and some sympathetic fibers innervate the ciliary muscle. However, controlling the regulation of the curvature and thus the refractive power of the lens via this muscle is essentially a parasympathetic function. This innervation allows focusing to occur when an object is close to the eye (accommodation). Of the total number of preganglionic fibers leaving the Edinger-Westphal nucleus, 94% travel to the ciliary muscle, whereas the remaining fibers supply the iris (Cross, 1993b). The accommodation-convergence reflex is necessary during near vision to correct for an unfocused image on the fovea (region of the retina associated with the most acute vision). The reflex response (mediated by CN III) results in an increase in lens curvature, pupillary constriction, and convergence of the eyes.

Knowledge of the innervation of the eye is important because pathologic conditions affecting the autonomic innervation can occur and because these eye functions can be tested in a neurologic examination. Pathologic conditions caused by disruption of parasympathetic fibers include the Argyll-Robertson pupil (associated with neurosyphilis), internal ophthalmoplegia, light-near dissociation, and Adie's pupil (Cross, 1993a). An example of a condition attributed to a lesion in the sympathetic system is Horner's syndrome (see the previous discussion).

Innervation of the Bladder

The bladder functions to store and evacuate urine. Control of bladder function occurs by a complex integration and coordination of bladder afferent fibers, sympathetic and parasympathetic efferent fibers, somatic efferent fibers (Fig. 10-18), pontine micturition centers, and hypothalamic and cortical areas (Abdel-Azim, Sullivan, & Yalla, 1991; Bradley, 1993; Carpenter & Sutin, 1983; de Groat & Steers, 1990). Sympathetic preganglionic neurons originate in cord segments T11 or T12 through L2 and synapse in corresponding ganglia and in small ganglia in the superior and inferior hypogastric plexuses. Postganglionic fibers course in the vesical plexus (anterior fibers of the inferior hypogastric plexus) to the bladder. Since the majority of these fibers are vasomotor (a few inhibit the smooth muscle [detrusor] of the bladder wall), it is speculated that sympathetic efferents have no essential role in micturition. Other sympathetic fibers richly supply (especially in the male) and stimulate the nonstriated muscle in the neck of the bladder (sphincter vesicae). Although this innervation may serve a minor function in maintaining urinary continence, its major role is to contract these muscle fibers during ejaculation (Carpenter & Sutin, 1983; Snell, 1992; Williams et al., 1989).

The more important autonomic efferent supply to the detrusor muscle of the bladder is the parasympathetic innervation. The parasympathetic fibers originate in S2 to S4, pass into the cauda equina, emerge from the S2 to S4 pelvic (ventral) sacral foramina, and form pelvic splanchnic nerves (Figs. 10-15 and 10-18). These nerves travel within the inferior hypogastric plexus and continue distally into the vesical plexus. These preganglionic fibers synapse with postganglionic neurons located in ganglia within the vesical plexus or within the bladder wall. The postganglionic fibers provide excitatory innervation to the detrusor muscle. (A few fibers supply and inhibit the nonstriated sphincter vesicae.)

Another important muscle involved with normal bladder function is the striated (voluntary) urethral sphincter muscle. The somatic motor neurons that innervate this muscle originate in Onuf's nucleus, which is located in the ventral horn of S2 to S4. These neurons course through the S2-4 ventral roots, spinal nerves, ventral

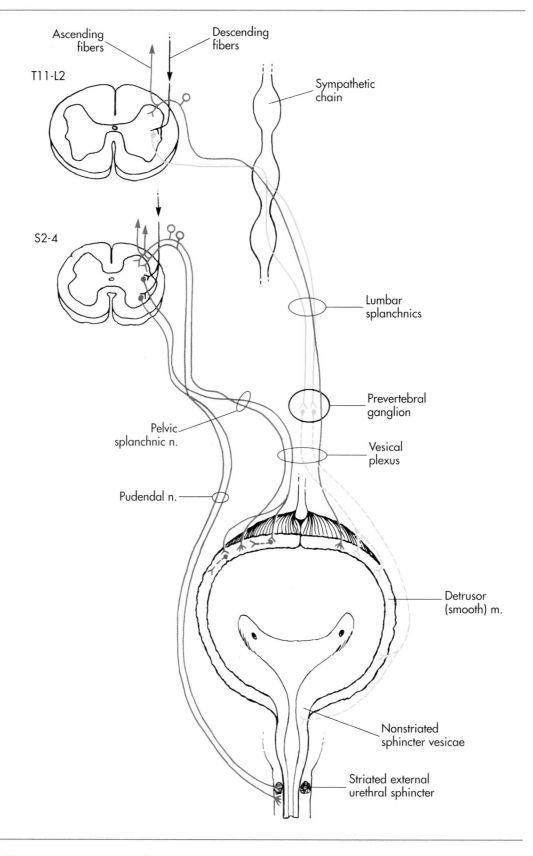

FIG. 10-18 The innervation of the bladder. Parasympathetic fibers *(red)* innervate the detrusor (smooth) muscle. Sympathetic fibers *(yellow)* are primarily vasomotor to the bladder wall but also supply the sphincter vesicae (nonstriated) muscle in the neck of the bladder, which functions to close the lumen of the neck during ejaculation. Somatic efferents *(blue)* coursing in the pudendal nerve also provide an important innervation to the external ventral sphincter (striated muscle). Afferent fibers *(green)* entering the cord may transmit information to higher centers, as well as provide the afferent arc for initiating the voiding response. Descending information from the hypothalamus and cerebral cortex may also modulate the spinal cord neurons.

rami, and travel in the pudendal nerve to reach the skeletal muscle fibers of the sphincter.

Sensory input is also important for micturition to occur. Afferents course in the pudendal nerves, sympathetic nerves, and parasympathetic nerves. The most important afferent fibers are the group A-delta and C fibers that convey information from stretch receptors in the bladder. As they approach the spinal cord, they travel in the pelvic splanchnic nerves and enter the sacral cord segments. This input is necessary to initiate the voiding response. To achieve efficient emptying, detrusor muscle contraction must be coordinated with relaxation of the striated external urethral sphincter muscle. Sensory information from the bladder ascends to higher centers, including the micturition centers of the pons. This center is also modulated by the cerebral cortex (frontal lobe) and diencephalic (primarily the hypothalamus) structures, which may also project directly to the spinal cord (Bradley, 1993; de Groat & Steers, 1990). These connections between the spinal cord and brain stem form a spinobulbospinal reflex, which is instrumental for sustaining detrusor muscle contraction and relaxing the striated sphincter during micturition. Additional descending cortical input allows for voluntary control of voiding and allows one to start and stop micturition on demand. Spinal cord lesions may disrupt the spinobulbospinal reflex, but spinal cord neurons can reorganize to allow group C afferent fibers to initiate a spinal reflex that produces an automatic reflex bladder (de Groat et al., 1990). This type of reflex results in voiding whenever the bladder is full.

Innervation of Sexual Organs

The innervation of sexual organs, which is similar to that of the bladder, consists of sympathetic, parasympathetic, and somatic fibers (de Groat & Steers, 1990; Seftel, Oates, & Krane, 1991; Stewart, 1993). This section is primarily concerned with the innervation of male sexual organs, although innervation to homologous female organs is somewhat similar.

The sympathetic preganglionic fibers take origin from approximately the T10 to L2 cord segments (Fig. 10-19). The route of these fibers varies. Some preganglionic fibers synapse with postganglionic neurons in the sympathetic chain. The axons of these postganglionic neurons enter into the hypogastric nerves and continue into the inferior hypogastric (pelvic) plexus. Other preganglionic fibers travel in the superior hypogastric plexus and synapse in ganglia scattered in the inferior hypogastric plexus (Seftel et al., 1991). In both cases the postganglionic fibers coursing within the inferior hypogastric plexus continue distally into the prostatic plexus (Williams et al., 1989). These fibers then leave the plexus as the cavernous nerve and innervate erectile tissue of the penis and smooth muscle in the seminal vesicles, prostate gland, vas deferens, and the nonstriated sphincter in the bladder neck. Parasympathetic preganglionic fibers originate from S2 to S4 and course in the pelvic splanchnic nerves (Fig. 10-19). The pelvic splanchnic nerves synapse in ganglia in the inferior hypogastric (pelvic) plexus. Postganglionic fibers, in conjunction with postganglionic sympathetic fibers, continue to (and are the primary innervation of) erectile tissue, as well as glandular tissue in the seminal vesicles, prostate, and urethra.

The somatic nervous system is also involved with sexual function. The pudendal nerve contains sensory fibers that course from the penis to sacral cord segments. It also contains motor fibers that travel from the spinal cord to the bulbocavernosus and ischiocavernosus skeletal muscles. The motor neurons originate in Onuf's nucleus, which is located in the ventral horn of the S2 to S4 cord segments. The erection phase of sexual function can be initiated by stimuli such as visual, auditory, imaginative, and tactile. Evidence from spinal cord–injured patients indicate that there are two types of erection reflexes: psychogenic and reflexogenic. In healthy individuals, both types of reflexes probably act synergistically. Reflexogenic erections are sacral spinal reflexes consisting of afferent fibers in the pudendal nerve activating sacral parasympathetic efferent fibers (a small number of afferent fibers ascend in the dorsal columns to higher centers). Psychogenic erections begin in supraspinal centers, including the limbic system and the hypothalamus. The hypothalamus has been implicated as the integration center for the erection response (de Groat & Steers, 1990; Stewart, 1993).

Fibers from these supraspinal centers descend through the brain stem and the lateral white column (funiculus) of the spinal cord to synapse on lower thoracic and lumbar preganglionic sympathetic neurons and the sacral preganglionic parasympathetic neurons. The parasympathetic fibers initiate the erectile response by causing dilation of the arteries within the erectile tissue. However, the sympathetic fibers contribute to this reflex because they can also initiate a psychogenic erection (possibly through the use of different neurotransmitters) when the parasympathetic preganglionic neurons are lesioned (de Groat & Steers, 1990; Seftel et al., 1991).

Emission and ejaculation are also a part of sexual function. Cortical modulation occurs, but the mechanism is complex and unclear. Emission is sympathetically controlled by neurons originating in the T10 to L2 or L3 cord segments (see previous discussion for the route of these sympathetic preganglionic and postganglionic fibers). This event includes the smooth muscle contraction of the vas deferens, seminal vesicles, prostate gland, and nonstriated sphincter vesicae (to prevent reflux of semen into the bladder during ejaculation) resulting in the

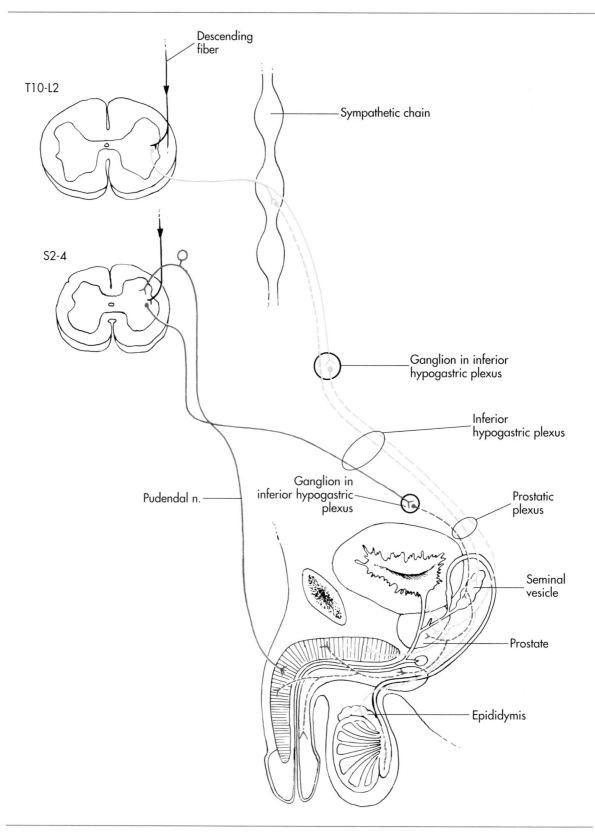

FIG. 10-19 The innervation of the male reproductive organs. Sympathetic fibers *(yellow)* are vasoconstrictive to the erectile tissue and also supply the glandular smooth muscle tissue. Parasympathetic fibers *(red)* are the major supply of the penile erectile tissue but also supply the glandular tissue. The pudendal nerve contains somatic efferent fibers (not pictured here) to the bulbocavernosus and ischiocavernosus muscles and afferent fibers *(green)* conveying sensory information from the penis. These afferent fibers form the sensory arc for reflexogenic erections. Descending fibers from the hypothalamus and limbic system structures send input to the spinal cord neurons, which initiate psychogenic erections.

deposition of semen into the prostatic urethra. The process of ejaculation consists of propelling the semen from the prostatic urethra through the membranous and penile parts of the urethra and out the urethral orifice. During this event the bulbocavernosus and ischiocavernosus skeletal muscles, which are innervated by the pudendal nerve, contract. The coordination of emission and ejaculation probably occurs by the integration of sensory afferent fibers, descending supraspinal input, and motor efferents in an ejaculation center located in the T12 to L2 cord segments (Seftel et al., 1991).

VISCERAL AFFERENTS
General Considerations

Although the ANS is considered by some to consist primarily of an efferent limb, visceral afferent fibers have an important relationship with the efferent fibers. Visceral afferent fibers, which have been known to accompany autonomic efferents since 1894 (Cervero & Foreman, 1990), function to provide information regarding changes in the body's internal environment. This input becomes integrated in the CNS and may participate in reflexes via autonomic and somatic efferents. These reflexes, such as the regulation of blood pressure and the chemical composition of the blood, aid the ANS in the control of homeostasis. However, visceral afferent fibers also mediate some conscious feelings, such as the visceral sensations of hunger, nausea, and distention. Although receptors of visceral afferent fibers do not respond to stimuli such as cutting or burning (as cutaneous receptors do), a pathologic condition or excessive distention produces visceral nociception. The continual barrage of impulses via visceral afferent fibers on the CNS is the probable cause of an individual's feeling of well-being or of discomfort.

Visceral afferent fibers convey information from peripheral receptors called interoceptors. These endings, which may be encapsulated or free nerve endings, are of variable shapes, such as knobs, loops, or rings (Williams et al., 1989). They are found in the walls of the viscera, glands, blood vessels, epithelium, mesentery, and serosa. Some are described as mechanoreceptors and include numerous pacinian corpuscles. These are located in the abdominal mesenteries. Other mechanoreceptors are found in the serosal covering of the viscera and also in the blood vessels, and they may be stimulated by movement or distention. Still others, found in smooth muscle such as that of the bladder, monitor both contraction and distention (Willis & Coggeshall, 1991). Nociceptors of two types have been located in the heart and GI tract. Both respond to mechanical, thermal, and chemical stimuli. One group is comparable to the cutaneous A-delta fiber type, whereas the other group is similar to the cutaneous C-fiber type (Willis & Coggeshall, 1991). In ad-

dition, chemoreceptors and baroreceptors are special interoceptors that are located specifically in the aortic arch and the bifurcation of the left and right common carotid arteries.

The visceral afferent fibers are similar to somatic afferent fibers in that just one neuron extends from the receptor into the CNS. The visceral afferent fibers are found in both the sympathetic and the parasympathetic divisions (the enteric nervous system afferent fibers have already been discussed) and travel with the autonomic efferents. The vast majority are unmyelinated, with the exception of those from the pacinian corpuscles located in the mesentery (see previous discussion). The cell bodies of visceral afferent fibers that travel with parasympathetic efferents in the glossopharyngeal (CN IX) and vagus (CN X) nerves are located in the inferior (petrosal) ganglion of CN IX and the inferior (nodose) ganglion of CN X. The dorsal root ganglia of the second, third, and fourth sacral roots house visceral afferent cell bodies of fibers that travel with pelvic parasympathetic efferents. Cell bodies of afferent fibers associated with sympathetic fibers are located in the dorsal root ganglia of the thoracic and upper lumbar dorsal roots. These fibers course from the periphery along with sympathetic efferent fibers, pass through the prevertebral ganglia without synapsing, and enter the sympathetic trunk (Fig. 10-20). Then they pass through the white rami communicantes into the dorsal root and terminate in the cord segment from which the accompanying preganglionic fibers originate.

Electron microscopic and retrograde tracing methods show that in comparison to the innervation of the skin, a low density of fibers innervates the viscera. Feline studies demonstrate that approximately 16,000 sympathetic afferent fibers exist, and 6000 to 7000 of these are found in the greater splanchnic nerves (Cervero & Foreman, 1990). However, the total number of afferent fibers represents less than 20% of all sympathetic fibers and approximately 2% of the fibers located in dorsal roots of thoracic and lumber spinal nerves. When the parasympathetic afferent fibers are enumerated, an obvious disparity is noticed. Feline visceral afferent fibers in the vagus nerve number about 40,000 and pelvic afferent fibers about 7500. Of the total number of fibers in the vagus, 80% are afferent. In the pelvic nerves 50% of the fibers are afferent (Cervero & Foreman, 1990). The specific functional differences between the afferent fibers associated with the sympathetic division and those associated with the parasympathetic division are not clear. The parasympathetic division afferent fibers are generally thought to transmit input concerning activity of the viscera, such as GI motility and secretion. By monitoring the activity, these afferent fibers are able to mediate reflexes necessary for the proper regulation of visceral function. The sympathetic division afferent fibers

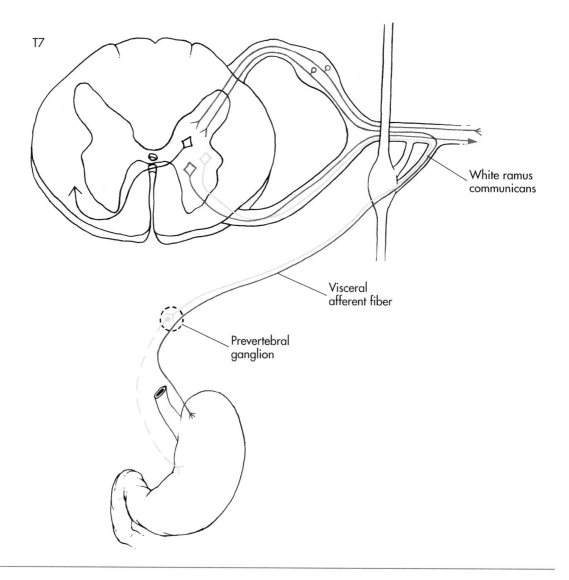

FIG. 10-20 The pathway of visceral afferent information into the spinal cord is shown using the stomach as an example. (Afferent fibers that travel in the vagus nerve and convey visceral information are not shown.) Note how the afferent fiber *(green)* travels with the sympathetic efferent fiber *(yellow)* but does not synapse in the prevertebral ganglion. Instead, the afferent fiber synapses in the dorsal horn and has the capability of influencing numerous neurons including preganglionic efferents, somatic efferents *(blue)*, or tract neurons *(black)*. In the case of visceral pain, the same tract neurons are also receiving input from cutaneous sources *(purple fiber)* thus providing a mechanism for pain referral.

appear to be concerned with sensations arising from the viscera, especially the sensation of pain (Cervero & Foreman, 1990).

Afferent Fibers Associated with the Parasympathetic Division

Afferent fibers coursing in the vagus nerve relay input from many sources (Williams et al., 1989). A partial list includes the following:

- ◆ Walls of the pharynx

- ◆ Thoracic structures
    Heart
    Walls of large vessels
    Mucosa and smooth muscle of the bronchial tree of the lung
    Connective tissue adjacent to the alveoli of the lung
- ◆ Abdominal structures
    Stomach and intestinal walls
    Digestive glands
    Kidneys

The glossopharyngeal nerve conveys visceral afferent information from the posterior region of the tongue, upper pharynx, tonsils, and the carotid sinus and carotid body.

The cell bodies of afferent fibers for both the vagus and the glossopharyngeal nerves are located in their respective inferior ganglia. These ganglia are located adjacent to the jugular foramen of the skull. The afferent fibers of both CNs IX and X synapse in the nucleus of the tractus solitarius, which is located in the medulla oblongata of the brain stem. From here, axons project to numerous areas in the central autonomic network of the brain stem and diencephalon (see Control of Autonomic Efferents and Fig. 10-23) and the cerebral cortex. The projections to the cerebral cortex travel by way of the thalamus. These cerebral projections allow for conscious awareness of sensations, such as hunger. When appropriate, reflexes may also be elicited. Examples include the swallowing, cough, cardiovascular, and respiratory reflexes.

Visceral afferent fibers from the pelvic viscera and distal colon enter the spinal cord via pelvic splanchnics. These fibers monitor stretch in the hollow viscera and possibly mediate nociception originating in the bladder and colon (Carpenter & Sutin, 1983; Cervero & Foreman, 1990).

Afferent Fibers Associated with the Sympathetic Division

As mentioned previously, input conveyed through sympathetic afferent fibers is concerned with visceral sensation, especially visceral nociception. The sensations that reach consciousness are poorly localized and, in the case of pain, may be referred. The cell bodies of these fibers are located in the dorsal root ganglia of the thoracic and upper lumbar dorsal roots. These visceral afferent fibers travel from the peripheral receptors in the cardiac, pulmonary, and splanchnic nerves and continue through the sympathetic trunk, white rami communicantes, dorsal roots, and finally terminate in the spinal cord.

Central Projections and the Referral of Pain

Visceral afferent fibers entering the spinal cord may initiate reflex responses or synapse on tract neurons. It has been shown through neuron tracing techniques that visceral afferent fibers synapse in numerous laminae, including I, V, VII, VIII, and X (Cervero & Foreman, 1990; Willis & Coggeshall, 1991). Limited information indicates that some large myelinated afferent fibers ascend in the dorsal column (Willis & Coggeshall, 1991). The more numerous unmyelinated fibers, such as those transmitting visceral nociception, enter the dorsolateral tract

of Lissauer. They immediately enter the dorsal horn as well as send collaterals up and down a few segments within Lissauer's tract before they also enter the dorsal horn. These fibers synapse in laminae I and V on tract neurons that form the spinothalamic tract and also in laminae VII and VIII on the spinoreticular tract neurons (Cervero & Foreman, 1990). The spinoreticular tract projects to the reticular formation of the brain stem, which in turn projects to the intralaminar thalamic nucleus. From here, fibers travel to the cerebral cortex and into the limbic system. The spinothalamic tract synapses in the ventral posterior and intralaminar thalamic nuclei, which project to the cerebral cortex. As the tract passes through the brain stem, it sends collateral fibers into the brain stem reticular formation (see Ascending Tracts in Chapter 9). Through the interconnections and terminations of these two tracts, higher centers are activated. This allows for a conscious perception of the nociception as pain and also allows the individual to respond to the pain. The spinothalamic tract helps to localize pain, although pain from the viscera is localized much less accurately than pain of somatic origin. Activating the reticular formation permits some localization and a conscious attentiveness to the pain. This is mediated not only by the reticular formation, but also by its connections with the thalamus and widespread areas of cerebral cortex. These three areas compose the ascending reticular activating system. Also, the accompanying discomfort and unpleasantness produce a particular affective mental state and subsequent behavioral patterns, which are mediated through the phylogenetically old limbic system.

The data that have demonstrated the termination of visceral afferent fibers in the spinal cord gray matter also lend credence to the convergence-projection theory of referred pain (Ruch, 1946). This theory maintains that referred pain occurs because of the convergence of visceral and somatic afferent fibers on the same pool of tract neurons (Fig. 10-20). Since somatic pain is more common than visceral pain, the higher centers misread the visceral input as originating from somatic afferent fibers. Therefore, pain is referred to the area of skin (muscle, bone, etc.) supplied by the somatic afferent fibers that have entered the same cord segments as the visceral afferent fibers.

A common example of pain referral occurs after a myocardial infarction or episode of angina pectoris. The relationship between visceral afferent fibers and the spinothalamic tract for pain originating from the heart was determined from data obtained from experiments on primates. These investigations were designed to demonstrate that cardiac ischemia stimulates cardiac afferent fibers, which in turn synapse on spinothalamic tract cells. Bradykinin, a peptide released from ischemic cells, was injected into cardiac tissue and resulted in stimulation of afferent fibers. By measuring tract neuron discharge rates, it was shown that 15 seconds after bradykinin injection (the time needed for receptor activation), 75% of the spinothalamic tract cells increased their firing rate (Cervero & Foreman, 1990). These data support the theory that visceral afferent fibers converge on the same tract cells on which somatic afferent fibers terminate. The peripheral distribution of these same somatic afferent fibers becomes the general location of the pain referral. The afferent fibers subserving nociception from the heart course primarily in the middle and inferior cardiac nerves (to the middle and inferior cervical sympathetic ganglia) and left thoracic cardiac branches (Barr & Kiernan, 1993) and eventually enter the first five thoracic cord segments. Pain is most frequently referred superficially to the left side of the chest and left inner arm, although this may vary depending on the exact segmental origin of the visceral afferent fibers.

Since pain is the most important clinical visceral sensation, knowledge of the spinal cord segments to which visceral afferent fibers project (which is the same location as the sympathetic preganglionic cell bodies) is extremely important. This knowledge allows a clinician to more effectively diagnose pathologic conditions occurring in the viscera (Table 10-2).

Autonomic Reflexes

Reflexes are common events mediated by the nervous system. A reflex can be simply described as an involuntary action that occurs fairly quickly, regulates some effector function, and has no direct involvement with the cerebral cortex. The components of a reflex arc include a peripheral receptor and its afferent fiber, which form the sensory limb; an efferent fiber that forms the motor limb; and an effector. Depending on whether the reflex arc is monosynaptic or polysynaptic, there may or may not be interneurons connecting the afferent and efferent fibers. Both types of afferents (somatic and visceral) and efferents (somatic and visceral) may be involved, thus creating four major kinds of reflex arcs. These are somatosomatic, viscerosomatic, viscerovisceral, and somatovisceral.

Somatosomatic Reflexes. Somatosomatic reflexes consist of somatic afferent fibers that influence somatic effectors, that is, skeletal muscle. Chapter 9 discusses examples of this type of reflex, which included the muscle stretch reflex and superficial reflexes (cremasteric and abdominal). The flexor (withdrawal) reflex and the crossed extensor reflex are also examples of somatosomatic reflexes.

Viscerosomatic Reflexes. The existence of polysynaptic viscerovisceral and viscerosomatic reflexes implies that visceral afferent fibers are involved not only

with the mediation of visceral functions, but also with the functions of somatic effectors, that is, skeletal muscles. Physiologic activities that exemplify viscerosomatic reflex responses concern respiratory function and GI activity. Regulation of respiratory rhythmicity is under the control of respiratory centers located in the medulla. However, in the initiation of expiration, the Hering-Breuer reflex may occur. Stretch receptors that lie in the bronchi and bronchioles of the lungs increase

Table 10-2	Origin of Preganglionic Autonomic Fibers	
Structure	**Sympathetic (cord segments)**	**Parasympathetic (nuclei/cord segments)**
Smooth muscle and glands of the head	T1-T3 (T4 or T5)	Edinger-Westphal nucleus (CN III), superior salivatory (CN VII), and inferior salivatory nuclei (CN IX)
Cutaneous effectors	T1-L2 or L3	None
Blood vessels of upper extremity skeletal muscles	T2-T6 or T7	None
Blood vessels of lower extremity skeletal muscles	T10-L2 or L3	None
Heart	T1-T4 or T5	Dorsal motor nucleus of CN X and nucleus ambiguus
Lungs	T2-T5	Dorsal motor nucleus of CN X
Stomach	T6-T10	Dorsal motor nucleus of CN X
Small intestine	T9-T10	Dorsal motor nucleus of CN X
Large intestine		
Ascending and transverse colon	T11-L1	Dorsal motor nucleus of CN X
Descending colon and rectum	L1-L2	S2-S4 cord segments
Liver and gallbladder	T7-T9	Dorsal motor nucleus of CN X
Spleen	T6-T10	Dorsal motor nucleus of CN X
Pancreas	T6-T10	Dorsal motor nucleus of CN X
Adrenal gland (medulla)	T8-L1	None
Kidney	T10-L1	Dorsal motor nucleus of CN X
Bladder	T11-L2	S2-S4 cord segments
Sex organs	T10-L2	S2-S4 cord segments

their firing rate as the lungs inflate. This information is conveyed via visceral afferent fibers in the vagus nerve to the nucleus of the tractus solitarius of the brain stem medulla. From this nucleus, neurons project into the respiratory center for expiratory activity. Descending fibers then inhibit the motor neurons that innervate the skeletal muscles of respiration and subsequently terminate the inspiration phase. Other visceral afferent fibers that reflexively influence respiratory skeletal muscles course in the glossopharyngeal and vagus nerves from chemoreceptors located in the carotid and aortic bodies. A change in the oxygen concentration causes a reflex change in the rate and depth of respiration. Abnormal stimuli such as visceral nociception can also produce skeletal muscle contractions. An example of this type of viscerosomatic reflex is the contraction of the abdominal skeletal musculature after excessive distention or the inflammation of peritonitis.

Experiments on rabbits have shown that stimulation of organs such as the renal pelvis and small intestine cause reflex paravertebral muscle contractions. In addition, some pathologic conditions (e.g., coronary artery disease) cause stimulation of afferent fibers that produce not only skeletal muscle contractions, but also concurrent activation of autonomic effectors in somatic tissue that results in cutaneous vasomotor and sudomotor changes (Beal, 1985).

Viscerovisceral Reflexes. Visceral afferent fibers also mediate visceral reflex responses. Viscerovisceral reflex responses are common occurrences and are best exemplified in the functioning of the cardiovascular and GI systems. Changes in blood pressure are monitored by baroreceptors of the carotid sinus and aortic arch. For example, an increase in blood pressure stimulates the baroreceptors. The visceral afferent fibers from these course in the glossopharyngeal and vagus nerves to the brain stem, causing a reflex slowing of the heart rate via visceral efferent fibers in the vagus nerve and peripheral vasodilation via inhibition of sympathetic efferent fibers. Visceral afferent fibers from the GI tract and bladder convey information allowing for the normal functioning of digestion, elimination, and voiding. Sensory input such as distention produces reflex responses, including contraction of smooth muscle (in the wall and in the sphincters) and mucosal secretion.

The enteric nervous system is intimately involved with viscerovisceral reflex responses. For example, a toxic microbial organism may stimulate the intrinsic sensory neurons of the submucosal plexus that innervate the epithelium of the gut. Although the circuitry is not completely understood, these neurons cause reflex secretion of water and ions, a decrease in absorption, and by means of the myenteric plexus, increased gut motility (Loewy, 1990a).

Somatovisceral Reflexes. The existence of somatovisceral reflexes indicates that visceral afferent fibers are not the sole initiators of visceral responses; somatic afferent fibers can also reflexively stimulate autonomic efferent fibers. This usually occurs when changes of skin temperature result in cutaneous vasomotor and sudomotor responses. Although evidence exists that stimulating the receptors of somatic afferent fibers produces changes in visceral activity, the exact neural circuitry for somatovisceral reflexes is not clearly understood.

Sato and his colleagues (Sato, 1992a; Sato, 1992b; Sato & Swenson, 1984; Sato, Sato, & Schmidt, 1984) have provided much evidence supporting the presence of somatovisceral reflexes. Using anesthetized rats, they stimulated the receptors of somatic afferent fibers from the skin, muscle, and knee joint and measured the reflex changes in heart rate, gut motility, bladder contractility, adrenal medullary nerve activity, and secretion of the adrenal medulla. Depending on the type of stimuli and organ involved, reflex responses to cutaneous stimuli produced the following varied responses:

1. Noxious and innocuous mechanical stimuli and thermal stimuli produced an increase in heart rate.
2. Noxious pinching of the abdominal skin resulted in inhibited gastric motility, although motility was sometimes facilitated when the hind paw was pinched.
3. Stimulation of the perianal area caused increased efferent firing to and reflex contractions in a quiescent (slightly expanded) bladder, but this caused the inhibition of bladder contractions in an expanded bladder.
4. Noxious pinching of the skin and noxious thermal stimuli resulted in an increase in the secretory activity of and neural activity to (via the greater splanchnic nerve) the medulla of the adrenal gland, whereas innocuous stimuli had the opposite effect.

Type III and IV muscle afferent fibers, stimulated by intraarterial injections of potassium chloride (KCl) and bradykinin (both of which are algesic agents), produced the following effects on heart rate and smooth muscle of the bladder:

1. "Injection of KCl regularly accelerates heart rate. With bradykinin, both accelerations and decelerations can be observed" (Sato, 1992a).
2. Both substances had effects on the bladder similar to those initiated by cutaneous stimuli, that is, excitation to the quiescent bladder and inhibition to the contractions of an expanded bladder.

Joint receptors from a normal knee joint and inflamed knee joint were stimulated by movements both within and beyond the joint's normal range of motion. Results showed that heart rate and secretory and nerve activity of the adrenal medulla increased when the normal knee joint was moved beyond its normal range and when the inflamed knee joint was moved within and beyond its normal range, with a greater increase occurring during the latter. These data indicated the variability that can occur in different effectors in response to various stimuli of somatic afferent fibers. These experiments showed that effectors could be mediated through both sympathetic or parasympathetic efferent fibers and that the response could be excitatory or inhibitory. Further, reflex responses may be integrated at the segmental level (spinal cord) or at the supraspinal level, and the data indicated both paths were used. For example, segmental integration occurred for the cutaneovesical reflex of the quiescent bladder, cutaneoadrenal reflex, and cutaneogastric reflex, and supraspinal integration was necessary for the cutaneocardiac reflex and cutaneovesical reflex of the expanded bladder.

In other experiments exploring somatovisceral reflexes, different forces were applied to the lateral aspect of two regions of immobilized spines of anesthetized rats (Fig. 10-21) to study the effect on heart rate, blood pressure, and activity in the nerve to the adrenal medulla and renal nerve to the kidney (Sato, 1992a; Sato & Swenson, 1984). Lateral flexion resulting from applied mechanical force stimulated afferent fibers supplying the vertebral column and produced the following results:

1. A consistently large decrease in blood pressure that returned to normal after the stimulus was removed
2. An inconsistently small decrease in heart rate
3. A decrease in blood flow to the gastrocnemius and biceps femoris muscles, with a concomitant decrease in systemic arterial blood pressure
4. An initial decrease in activity in the renal nerve and subsequent recovery, both during the period of stimulation
5. An initial decrease in activity in the adrenal nerve with a gradual return to baseline activity, which was followed by an additional increase in activity (likely caused by a baroreceptor-mediated reflex response)

In summary, these experiments show that a stress applied to the spine initiates reflex arcs resulting in changes in heart rate, blood pressure, and activity in sympathetic efferents to the kidney and medulla of the adrenal gland. Based on this evidence, the neural components for this type of somatovisceral reflex do exist, and spinal manipulation may stimulate somatic afferent fibers to create similar somatovisceral reflex responses. Pathologic processes affecting the spine may also result in reflex changes in visceral activity (Sato, 1992a).

NEUROTRANSMITTERS

The chemical mediation that occurs in autonomic ganglia and at the effector is important for both neurotransmission and for pharmacologic intervention. The two major neurotransmitters involved in the ANS are acetylcholine (ACh) and norepinephrine (NE), also called noradrenaline. Since 1935 the fibers releasing these neurotransmitters have been functionally classified as cholinergic and adrenergic, respectively (Dale, 1935).

Acetylcholine

All preganglionic fibers (both parasympathetic and sympathetic) release ACh at the level of the ganglion. Parasympathetic postganglionic fibers also release ACh at the level of the effector (Fig. 10-22). Research in the early 1900s found that ACh would bind to two types of receptors, one on postganglionic neurons and one on the effector. These were called nicotinic and muscarinic receptors, respectively, because the administration of the drug nicotine and the alkaloid muscarine (derived from the *Amanita* mushroom) mimicked specific actions of

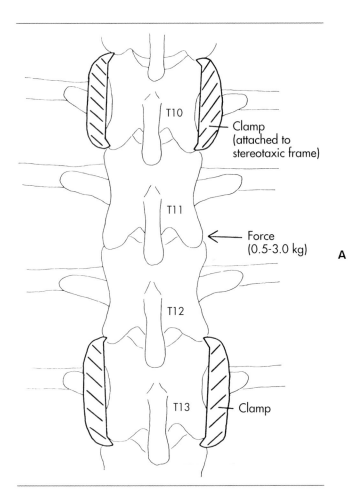

A

FIG. 10-21 **A,** Illustration of the stimulation procedure (thoracic spine shown). Segments isolated from skin and muscle, upper and lower segments fixed in a spinal stereotaxic device, force exerted (0.5-3.0 kg) on mobile segments. (From Sato, A. & Swenson, R.S. [1984]. *J Manipulative Physiol Ther,* 7[3], 141-147.)

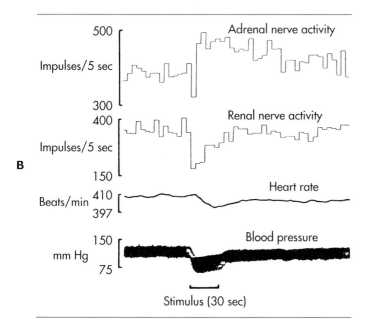

B

FIG. 10-21, cont'd.   **B,** Sample record from a CNS intact animal with thoracic spine stimulation. Force (3.0 kg) delivered during the period marked by the dark bar below the blood pressure trace.

the stimulated parasympathetic system. Since then a minimum of three functional muscarinic receptors and at least three nicotinic receptors have been found. One of the nicotinic receptors described is the receptor that binds ACh at the neuromuscular junction (Parkinson, 1990b).

ACh is rapidly broken down within the synaptic cleft. More specifically, ACh is hydrolyzed by the enzyme acetylcholinesterase into choline and acetate. Subsequent reuptake returns choline to the nerve terminal. Because of the rapid inactivation, the time span of parasympathetic discharge is brief.

Norepinephrine

Sympathetic postganglionic fibers release NE at the effector membrane (Fig. 10-22). (However, postganglionic fibers that innervate sweat glands are cholinergic.) NE is capable of binding to two categories of receptors, alpha or beta. However, its major site of action is the alpha receptor. Beta receptors may also be activated by epinephrine (released by the adrenal medulla) and, in addition, strongly react to the agent isoproterenol, which consists of epinephrine and a propyl group. Each of the adrenergic receptors is subdivided into two types: alpha 1 and alpha 2 and beta 1 and beta 2 (Parkinson, 1990a). Thus, four varieties of adrenergic receptors exist to which NE (and epinephrine) can bind. This allows for a diversity of sympathetic responses. In general, activation of alpha receptors produces excitatory responses such

as smooth muscle contraction. Activation of beta receptors results in inhibitory responses, such as the contractile inhibition seen in vasodilation. NE is slowly deactivated by various mechanisms. Substances that deactivate NE include intracellular monoamine oxidase and extracellular catechol-o-methyltransferase. NE is also deactivated by its active reuptake into the presynaptic nerve terminal.

Neuropeptides

Although ACh and NE are the main neurotransmitters of the ANS, it has been shown that neuropeptides are also found in the same neurons and probably modify neurotransmission at the synapse. For example, postganglionic sympathetic fibers innervating the submucosal ganglia and GI mucosa contain the neuropeptide somatostatin, and those supplying sweat glands contain both calcitonin gene-related peptide and vasoactive intestinal polypeptide (Loewy, 1990a). Neuropeptides are also found in the region of the preganglionic cell columns of the spinal cord. They include substance P, somatostatin, enkephalins, and neuropeptide Y (primarily in the sympathetic column). Also, vasoactive intestinal polypeptide and calcitonin gene-related peptide are both located primarily in the sacral cell column. All these may be involved with the integration and modulation of both autonomic reflexes and the descending input from higher centers (Harati, 1993).

Pharmacologic Applications

The synapse between preganglionic and postganglionic neurons and postganglionic fibers and effectors is of interest pharmacologically. Various agents, some of which are produced synthetically, can produce numerous effects. Some mimic the actions of sympathetic (sympathomimetic) stimulation, and others mimic the actions of parasympathetic (parasympathomimetic) stimulation. Many agents block receptor sites or alter the deactivation mechanism of the neurotransmitter. Examples of blocking agents are high concentrations of nicotine, which act at the ganglion level and sustain postganglionic depolarization; atropine, which binds to muscarinic receptors (used to dilate the pupils and increase heart rate); phenoxybenzamine, which blocks alpha-adrenergic receptors; propranolol, which blocks beta-adrenergic receptors (used to treat hypertension); and reserpine, which inhibits NE synthesis and storage (Snell, 1992).

Some pharmacologic agents can also inhibit or inactivate acetylcholinesterase. Because ACh is not deactivated, it continues to stimulate cholinergic fibers. Examples of these reversible anticholinesterase drugs are physostigmine and neostigmine, used in treating

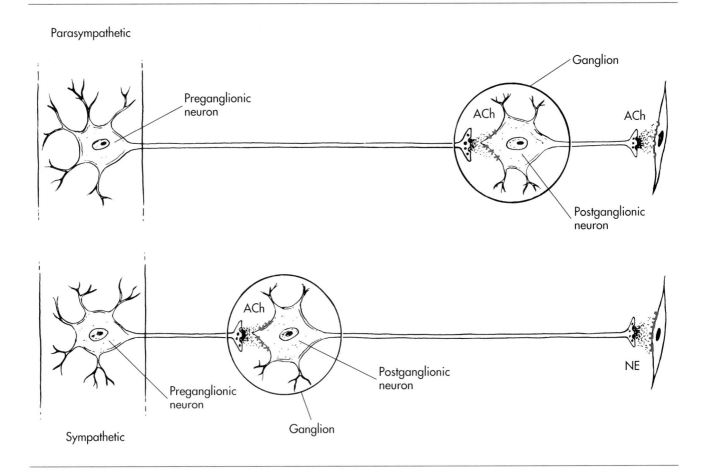

FIG. 10-22   The major neurotransmitters released by parasympathetic and sympathetic neurons. Note the receptors (nicotinic, *green*; muscarinic, *purple*; alpha, *blue*) to which the neurotransmitters bind. Preganglionic neurons of both systems and postganglionic parasympathetic neurons release acetylcholine (ACh). Postganglionic sympathetic neurons typically release norepinephrine (NE). (Those to sweat glands release acetylcholine.)

glaucoma and myasthenia gravis. Irreversible anticholinesterase drugs are also produced. Some of these are toxic, such as "nerve gas" (Carpenter & Sutin, 1983). Pharmacologic agents can also mimic autonomic function by stimulating receptors. Phenylephrine (Neo-Synephrine; used to decrease nasal secretions) and isoproterenol (Isuprel; used as a bronchodilator during attacks of asthma) activate alpha and beta receptors, respectively. Pilocarpine can mimic parasympathetic activity and is also used in the treatment of glaucoma (constriction of the sphincter pupillae muscle allows for drainage of the anterior chamber of the eye by opening the canals of Schlemm).

CONTROL OF AUTONOMIC EFFERENTS
Hypothalamus

The results of much investigation have clarified the components, neurotransmitters, and functions of the sympathetic and parasympathetic divisions of the ANS. However, not until the past 15 years have the results of research begun to elucidate the complex neural circuitry that integrates and regulates autonomic efferents. This circuitry is located in the brain stem and in more rostral structures. The hypothalamus has been considered to be the major controller of the ANS. It is also considered to be an integrator of both the ANS and endocrine systems, which are essential for maintaining homeostasis. In fact, stimulating the anterior and posterior hypothalamic nuclei produces parasympathetic and sympathetic responses, respectively. In addition to input from numerous regions of the CNS, some hypothalamic neurons are sensitive to information conveyed by the blood, including temperature, osmolarity, and glucose and hormone concentrations. The hypothalamus is also intimately involved with the limbic system, which is a phylogenetically old system concerned with behaviors and visceral responses necessary for survival. Although important, the hypothalamus is just one part of the central autonomic network.

Nucleus of the Tractus Solitarius

Another integral component of this circuitry is the nucleus of the tractus solitarius (NTS) (Barron & Chokroverty, 1993; Loewy, 1990c). This nucleus lies adjacent to the dorsal motor nucleus of the vagus in the dorsomedial aspect of the brain stem medulla (Fig. 10-23). Studies performed on rats show that the NTS is the major brain stem integrator of visceral afferent fibers, including those conveying cardiovascular, respiratory, GI, and taste information. It also receives somatic information from the spinal cord and trigeminal system, paving the way for integration and possibly somatovisceral and viscerovisceral reflex responses (Menetrey & Basbaum, 1987).

The NTS is uniquely organized. Some afferent fibers terminate in organ-specific subnuclei, which in turn connect with appropriate preganglionic neurons and make reflex adjustments on effector organs. Other afferent fibers synapse on a common region of the NTS called the commissural nucleus (Loewy, 1990c). This nucleus is reciprocally connected to brain stem nuclei and forebrain nuclei such as the thalamus, hypothalamus, amygdala, caudal raphe nuclei, and bed nucleus of the stria terminalis. These connections form the central autonomic network. This network integrates the input it receives and subsequently activates numerous structures that are responsible for widespread autonomic, endocrine, and behavioral effects. For the visceral effectors to produce a response, the central autonomic network sends input to the preganglionic parasympathetic (primarily the vagal system) and sympathetic neurons.

Other ANS Influences

Preganglionic sympathetic neurons receive descending input from the hypothalamus (paraventricular nucleus), pontine noradrenergic cell group (A5), caudal raphe nuclei, and the rostral ventrolateral and ventromedial medullary reticular formation. Interneuronal circuits in the intermediate gray matter of each sympathetic spinal cord level also can influence sympathetic output, although the exact mechanism is unclear (Loewy, 1990c).

In addition to the central autonomic network, the cerebellum and the cerebral cortex have been implicated in playing a role in the production of autonomic responses. Data gathered from stimulation and ablation studies of the cerebellum suggest the cerebellum is involved at least with cardiovascular functions. On stimulation of the cerebral cortex (superior frontal gyrus, insula, and sensorimotor strip), changes in cardiovascular and respiratory functions, GI motility, and pupillary dila-

tion are produced. These changes are caused by cortical projections that are likely channeled through the hypothalamus. The cerebellar and cerebral pathways mediating these autonomic responses are, as yet, unknown (Barron & Chokroverty, 1993).

Because the majority of this information was gathered from experiments performed on lower mammals, much research needs to be done to clarify the central autonomic circuitry of the human brain. Sympathetic and parasympathetic efferents are certainly under the control of numerous CNS structures that have formed a complex network. This network is linked in such a way that integration and modulation of the autonomic and endocrine systems are possible and behavioral responses can even be affected.

CLINICAL APPLICATIONS

A discussion of the vast number of lesions that can alter autonomic activity is beyond the scope of this chapter. Therefore the following are just a few examples of various pathologic processes that may cause autonomic dysfunction.

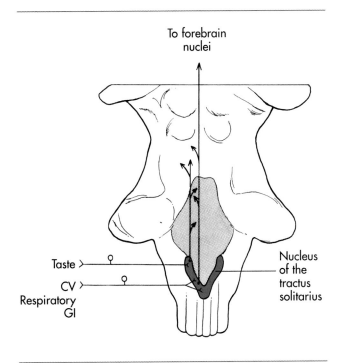

FIG. 10-23 The nucleus of the tractus solitarius. This nucleus is an integrative center and a major component of the central autonomic network of the brain. The nucleus receives various afferent input, such as taste, cardiovascular (CV), respiratory, and gastrointestinal. The output *(arrows)* is dispersed to numerous areas, including brain stem nuclei and forebrain nuclei (e.g., the thalamus and hypothalamus), resulting in reflex responses, as well as autonomic, endocrine, and behavioral responses.

Denervation Hypersensitivity

Although total disruption of the innervation to skeletal muscles prohibits contraction from occurring, many viscera are autoregulated, and lesions of preganglionic and postganglionic fibers to these autonomic effectors may not cause total cessation of function. However, under these circumstances the autonomic effector may not function in the most efficient manner. Depending on its location, a lesion would likely eliminate the release of neurotransmitters either between the preganglionic and postganglionic neurons or between the postganglionic neuron and the effector. When this occurs, the denervated structures show an increase in sensitivity to their neurotransmitters, which at times may be found in the circulation. This hypersensitivity is possibly caused by an increase in the number of cell membrane adrenergic receptor sites or by alterations in the reuptake mechanism of certain neurotransmitters (e.g., epinephrine) (Carpenter & Sutin, 1983; Snell, 1992). The effectors show greater sensitization as a result of sectioning postganglionic fibers rather than sectioning preganglionic fibers (Carpenter & Sutin, 1983).

An example of the effects of denervation hypersensitivity may be observed in the pupils of individuals who have Horner's syndrome, which is caused by a disruption of sympathetic fibers (see following discussion). If the individual's sympathetic nervous system is stimulated (e.g., overexcitement), epinephrine and NE are released from the medulla of the adrenal gland into the blood and cause the pupil to dilate (paradoxic pupillary response), even though the sympathetic innervation to the iris has been interrupted (Noback et al., 1991). Administration of sympatheticomimetic agents to individuals with Horner's syndrome also produces this same pupillary response (Cross, 1993a).

Horner's Syndrome

Horner's syndrome is primarily an acquired pathologic condition but rarely may occur as a congenital condition. This syndrome is caused by the interruption of the sympathetic innervation to effectors located in the head. Characteristic signs seen in Horner's syndrome are those associated with the ipsilateral loss of sympathetic innervation to the following structures: smooth muscle of the dilator pupillae muscle of the iris, producing pupillary constriction (miosis), which is more apparent in dim light; smooth muscle (Müller's) of the upper eyelid, producing ptosis; sweat glands of the face, causing anhidrosis; and smooth muscle of the blood vessels, resulting in vasodilation (this makes the skin flushed and warm to the touch). The patient may also appear to have enophthalmos ("sunken eye"). This feature is actually caused by the narrowed palpebral fissure following denervation

of the upper eyelids. Because of its denervation, the dilator pupillae muscle is also hypersensitive to circulating adrenergic neurotransmitters (see previous discussion).

One area of the CNS that can be lesioned to produce Horner's syndrome is in the brain stem (Fig. 10-24, A). Fibers originating in the hypothalamus and destined for the intermediolateral cell column of the spinal cord descend in the lateral aspect of the brain stem. Interruption of these fibers can be caused by tumors, multiple sclerosis, trauma, or vascular insufficiency, such as that seen in lateral medullary (Wallenberg's) syndrome. Preganglionic and postganglionic sympathetic fibers can also be disrupted, resulting in a Horner's syndrome. Preganglionic fibers originating from the upper three thoracic segments enter the sympathetic chain, ascend, and synapse in the superior cervical ganglion. Postganglionic fibers to the effectors travel with the external and internal carotid arteries. Therefore an interruption of preganglionic fibers (in the ventral roots or in the cervical sympathetic chain) or postganglionic fibers may also result in Horner's syndrome (Fig. 10-24, A).

Some causes of interruption of preganglionic sympathetic fibers include an apical lung (Pancoast) tumor pressing on the stellate ganglion (Fig. 10-24, B), surgical trauma to the thorax or neck, and a cervical spine fracture or dislocation (Cross, 1993a). Postganglionic fibers may be disrupted in the neck or within the cranium. A lesion distal to the superior cervical ganglion may produce variation in the clinical signs and symptoms presented by the patient, since the postganglionic fibers use several different arteries to travel to their effectors. Therefore the signs and symptoms depend on which postganglionic fibers have been damaged.

Raynaud's Disease

Raynaud's disease is the result of vasospasms in the digital arteries and arterioles of the fingers (most frequently). Although rarely affected alone, the toes may become involved in conjunction with the fingers. Induced by cold, this painful episodic condition presents bilaterally as changes in skin color caused by vasoconstriction and later a reactive hyperemia. This phenomenon may also be present secondary to other disorders, such as thoracic outlet syndrome, carpal tunnel syndrome, connective tissue disorders, and occupational trauma (e.g., operating air hammers or chain saws). Although conservative treatment should be attempted first, in serious cases the administration of sympathetic pharmacologic blockers (e.g., reserpine) or even sympathectomy may be necessary to treat this condition (Carpenter & Sutin, 1983; Khurana, 1993; Snell, 1992).

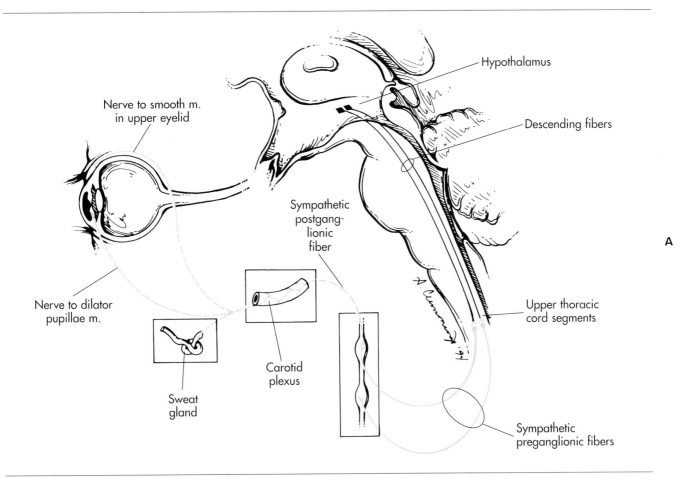

Nerve to smooth m. in upper eyelid

Hypothalamus

Descending fibers

A

Sympathetic postganglionic fiber

Nerve to dilator pupillae m.

Carotid plexus

Sweat gland

Upper thoracic cord segments

Sympathetic preganglionic fibers

FIG. 10-24 Sites of lesions that may cause Horner's syndrome. **A,** An interruption of descending hypothalamic fibers within the brain stem, of sympathetic preganglionic, or of sympathetic postganglionic fibers may produce the symptoms associated with Horner's syndrome.

Continued.

Hirschsprung's Disease

Hirschsprung's disease (megacolon) is a congenital condition affecting the enteric nervous system. It occurs when the myenteric plexus of a segment of the distal colon does not develop, leaving that segment of colon in a state of constriction. This subsequently blocks evacuation of the bowel and causes the region proximal to the constriction to become immensely dilated.

Spinal Cord Injury

General Considerations. As mentioned in Chapter 9, an injury to the spinal cord may cause dysfunction in somatic motor activity and may impair somatic sensory input. This same type of lesion may also have widespread and disastrous effects on the ANS. These effects may occur by destroying the preganglionic neuron cell bodies or by removing the descending influence on preganglionic neurons from higher centers.

The latter scenario would result in loss of input from the hypothalamus, medullary centers, and other centers on the preganglionic neurons below the level of the lesion.

The specific level of the lesion and the amount of neuronal loss determine which functions of the ANS are lost and which are retained. High lesions of upper thoracic or cervical segments are especially detrimental because they can eliminate all brain control on essential homeostatic mechanisms. These mechanisms are extremely important in permitting the body to respond to such events as environmental changes (e.g., temperature) or emotional stresses. For example, with complete lesions of the lower cervical spinal cord, all integration between segmental autonomic reflexes and descending influences is eliminated. This leaves any remaining control of bladder and bowel function, sexual function, cardiovascular regulation, and thermoregulation to the uninhibited reflex arcs formed by visceral afferent fibers and

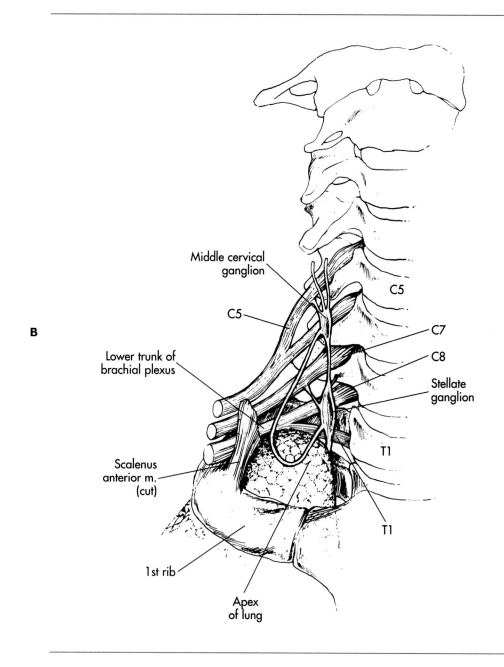

B

Middle cervical ganglion

C5

C5

C7

C8

Stellate ganglion

Lower trunk of brachial plexus

Scalenus anterior m. (cut)

T1

T1

1st rib

Apex of lung

FIG. 10-24, cont'd.   B, Because of the location of the lung apex, stellate ganglion, and lowest trunk of the brachial plexus, a tumor in the lung apex may result in a Horner's syndrome and in lesion signs in the upper extremity (as a result of pressure on the stellate ganglion and lowest trunk of the brachial plexus, respectively).

preganglionic sympathetic and sacral parasympathetic efferent fibers. This can be life-threatening in the case of regulation of vasomotor tone and thermoregulation. The dysfunctions resulting from spinal cord injuries are usually most apparent in effectors that normally function automatically, are usually taken for granted (e.g., bladder and bowel function), but are an extremely important part of daily living.

Spinal Shock and Other Consequences. The initial reaction to a complete transection of the spinal cord is spinal shock, which affects somatic (see Chapter 9) and autonomic functions. Removing supraspinal input causes loss of all autonomic reflexes below the level of the lesion. This results in an areflexic, atonic bladder that is characterized by acute retention (Abdel-Azim et al., 1991) with overflow incontinence and in a paralytic ileus (Adams & Victor, 1989; Hanak & Scott, 1983; Snell, 1992). High thoracic or cervical transections can also result in the following: profound hypotension from loss of vasomotor tone, loss of thermoregulation also caused by impaired vasomotor tone, and possible loss of sweating and piloerection.

After the effects of spinal shock have worn off, autonomic functions and homeostatic control rely on the integrity of the afferent and efferent neurons below the level of the lesion, and a stage of heightened reflex activity ensues. This stage is characterized by hyperactivity in deep tendon reflexes, a spastic bladder (see Effects on Bladder Function), and heightened vasoconstrictor and sweating responses to epinephrine (see Denervation Hypersensitivity).

In addition to bladder, bowel, and sexual functions being disrupted, lesions causing quadriplegia continue to produce serious impairment of other ANS functions, since descending input to sympathetic efferents destined for the heart, peripheral blood vessels, sweat glands, and arrector pili muscles is severed. A specific example of a difficulty that arises from the loss of descending input to preganglionic sympathetic neurons is a marked decrease in the ability to regulate blood pressure. Normally a decrease in cerebral blood pressure, such as would occur when sitting up from a supine position, is easily corrected. In patients with cervical cord injuries, the decrease in blood pressure stimulates baroreceptors, but the stimulation does not result in reflex sympathetic vasoconstriction. Therefore the patient is prone to orthostatic hypotension, and if the drop in blood pressure is severe enough, consciousness may be lost. Also, the regulation of vasomotor tone in response to temperature changes or emotional stress (which usually acts as a sympathetic stimulus) is absent in dermatomes below the level of the lesion. For example, with an injury of the upper thoracic spinal cord (about T3) the face and neck may demonstrate flushing and sweating in response to a rise in temperature, but reflex vasodilation of the rest of the body does not occur (Adams & Victor, 1989; Appenzeller, 1986). These patients have difficulty controlling their body temperature.

Effects on Bladder Function. The normal functioning of the bladder is regulated by numerous areas in the CNS (see Fig. 10-18). The involvement of higher centers with sacral afferent and efferent neurons generates a sense of fullness and the need to void. These connections also allow the suppression of voiding until an appropriate time, and also provide the ability to start and stop voiding and to evacuate the bladder completely. Lesions in the spinal cord disrupt this type of voluntary control.

A complete lesion above the lumbosacral cord segments severs ascending sensory input to the brain and descending information from the brain and results in a reflex neurogenic (spastic) bladder. The bladder is hyperreflexic, and stretch receptors initiate reflex contraction on filling. However, incomplete emptying occurs because of "detrusor-striated sphincter dyssynergia" (lack of coordination between the detrusor muscle and the external urethral sphincter, caused by the disruption of descending fibers) (Abdel-Azim et al., 1991; Bradley, 1993; de Groat et al., 1990). A lesion in sacral cord segments (conus medullaris) or the cauda equina destroys the innervation to the bladder and produces a nonreflex, autonomous (flaccid) bladder. The detrusor muscle is areflexic and atonic, and the bladder fills and overflows (overflow incontinence). It is possible for patients to manage bladder function by learning and maintaining a routine of consistent fluid intake and by catheterization (preferably intermittent). In some instances, pharmacologic therapy may also be necessary. In patients with supraspinal lesions, surgical enlargement of the bladder (augmentation cystoplasty) may also become an option. In individuals with sacral cord lesions, micturition is possible by using the Credé (applying manual pressure to the suprapubic region) and Valsalva maneuvers (Abdel-Azim et al., 1991).

Effects on Bowel Function. Lesions that result in bladder dysfunction also affect bowel activity. The types of effectors involved with normal bowel function (i.e., smooth muscle and striated sphincters) are similar to those involved with bladder functions. The pattern of innervation of the bowel is also similar to that of the bladder. Thus, similarities exist between the effects of spinal cord lesions on bowel function and the effects on bladder function. Loss of descending input from the brain eliminates the voluntary control of defecation, the awareness of the sensation to defecate, and the knowledge that defecation is occurring. Instead, the bowel is automatic, which means that it contracts in response to local reflexes. These reflexes are initiated by distention, irritation (e.g., suppositories), and in some instances digital anal stimulation. Management of bowel, as well as bladder, function is of great concern for the patient, and helping the patient become as independent as possible is a psychologic advantage. Setting aside a routine time for reflex bowel action is important for bowel training. Proper diet, fluid intake, positioning, and medication can also help to maximize the success of such training (Sutton, 1973).

Effects on Sexual Function. Of great importance to many patients with spinal cord injuries is the extent to which their sexual functions are impaired. As with the urinary system, the genitalia receive parasympathetic, sympathetic, and somatic innervation (see Fig. 10-19). Male sexual dysfunction has been extensively studied, more so than dysfunction in females, most likely because fewer females experience spinal cord injuries and their functional loss is less detrimental. Similar to the effects seen in other organs, the degree of dysfunction depends on the completeness of the lesion and the level of the injury.

Erections can be psychogenic or reflexogenic (see earlier discussion). The former are initiated by supraspinal input channeled through the hypothalamus and limbic systems to descend ultimately to parasympathetic and sympathetic efferents (de Groat & Steers, 1990). Reflexogenic erections are elicited by exteroceptive stimuli and are mediated by a reflex arc that uses sacral cord segments. In healthy individuals, both supraspinal and reflex connections probably work in concert.

Patients with spinal cord injuries are usually still capable of having erections (Seftel et al., 1991). Patients with complete lower motor neuron lesions in the sacral cord (conus medullaris) or cauda equina may still retain psychogenic erections via the sympathetic innervation of the penis, although reflexogenic erections are absent (de Groat & Steers, 1990; Seftel et al., 1991). However, patients with complete upper motor neuron lesions, above the T12 cord segment, are incapable of psychogenic erections, although reflexogenic erections are usually present (Seftel et al., 1991). Tactile stimulation of the genital area is the initiator of this reflex response. Incomplete lower or upper motor neuron lesions increases the chances of being able to have psychogenic erections.

Although erections occur frequently in spinal cord–injured patients, ejaculation is uncommon in patients with complete upper motor neuron lesions. The CNS mediation of ejaculation is highly complex, involving an ejaculatory center in the lower thoracolumbar spinal cord segments and in supraspinal areas, such as the cerebral cortex. Although the circuitry is not completely understood, these centers are thought to be vulnerable to injury. Because of the failure to ejaculate, infertility is a major problem among patients with spinal cord lesions (Seftel et al., 1991).

Conus Medullaris Syndrome. As mentioned previously, the pattern of innervation to the bladder, bowel, and genitalia is similar and involves sympathetic, parasympathetic, and somatic neurons. Lesions in the sacral segments produce a conus medullaris syndrome affecting the bladder, bowel, and genitalia in a manner described previously. Conus medullaris syndrome also results in anesthesia in the perianal region. Of diagnostic value is that this syndrome results in perianal sensory loss and autonomic disturbances, but the lower extremities retain their normal sensory and motor functions (Carpenter & Sutin, 1983).

Autonomic Dysreflexia. Spinal cord lesions of midthoracic and cervical segments also produce a condition called autonomic dysreflexia, also known as autonomic hyperreflexia. This syndrome is a widespread autonomic reflex reaction to afferent stimuli that is normally modulated by descending supraspinal input. The initiation of autonomic dysreflexia occurs when a noxious stimulus causes afferent fibers to fire and send input into the spinal cord below the level of the lesion. Common stimuli are distention of the bladder, urinary tract infection, blockage or insertion of a catheter, rectal distention, and occasionally cutaneous stimulation and flexion contractures (Appenzeller, 1986; Benarroch, 1993). Without normal supraspinal inhibition, sympathetic efferents cause widespread reflex vasoconstriction in areas innervated by cord segments below the lesion. This results in hypertension. Baroreceptors monitoring the increase in blood pressure send information to vasomotor centers, which in turn attempt to correct this threatening situation. This results in bradycardia, and above the level of the lesion (usually in the face and neck), vasodilation, flushing, and profuse sweating occur.

However, because of the lesion, no corrective message reaches the sympathetic fibers below the spinal cord blockage, and therefore vasoconstriction continues and is accompanied by piloerection and skin pallor (Naftchi et al., 1982b). Patients monitored during a hypertensive crisis exhibit an increase of their mean arterial pressure from 95 to 154 mm Hg (Naftchi et al., 1982a). Others demonstrate a systolic pressure that may exceed 200 mm Hg (Ropper, 1993). This hypertension usually produces a throbbing headache and is extremely serious because it can result in seizures, localized neurologic deficits, myocardial infarction, visual defects, and cerebral hemorrhaging (Adams & Victor, 1989; Benarroch, 1993; Hanak & Scott, 1983). Immediate alleviation of this condition by identifying and removing the cause of the stimulus, which can produce a decrease in blood pressure within 2 to 10 minutes (Ropper, 1993), is imperative.

Conclusion. Lesions of the spinal cord producing dysfunction of normal sexual, bowel, and bladder activities cause not only considerable physical impairment, but also significant psychologic concern for the patient. Rehabilitation of the patient to as much independent control as possible with as little reliance on others as possible is extremely important. The location of the lesion determines the amount and type of function that remain, and the amount of remaining function determines the methods that may be used to achieve self-reliance.

As can be seen from the previous discussion, the effects of spinal cord injury to the somatic (see Chapter 9) and autonomic nervous systems can be considerable and in some cases life-threatening. The resulting loss of sensory and motor functions serves as a continual reminder of the importance of the intricate and complex neural circuitry that is necessary for the normal functioning of the human body.

REFERENCES

Abdel-Azim, M., Sullivan, M., & Yalla, S.V. (1991). Disorders of bladder function in spinal cord disease. *Neurol Clin, 9*(3), 727-740.

Adams, R.D. & Victor, M. (1989). *Principles of neurology* (4th ed.). St. Louis: McGraw-Hill.

Appenzeller, O. (1986). *Clinical autonomic failure*. New York: Elsevier.

Barr, M.L. & Kiernan, J.A. (1993). *The human nervous system* (6th ed.). Philadelphia: JB Lippincott.

Barron, K.D. & Chokroverty, S. (1993). Anatomy of the autonomic nervous system: Brain and brainstem. In P.A. Low (Ed.), *Clinical autonomic disorders*. Boston: Little, Brown.

Beal, M.C. (1985). Viscerosomatic reflexes: A review. *J Am Osteopath Assoc, 85*(12), 53-68.

Benarroch, E.E. (1993). Central autonomic disorders. In P.A. Low (Ed.), *Clinical autonomic disorders*. Boston: Little, Brown.

Bradley, W.E. (1993). Autonomic regulation of the urinary bladder. In P.A. Low (Ed.), *Clinical autonomic disorders*. Boston: Little, Brown.

Cabot, J.B. (1990). Sympathetic preganglionic neurons: Cytoarchitecture, ultrastructure, and biophysical properties. In A.D. Loewy & K.M. Spyer (Eds.) *Central regulation of autonomic functions*. New York: Oxford University Press.

Camilleri, M. (1993). Autonomic regulation of gastrointestinal motility. In P.A. Low (Ed.), *Clinical autonomic disorders*. Boston: Little, Brown.

Carpenter, M.B. & Sutin, J. (1983). *Human neuroanatomy* (8th ed.). Baltimore: Williams & Wilkins.

Cervero, F. & Foreman, R.D. (1990). Sensory innervation of the viscera. In A.D. Loewy & K.M. Spyer (Eds.), *Central regulation of autonomic functions*. New York: Oxford University Press.

Cross, S.A. (1993a). Autonomic disorders of the pupil, ciliary body, and lacrimal apparatus. In P.A. Low (Ed.), *Clinical autonomic disorders*. Boston: Little, Brown.

Cross, S.A. (1993b). Autonomic innervation of the eye. In P.A. Low (Ed.), *Clinical autonomic disorders*. Boston: Little, Brown.

Dale, H. (1935). Pharmacology and nerve endings. *Proc R Soc Med, 28*, 319-332.

de Groat, W.C. & Steers, W.D. (1990). Autonomic regulation of the urinary bladder and sexual organs. In A.D. Loewy & K.M. Spyer (Eds.), *Central regulation of autonomic functions*. New York: Oxford University Press.

de Groat, W.C. et al. (1990). Mechanisms underlying the recovery of urinary bladder function following spinal cord injury. *J Auton Nerv Syst, 30*, S71-S78.

Dodd, J. & Role, L.W. (1991). The autonomic nervous system. In E.R. Kandel, J.H. Schwartz, & T.M. Jessell (Eds.), *Principles of neural science* (3rd ed.). New York: Elsevier.

Gershon, M.D. (1981). The enteric nervous system. *Annu Rev Neurosci, 4*, 227-272.

Guyton, A.C. (1991). *Textbook of medical physiology* (8th ed.). Philadelphia: WB Saunders.

Hanak, M. & Scott, A. (1983). *Spinal cord injury*. New York: Springer.

Harati, Y. (1993). Anatomy of the spinal and peripheral autonomic nervous system. In P.A. Low (Ed.), *Clinical autonomic disorders*. Boston: Little, Brown.

Jänig, W. (1990). Functions of the sympathetic innervation of the skin. In A.D. Loewy & K.M. Spyer (Eds.). *Central regulation of autonomic functions*. New York: Oxford University Press.

Jänig, W. (1988). Integration of gut function by sympathetic reflexes. *Baillieres Clin Gastroenterol, 2*(1), 45-62.

Khurana, R.K. (1993). Acral sympathetic dysfunctions and hyperhidrosis. In P.A. Low (Ed.), *Clinical autonomic disorders*. Boston: Little, Brown.

Loewy, A.D. (1990a). Anatomy of the autonomic nervous system: An overview. In A.D. Loewy & K.M. Spyer (Eds.). *Central regulation of autonomic functions*. New York: Oxford University Press.

Loewy, A.D. (1990b). Autonomic control of the eye. In A.D. Loewy & K.M. Spyer (Eds.), *Central regulation of autonomic functions*. New York: Oxford University Press.

Loewy, A.D. (1990c). Central autonomic pathways. In A.D. Loewy & K.M. Spyer (Eds.), *Central regulation of autonomic functions*. New York: Oxford University Press.

Loewy, A.D. & Spyer, K.M. (1990). Vagal preganglionic neurons. In A.D. Loewy & K.M. Spyer (Eds.). *Central regulation of autonomic functions*. New York: Oxford University Press.

Menetrey, D. & Basbaum, A.I. (1987). Spinal and trigeminal projections to the nucleus of the solitary tract: A possible substrate for somatovisceral and viscerovisceral reflex activation, *J Comp Neurol, 255*, 439-450.

Moore, K.L. (1980). *Clinically oriented anatomy*. Baltimore: Williams & Wilkins.

Naftchi, N.E. et al. (1982a). Autonomic hyperreflexia: Hemodynamics, blood volume, serum dopamine-β-hydroxylase activity, and arterial prostaglandin PGE2. In N.E. Naftchi (Ed.), *Spinal cord injury*. New York: Spectrum.

Naftchi, N.E. et al. (1982b). Relationship between serum dopamine-β-hydroxylase activity, catecholamine metabolism, and hemodynamic changes during paroxysmal hypertension in quadriplegia. In N.E. Naftchi (Ed.), *Spinal cord injury*. New York: Spectrum.

Noback, C.R., Strominger, N.L., & Demarest, R.J. (1991). *The human nervous system* (4th ed.). Philadelphia: Lea & Febiger.

Nolte, J. (1993). *The human brain* (3rd ed.). St. Louis: Mosby.

Ogawa, T. & Low, P.A. (1993). Autonomic regulation of temperature and sweating. In P.A. Low (Ed.), *Clinical autonomic disorders*. Boston: Little, Brown.

Parkinson, D. (1990a). Adrenergic receptors in the autonomic nervous system. In A.D. Loewy & K.M. Spyer (Eds.), *Central regulation of autonomic functions*. New York: Oxford University Press.

Parkinson, D. (1990b). Cholinergic receptors. In A.D. Loewy & K.M. Spyer (Eds.), *Central regulation of autonomic functions*. New York: Oxford University Press.

Ropper, A.H. (1993). Acute autonomic emergencies in autonomic storm. In P.A. Low (Ed.), *Clinical autonomic disorders*. Boston: Little, Brown.

Ruch, T.C. (1946). Visceral sensation and referred pain. In J.F. Fulton (Ed.), *Howell's textbook of physiology* (15th ed.). Philadelphia: WB Saunders.

Sato, A. (1992a). The reflex effects of spinal somatic nerve stimulation on visceral function. *J Manipulative Physiol Ther, (15)*(1), 57-61.

Sato, A. (1992b). Spinal reflex physiology. In S. Haldeman (Ed.), *Principles and practice of chiropractic* (2nd ed.). East Norwalk, Conn: Appleton & Lange.

Sato, A. & Swenson, R.S. (1984). Sympathetic nervous system response to mechanical stress of the spinal column in rats. *J Manipulative Physiol Ther, 7*(3), 141-147.

Sato, A., Sato, Y., & Schmidt, R.F. (1984). Changes in blood pressure and heart rate induced by movements of normal and inflamed knee joints. *Neurosci Lett, 52*, 55-60.

Seftel, A.D., Oates, R.D., & Krane, R. J. (1991). Disturbed sexual function in patients with spinal cord disease. *Neurol Clin, 9*(3), 757-778.

Snell, R.S. (1992). *Clinical neuroanatomy for medical students* (3rd ed.). Boston: Little, Brown.

Stewart, J.D. (1993). Autonomic regulation of sexual function. In P.A. Low (Ed.), *Clinical autonomic disorders.* Boston: Little, Brown.

Sutton, N.G. (1973). *Injuries of the spinal cord.* Toronto: Butterworth.

Taylor, G.S. & Bywater, R.A. (1988). Intrinsic control of the gut. *Baillieres Clin Gastroenterol, 2*(1), 1-22.

Williams, P.L. et al. (1989). *Gray's anatomy* (37th ed.). Edinburgh: Churchill Livingstone.

Willis, W.D. & Coggeshall, R.E. (1991). *Sensory mechanisms of the spinal cord* (2nd ed.). New York: Plenum Press.

CHAPTER 11

Pain of Spinal Origin

Gregory D. Cramer
Susan A. Darby

The purpose of this chapter is to apply much of the information discussed in previous chapters to the clinical setting. This is accomplished by discussing the case of a typical patient with low back pain. In addition, structural features of other regions of the spine particularly susceptible to injury or pathologic conditions are also briefly mentioned. The aspects of pain discussed in this chapter are meant to include the most common causes of discomfort. Exhaustive lists are beyond the scope of this chapter. It is not our intention in this chapter to cover the topic of back pain thoroughly. Fortunately,

this subject has been reported thoroughly elsewhere (see Bogduk & Twomey, 1991; Haldeman, 1992; and Kirkaldy-Willis, 1988a). Rather, the primary purpose of this chapter is to apply the previously covered gross anatomic and neuroanatomic information to clinical practice. To accomplish this purpose, we have chosen to discuss a challenging problem that faces clinicians continuously, their patients' pain.

PATIENT BACKGROUND

On a bright Monday afternoon in January, Mr. S, a 40-year-old male, enters your waiting room. The receptionist recognizes Mr. S as a previous patient. As she hands him a form inquiring about the details of his chief complaint, she notices his extremely slow gait and very guarded stance. While Mr. S diligently fills out the form, the receptionist retrieves his previous records. At the earliest opportunity, she hands you the file previously compiled on Mr. S and mentions that he appears to have "a nasty case of low back pain." As you review the records, you immediately recall Mr. S as a patient from 3 years earlier. He had strained the muscles of his low back while unloading bags of dry cement mix, which he was planning to use for a home improvement project. You suspect his complaint today may be related to this prior incident, and you begin to analyze the perception of pain.

PERCEPTION OF PAIN

Your general approach to patients complaining of pain is that their pain is real. It has both physical and psychologic components, one of which may predominate, and the pain always alters the personality of the individual (Kirkaldy-Willis, 1988b). This alteration of personality usually returns to the prepain state when the physical cause of the discomfort has sufficiently healed. In addition, pain always has a subjective component and is perceived by patients in relation to previous experiences with pain, usually from their early years (Weinstein, 1988).

Pain has been defined by the International Association for the Study of Pain as "an unpleasant sensory and emotional experience associated with actual or potential tissue damage, or described in terms of such damage" (Merskey, 1979). This group's committee on taxonomy goes on to state, "If a patient regards their experience as pain and if they report it in the same ways as pain caused by tissue damage, it should be accepted as pain" (Merskey, 1979). Therefore, not all pain is the result of a nociceptive stimulus received and transmitted by a sensory receptor of a peripheral nerve (Weinstein, 1988).

Many other factors may influence the patient's perception of pain, including the following: the individual's general health, the nervous system's overall status, the pain's chronicity, and even the environment in which the patient lives (Haldeman, 1992). In addition, the dorsal root ganglia, the spinal cord, and higher centers are all capable of adjusting and regulating (modulating) painful stimuli. Therefore, to continue with our example of Mr. S, the clinician may not fully appreciate and understand the severity of Mr. S's pain until he or she has had an opportunity to observe him on several different occasions (Kirkaldy-Willis, 1988b).

The characteristics and quality of pain, such as that experienced by Mr. S, can be important. For example, diffuse burning pain, which may or may not radiate into the lower extremity, is usually of sympathetic origin. Peripheral receptors of the recurrent meningeal nerve carry afferents that travel with sympathetic fibers. These receptors may be stimulated by arachnoiditis and postoperative fibrosis and could possibly be a source of diffuse burning pain of sympathetic origin (Kirkaldy-Willis, 1988b). However, aching is usually the result of muscle tightness or soreness and is frequently relieved by stretching and short periods of rest. Other generalized lower extremity pain, excluding aching pain, is often associated with a vascular or neurogenic cause (Weinstein, 1988).

PAIN OF SOMATIC ORIGIN

You now begin to consider the possible causes of Mr. S's current discomfort. You know that even though low back pain is one of the most common complaints seen by physicians, it is also one of the most difficult to understand (Weinstein, 1988). Recall that an anatomic structure must be supplied by nociceptive nerve endings (nerve endings sensitive to tissue damage; see Chapter 9) to be a cause of low back pain, and that Mr. S's perception of his low back pain greatly depends on the factors described previously. Also recall that nociceptors may be stimulated by mechanical, thermal, or chemical means, and because the structures that receive nociceptive innervation are able to "generate pain," they are sometimes referred to as pain generators.

Once a nociceptor has depolarized, it changes its properties, frequently becoming more sensitive to subsequent noxious stimuli. This increased sensitivity is known as hyperalgesia. The central nervous system (CNS) also has several mechanisms by which it, too, may create hyperalgesia in an area of injury. Therefore, after tissue is damaged, it is usually more sensitive to further nociception until healing has occurred. After pathologic conditions or injury, hyperalgesia may also be present in the healthy tissues surrounding the site of the lesion.

Frequently, nociception of spinal origin is the result of damage to several structures, and the effects of hyperalgesia allow for nociception to be felt from tissues that, if injured to the same degree independently, might have gone unnoticed (Haldeman, 1992).

Most pain has a physical cause, even though not all the structures supplied by nociceptors, and therefore capable of producing "pain," are known (Haldeman, 1992). Also, those tissues that are supplied by nociceptive nerve endings can usually undergo a number of different pathologic processes that can lead to stimulation of nociceptors (Haldeman, 1992).

One of the best ways to organize Mr. S's possible "pain generators" is by listing them according to the four main sources of neural innervation to spinal structures: the anterior primary division (APD, ventral ramus), the posterior primary division (PPD, dorsal ramus), the recurrent meningeal nerve, and sensory fibers that course with the sympathetic nervous system (Fig. 11-1). All these afferent nerves have their cell bodies in the dorsal root ganglia (DRGs), which, with the exception of C1 and C2 (see Chapter 5), are located within the intervertebral foramina (IVFs) of the spine. Note that the sensory fibers, which are associated with the recurrent meningeal nerve and the sympathetic nervous system, provide a route for the transmission of nociception from somatic structures of the vertebral column's anterior aspect. Fibers arising from these sources pass through the APD for a short distance before reaching the mixed spinal nerve. They then enter the dorsal root. Even though these nerves briefly pass through the ventral ramus, they are best considered separately because they are important with regard to nociception of spinal origin.

Anterior Primary Divisions (Ventral Rami)

To approach the cause of the discomfort experienced by Mr. S, let us first consider those structures innervated by

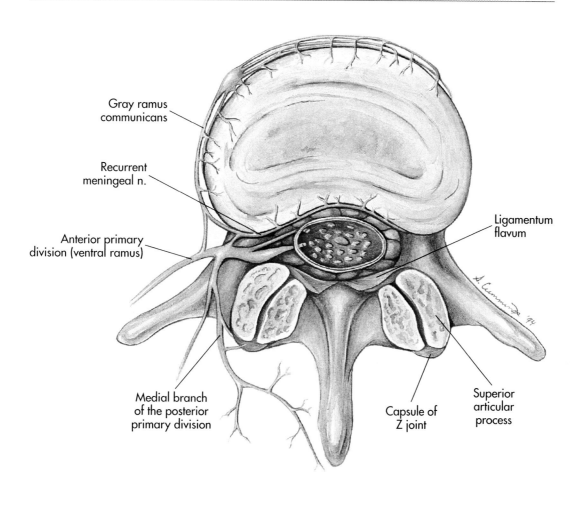

Gray ramus communicans

Recurrent meningeal n.

Anterior primary division (ventral ramus)

Ligamentum flavum

Medial branch of the posterior primary division

Capsule of Z joint

Superior articular process

FIG. 11-1 Horizontal view of a lumbar vertebra, the intervertebral foramina, the vertebral foramen, and the nerves associated with this region. Notice the innervation to the zygapophyseal joint by the medial branch of the posterior primary division. Also notice the recurrent meningeal nerve innervating the posterior aspect of the intervertebral disc. The recurrent meningeal nerve also innervates the posterior longitudinal ligament and the anterior aspect of the spinal dura mater.

the lumbar APDs (see the box at right). The APDs of the lumbar region innervate much of the gluteal and inguinal regions, as well as the entire lower extremity. Although these regions may refer to the low back, they usually are accompanied by more localized pain from the structure that is either injured or is affected by some form of pathologic process. More likely causes of back pain originating from structures innervated by APDs (ventral rami) are several muscles, including the psoas major, the quadratus lumborum, and the lateral intertransversarii. Strain or possibly increased tightness (what some would call "spasm") of these muscles can be a source of back pain. Abscess within the psoas muscle is also a possible source of pain. The transverse processes

(TPs) are also innervated by the APD, and a fracture of a TP or a bruise to its periosteum may result in pain (Bogduk, 1983).

SPINE-RELATED STRUCTURES INNERVATED BY THE VENTRAL RAMUS

Possible pain generators
- Referred pain from structures innervated by nerves of the lumbar plexus
- Psoas muscle
- Quadratus lumborum muscle
- Intertransversarii muscles (lateral divisions)

Posterior Primary Divisions (Dorsal Rami)

Discomfort such as that experienced by Mr. S may also arise from structures innervated by the PPDs (dorsal rami). These are listed in the box below. This list contains some of the most frequent causes of low back pain, including the deep back muscles, which receive nociceptive innervation by means of nerves accompanying the vessels that supply these muscles; spinal ligaments (nociceptors are most numerous in the posterior longitudinal ligament [innervated by the recurrent meningeal nerve] and fewest in the interspinous ligament and the ligamentum flavum); and the zygapophyseal joints (Z joints). These are all high on the list of possible causes of pain similar to that experienced by Mr. S. Each of these groups of structures may be affected by a number of pathologic conditions or injuries. The muscles may be strained or may be affected by areas of myofascial tenderness ("trigger points") (Bogduk, 1983; Hubbard & Berkoff, 1993). The ligaments may be sprained. Pain from the Z joints may be difficult to localize because each Z joint receives innervation from the PPD of the same level and also from the PPD of the level above (Bogduk, 1976). The Z joints may be fractured or they may be inflamed as a result of arthritic changes. Discomfort can also arise from a Z joint articular capsule or a Z joint synovial fold that has become entrapped within the Z joint or pinched between the articular surfaces (see Chapter 7). Degeneration of articular cartilage may produce inflammatory agents that may stimulate nociceptors of the Z joint articular capsules. Inactivity of the spinal joints, even if this inactivity is imposed on these joints by muscle guarding, may promote pain (Kirkaldy-Willis, 1988b). In addition, the spinous processes may be fractured or may repeatedly collide with one another (Bastrup's syndrome).

Recurrent Meningeal Nerve

Structures innervated by the recurrent meningeal (sinuvertebral) nerve may also be a source of back pain. The list in the box below identifies the structures supplied by these nerves. The periosteum of a vertebral body may be affected by fracture or neoplasm within the vertebral body. The basivertebral veins may possibly be affected by intraosseous hypertension, crush fractures, or neoplasms of the vertebral body (Bogduk, 1983). The epidural veins may be affected by venous engorgement. The posterior aspect of the intervertebral disc (IVD) can be affected by internal disc disruption, protrusion of the nucleus pulposus through the outer layers of the anulus fibrosus, or tearing (sprain) of the outer layers of the anulus fibrosus. The posterior longitudinal ligament can be torn (sprain) during severe hyperflexion injuries or may be pierced by an IVD protrusion. The anterior aspect of the dura mater may be compressed by an IVD protrusion or may be irritated by the release of chemical mediators associated with internal disc disruption (see Chapter 7).

STRUCTURES INNERVATED BY THE RECURRENT MENINGEAL NERVE

Possible pain generators

- Periosteum of posterior aspect of vertebral bodies
- Internal vertebral (epidural) veins *and* basivertebral veins
- Epidural adipose tissue
- Posterior aspect of intervertebral disc
- Posterior longitudinal ligament
- Anterior aspect of spinal dura mater

Nerves Associated With the Sympathetic Nervous System

Finally, recall that several structures are innervated by nerves that arise directly from the sympathetic trunk and the gray communicating rami (see the box on p. 359). The sensory fibers of these nerves follow the gray rami to the APD, where they enter the mixed spinal nerve. They then reach the spinal cord by coursing through the dorsal roots. Pathologic conditions of the periosteum of the anterior and lateral aspects of the vertebral body, which are innervated by sensory fibers traveling with gray rami, may result in pain. Some of the most common causes of this type of pathologic condition include fracture, neoplasm, and osteomyelitis (Bogduk, 1983). Sprain of the anterior longitudinal ligament or the outer layers of the anterior or lateral part of the anulus fibrosis

---

STRUCTURES INNERVATED BY THE DORSAL RAMUS

Possible pain generators

Medial branch of the dorsal ramus innervates:
- Deepest back muscles
- Zygapophyseal joints
- Periosteum of posterior vertebral arch
- Interspinous, supraspinous, and intertransverse ligaments, ligamentum flavum
- Skin (in the case of upper cervical, middle cervical, and thoracic dorsal rami)

Lateral branch of the dorsal ramus innervates:
- Erector spinae muscles
- Splenius capitis and cervicis muscles (cervical region)
- Skin

may also result in nociception conducted by fibers that course with the gray communicating rami.

STRUCTURES INNERVATED BY NERVES ASSOCIATED WITH THE SYMPATHETIC TRUNK AND THE GRAY RAMI COMMUNICANTES

Possible pain generators

◆ Periosteum of the anterior and lateral aspects of the vertebral bodies
◆ Lateral aspect of the intervertebral disc
◆ Anterior aspect of the intervertebral disc
◆ Anterior longitudinal ligament

Pain Generators Unique to the Cervical Region

If Mr. S was presenting with pain in the cervical region, other structures would be included on the list of possible pain generators. These include irritation of the nerves surrounding the vertebral artery and nociception arising from uncovertebral "joints."

Nociception arising from almost any structure innervated by the upper four cervical nerves may refer to the head, resulting in head pains and headaches (Aprill, Dwyer, & Bogduk, 1990; Bogduk, 1984; Bogduk, Lambert, & Duckworth, 1981; Campbell & Parsons, 1944; Dwyer, Aprill, & Bogduk et al., 1990; Edmeads, 1978). Pain originating from the region of the basiociput and occipital condyles frequently refers to the orbital and frontal regions (Campbell & Parsons, 1944). Autonomic reactions such as sweating, pallor, nausea, alterations of pulse, and other autonomic disturbances have frequently been observed in association with disturbances of the suboccipital and upper cervical spine. The intensity of these autonomic reactions seems to be proportional to the stimulus and the proximity of the stimulus to the suboccipital region. The autonomic response ranges from mild subjective discomforts to measurable objective signs (Campbell & Parsons, 1944).

Pain Generators Unique to the Thoracic Region

If Mr. S should present with discomfort of the thoracic region, the costocorporeal and costotransverse articulations would be added to the list of possible pain generators (see Chapter 6). Also, a compression fracture of one or more of the thoracic vertebral bodies would be a realistic source of acute pain arising from the thoracic region.

Dorsal Root Ganglia

The DRGs serve as modulators of spinal nociception. They contain many neuropeptides (see Chapter 9) associated with the transmission of nociception (substance P, calcitonin, gene-related peptide, vasoactive intestinal peptide) (Weinstein, 1988). These substances may be released from the peripheral terminals of sensory nerves that transmit nociception. The neuropeptides may reach these peripheral terminals (receptors) by axonal transport mechanisms. The presence of neuropeptides in and around the receptors may "prime" the receptors, making them more susceptible to depolarization (Weinstein, 1988).

SOMATIC REFERRED PAIN

Nociception arising from any of the somatic structures previously listed may be perceived by Mr. S or a similar patient as being a considerable distance from the pain generator. This is known as pain referral, and the term *somatic referred pain* has been used to describe this type of back pain (Bogduk & Twomey, 1991).

Several possible mechanisms of pain referral exist. Perhaps one of the most important mechanisms is the result of the internal organization of the spinal cord. The nociceptive information coming in from a pain generator is dispersed by either ascending or descending fibers that make up the dorsolateral tract of Lissauer (see Chapter 9). These fibers may ascend or descend several cord segments before synapsing. Thus, nociceptive information, entering from several different spinal cord segments, converges on the same interneuronal pool. Therefore, this interneuronal pool receives primary sensory information from different somatic regions (Fig. 11-2). The dispersal of incoming afferents onto different-tract neurons, in combination with the convergence of several different afferents onto single-tract neurons, may decrease the ability of the CNS to localize nociception (Darby & Cramer 1994; Haldeman, 1992). This type of dispersal and convergence may also be found at the second synapse along the nociceptive pathway. This synapse occurs in the ventral posterior lateral nucleus of the thalamus (see later discussion on pain pathway).

The ventral posterior lateral thalamic nucleus projects to the postcentral gyrus of the cerebral cortex. The region of the back is represented on a small area of the postcentral gyrus (sensory homunculus) of the cerebral cortex. This may also contribute to the poor localization of nociception of spinal origin (Haldeman, 1992). In addition, the tract neurons for ascending pain pathways most frequently carry nociceptive information from cutaneous areas. Therefore, when the tract neurons are stimulated to fire, the cerebral cortex (where conscious

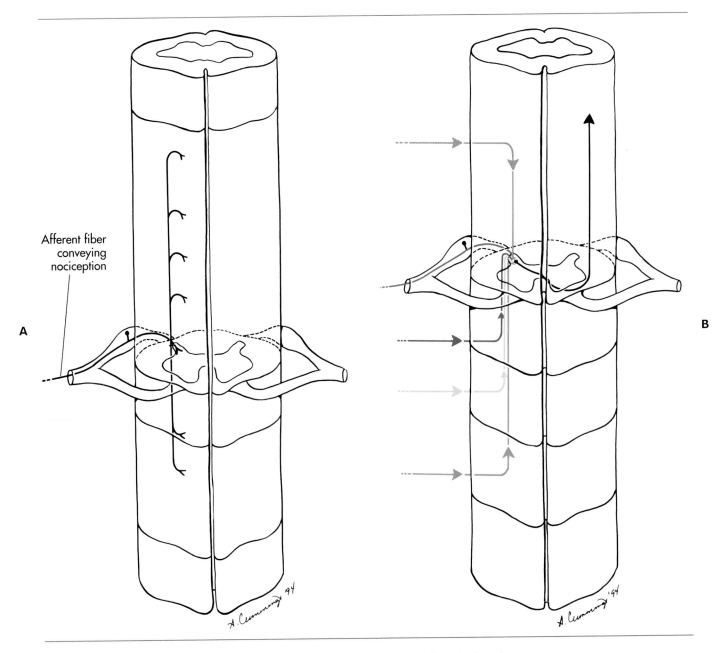

Afferent fiber
conveying
nociception

A

B

FIG. 11-2 **A,** Dispersion of afferents conducting nociception as they enter the spinal cord.
B, Convergence of afferents conducting nociception onto a tract neuron.

awareness of nociception occurs) may interpret the impulse as originating from a cutaneous region or from another recently injured region. Either of these regions may be distant to the structure that is currently damaged or inflamed. This phenomenon is sometimes referred to as pain memory (Carpenter & Sutin, 1983; Nolte, 1988; Wyke, 1987).

The existence of pain referral between somatic structures has been documented for some time (Hockaday & Whitty, 1967; Inman & Saunders, 1944; Kellgren, 1938; McCall, Park, & O'Brien, 1979). The term *somatic re-*

ferred pain is currently used when discussing pain of somatic origin that is felt distant to the structure generating the nociception (see the boxed definition on p. 361). This type of pain is characterized as being dull and aching, difficult to localize, and fairly constant in nature (Bogduk & Twomey, 1991). For future reference, these characteristics of somatic referred pain are highlighted in the boxes on p. 361.

Increased tenderness to deep palpation of the back muscles and hyperalgesia of all innervated tissues may occur in areas of referred pain (Weinstein, 1988). An

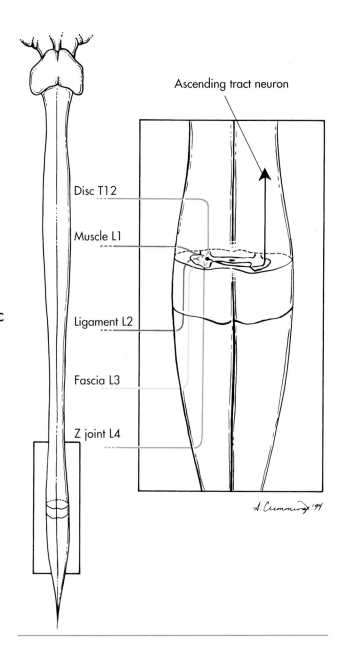

Ascending tract neuron

Disc T12

Muscle L1

Ligament L2

Fascia L3

Z joint L4

C

A. Cummings '94

FIG. 11-2, cont'd. **C,** Nociception from a variety of sources may influence the same pool of tract neurons.

example of somatic referred pain is the pain arising from an inflamed Z joint, which may refer to the groin, buttock, greater trochanter of the femur, and the posterior aspect of the thigh, extending to the knee and occasionally extending inferiorly to the leg's posterior and lateral calf (Weinstein, 1988).

Activity of the muscles and the Z joints, as well as spinal manipulation of the Z joints, tends to decrease pain via a "gate control" type of mechanism (Kirkaldy-Willis, 1988b; Melzack & Wall, 1965). Therefore, if the

pain was of somatic origin, Mr. S might benefit most from treatment designed to promote activity and movement (Kirkaldy-Willis, 1988b). At the same time, precautions should also be taken to avoid further compromise of the damaged tissue.

SOMATIC REFERRED PAIN

Nociception generated by a skeletal or related structure (muscle, ligament, zygapophyseal joint), which is felt in an area *distant* to the structure generating the nociception

---

DISTINGUISHING FEATURES OF SOMATIC REFERRED PAIN

◆ Dull ache
◆ Difficult to localize
◆ Rather constant in nature

◆ ◆ ◆

All the previously discussed information was quickly recalled even before you entered the examination room to see Mr. S. Just as you step into the room, you quickly remember the pathways for the transmission of pain.

CENTRAL TRANSMISSION OF NOCICEPTION

"Pain" is the perception that results from the interpretation of nociceptive input by a variety of CNS structures (Jessell & Kelly, 1991). Some of the CNS structures that have been implicated in this process include the dorsal horn of the spinal cord, ascending pathways, reticular formation of the brain stem, thalamus, and cerebral cortex. The interconnections of these areas and subsequent integration of the information result in the components associated with the sensation of pain. These components include discriminatory qualities, emotions, attentiveness to the painful area, and reflex responses involving both the autonomic and the endocrine systems (Haldeman, 1992).

The afferent fibers that convey nociception are group A-delta and group C fibers. These fibers enter the dorsolateral tract of Lissauer, located at the tip of the cord's dorsal horn. Some fibers continue directly into the gray matter of the dorsal horn, whereas their collateral branches ascend or descend numerous cord segment levels before entering the dorsal horn (Fig. 11-2, *A*). The A-delta fibers convey nociception quickly and rapidly and terminate in lamina I and laminae IV through VI. The group C fibers convey a dull sensation of pain at a slow rate and terminate in lamina II. The neurons that transmit the information to higher centers are located in various laminae of the gray matter (see Chapter 9). Surgical cordotomy procedures that relieve pain have shown that the most important fibers transmitting nociception to higher centers decussate in the ventral white commissure and then ascend in the anterolateral quadrant of the cord's white matter (Hoffert, 1989). Alternative pathways may also be involved, although their course and function in humans remain unclear (Besson, 1988; Hoffert, 1989).

Neospinothalamic Tract

One of the tracts in the anterolateral quadrant is the neospinothalamic tract. This tract ascends through the brain stem to the ventral posterior lateral nucleus and also to the posterior nucleus of the thalamus with little or no input to the brain stem (Fig. 11-3, *A*). From the thalamus, axons course to the somesthetic region of the cortex, which is the postcentral gyrus and the posterior part of the paracentral lobule of the parietal lobe. As the axons ascend, body parts are represented in specific regions of the tract. This specific pattern is retained in the cerebral cortex such that a specific area of cortex corresponds to the region of the body from which the sensory fibers originate. This cortical representation is referred to as the sensory homunculus. The size of the body part represented on the homunculus reflects the amount of sensory innervation devoted to that body area. As previously mentioned, this unequal neuronal representation may be one reason that localization of sensations, such as pain, is more difficult in one region (e.g., back) than in another (e.g., finger tips or lips). The neospinothalamic tract ends by synapsing in the region of the sensory homunculus. This tract and the region of the sensory homunculus provide the basis for the discriminatory qualities of pain sensation. These qualities include stimulus intensity and spatial localization.

Paleospinothalamic and Spinoreticular Tracts

Two additional tracts that ascend in the anterolateral quadrant are the paleospinothalamic and spinoreticular tracts (Fig. 11-3, *B* and *C*). The paleospinothalamic tract, which ascends through the brain stem and probably contributes collateral branches to the reticular formation, terminates in the midline and intralaminar thalamic

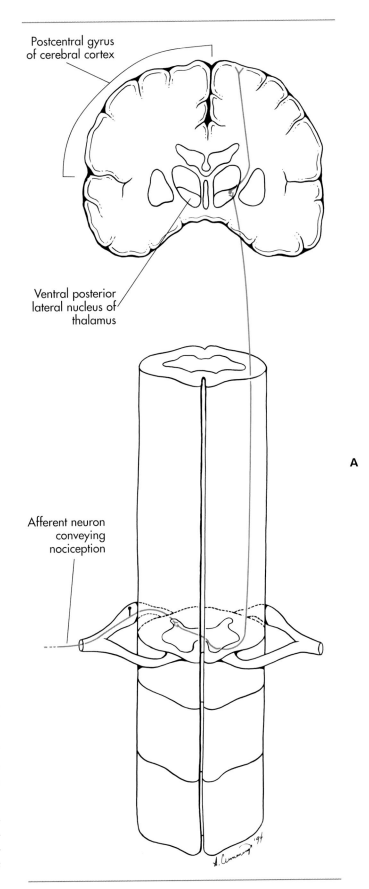

Postcentral gyrus of cerebral cortex

Ventral posterior lateral nucleus of thalamus

A

Afferent neuron conveying nociception

FIG. 11-3   Ascending spinal cord tracts associated with nociception. The neospinothalamic tract, **A,** is associated with localization of nociceptive stimulation. This pathway is also associated with the evaluation of the intensity of nociceptive stimulation.

B

C

Midline and intralaminar thalamic nuclei

Reticular formation

FIG. 11-3, cont'd. The paleospinothalamic tract, **B,** which sends collateral branches into the brain stem reticular formation, and spinoreticular tract, **C,** are most likely associated with the evaluation of nociceptive input as being unpleasant (painful). They both project to widespread areas of cerebral cortex and are associated with the body's autonomic response to nociceptive stimuli (e.g., increased sympathetic stimulation).

nuclei. From these nuclei, thalamic fibers travel to regions associated with the limbic system and to widespread areas of cerebral cortex, including the orbitofrontal region.

The spinoreticular tract ascends to the reticular formation of the brain stem. The reticular formation is a complex network of neurons located throughout the core of the brain stem. It has numerous functions and is a major component, along with the thalamus and the cerebral cortex, of the ascending reticular activating system (ARAS). The ARAS provides the circuitry through which arousal and attentiveness are maintained. The tract neurons synapsing in the reticular formation form complex connections within this region and subsequently project to brain stem nuclei, the hypothalamus, and the midline and intralaminar nuclei of the thalamus. Subsequent thalamic projections course to widespread areas of cerebral cortex.

The paleospinothalamic and spinoreticular tracts possess similar characteristics, including projections to the same regions of the thalamus. These thalamic regions, in turn, project to nonspecific areas of cerebral cortex. Another similarity is that neither tract is somatotopically organized. Both the spinoreticular and the paleospinothalamic tracts may be involved with the generation of chronic pain and the qualities associated with that sensation. The response of the brain to painful stimuli is quite intricate.

The perception of pain takes place in the thalamus, postcentral gyrus, frontal cortex (affective component), and temporal cortex (memory of previous pain component) (Kirkaldy-Willis, 1988b). The unpleasant emotional response associated with pain seems to be associated with the limbic system. The limbic system allows an individual to perceive a sensation as being uncomfortable, aching, or hurting (Haldeman, 1992). The focusing of the individual's attention on the painful area is most likely a function of the ARAS.

CONTROL OF NOCICEPTION
Segmental Control

The neurotransmission of nociception can be modulated at the segmental level (Fig. 11-4). This mechanism has been known to exist since Melzack and Wall (1965) proposed the gate control theory. Since then the dorsal horn, and especially the superficial dorsal horn, has been extensively investigated. The data from this research have led to numerous questions concerning the details of the gate control theory, and subsequently the theory was revised. However, the general concept of the gate control theory appears to be accepted (McMahon, 1990; Willis & Coggeshall, 1991). Briefly, this theory states that increased activity of large-diameter low-threshold afferents, relative to the activity of small-diameter affer-

ent fibers, competitively inhibits the transmission of nociception to higher centers. This concept has led to effective therapies for relief of pain, such as transcutaneous nerve stimulation and dorsal column stimulation (McMahon, 1990).

The inhibition of the tract neurons conducting nociception most likely comes from a population of interneurons located in lamina II (substantia gelatinosa). Many of these interneurons use enkephalins as neurotransmitters. These interneurons receive excitatory input (possibly indirectly) from large-diameter fibers. The interneurons, in turn, inhibit the projection (tract) neurons (Basbaum, 1984). A balance between this inhibitory input and the excitatory input from small-diameter fibers is likely to be required for the normal processing of nociception (McMahon, 1990). This balance is probably the result of modulation originating from the complex circuitry of the superficial dorsal horn. Further research is necessary to clarify this circuitry and its relationship to the descending input from regions in the brain stem (see following discussion).

Supraspinal Control

Evidence from studies in which electrical stimulation of regions of the brain stem produced analgesia (Basbaum & Fields, 1978) indicates that descending pathways can modulate nociceptive signals. One of the components of this endogenous pain control system is the periaqueductal gray matter (PAG) of the midbrain. This region has a major projection to the nucleus raphe magnus, which is located in the midline of the rostroventral medulla (Fig. 11-4). This nucleus is rich in the neurotransmitter serotonin. From this region, serotonergic fibers course into the dorsolateral funiculus of the spinal cord (raphespinal tract) and many fibers synapse on neurons in the superficial dorsal horn (laminae I and II). The superficial dorsal horn is also the region that receives input from afferent fibers conveying nociception. In addition, it is the location of the origin of the spinothalamic tracts (Basbaum & Fields, 1978; Jessell & Kelly, 1991) and the area involved with the segmental modulation of nociception (see previous discussion). Descending fibers synapse on several types of neurons. These include enkephalin (an opioid peptide) containing inhibitory interneurons and also the nociceptive projection neurons. The opioid-containing inhibitory interneurons are close to both primary nociceptive afferents and the tract neurons. In fact, the afferent endings and the dendrites of the tract neurons both contain opioid receptors (Jessell & Kelly, 1991). Pharmacologic studies have shown that the release of opioid peptides from the inhibitory interneurons block transmission of nociception by two mechanisms (Fig. 11-4). One mechanism is by binding to receptors and blocking the release of neurotransmitters,

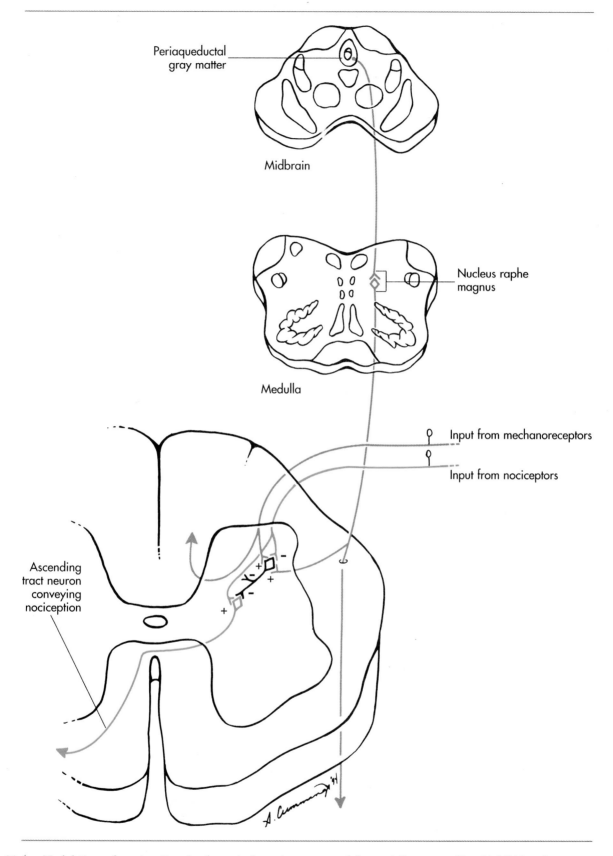

Periaqueductal
gray matter

Midbrain

Nucleus raphe
magnus

Medulla

Input from mechanoreceptors

Input from nociceptors

Ascending
tract neuron
conveying
nociception

FIG. 11-4 Modulation of nociception in the spinal cord. Notice that local afferents conducting impulses from mechanoreceptors and descending fibers from the nucleus raphe magnus of the medulla are capable of inhibiting the tract neurons that conduct nociception. This modulation of nociception is accomplished by means of interneurons.

such as substance P, from the primary afferent fibers. Although direct axoaxonic synapses between enkephalin neurons and the primary afferent fibers have not yet been found, enkephalins may possibly bind to receptors by diffusing from their site of release to the presynaptic membrane of the primary afferent fiber (Basbaum, 1987; Besson, 1988; Jessell & Kelly, 1991).

The second mechanism by which inhibitory interneurons can mediate spinal neurotransmission of nociception is by directly synapsing with the postsynaptic membrane of the tract neuron (Fig. 11-4). This occurrence has been well documented (Basbaum, 1987; Besson, 1988; Jessell & Kelly, 1991). Through these connections, nociceptive transmission is prevented. Therefore analgesia can be produced by neural stimulation. Analgesia can also be produced by the administration of opiates into the CNS. The areas activated by the opiates are the same as those that produce analgesia when electrically stimulated, that is, the PAG and the rostroventral medulla. This lends credence to the theory that endogenous opioid peptides, which have been found in the brain, can activate the descending system (Jessell & Kelly, 1991).

In addition to the serotonergic descending pathway, other fibers descend from the pons (Basbaum, 1987; Hoffert, 1989) and appear to be involved with control of the nociceptive system. These descending fibers contain norepinephrine and also appear to inhibit nociception at the dorsal horn level. However, at the same time, collateral branches of these fibers synapse on the serotonergic neurons of the raphe nuclei. The subsequent release of norepinephrine at this level results in "tonic inhibition" of the raphe-spinal neurons (Basbaum, 1987). Thus both systems provide a descending component to the mechanism for controlling pain. Feeding into these two systems is the nociceptive information transmitted through the ascending pathways (Basbaum & Fields, 1978). These ascending pathways possibly include the spinomesencephalic tract and input from the reticular formation (see Chapter 9). Also possibly feeding into the two descending systems is stress-induced input channeled through the limbic system and hypothalamus (Jessell & Kelly, 1991).

◆   ◆   ◆

After a brief pause to review the nature of mechanical back pain, you enter the room to greet Mr. S. You are now mentally prepared to consider the pain that has bothered him for the past 3 years.

DIFFERENTIATION BETWEEN PAIN OF SOMATIC ORIGIN AND RADICULAR PAIN

On meeting Mr. S, you notice that he is not seated in your consultation room but instead is standing and is partially supporting himself on the edge of the desk located near the center of the room. Mr. S appears to be in great pain. As you approach, he lets go of the desk and slowly reaches to shake your hand. You notice that in doing so, he leans dramatically to the right and has his left hand placed along his left buttock. You have read Mr. S's account of his chief complaint and have noted that he has been experiencing rather mild low back pain on and off over the past 2 years. However, this morning while unloading his truck (Mr. S drives a truck for a prominent soft drink manufacturer, and his job requires him to deliver the soda to grocery and convenience stores), he heard a "pop," and shortly thereafter felt extreme pain in his back that shot "like a lightning bolt" down his left leg (Fig. 11-5). During your questioning, Mr. S states the pain is a dull ache in his low back region (he moves his hand around a rather large area of his lower lumbar region and into his left buttock). He goes on to say that the lightning bolt pain is "on and off" and extends (he points) into his left posterior thigh and leg and the lateral aspect of the sole of his left foot. You carefully question Mr. S about somatic and visceral symptoms of the head and neck, thorax, abdomen, and pelvis and other possible injury to his lower extremity. Your inquiries reveal that he has had no significant difficulties or symptoms arising from these regions.

Your physical examination reveals Mr. S to be an individual who, his present state excluded, is physically fit. His vital signs are normal. Chest and abdomen are normal to palpation, percussion, and auscultation, and he has no palpable inguinal hernia. Rectal examination is normal. Examination of his head, anterior neck, and cervical and upper thoracic regions are normal. Cranial nerves and upper extremity sensation, reflexes, and muscle strength are all normal.

Mr. S has a great deal of muscle guarding during your examination of his lumbar region. You note marked tightness of his erector spinae muscles (possibly hyperalgesia), and he is particularly sensitive to percussion over the L5 spinous process. Reflexes, sensory findings (pinprick, ability to identify touch from a cotton swab, vibration sense), and motor strength of his right lower extremity are all normal. His left extremity reveals very slight weakness of plantar flexion, slightly diminished Achilles reflex, and diminished sensation to pinprick and to a wisp of cotton along the posterior leg and lateral aspect of the sole of the left foot. Nerve tension signs (straight leg raising and well leg raising) are positive (40° on the left and 60° on the right), reproducing the lightning bolt pain that extends down the left lower extremity into the sole of the left foot.

Because of his antalgic posture, description of a sharp stabbing pain, positive nerve tension signs, decreased sensation, and diminished Achilles reflex, you strongly suspect that Mr. S has a disc bulge or possibly a disc herniation of the L5-S1 disc. You believe the disc is

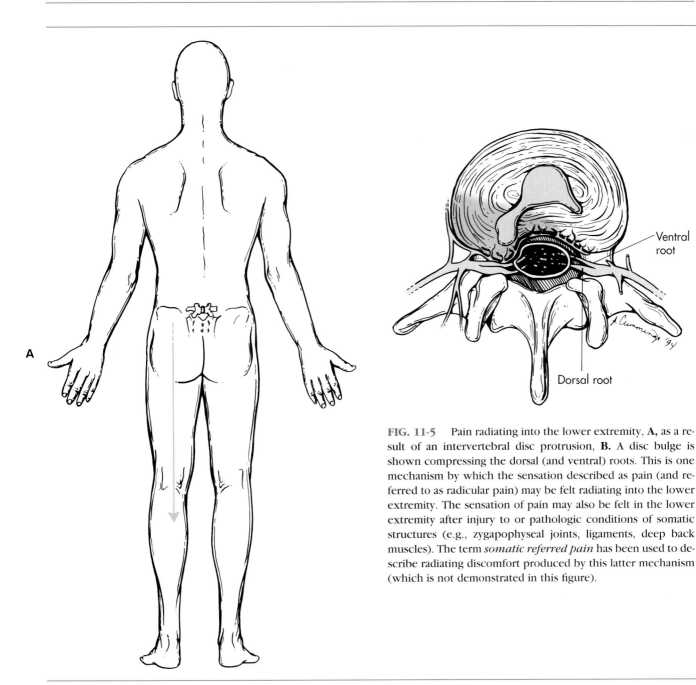

FIG. 11-5   Pain radiating into the lower extremity, **A,** as a result of an intervertebral disc protrusion, **B.** A disc bulge is shown compressing the dorsal (and ventral) roots. This is one mechanism by which the sensation described as pain (and referred to as radicular pain) may be felt radiating into the lower extremity. The sensation of pain may also be felt in the lower extremity after injury to or pathologic conditions of somatic structures (e.g., zygapophyseal joints, ligaments, deep back muscles). The term *somatic referred pain* has been used to describe radiating discomfort produced by this latter mechanism (which is not demonstrated in this figure).

compressing the S1 dorsal and ventral nerve roots (Figs. 11-5, 11-6, and 11-7). Compression of this kind results in a type of pain frequently encountered in clinical practice, known as radicular pain. Radicular pain is caused by activation of sensory fibers at the level of the dorsal root or DRG. It is experienced as a thin band of sharp, shooting pain along the distribution of the nerve or nerves supplied by the affected dorsal root (see boxed definition).

Some of the causes of radicular pain include IVD protrusion, spinal (vertebral) canal stenosis (see Chapter 7),

and other space-occupying lesions. The list in the box on p. 368 shows several additional **causes** of radicular pain,

RADICULAR PAIN
Pain arising from the *dorsal root* or the *dorsal root ganglion;* Usually causes pain to be referred along a portion of the course of the nerve or nerves formed by the affected dorsal root. This is known as a dermatomal pattern.

Intervertebral disc protrusion

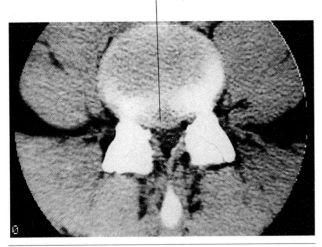

FIG. 11-6 Computed tomography scan of the lower lumbar region. Notice that a protrusion of the intervertebral disc can be seen on this horizontal image.

and the most likely **mechanism** of radicular pain is shown in the box on p. 369. Note that pressure on the DRG eventually results in decreased blood flow to sensory nerve cell bodies, which results in neural ischemia, and the neural ischemia is perceived as radicular pain (Rydevik, Myers, & Powell, 1989).

STRUCTURES AND CONDITIONS THAT CAN IRRITATE THE DORSAL ROOTS (OR GANGLIA)

- ◆ Disc lesion
- ◆ Abscess (osteomyelitis and tuberculosis)
- ◆ Tumor of the spinal canal
- ◆ Spondylolisthesis
- ◆ Malformation of the vertebral canal
- ◆ Malformation of the spinal nerve root and its sheath
- ◆ Miscellaneous diseases of bone
- ◆ Histamine-like chemicals released from degenerating intervertebral disc

Modified from Bogduk. (1976) *Med J Aust, 1,* 878-881.

However, mechanical deformation affects not only the nerve fibers within the dorsal root, but also the blood vessels and connective tissue elements associated with the root (Dahlin et al., 1992). The spinal cord and nerve roots are more susceptible to compression than the peripheral nerves. Weinstein (1988) has stated, "The intensity of the pain and its radicular nature are dependent on the strength of the stimulus" (i.e., amount of compression).

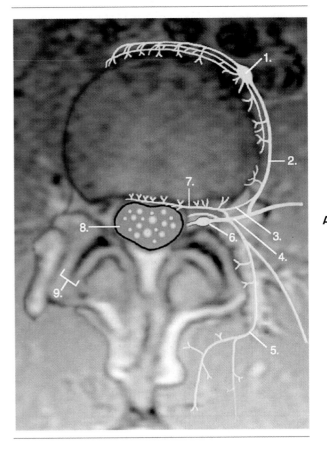

A

FIG. 11-7 The innervation of the intervertebral disc in horizontal section. **A,** Neural elements have been drawn onto a horizontal magnetic resonance imaging scan. The top of the illustration is anterior and the bottom is posterior. Numbers indicate the following: *1,* sympathetic ganglion; *2,* gray ramus communicans; *3,* branch of the gray ramus coursing toward the intervertebral foramen to contribute to the recurrent meningeal (sinuvertebral) nerve; *4,* anterior primary division (ventral ramus); *5,* medial branch of posterior primary division (the lateral branch is seen coursing to the reader's right of the medial branch; *6,* dorsal root (spinal) ganglion and dural root sleeve (red) within the intervertebral foramen; *7,* recurrent meningeal (sinuvertebral) nerve; *8,* cauda equina (yellow) within the cerebrospinal fluid (blue) of the lumbar cistern of the subarachnoid space; *9,* zygapophyseal joint. Notice that the intervertebral disc is receiving innervation from branches of the sympathetic ganglion (anteriorly), gray communicating ramus (laterally and posterolaterally), and the recurrent meningeal nerve (posteriorly). Also notice that the zygapophyseal joint is receiving innervation from the medial branch of the posterior primary division. (Photograph by Ron Mensching and illustration by Dino Juarez, The National College of Chiropractic.)

The IVF nerve roots may respond to pressure differently than those comprising the cauda equina of the spinal canal. The cauda equina may be more sensitive to compression than the dorsal roots (Dahlin et al., 1992), and even a small amount of pressure (compression) may

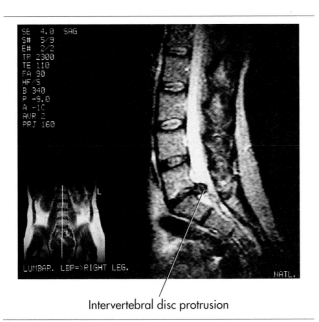

B

Intervertebral disc protrusion

FIG. 11-7, cont'd. **B,** Magnetic resonance imaging scan performed in the horizontal plane, showing an intervertebral disc protrusion.

MECHANISM OF RADICULAR PAIN

Pressure on dorsal root or dorsal root ganglion
↓
Edema within the nerves
↓
Further edema and hemorrhage within
the dorsal root ganglion
↓
Decreased blood flow to sensory nerve cell bodies
↓
Ischemia of neural elements
Ischemia perceived as PAIN

Modified from Rydevik et al. (1989) *Spine, 14,* 574-576.

---

produce venous congestion of the intraneural microcirculation of nerve roots in the cauda equina (Olmarker, et al., 1989). Kirkaldy-Willis (1988b) stated:

Compromise of the cauda equina as a result of spinal stenosis may result in unusual sensations which may be "bizarre" in nature and may affect one or both limbs. . ... He may say that the legs feel as though they do not belong to him . . . or are made of rubber.

When a dorsal nerve root is affected, other sensory and even motor modalities are also influenced (see the box at upper right). Therefore, radicular pain usually is accompanied by paresthesia, hypesthesia, and decreased

reflexes (because the sensory limb of the deep tendon reflex is affected). Because the dorsal root and ventral nerve root are adjacent to each other, compression of the dorsal root is usually accompanied by compression of the ventral nerve root as well. Compression of the ventral root results in motor weakness. Therefore, radicular pain may be accompanied by motor weakness (see the box below).

**DISTINGUISHING FEATURES
OF RADICULAR PAIN**

◆ Sharp, shooting type of pain along the distribution of the nerve(s) supplied by the affected dorsal root
◆ Long radiation into the upper or lower extremity (although this does not necessarily have to be the case)
◆ Pain coursing along a fairly thin band
◆ Pain accompanied by paresthesia, hypesthesia, and decreased reflexes
◆ Pain may be accompanied by motor weakness (as a result of compromise of the ventral roots)

In addition to the radicular signs and symptoms just discussed, Mr. S also has diffuse low back pain. This leads you to suspect he may be experiencing two different types of pain, somatic referred and radicular pain.

Recall that pain of somatic origin displays certain characteristics. Some of the generalized discomfort experienced in a patient exemplified by Mr. S may be emanating from a lesion of a somatic structure. Since only those structures innervated by nociceptive nerve endings are capable of producing pain, a review of possible somatic pain generators is useful (see previous boxes).

Our prototypical patient, Mr. S, also appears to be experiencing pain and some loss of function resulting from irritation of the S1 nerve roots. Therefore, Mr. S is simultaneously experiencing both radicular pain and pain arising from somatic structures. This is not unusual. Pain of spinal origin frequently arises from more than one pain generator. In addition, the referral zones of somatic referred pain and radicular pain frequently overlap. A patient with the symptoms and signs described for Mr. S could be experiencing somatic referred pain originating from the posterior aspect of the anulus fibrosus, the posterior longitudinal ligament, and the anterior aspect of the dural root sleeve. The nociceptive input from these structures is carried by the recurrent meningeal nerve to the dorsal horn of the spinal cord and then follows the previously described pathways to higher centers.

The radicular pain and functional deficits (decreased Achilles reflex and loss of plantar flexion) of the left lower extremity described in this particular case are caused by compression of the S1 nerve roots between the bulging L5 IVD and the left superior articular process of S1. The mechanism of nociception arising from compression of the dorsal root, as well as the mechanism of the loss of motor function from compression of the ventral root, are described earlier in this section.

Interaction Between the Zygapophyseal Joints and the Intervertebral Discs

Even though the zygapophyseal joints are probably not the primary source of back pain, in the case of Mr. S, the structures of the posterior vertebral arch, and particularly the Z joints, may also contribute to radicular pain of discal origin. This is because Z joint facet arthrosis may further decrease the space available for the exiting nerve roots (Kirkaldy-Willis, 1988a) (Fig. 11-8). Chapter 7 discusses the role that may be played by facet arthrosis in the development of spinal (vertebral) canal stenosis and of IVF stenosis.

The reverse is also true. Disc degeneration may lead to increased stress on the Z joints. This can result in somatic pain, not originating from the articular cartilage but from pressure on the subchondral bone underlying the articular cartilage. The added pressure on the Z joints secondary to disc degeneration may also result in a small piece of soft tissue (articular capsule or zygapophyseal joint synovial fold) being nipped between the facets (Hutton, 1990).

Recall that lumbar radiculopathy may be caused by chemical irritation (see Chapter 7). This has been reproduced by selective nerve sheath injection with hypertonic saline (Rauschning, 1987). In addition, escape of radiopaque contrast medium into the nerve root canals has been repeatedly observed during facet joint arthrography. Since extraarticular synovial fluid is known to have strong tissue-irritating properties, Rauschning (1987) believes that "leakage of synovial fluid from ruptured intraspinal synovial cysts or weakened facet joint capsules may cause pain and possibly transient nerve root dysfunction."

Therefore, simultaneous radicular pain and somatic pain arising from the Z joints are a real possibility (Fig. 11-8).

Other Considerations

Pain referral is related to the embryologic origin of pain generators. Recall that paraxial mesoderm, which surrounds the embryonic neural tube, condenses to form paired somites. Each somite subdivides into a dermatome (to form dermis), myotome (to form muscle), and sclerotome (to form the vertebrae, Z joints, the ligaments between the vertebrae, and the anulus fibrosus of the IVDs). Some authors state that in addition to typical dermatomal referral patterns, pain arising from DRGs or dorsal roots may also refer along myotomal or sclerotomal distributions (Weinstein, 1988). Some embryologic myotomes migrate and fuse with one another. Therefore, myotomal patterns of pain referral may be quite large. This is exemplified by the large erector spinae muscles. The deeper muscles, such as the transversospinalis group, interspinales, and intertransversarii muscles, remain more segmental in distribution and innervation. However, even the smaller muscles and the small joints of the spine frequently receive innervation from more than one spinal nerve. This overlap of segmental innervation contributes to broad referral patterns of somatic pain arising from the deep back structures.

◆ ◆ ◆

You focus your care of Mr. S on his disc protrusion with radiculopathy, and during the next few weeks, he responds well to your treatment. After your investigation and treatment of Mr. S's pain, you decide that, by reigniting your interest in the mechanism of back pain, Mr. S has provided a service to you almost of equal value to the help you have been to him.

Suggested Readings

The work of Bogduk and Twomey (1991) provides a clear, well-organized, and well-referenced account of structures of the spine receiving nociceptive innervation. It also describes the mechanisms, as best as they are understood, of somatic referred and radicular pain. The books of Kirkaldy-Willis (1988) and Haldeman (1992) provide excellent correlations between the basic science considerations of pain of spinal origin and clinical practice.

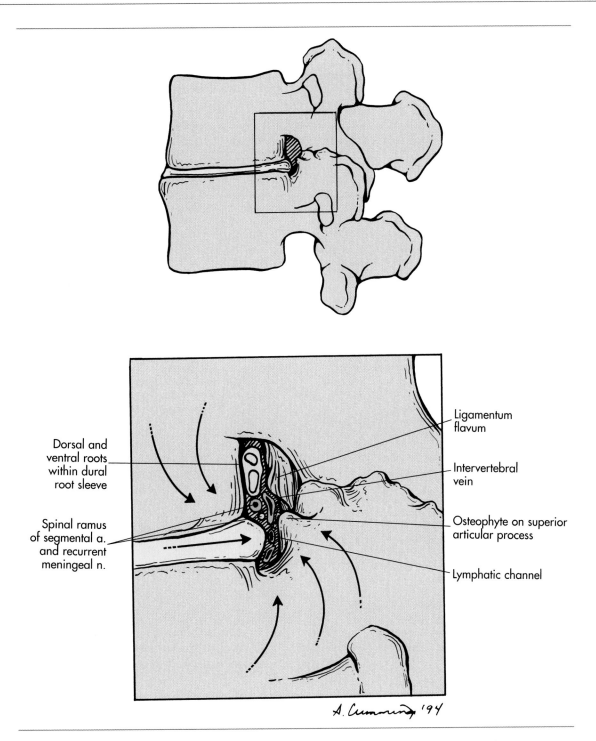

Dorsal and
ventral roots
within dural
root sleeve

Spinal ramus
of segmental a.
and recurrent
meningeal n.

Ligamentum
flavum

Intervertebral
vein

Osteophyte on superior
articular process

Lymphatic channel

A. Cummings '94

FIG. 11-8   Foraminal encroachment from a variety of sources *(arrows)*, intervertebral disc narrowing, intervertebral disc bulge, and zygapophyseal joint arthrosis. Notice that as the two vertebrae approximate each other, because of the disc narrowing, the more superior body also shifts slightly posteriorly.

REFERENCES

Aprill, C., Dwyer, A., & Bogduk, N. (1990). Cervical zygapophyseal joint pain patterns. II. A clinical evaluation. *Spine, 15*(6), 458-461.

Basbaum, A.I. (1984). Anatomical substrates of pain and pain modulation and their relationship to analgesic drug action. In M. Kuhar & G. Pasternak (Eds.), *Analgesics: neurochemical, behavioral, and clinical perspectives.* New York: Raven Press.

Basbaum A.I. (1987). Cytochemical studies of the neural circuitry underlying pain and pain control. *Acta Neurochir,* Suppl (Wein), *38,* 5-15.

Basbaum, A.I. & Fields, H.L. (1978). Endogenous pain control mechanisms: Review and hypothesis, *Ann Neurol, 4,* 451-462.

Besson, J.M. (1988). The physiological basis of pain pathways and the segmental controls of pain, *Acta Anaesth Belg, 39*(Suppl. 2), 47-51.

Bogduk, N. (1976). The anatomy of the intervertebral disc syndrome, *Med J Aust, 1,* 878-881.

Bogduk, N. (1983). The innervation of the lumbar spine, *Spine, 8,* 286-293.

Bogduk, N. (1984). The rationale for patterns of neck and back pain, *Patient Management, 13,* 17-28.

Bogduk, N. & Twomey, L.T. (1991). *Clinical anatomy of the lumbar spine.* London: Churchill Livingstone.

Bogduk, N., Lambert, G.A., & Duckworth, J.W. (1981). The anatomy and physiology of the vertebral nerve in relation to cervical migraine, *Cephalalgia, 1,* 11-24.

Carpenter, M.B. & Sutin, J. (1983). *Human neuroanatomy* (8th ed.). Baltimore: Williams & Wilkins.

Campbell, D. & Parsons, C. (1944). Referred head pain and its concomitants, *J Nerv Ment Dis, 99,* 544-551.

Dahlin, L.B. et al (1992). Physiology of nerve compression. In S. Haldeman (Ed.), *Principles and practice of chiropractic* (2nd ed.). East Norwalk, Conn: Appleton & Lange.

Darby, S. & Cramer, G. (1994). Pain generators and pain pathways of the head and neck. In D. Curl (Ed.), *Chiropractic approach to head pain.* Baltimore: Williams & Wilkins.

Dwyer, A., Aprill, C., & Bogduk, N. (1990). Cervical zygapophyseal joint pain patterns. I. A study in normal volunteers, *Spine, 15*(6), 453-457.

Edmeads, J. (1978). Headaches and head pains associated with diseases of the cervical spine, *Med Clin North Am, 62*(3), 533-544.

Haldeman, S. (1992). The neurophysiology of spinal pain. In S. Haldeman (Ed.), *Principles and practice of chiropractic.* (2nd ed.). East Norwalk, Conn: Appleton & Lange.

Hockaday, J.M. & Whitty, C.M. (1967). Patterns of referred pain in the normal subject, *Brain, 90*(3), 481-496.

Hoffert, M.J. (1989). The neurophysiology of pain, *Neurol Clin, 7*(2), 183-203.

Hubbard, D.R. & Berkoff, G.M. (1993). Myofascial trigger points show spontaneous needle EMG activity, *Spine, 18,* 1803-1807.

Hutton, W.C. (1990). The forces acting on a lumbar intervertebral joint, *J Manual Med, 5,* 66-67.

Inman, V.T. & Saunders, J.B. (1944). Referred pain from skeletal structures, *J Nerv Ment Dis, 996,* 660-667.

Jessell, T.M. & Kelly, D.D. (1991). Pain and analgesia. In E.R. Kandel, J.H. Schwartz, & T.M. Jessell (Eds.), *Principles of neural science* (3rd ed.). New York: Elsevier.

Kellgren, J.H. (1938). Observations on referred pain arising from muscle, *Clin Sci, 3,* 175-190.

Kirkaldy-Willis, W.H. (1988a). The pathology and pathogenesis of low back pain. In W. Kirkaldy-Willis (Ed.), *Managing low back pain* (2nd ed.). New York: Churchill Livingstone.

Kirkaldy-Willis, W.H. (1988b). The mediation of pain. In W. Kirkaldy-Willis (Ed.), *Managing low back pain* (2nd ed.). New York: Churchill Livingstone.

Melzack, R. & Wall, P.D. (1965). Pain mechanism: A new theory, *Science, 150,* 971-979.

McCall, I.W., Park, W.M., & O'Brien, J.P. (1979). Induced pain referral from posterior lumbar elements in normal subjects, *Spine, 4*(5), 441-446.

McMahon, S. (1990). The spinal modulation of pain. In J.K. Paterson, L. Burn (Eds.), *Back pain: An international review.* Dordrecht, Netherlands: Klumer Academic Publishers.

Merskey, H. (1979). Pain terms: A list with definitions and notes on usage. Recommended by the IASP subcommittee on taxonomy. *Pain, 6,* 249-252.

Nolte, J. (1988). *The human brain* (2nd ed.). St. Louis: Mosby.

Olmarker, K. et al. (1989). Effects of experimental graded compression on blood flow in spinal nerves roots: A vital microscopic study on the porcine cauda equina. *J Orthop Res, 7,* 817-823.

Rauschning, W. (1987). Normal and pathologic anatomy of the lumbar root canals. *Spine, 12,* 1008-1019.

Rydevik, B.L., Myers, R.R., & Powell, H.C. (1989). Pressure increase in the dorsal root ganglion following mechanical compression. *Spine, 14*(6), 574-576.

Weinstein, W.H. (1988). The perception of pain. In W. Kirkaldy-Willis (Ed.), *Managing low back pain* (2nd ed.). New York: Churchill Livingstone.

Willis, Jr., W.D. & Coggeshall, R.E. (1991). *Sensory mechanisms of the spinal cord* (2nd ed.). New York: Plenum Press.

Wyke, B. (1987). The neurology of low back pain. In M. Jayson (Ed.), *The lumbar spine and back pain* (3rd ed.). New York: Churchill Livingstone.

PART III

SPINAL DEVELOPMENT AND MICROSCOPIC ANATOMY

CHAPTER 12

Development of the Spine and Spinal Cord

William E. Bachop

In the early human embryo, the back can be defined operationally as what lies displayed by a plane passed from side to side, or from head to tail, between the floor of the amnionic cavity and the roof of the yolk sac cavity (Fig. 12-1). As yet, no complete body wall (no sides, no front) exists, only the back (Brash, 1951b). The primitive back is present from the beginning of the embryo, and it contains all the primordia that make up the definitive back: the surface ectoderm; the neural tube; the neural crest; and the mesoderm, which consists of the notochordal, paraxial, intermediate, lateral plate, and mesenchyme. Its posterior boundary is the surface ectoderm flooring the amnionic cavity, and its anterior boundary is the endoderm roofing the yolk sac cavity.

THE BLASTOCYST

The human begins as the fertilized egg, which cleaves itself into smaller and smaller units, each carrying all the genetic information needed to build any tissue or organ in the body (Williams et al., 1989). The resulting cells at first form a solid sphere, but rearrangement and continued cell division produce a hollow sphere known as the blastocyst (Patten, 1964). The latter is a single cell layer thick except at one pole, where the cells form into a disc that is several cell layers thick (Brash, 1951b) (Fig. 12-2, A). This disc is called the inner cell mass to distinguish it from all the other cells, which are referred to collectively as the trophoblast (Mossman, 1987).

The inner cell mass and the trophoblast have different fates. The former go on to form the embryo proper. The latter can be likened to an embryonic scaffolding that eventually is dismantled or discarded. Before that happens, trophoblast cells proliferate by mitosis until they are several cell layers thick. The innermost layer of the trophoblast mentioned earlier is still lining the blastocyst cavity. It remains cellular and is called the cytotrophoblast (Baxter, 1953). The cells in the outermost layer begin to lose their cell membranes, thus forming a syncytium known as the syncytiotrophoblast (Williams et al., 1989) (Fig. 12-2, B). This syncytium releases proteolytic enzymes that enable the blastocyst to digest its way into the lining of the uterus, called the endometrium. Once the blastocyst has sunk into the uterine wall and is completely surrounded by endometrial tissue, it has left forever the cavity of the uterus. That cavity is itself soon obliterated by the walls of the uterus fusing with each other (Moore, 1988). The implanted blastocyst does not leave that uterine wall until it bursts out in the form of a newborn (Beck, Moffat, & Davies, 1985).

Meanwhile, the inner cell mass also has been changing (Williams et al., 1989). A space, the first sign of the amnionic (amniotic) cavity, has appeared within it (Fig. 12-2, B). The latter can be thought of as being enclosed by walls, a roof, and a floor (Langebartel, 1977). The roof and walls become the amnion. The floor becomes the dorsal surface of the embryo and later transforms into

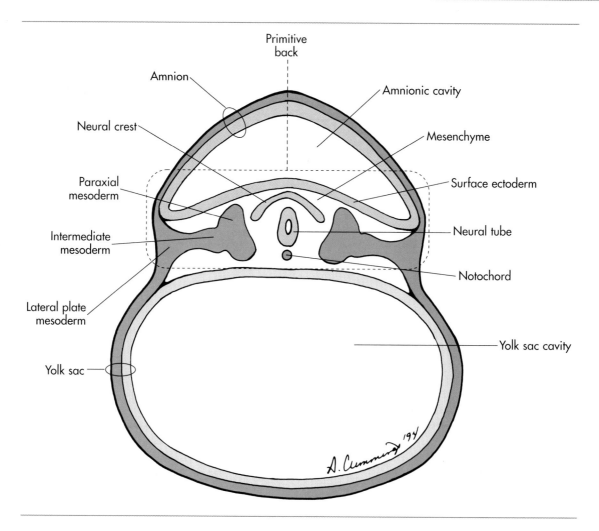

FIG 12-1   Cross section of the primitive back.

the outer layer of the skin on the newborn's back (Sadler, 1990). By this time the inner cell mass is attached to the cytotrophoblast by only a narrow bridge of cells that is called the connecting stalk (Fig. 12-3). The connecting stalk marks the tail or caudal end of the embryo just as the amnion marks its dorsal surface. A close observer would note that cells in the inner cell mass have grouped themselves into two layers (Fig. 12-2, *B*). One layer floors the amnionic cavity and is called the ectoderm. The other layer roofs the blastocyst cavity and is called endoderm (Robertson, 1966). This endodermal layer becomes continuous with a thin transient layer of cells that by some arcane process has come to line the blastocyst cavity. All these cells separate from the cytotrophoblast, and the end result is the formation of a sac made up of endodermal cells. This sac is suspended from the endodermal layer of the bilaminar embryonic disc and is called the yolk sac even though it contains a negligible amount of yolk (Scammon, 1953). The yolk sac is composed of a single layer of

cells that separates the yolk sac cavity inside it from what remains of the blastocyst cavity outside it (Snell, 1975) (Fig. 12-3).

The cytotrophoblast next buds off cells that deposit themselves on the outside of the yolk sac, where they make up a layer called extraembryonic splanchnic mesoderm (Moore, 1988). They settle on the outside of the amnion as well, and there they form the layer called extraembryonic somatic mesoderm. Other cells produced by the cytotrophoblast remain adherent to it as a lining layer likewise called extraembryonic somatic mesoderm (Fig. 12-4). The triple layer, consisting of the cytotrophoblast sandwiched between the syncytiotrophoblast and the extraembryonic somatic mesoderm, is called the chorion and is derived completely from the trophoblast (Goss, 1966). That means the cavity inside the chorion actually corresponds to the previous blastocyst cavity (Sadler, 1990). To recognize the changes that have occurred, such as the appearance of the yolk sac and the extraembryonic mesoderm, the cavity within is

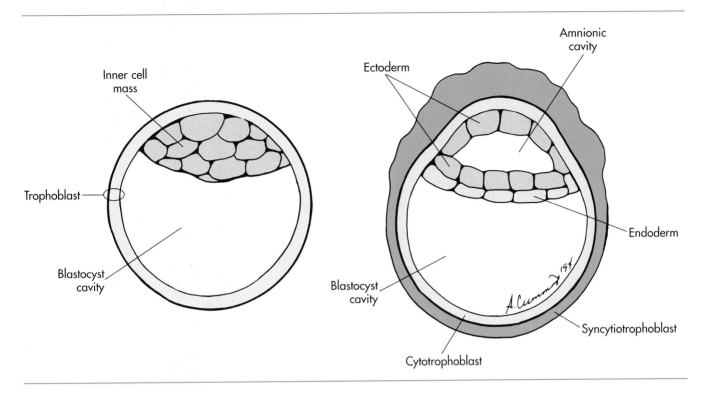

FIG 12-2   Cross section of the early blastocyst.

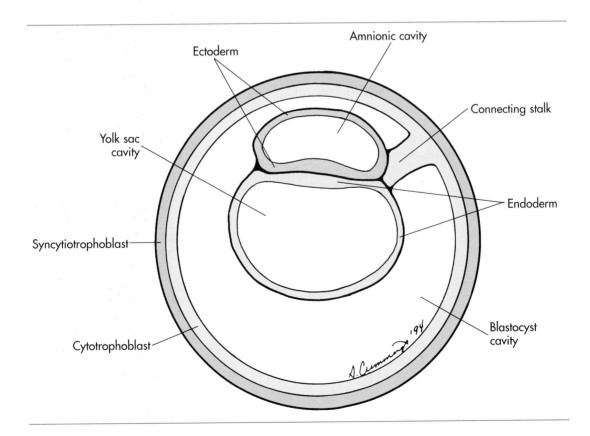

FIG 12-3   Longitudinal section of the later blastocyst.

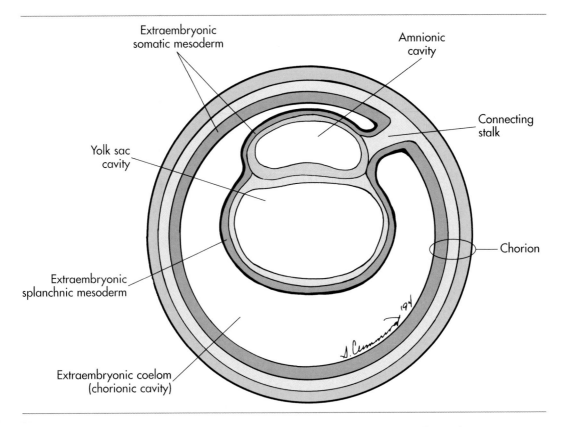

FIG 12-4   Longitudinal section through bilaminar embryo before appearance of mesoderm.

renamed the extraembryonic coelom and is also referred to as the chorionic cavity (Goss, 1966) (Fig. 12-4).

While all the foregoing changes have been taking place, the floor of the amnionic cavity has been changing as well (Williams et al., 1989). The ectodermal floor has been thickening along its length in the midline into what is called the neural plate, that is, the primordium of the entire nervous system (Arey, 1965). A groove runs the length of the neural plate, with two folds flanking it. This neural groove deepens and sinks below the surface, and the neural folds close over it, thus forming a hollow tube of ectoderm called the neural tube (Scothorne, 1976) (Fig. 12-5). The neural tube is the primordium of the brain and spinal cord and some motor neuroblasts. Some of these neuroblasts develop processes that grow out from the neural tube as components of the peripheral nervous system to reach skeletal muscle. Processes of other motor neuroblasts grow out toward smooth muscle, cardiac muscle, and glands and form elements of the autonomic nervous system (Langebartel, 1977). The amnionic cavity still has a floor, but the cells of the floor now have different fates. Some are destined to form the epidermis (the surface layer of the skin) and are named, appropriately, surface ectoderm. Others are destined to form mesoderm and must invaginate (Allan, 1969).

Lying between the amnionic floor cells and the neural tube are some ectodermal cells that had invaginated along with the neural tube but had remained apart from it (Romanes, 1972a and b). They are known collectively as the neural crest (Fig. 12-5) and give rise to many important components of the nervous system: all sensory neurons, all postganglionic autonomic neurons, and all ganglia, both sensory and motor (Scothorne, 1976).

DEVELOPMENT OF THE NOTOCHORD AND ASSOCIATED STRUCTURES

The cells of the neural crest and neural tube are not the only cells that have been invaginating through the floor of the amnionic cavity. More caudally, other cells have also been disappearing below the surface near the connecting stalk at a site known as the primitive streak (Hamilton & Mossman, 1972) (Fig. 12-6). As if on a down escalator, these cells disappear from view, but then move in all directions between the ectoderm above them and the endoderm below them. This process is known as gastrulation. These in-between cells form a middle layer called mesoderm, or middle layer, since they lie dorsal to the roof of the yolk sac and ventral to the floor of the amnionic cavity. Those moving superiorly in the midline toward the future head turn into a structure known as the notochord (Figs. 12-1 and 12-8). The notochord marks the longitudinal axis of the embryonic body. The vertebral column later occupies this

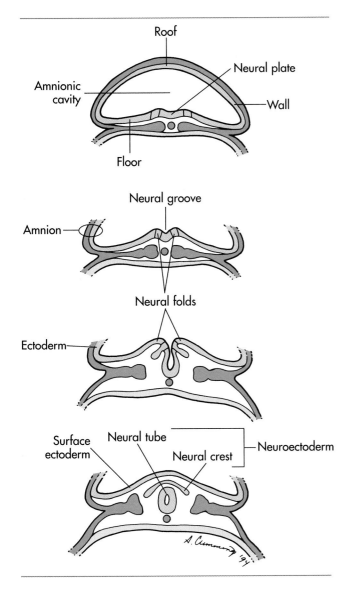

FIG 12-5   Cross section through the amnionic (amniotic) cavity showing the formation of the neural tube and neural crest from its floor.

site, and by then the notochord has turned into the part of the intervertebral disc known as the nucleus pulposus. The mesoderm lying just lateral to the notochord parallels the embryonic axis and is called the paraxial mesoderm. The paraxial mesoderm soon subdivides into segments known as somites, which are major contributors to muscles, bones, and skin. Just lateral to the somites on both sides of the embryo, other mesodermal cells have formed into a structure referred to as intermediate mesoderm. Its other name, nephrotome, alludes to its eventual role in kidney formation (Figs. 12-1 and 12-9).

During the next several weeks, the amnion undergoes a series of folds creating the embryo's body wall (Fig. 12-7). At the same time, the embryo's primitive gut is

formed from derivatives of the yolk sac. The embryo's body cut in cross section now appears as two concentric rings. The inner ring is splanchnopleure; the outer is somatopleure (Goss, 1966) (Fig. 12-9). The outer ring actually has the shape of a jeweler's signet ring. Tucked close together inside the signet part are the neural tube, neural crest, notochord, somites, intermediate mesoderm, and mesenchyme (Fig. 12-9). The signet part corresponds to what is variously called the back, the posterior body wall, and the posterior abdominal/posterior thoracic wall (Callander, 1939; Davenport, 1966; Grant, 1952).

During the same time, morphogenesis has progressed to the point that the primordia for the spinal cord, vertebral column, associated soft tissues, and the sympathetic nervous system are all in place.

NEURAL TUBE

One of these primordia, the neural tube, has already organized itself into a brain and spinal cord. The component cells are called neuroectoderm as a way of distinguishing them from the ectodermal cells that remained on the floor of the amnionic cavity (the surface ectoderm). Some neuroectodermal cells differentiate into macroglioblasts and others into neuroblasts (Clark, 1951). The latter soon take on the characteristics of a neuron-to-be (Williams et al., 1989). A blob of protoplasm, the future nerve cell body, contains the chromosomes. The cytoplasm streams out into fingerlike projections that become axons and dendrites (Sadler, 1990). Sometimes the cytoplasmic processes merely connect one side of the neural tube with the other, never leaving the tube (Noback & Demarest, 1975). At other times, one cytoplasmic process travels down or up the cord, even to the brain stem itself, while other processes remain at the same level of the neural tube at which they originated (Williams et al., 1989).

A cytoplasmic process of one neuroblast usually travels with others having a common origin and a common destination (Williams et al., 1989). Such a bundle of cytoplasmic processes inside the neural tube is called a tract (Barr & Kiernan, 1988). The cytoplasmic processes traveling together originate from a group of nerve cell bodies in the primitive spinal cord and, for example, may terminate in the thalamus. These cytoplasmic processes form the spinothalamic tract (Goss, 1966). Sometimes the cytoplasmic process from a neuroblast leaves the spinal cord altogether (Durward, 1951) and, with many others, forms an aggregate known as the ventral root of the spinal nerve (Goss, 1966). An individual cytoplasmic process of this type finds its way to a particular region of a particular skeletal muscle. Along the way it has passed through a spinal nerve, the dorsal or ventral ramus of the spinal nerve, perhaps

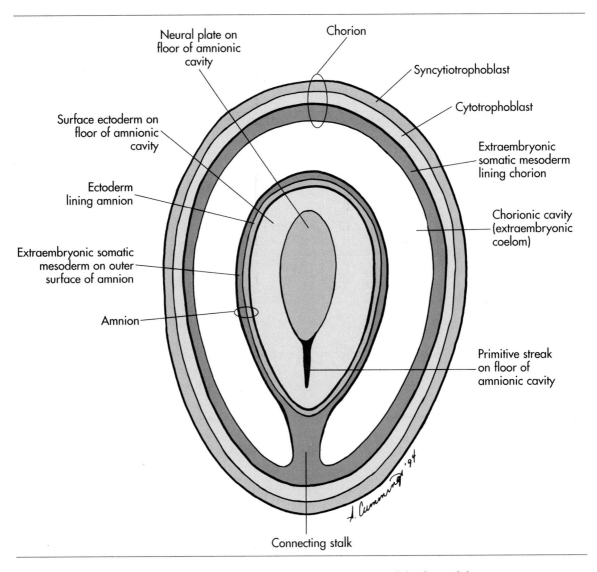

FIG 12-6   Frontal section through chorion and amnion revealing a view of the floor of the amnionic cavity as would be seen by an observer positioned on the roof of that cavity.

through a nerve plexus, and finally through a peripheral nerve (Larsell, 1953).

DEVELOPMENT OF THE AUTONOMIC NERVOUS SYSTEM

Other neuroblasts are located elsewhere in the gray matter, in an area known as the lateral horn (Romanes, 1972a). Each neuroblast sends one of its cytoplasmic processes into the closest ventral root, not heading for skeletal muscle but rather toward nonskeletal muscle and glands (Sadler, 1990). Each process can change course, leave the spinal nerve it has entered, and travel to a nearby structure known as a sympathetic chain ganglion (Goss, 1966) (see Fig. 10-5). In so doing, the processes create a bridgelike structure that appears whitish in vivo and is called a white ramus communicans (Ellis, 1983).

These neuroblasts, stretching from the lateral horn (the future intermediolateral cell column) to a sympathetic chain ganglion, are myelinated and are referred to as preganglionic neuroblasts (Romanes, 1972a and b). They function as motor neurons, which means the white ramus is made up of axons derived from the neural tube. As a rule, white rami are found attached only to the T1 through L2 spinal nerves (Crafts, 1966). The lateral horn corresponds to the nerve cell bodies, and the white ramus corresponds to the axons of the same neuroblasts, or preganglionic sympathetic neuroblasts (Durward, 1951). Above and below these spinal levels, there is no lateral horn, no white rami exist, and the ventral roots do not contain myelinated axons of preganglionic sympathetic neuroblasts (Bruce & Walmsley, 1939).

Some axons of preganglionic neuroblasts cross over a white ramus to a sympathetic chain ganglion but do not terminate within the ganglion (Francis & Voneida,

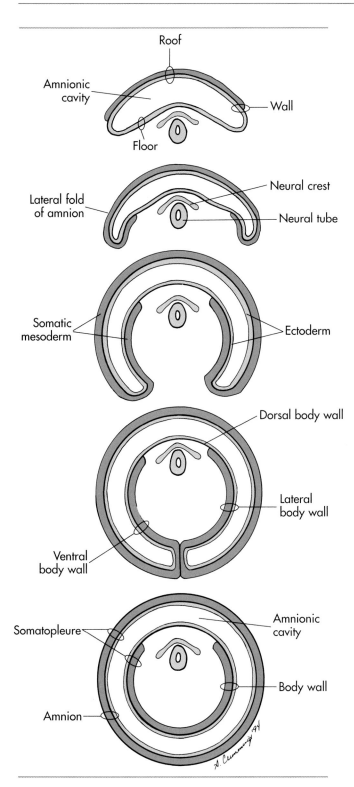

FIG 12-7 Cross section through the amnionic cavity and neural tube showing how the original amnion transforms itself into two concentric tubes. The inner tube is the embryo's body wall; the outer is the definitive amnion.

1966). Instead, they pass through the ganglion and continue up the sympathetic chain or down the chain to a sympathetic chain ganglion at a different spinal level,

where they terminate (Langebartel, 1977). Inside they synapse with neuroblasts known as postganglionic sympathetics (Goss, 1966). Some axons of preganglionic neuroblasts reach sympathetic chain ganglia by way of white rami, but they do not terminate in any sympathetic chain ganglion (Goss, 1966). Instead, these preganglionic axons pass through the sympathetic chain ganglion without synapsing and continue on their way to a sympathetic ganglion in the abdominal cavity, where they terminate, for example, in the celiac ganglion (Francis & Voneida, 1966). These are called splanchnic nerves (see Chapter 10). Some preganglionic neuroblasts have nerve cell bodies located in the gray matter of the sacral region of the neural tube. That means they are classified as parasympathetic. Their axons travel long distances and terminate in parasympathetic ganglia located close to the pelvic organs they innervate (Scothorne, 1976). They synapse inside these parasympathetic ganglia with postganglionic parasympathetic neuroblasts located within or close to the organs (Romanes, 1972b).

All sympathetic and parasympathetic postganglionic neuroblasts, as well as the ganglia they help to form, derive from the neural crest (O'Rahilly & Muller, 1992). These motor ganglia are made up of the nerve cell bodies of postganglionic neuroblasts that migrated from the original site of the neural crest (i.e., dorsolateral to the neural tube) to the site of the ganglion. Most, if not all, postganglionic neuroblasts in a sympathetic chain ganglion send their cytoplasmic processes out of the ganglion to the closest spinal nerve and, in so doing, form a bridge called a gray ramus communicans, gray because in vivo their unmyelinated axons appear grayish (Romanes, 1972a). Once in the spinal nerve, the postganglionic axons twist their way through the branches of the spinal nerves. These include dorsal and ventral rami, nerve plexuses when present, and peripheral nerves (Woodburne, 1983). The postganglionic axons terminate in the smooth muscle of blood vessels or in glands (Hollinshead & Rosse, 1985).

Although all spinal nerves have gray rami, sometimes the axons of postganglionic sympathetic neuroblasts shun the gray rami and are not distributed by a spinal nerve (Larsell, 1953). Instead, they travel directly to the organ they innervate (Durward, 1951). This is the case with the heart, where the axons of postganglionic sympathetic neuroblasts to the heart make up the cardiac sympathetic nerves (Francis & Voneida, 1966). The nerve cell bodies for these postganglionic neuroblasts lie in cervical sympathetic chain ganglia (Durward, 1951).

Not all neural crest cells migrate away from their early location to transform into postganglionic neuroblasts. Some migrate toward the skin to become melanoblasts. Others migrate to the intermediate mesoderm, which is forming the adrenal cortex, and they burrow inside to become the adrenal medulla (Coupland, 1976). Still

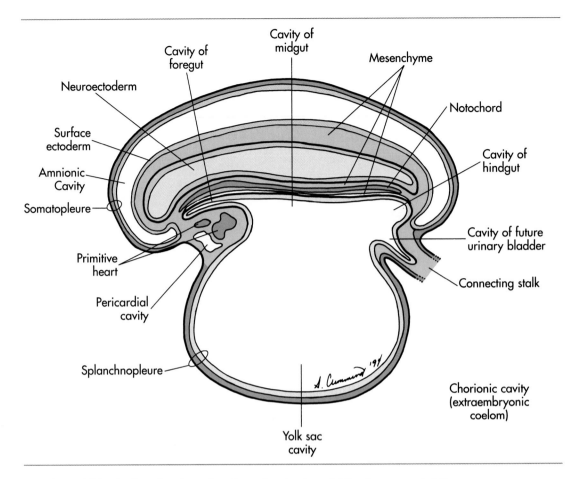

FIG 12-8   Midsagittal section through embryo showing how folding has converted the proximal part of the yolk sac into a foregut (at the head end), a hind gut (at the tail end), and a midgut (which still lacks a floor and is confluent with the yolk sac cavity).

others rearrange themselves into discrete clusters not far from their original location dorsolateral to the neural tube (Romanes, 1972a).

DEVELOPMENT OF THE DORSAL AND VENTRAL ROOTS

Two cytoplasmic processes issue forth in opposite directions from most of these clustered neural crest cells. One process travels dorsomedially into the neural tube, where as an axon (central process), it terminates in the region that becomes the dorsal horn of the gray matter (see Chapters 3 and 9). In the dorsal horn the central process synapses with neuroblasts derived from the neural tube. The second cytoplasmic process travels ventrolaterally, where as a dendrite (peripheral process), it enters a spinal nerve. The cytoplasmic process going dorsomedially and the one going ventrolaterally, as well as the nerve cell body they are both attached to, are said to lie in the dorsal root of the spinal nerve. Such a dorsal root contains many other neuroblasts with the same shape and spatial configuration, and all their nerve cell

bodies together form the spinal ganglion, also known as the dorsal root ganglion (Clark, 1951). It is a sensory ganglion, and no synapses occur within it. The dorsal root is called a sensory root because the current consensus holds that it contains only fibers of afferent neuroblasts derived from neural crest (Scothorne, 1976). The consensus also holds that the ventral root is a motor root and contains only axons of efferent neuroblasts derived from the neural tube (Cohen et al., 1992). That means that the spinal nerve formed by the intersection of the sensory and motor roots is a mixed nerve, and that the cell bodies of the nerve fibers are derived from both neural tube and neural crest (Clark, 1976) (see Fig. 3-9).

The dorsal and ventral roots are attached to the neural tube at one end and converge to form the spinal nerve at the other end (Clark, 1976). In the early embryo, the roots on one side are not much different in length from the roots on the opposite side and from one spinal level to another (Francis & Voneida, 1966). With time, however, these relationships change (Sadler, 1990).

Each dorsal root and the corresponding ventral root grow laterally toward the paraxial mesoderm before the

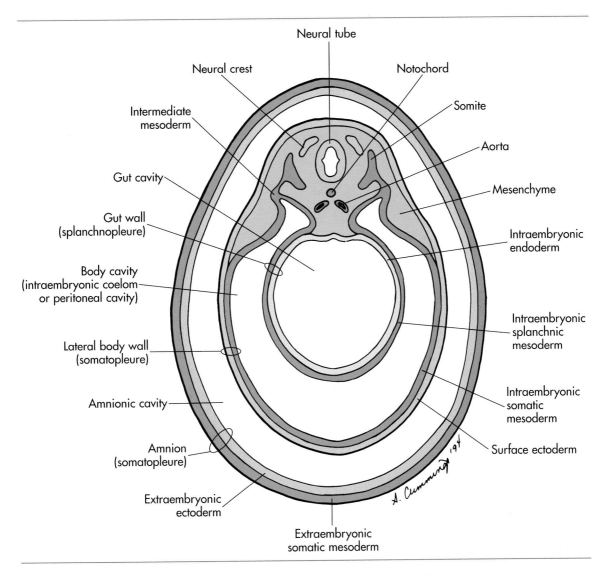

Neural tube

Neural crest

Notochord

Intermediate mesoderm

Somite

Aorta

Gut cavity

Mesenchyme

Gut wall (splanchnopleure)

Intraembryonic endoderm

Body cavity (intraembryonic coelom or peritoneal cavity)

Intraembryonic splanchnic mesoderm

Lateral body wall (somatopleure)

Intraembryonic somatic mesoderm

Amnionic cavity

Surface ectoderm

Amnion (somatopleure)

Extraembryonic ectoderm

Extraembryonic somatic mesoderm

FIG 12-9   Cross section through the two concentric tubes that run the length of the embryonic body: the inner primitive gut tube (splanchnopleure) and the outer body wall tube (somatopleure). The space between them becomes the body cavity.

vertebrae have formed (Beck et al., 1985). Both eventually become trapped between the vertebra formed cephalic to them and the vertebra formed caudal to them (Hollinshead & Rosse, 1985) (see Fig. 12-12). When first formed, all these roots at all spinal levels have approximately the same length, and they all extend out laterally from the neural tube at about the same angle, close to 90°. When these roots become trapped, however, they do not all remain the same length and do not all continue to make the same angle with the neural tube (Cohen et al., 1992). The dorsal and ventral roots that are trapped between a pair of vertebral primordia must elongate when the neural tube stays fixed in place, since the vertebral primordia seem to be moving caudally. If the roots did not lengthen, they would be torn, that is, avulsed from the neural tube. The vertebral primordia

trapping cervical and thoracic roots move caudally the least, if at all, and thus their nerve roots elongate the least (Romanes, 1972a and b). By contrast, the vertebral primordia trapping lumbar and sacral roots move caudally the most, which means their nerve roots elongate the most (Snell, 1981) (see Fig. 3-6). The angle the elongated roots make with the neural tube has also been reduced less than 90° to an acute angle, and the more elongated the root, the more acute the angle (Clark, 1976). The longest roots have had their angle reduced to 0°, so they hang down vertically, paralleling the neural tube itself (Parke, 1992b). Early anatomists thought the dozens of nerve roots hanging down together caudal to the neural tube resembled a horse's tail, thus the name in Latin, *cauda equina* (Hollinshead, 1982) (see Fig. 3-8).

Development of the Meninges

Each root is ensheathed in epithelium called the pia mater, and there has been uncertainty as to whether the pia traces back to mesoderm or to neural crest (Williams et al., 1989). A similar uncertainty exists about the origin of the arachnoid mater, which faces the pia mater across the subarachnoid space (Carlson, 1981). It is generally agreed that the outermost meninx, the dura mater, derives from mesoderm (Williams et al., 1989).

SOMITES AND DEVELOPMENT OF THE BACK MUSCLES

Mesodermal cells had earlier filled the entire space between the surface ectoderm of the body wall, the neuroectoderm of the neural tube, and the endoderm of the primitive gut, that is, the space between the three tubes that run the length of the embryonic body. The only space unfilled was the body cavity (Allan, 1969). In many locations each mesodermal cell was separated from its neighbors by a large intercellular space, and such locations were said to be occupied by mesenchyme (Harrison, 1972). In other places the mesodermal cells aggregated into tightly packed clumps, similar to the paraxial, intermediate, and lateral plate mesoderm. Each of these three mesodermal types has a subsequent history of its own.

The paraxial mesoderm segments into somites that turn into staging areas from which somite cells deploy to new locations (Sadler, 1990). For example, some somite cells migrate toward the undersurface of the surface ectoderm, where they become the dermis of the skin (Beck et al., 1985). The part of the somite from which they arise is called the dermatome (Fig. 12-10). Other somite cells migrate toward the notochord and neural tube. These cells eventually produce hard tissues, such as bone and cartilage, so the part of the somite from which they are derived is appropriately called sclerotome (Harrison, 1972) (Fig. 12-10). The somite cells that have not migrated form the myotome, and these cells eventually form skeletal muscle (Fischman, 1972). Some myotome cells move dorsally into the space between the developing skin, the developing neural tube, and the developing vertebral column (Beck et al., 1985). These cells and the part of the myotome from which they arise are referred to as an epimere. The epimere from one myotome soon encounters the epimeres from the myotomes cephalic and caudal to it. The epimeres lose their individual identities, and transform into the deep muscles of the back (Lockhart, 1951). The deep back muscles are also called the intrinsic or "true" muscles of the back and include the erector spinae and transversospinalis groups, the two splenius muscles, and the suboccipital muscles. The muscles are all derived from epimeres and innervated by the dorsal rami of spinal nerves (Joseph, 1976) (see Figs. 4-2 to 4-4).

Development of Other Muscles Related to the Spine

During this time, other myotome cells have been moving ventrolaterally between the two layers making up the lateral and ventral body wall, that is, the surface ectoderm and the somatic mesoderm (Sadler, 1990). These migrating cells and the part of the myotome from which they originate are referred to as a hypomere (Langebartel, 1977). The hypomeres from adjacent myotomes run into one another, lose their individual iden-

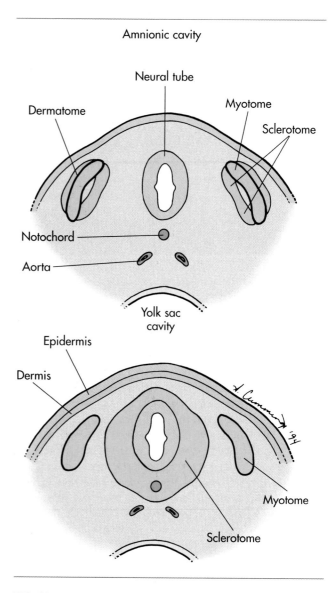

FIG 12-10   Cross section through two stages in somite differentiation: before and after dermatome cells and sclerotome cells have migrated to the destinations shown by the arrows.

tities, and form the muscles of the thoracic and abdominal body wall (Williams et al., 1989). These include many muscles that can be seen from the back, such as the intercostal, subcostal, levator costarum, the two serratus posterior, and the external abdominal oblique muscles (Sinclair, 1972).

All the muscles derived from hypomeres are innervated by the ventral rami of spinal nerves (Sadler, 1990). Hypomeres also send myoblasts ventromedially toward the vertebral column, where myoblasts from adjacent hypomeres form muscles located at the sides and front of the vertebral column (Lockhart, 1951). These muscles include the three scalenes, the two longus (colli and capitis), the two psoas, and the two quadratus lumborum (Snell, 1975). Hypomeres also form the two muscular sheets that roof and floor the abdominal cavity, the thoracoabdominal and pelvic diaphragms (Arey, 1965; Moore, 1988), both of which intersect the posterior body wall. Still other hypomere cells move posteriorly to form the muscles that hold the scapula to the vertebral column or ribs (Corliss, 1976). These muscles include the rhomboids, levator scapulae, and serratus anterior, all of which are innervated by ventral rami that have been channeled through the brachial plexus (Leeson & Leeson, 1972) (see Fig. 4-1).

The scapula is somewhat of an intermediary between the bones visible from the back (spine and ribs) and the bone that extends from the elbow to the shoulder (humerus) (Breathnach, 1958). The shoulder muscles that connect the scapula to the humerus include the supraspinatus, infraspinatus, teres major, teres minor, subscapularis, and deltoid (Romanes, 1976). All but the subscapularis can be seen from behind (Crafts, 1966), but the gross anatomist does not regard them as back muscles, even though the average person might (Hollinshead, 1982). All these muscles develop from hypomeres and consequently are innervated by ventral rami of spinal nerves through the brachial plexus (Langebartel, 1977). One muscle, however, connects the humerus directly to the posterior aspect of the trunk, largely bypassing the scapula (Sinclair, 1972). This muscle is the latissimus dorsi, and its origin also can be traced back to hypomeres innervated by ventral rami through the brachial plexus (Lockhart, 1951).

The previously mentioned derivatives of hypomeres that migrated toward the back can be regarded as making up the extrinsic muscles of the back just as the derivatives of epimeres make up the intrinsic musculature of the back (Mortenson & Pettersen, 1966). The extrinsic muscles, with one exception (trapezius), are innervated by ventral rami; the intrinsic muscles, with no exception, are innervated by dorsal rami (Lockhart, 1951). The hypomere derivatives migrate dorsally and eventually come to overlie the epimere derivatives, and in so doing, they bring branches of the brachial plexus to the superficial back (Scothorne, 1976).

Trapezius Muscle. One superficial, or extrinsic, back muscle, however, may derive from neither epimere nor hypomere but overlies those that do (Zuckerman, 1961). This muscle, the trapezius, may derive from the mesoderm located in the transition zone between the pharyngeal (branchial) arches and the cervical somites (Lockhart, 1951). Its motor innervation comes from the same cranial nerve that innervates the most caudal branchial arches, the (spinal) accessory or eleventh, and its sensory innervation may come from cervical spinal nerves (Williams et al., 1989). However, some disagreement exists about how to interpret this dual innervation (Hollinshead, 1982).

THE SCLEROTOME

The cells previously referred to as sclerotome migrate medially from the somite to surround the neural tube and notochord. Instead of forming a continuous tunnel of cells, they form a series of discrete arches called neural arches (Williams et al., 1989). Each neural arch rests on a base of sclerotome cells called the centrum, and out of these primordia (neural arch and centrum), the primitive vertebra is built (O'Rahilly, 1986) (Fig. 12-11).

Development of the Vertebrae

For years the accepted view has been that the sclerotome cells forming a centrum derived from two contiguous somites (Beck et al., 1985). This dual origin supposedly accounted for the staggered position of myotomes and centra (Sadler, 1990). This accepted view was challenged not long ago (Verbout, 1985) and may eventually be replaced (Williams et al., 1989). On the other hand, experimental support for the accepted view has recently been adduced (Bagnall et al., 1987).

Regardless of their origin, the sclerotome cells shape themselves into a primitive centrum, and soon after some of them begin laying down an extracellular cartilaginous matrix (Hall, 1978). Several chondrification centers appear in each centrum and the attached neural arch (Williams et al., 1989) (Fig. 12-11). By the time the vertebra, made only of cells, has been succeeded by a vertebra made of cells and cartilage, an ossification center appears in the centrum and two more appear in the neural arch (O'Rahilly & Muller, 1992) (Fig. 12-11). The cartilage is broken down and seemingly removed in many places but is left in many others, even after birth (Patten, 1964). In time, secondary ossification centers appear in the remaining cartilage (Sinclair, 1972) (Fig. 12-11). The number and distribution of these centers vary from vertebra to vertebra, so the eventual size and

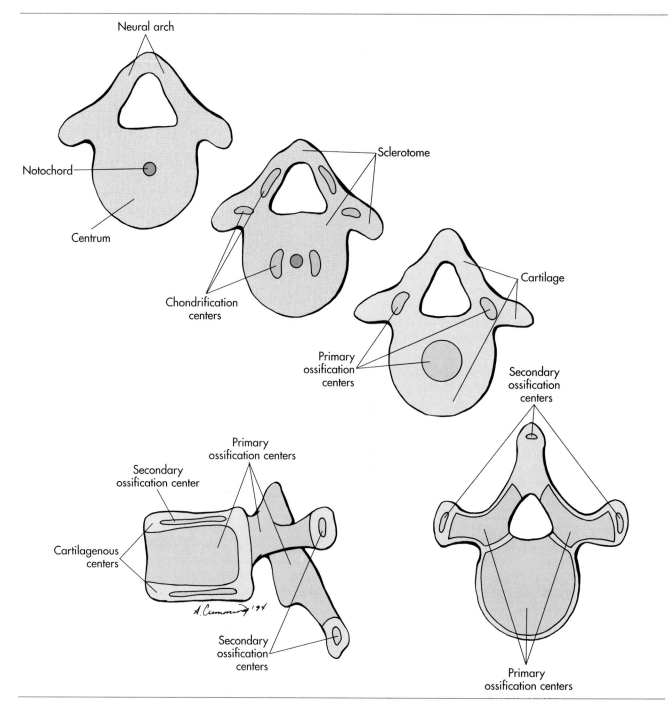

FIG 12-11   Four cross-sectional views and a lateral view of a vertebra composed at first almost entirely of sclerotome cells, which are gradually replaced by cartilage, which is almost entirely replaced by bone.

shape of the definitive bony vertebra differs accordingly (Inkster, 1951). A vertebra can increase in height and diameter before and after birth by employing intrinsic bone-depositing mechanisms around the circumference, or periosteum, and at the ends, or anular epiphyses (Bogduk & Twomey, 1987).

Each primitive vertebra has, in addition to the centrum and neural arch, a costal element that becomes a rib in the thoracic region and a part of the transverse process in the cervical and lumbar regions. In the sacral region, it becomes incorporated into the lateral part of the sacrum, which itself derives from the fusion of sacral vertebrae (Robertson, 1966).

For the sake of clarification, it should be mentioned that part of the fetal neural arch fuses with the fetal centrum to produce a postpartum structure known as the vertebral body (Trotter & Peterson, 1966). The arch now joined to the postpartum vertebral body is less extensive than the fetal neural arch, so it receives a new name, the vertebral arch (O'Rahilly, 1986).

Hemivertebra and Spina Bifida

Hemivertebra. Vertebral centra have been known to grow much more on one side than the other, with the result that the centrum appears wedge shaped when viewed from the front. Lateral deviation of the spine cephalic to the wedge can ensue, that is, scoliosis, and the wedge is referred to as a hemivertebra. Explanations offered for this asymmetric growth remain speculative (Rothman & Simeone, 1992).

Spina Bifida. If mesoderm does not migrate between the surface ectoderm flooring the early amniotic cavity and the neuroectoderm, the tissues that would have derived from that mesoderm are missing. The absence of mesoderm may be partial or complete. Why mesoderm fails to migrate or why it fails to differentiate once it has proliferated are questions that still await satisfactory answers.

Sometimes the mesoderm forms vertebral laminae and spinous processes made of cartilage that does not differentiate further into bone, the clinician's spina bifida occulta. Sometimes the mesoderm forming the vertebral laminae and spinous processes does not even differentiate into cartilage but remains a soft tissue that can be displaced or deformed. Then the meninges unrestrained dorsally by hard tissue may balloon toward the embryo's dorsal surface, and sometimes the neural tube also may bulge dorsally, the clinician's spina bifida cystica. Sometimes the neural tube and meninges may bulge so far dorsally they meld with the surface ectoderm flooring the early amnionic cavity, the clinician's spina bifida aperta. Worst of all, the neural tube itself may never form, and the neural plate remains open on the floor of the amnionic cavity, the clinician's myeloschisis (O'Rahilly & Muller, 1992).

Notochord and Intervertebral Discs

The notochord had once formed the core of every centrum, since the sclerotome cells had condensed around it (Breathnach, 1958). However, changes occur such that the notochord disappears from the core and is replaced, first by cartilage, then bone (Parke, 1992b). In the space between centra, however, the notochord persists and becomes the nucleus pulposus of the intervertebral disc (IVD) (Williams et al., 1989) (see Fig. 12-10). The sclerotome cells that come to surround the nucleus pulposus become the anulus fibrosus of that IVD between two centra (Moore, 1988) (Fig. 12-12). Variant interpretations of the roles of the nucleus pulposus and

the sclerotome cells have been offered by Williams and colleagues (1989) and Walmsley (1972).

Spinal Ligaments, Zygapophyseal Joints, and Sacroiliac Joints

All the ligaments that connect the vertebrae to each other, to the skull, and to the pelvic girdle trace their origin back to the mesoderm, as do the bones to which they attach (Walmsley, 1972). The same is true of intervertebral joints and their capsules, for example, zygapophyseal joints (Bogduk & Twomey, 1987). The sacroiliac joint likewise traces back to mesoderm that differentiates in situ (Salsabili & Hogg, 1991).

VESSELS OF THE BACK AND SPINAL CORD

While all the previously mentioned embryonic and fetal events have been taking place, the ubiquitous mesoderm has been constructing the cardiovascular system (Brash, 1951a). On the surface of the yolk sac, reddish spots develop called blood islands. The redness is caused by hemoglobin in erythroblasts that appear inside these blood islands as they hollow out and become confluent with each other. Other vascular plexuses are formed in the same way throughout the embryo, but certain channels begin to predominate while others disappear (Yoffey, 1976). Two large channels located ventral to the foregut turn out to be the mesodermal rudiments of the heart. This primitive heart drains into vascular channels that have derived from the mesoderm that lies on either side of the nearby pharyngeal arches (Patten, 1953). These paired channels carry blood dorsally away from the heart to the left and right dorsal aortae, and they are called aortic arches (Yoffey, 1976) or aortic arch arteries (Moore, 1988).

The blood entering the paired dorsal aortae moves into all the branches from this pair of arteries, which are the largest of the embryonic body. The paired branches going to the back have been called segmental arteries (Hollinshead, 1982). The capillaries of the back return that blood to segmental veins that empty into paired anterior and posterior cardinal veins (Brash, 1951a). The anterior and posterior cardinals on each side empty into a common cardinal vein, and the two of these empty into the primitive heart (Sadler, 1990). The circulatory pathway is now complete, but restructuring of that vasculature commences almost at once (Hollinshead & Rosse, 1985).

Arteries of the Back

The aortic arches largely disappear, except for the third, fourth, and sixth pairs, and those that remain are modified (Oelrich, 1966). The third pair is used to help build the carotid artery system (Walls, 1972). One component

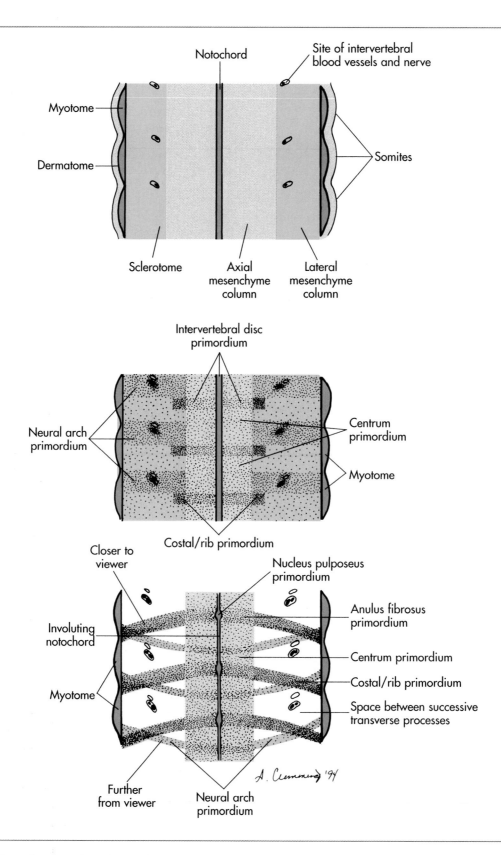

FIG 12-12 Frontal section through notochord and somites depicting three stages in formation of intervertebral discs and vertebrae. Cells migrate from the sclerotome to surround the notochord, but cell density is not the same everywhere along the notochordal length. Cell condensations mark the sites where intervertebral discs will appear. The vertebral centra will develop in the spaces between cell condensations. Other sclerotome cells located dorsolaterally form condensations that mark the sites where neural arches will appear. The spinal nerve and intervertebral blood vessels appear in the spaces between the developing neural arches. Other sclerotome cells located laterally condense next to the disc at the site where the costal element will appear.

of that system, the external carotid artery, serves the back through two of its branches, the ascending pharyngeal and the occipital (Williams et al., 1989).

The fourth pair of aortic arches also helps shunt blood toward the back by contributing to the formation of the subclavian artery and the arch of the aorta. The subclavian artery sends blood through many of its branches to the back (Oelrich, 1966). A list of these branches would include the vertebral artery, branches of the costocervical trunk (the deep cervical and highest intercostal arteries), and branches of the thyrocervical trunk (the ascending cervical, transverse cervical, and suprascapular arteries) (Romanes, 1966).

As development proceeds, the two dorsal aortae fuse into a single aorta, located caudally, and the paired segmental arteries branching from this single aorta proceed to designations that vary depending on the body region they serve. These segmental branches include intercostals, subcostals, and lumbars, and all these send branches to the back (Williams et al., 1989). Those paired segmental arteries supplying paired organs embedded retroperitoneally in the embryo's posterior body wall are named after the organ they serve, that is, renal, adrenal, and gonadal (Brash, 1951a).

Before attenuation of the single dorsal aorta into an unpaired terminal artery known as the median sacral, the dorsal aorta gives off a pair of umbilical arteries that help to form the common iliac trunk on each side (Walls, 1972). The segmental arteries referred to as the fifth lumbars may also help to form this trunk (Williams et al., 1989). One artery that branches from the common iliac trunk is the internal iliac artery, and it gives rise to two arteries that serve the back: the iliolumbar and lateral sacral (Parke, 1992a).

The aortic arches and dorsal aorta have been sending branches to the embryo's intervertebral foramina (IVFs) (Williams et al., 1989). By the time arterial differentiation is complete, the arteries supplying branches to the IVFs have undergone changes that vary according to the spinal level (Woodburne, 1983). In the cervical region, they branch from the ascending cervical, deep cervical, and vertebral arteries; in the thoracic region, they branch from the posterior intercostals and subcostal arteries; and in the abdominal region, they branch from the lumbar, iliolumbar, lateral sacral, and median sacral arteries (Oelrich, 1966). Once inside the IVF, they rebranch (Hollinshead, 1982) and in the process intersect three arteries that run the length of the spinal cord: the single anterior spinal and the two posterior spinal arteries (see Chapter 3).

The anterior spinal artery had formed near the juncture of the brain and spinal cord by the union of a branch from one vertebral artery with a branch from the other vertebral artery to form an artery that extends caudally on the cord's anterior aspect (Yoffey, 1976) (see Fig. 3-12). Each posterior spinal artery had branched

from a vertebral and sometimes a posterior inferior cerebellar artery. The posterior spinal artery extends caudally on the posterior aspect of the spinal cord (Walls, 1972). The posterior inferior cerebellar arteries were themselves branches from the vertebral arteries, which branch from the subclavian arteries (Goss, 1966). Thus the blood supply for the spinal cord and its adnexa (hard and soft tissues) originates from within the cranium by way of the vertebral arteries and, periodically all along the spine's length, by way of feeder arteries, that is, tributaries of arteries that enter IVFs (Parke, 1992a). Chapter 3 discusses the arterial supply of the spinal cord in further detail.

The previous account has related how the embryo constructs mesodermal channels delivering blood to those back muscles that are called intrinsic, deep, or true. The embryo develops different channels to the other back muscles that have been designated extrinsic or superficial. These latter arteries branch from the subclavian or axillary and include the following: transverse cervical, suprascapular, scapular circumflex, posterior humeral circumflex, and thoracodorsal (Crafts, 1966). Their synonymy and variability are complex (Goss, 1966). Mesoderm has also formed channels returning blood from these superficial back muscles, and often these veins retrace the route of the arteries and also bear the same names (Hollinshead & Rosse, 1985). Their variability is even greater than that of the arteries (Brash, 1951a).

Veins of the Back

While all the arterial development has been happening, the mesoderm in the epidural space surrounding the spinal cord has been forming a network of veins (Romanes, 1966) (see Fig. 3-14). This plexus lies between the meninges and the vertebrae and is known as the internal (epidural) vertebral venous plexus. This plexus receives blood from the spinal cord and the vertebrae and channels it into the intervertebral veins (Walls, 1972). These veins exit the IVFs and ventral sacral foramina (Woodburne, 1983).

Outside the foramina, the intervertebral veins drain into veins called segmental by some (Hollinshead, 1982) and intersegmental by others (Brash, 1951a). These segmental/intersegmental veins receive specific names according to their spinal level, for example, vertebrals, intercostals, lumbars, and lateral sacrals (Brash, 1951a). These veins carry the blood back to the heart by different routes. The vertebral veins drain into the brachiocephalic veins, which pass the blood to the superior vena cava (Romanes, 1966). The intercostal veins drain into the azygos system of veins (Gosling et al., 1990), and this variable system also drains the blood to the superior vena cava. The superior vena cava empties into the right atrium of the heart (Romanes, 1968).

The lumbar veins are even more variable in their drainage pattern (Brash, 1951a). The first and second lumbar veins drain into a vein called the ascending lumbar, which in turn drains into the subcostal vein. The subcostal vein drains into the azygos system, and the venous blood continues on to the heart by way of the superior vena cava (Oelrich, 1966). The third and fourth lumbar veins are tributaries to the inferior vena cava, which empties into the right atrium of the heart (Brash, 1951a). The fifth lumbar vein drains into the iliolumbar vein. The iliolumbar vein drains into the common iliac vein, itself a tributary of the inferior vena cava, which empties into the heart (Romanes, 1968). The intervertebral veins exiting from the ventral sacral foramina drain into the lateral sacral veins (Oelrich, 1966). From there the blood passes to the internal iliac vein, then to the common iliac vein, and finally into the inferior vena cava, which drains into the right atrium of the heart (Goss, 1966).

The intervertebral veins draining into veins in the neck, thorax, and abdomen have a common pattern. In each case they intersect a vein running lengthwise. In the cervical region the intervertebral veins are linked vertically by the vertebral vein, since they are all tributaries to it (Brash, 1951a). In the thoracic region they are connected to the vertically running azygos system of veins (Goss, 1966). In the abdominal region they drain to the ascending lumbar vein (Romanes, 1968). In the pelvic region they are linked vertically by the lateral sacral vein (Brash, 1951a). At least one authority has regarded the azygos vein as a cephalic continuation of the ascending lumbar vein (Goss, 1966).

When the mesoderm constructed a venous plexus inside the vertebral canal, it also constructed one on the outside, the external vertebral venous plexus (Parke, 1992). This external plexus of veins drains the soft and hard tissues contiguous to it (Oelrich, 1966). This external plexus also anastomoses with the internal plexus of veins inside the vertebral canal (Hollinshead, 1982). Both venous plexuses drain into the segmental veins (Goss, 1966). (The latter include the posterior intercostal, lumbar, and lateral sacral veins [Walls, 1972].) Thus the segmental veins receive blood from the vertebrae and the soft tissues that envelop them by way of the external venous plexus (O'Rahilly, 1986). All the blood from the two plexuses is added to the blood already in the segmental veins, blood that was returning from the deep muscles and skin of the back (Romanes, 1968). The blood next flows from these segmental veins into various definitive veins that the fetus has fashioned out of various precursor veins of the early embryo (Brash, 1951a).

The definitive vein that the blood from segmental veins in the cervical region ultimately drains into is known as the superior vena cava (Oelrich, 1966). It is derived from the right common cardinal vein and a part of the right anterior cardinal vein (Patten, 1953). Blood from segmental veins in the thoracic region drains into the azygos system of veins: the azygos, hemiazygos, and accessory hemiazygos veins (Walls, 1972). This azygos system forms from the embryo's posterior cardinal veins (Goss, 1966). According to Patten (1953), the embryo's supracardinal veins may also contribute. Blood from segmental veins in the lower lumbar and sacral regions drains into the inferior vena cava, which forms from the posterior cardinal, subcardinal, and supracardinal veins of the embryo (Patten, 1953). Blood from the embryonic gonads, kidneys, and adrenal glands is delivered to the inferior vena cava by veins named after the organ they serve. They are all derived from the subcardinal veins of the embryo (Williams et al., 1989).

Virtually all the tissues making up the bulk of the posterior body wall are derived from mesoderm, for example, the thoracic duct and its lymphatic tributaries and the various fasciae: superficial, deep, endothoracic, transversalis, and thoracolumbar (Goss, 1966). However, the neural elements, such as the lumbosacral plexus, develop from ectoderm (Larsell, 1953).

Suggested Readings

Space limitations and other considerations do not allow discussion of the appearance of supernumerary structures, such as cervical and lumbar ribs, or persistent embryonic tissue, as in chordoma (O'Rahilly & Muller, 1992). Detailed description of the normal development of complex structures such as the dens (see Chapter 5) and sacrum (see Chapter 8) are likewise absent (Goss, 1966; Inkster, 1951; Larsell, 1953; Trotter & Peterson, 1966; Williams et al., 1989). Accounts of investigative studies on the development of frog, chick, and mouse embryos as related to the human embryo have also been excluded (Ballard, 1964; Rugh, 1964). However, the reader has been provided a substantial amount of background information with which to continue the study of the enormous amount of information available in the field of human development (Rothman & Simeone, 1992). Readers requiring more depth and breadth than given in this chapter are recommended to consult the scholarly treatises of Parke (1992a and 1992b) and O'Rahilly and Muller, (1992), both authorities in the field. They fill in the lacunae, sort through the controversies, and are reliable guides to primary sources in the literature.

REFERENCES

Allan, F.D. (1969). *Essentials of human embryology* (2nd ed.). New York: Oxford University Press.
Arey, L.B. (1965). *Developmental anatomy* (7th ed.). Philadelphia: WB Saunders.

Bagnall, K. et al. (1987). Some experimental data to support the theory of resegmentation in vertebral formations. *Anat Rec, 218*(1), 12A.

Ballard, W.W. (1964). *Comparative embryology and embryology.* New York: Ronald Press.

Barr, M.L. & Kiernan, J.A. (1988). *The human nervous system* (5th ed.). Philadelphia: JB Lippincott.

Baxter, J.S. (1953). *Frazer's manual of embryology.* London: Bailliere, Tindall & Cox.

Beck, F., Moffat, D.B., & Davies, D.P. (1985). *Human embryology* (2nd ed.). Oxford: Blackwell Scientific Publications.

Bogduk, N. & Twomey, L.T. (1987). *Clinical anatomy of the lumbar spine.* Melbourne: Churchill Livingstone.

Brash, J.C. (1951a). Blood vascular and lymphatic systems. In J.C. Brash (Ed.), *Cunningham's textbook of anatomy* (9th ed.). London: Oxford University Press.

Brash, J.C. (1951b). Human embryology. In J.C. Brash (Ed.), *Cunningham's textbook of anatomy* (9th ed.). London: Oxford University Press.

Breathnach, A.S. (1958). *Frazer's anatomy of the human skeleton* (5th ed.). London: Churchill.

Bruce, J. & Walmsley, R. (1939). *Beesly and Johnston's manual of surgical anatomy.* London: Oxford University Press.

Callander, C.L. (1939). *Surgical anatomy* (2nd ed.). Philadelphia: WB Saunders.

Carlson, B.M. (1981). *Patten's foundations of embryology* (4th ed.). New York: McGraw-Hill.

Clark, W.E. (1951). Central nervous system. In J.C. Brash (Ed.), *Cunningham's textbook of anatomy* (9th ed.). London: Oxford University Press.

Clark, W.E. (1976). Central nervous system. In W.J. Hamilton (Ed.), *Textbook of human anatomy* (2nd ed.). St. Louis: Mosby.

Cohen, M.S. et al. (1992). Anatomy of the spinal nerve roots in the lumbar and lower thoracic spine. In R.R. Rothman & F.A. Simeone (Eds.), *The spine* (Vol. 2). (3rd ed.). Philadelphia: WB Saunders.

Corliss, C.E. (1976). *Patten's human embryology.* New York: McGraw-Hill.

Coupland, R.E. (1976). Endocrine system. In W.J. Hamilton (Ed.), *Textbook of human anatomy* (2nd ed.). St. Louis: Mosby.

Crafts, R.C. (1966). *A textbook of human anatomy.* New York: Ronald Press.

Davenport, H.A. (1966). Introduction and topographic anatomy. In B.J. Anson (Ed.), *Morris' human anatomy* (12th ed.). New York: McGraw-Hill.

Durward, A. (1951). Peripheral nervous system. In J.C. Brash (Ed.), *Cunningham's textbook of anatomy* (9th ed.). London: Oxford University Press.

Ellis, H. (1983). *Clinical anatomy* (7th ed.). Oxford: Blackwell Scientific Publications.

Fischman, D.A. (1972). Development of striated muscle. In G.H. Bourne (Ed.), *The structure and function of muscle* (Vol. 2). (2nd ed.). New York: Academic Press.

Francis, C.C. & Voneida, J.J. (1966). The nervous system. In B.J. Anson (Ed.), *Morris' human anatomy* (12th ed.). New York: McGraw-Hill.

Gosling, J.A. et al. (1990). *Human anatomy* (2nd ed.). London: Gower Medical Publishing.

Goss, C.M. (1966). *Gray's anatomy of the human body* (28th ed.). Philadelphia: Lea & Febiger.

Grant, J.C.B. (1952). *A method of anatomy* (5th ed.). Baltimore: Williams & Wilkins.

Hall, B.K. (1978). *Developmental and cellular skeletal biology.* New York: Academic Press.

Hamilton, W.J. & Mossman, H.W. (1972). *Human embryology* (4th ed.). Baltimore: Williams & Wilkins.

Harrison, R.G. (1972). Introduction to human embryology. In G.J. Romanes (Ed.), *Cunningham's textbook of anatomy* (11th ed.). London: Oxford University Press.

Hollinshead, W.H. (1982). *The back and limbs: Vol 3. Anatomy for surgeons* (3rd ed.). Philadelphia: Harper & Row.

Hollinshead, W.H. & Rosse, C. (1985). *Textbook of anatomy* (4th ed.). Philadelphia: Harper & Row.

Inkster, R.G. (1951). Osteology. In J.C. Brash (Ed.), *Cunningham's textbook of anatomy* (9th ed.). London: Oxford University Press.

Joseph, J. (1976). Locomotor system. In W.J. Hamilton (Ed.), *Textbook of human anatomy* (2nd ed.). St. Louis: Mosby.

Langebartel, D.A. (1977). *The anatomical primer.* Baltimore: University Park Press.

Larsell, O. (1953). The nervous system. In J.P. Schaeffer (Ed.), *Morris' human anatomy* (11th ed.). New York: McGraw-Hill.

Leeson, C.R. & Leeson, T.S. (1972). *Human structure.* Philadelphia: WB Saunders.

Lockhart, R.D. (1951). Myology. In J.C. Brash (Ed.), *Cunningham's textbook of anatomy* (9th ed.). London: Oxford University Press.

Moore, K.L. (1988). *The developing human* (4th ed.). Philadelphia: WB Saunders.

Mortenson, O. & Pettersen, J.C. (1966). The musculature. In B.J. Anson (Ed.), *Morris' human anatomy* (12th ed.). New York: McGraw-Hill.

Mossman, H.W. (1987). *Vertebrate fetal membranes.* New Brunswick: Rutgers University Press.

Noback, C.R. & Demarest, R.J. (1975). *The human nervous system* (2nd ed.). New York: McGraw-Hill.

Oelrich, T.M. (1966). The cardiovascular system—arteries and veins. In B.J. Anson (Ed.), *Morris' human anatomy* (12th ed.). New York: McGraw-Hill.

O'Rahilly, R. (1986). *Gardner-Gray-O'Rahilly anatomy: A regional study of human structure* (5th ed.). Philadelphia: WB Saunders.

O'Rahilly, R. & Muller, F. (1992). *Human embryology and teratology.* New York: John Wiley & Sons.

Parke, W.W. (1992a). Applied anatomy of the spine. In R.R. Rothman, F.A. Simeone (Eds.), *The spine* (Vol. 2). (3rd ed.). Philadelphia: WB Saunders.

Parke, W.W. (1992b). Development of the spine. In R.R. Rothman, F.A. Simeone (Eds.), *The spine* (Vol. 2). (3rd ed.). Philadelphia: WB Saunders.

Patten, B.M. (1953). The cardiovascular system. In J.P. Schaeffer (Ed.), *Morris' human anatomy* (11th ed). New York: McGraw-Hill.

Patten, B.M. (1964). *Foundations of embryology* (2nd ed.). New York: McGraw-Hill.

Robertson, G.G. (1966). Developmental anatomy. In B.J. Anson (Ed.), *Morris' human anatomy* (12th ed.). New York: McGraw-Hill.

Romanes, G.J. (1966). *Cunningham's manual of practical anatomy* (Vol. 3). (13th ed.). London: Oxford University Press.

Romanes, G.J. (1968). *Cunningham's manual of practical anatomy* (Vol. 2). (13th ed.). London: Oxford University Press.

Romanes, G.J. (1972a). The central nervous system. In G.J. Romanes (Ed.), *Cunningham's textbook of anatomy* (11th ed.). London: Oxford University Press.

Romanes, G.J. (1972b). The peripheral nervous system. In G.J. Romanes (Ed.), *Cunningham's textbook of anatomy* (11th ed.). London: Oxford University Press.

Romanes, G.J. (1976). *Cunningham's manual of practical anatomy* (Vol. 1). (14th ed.). London: Oxford University Press.

Rothman, R.R. & Simeone, F.A. (1992). *The spine* (Vols. 1 and 2). (3rd ed.). Philadelphia: WB Saunders.

Rugh, R. (1964). *Vertebrate embryology.* New York: Harcourt, Brace, & World.

Sadler, T.W. (1990). *Langman's medical embryology* (6th ed.). Baltimore: Williams & Wilkins.

Salsabili, N. & Hogg, D.A. (1991). Development of the human sacroiliac joint, *Clin Anat, 4*(2), 199-208.

Scammon, R.E. (1953). Developmental anatomy. In J.P. Schaeffer (Ed.), *Morris' human anatomy* (11th ed.). New York: McGraw-Hill.

Scothorne, R.J. (1976). Peripheral nervous system. In W.J. Hamilton

(Ed.), *Textbook of human anatomy* (2nd ed.). St. Louis: Mosby.

Sinclair, D.C. (1972). Muscles and fasciae. In G.J. Romanes (Ed.), *Cunningham's textbook of anatomy* (11th ed.). London: Oxford University Press.

Snell, R.S. (1975). *Clinical embryology for medical students* (2nd ed.). Boston: Little, Brown.

Snell, R.S. (1981). *Clinical anatomy for medical students* (2nd ed.). Boston: Little, Brown.

Trotter, M. & Peterson, R.R. (1966). Osteology. In B.J. Anson (Ed.), *Morris' human anatomy* (12th ed.). New York: McGraw-Hill.

Verbout, A.J. (1985). The development of the vertebral column. *Adv Anat Embryo Cell Biol, 90,* 1-122.

Walls, E.W. (1972). The blood vascular and lymphatic systems. In G.J. Romanes (Ed.), *Cunningham's textbook of anatomy* (11th ed.) London: Oxford University Press.

Walmsley, R. (1972). Joints. In G.J. Romanes (Ed.), *Cunningham's textbook of anatomy* (11th ed.) London: Oxford University Press.

Williams, P.L. et al. (Eds.). (1989). *Gray's anatomy* (37th ed.). Edinburgh: Churchill Livingstone.

Woodburne, R.T. (1983). *Essentials of human anatomy* (7th ed.). New York: Oxford University Press.

Yoffey, J.M. (1976). Cardiovascular system. In W.J. Hamilton (Ed.), *Textbook of human anatomy* (2nd ed) St. Louis: Mosby.

Zuckerman, S. (1961). *A new system of anatomy.* London: Oxford University Press.

CHAPTER 13

Microscopic Anatomy of the Zygapophyseal Joints and Intervertebral Discs

Peter C. Stathopoulos
Gregory D. Cramer

Much of the current anatomic research related to the spine is concerned with the zygapophyseal joints (Z joints) and the intervertebral discs (IVDs). The gross anatomy of these structures is covered in detail in Chapter 2. The characteristics of these structures unique to the cervical, thoracic, and lumbar regions are covered in Chapters 5, 6, and 7, respectively. Because much of the current investigation related to the Z joints and the IVDs has been carried out in the lumbar region, Chapter 7 describes the Z joints and IVDs in significant detail. However, a considerable amount of the research on these two tissues is associated with their microscopic anatomy (Giles, 1992a, 1992b), and molecular structure (Buckwalter et al., 1989). The results of these investigations provide a greater understanding of normal, as well as pathologic, structure and function at the microscopic, ultrastructural (electron microscopic), and molecular levels.

As more information becomes available on the precise composition and arrangement of the tissues of normal and diseased Z joints and IVDs, a better understanding of the biologic basis for current treatment develops (Giles & Taylor, 1987). Continued investigation should lead to an increase in the understanding of spinal dysfunction. With changing concepts on the mechanisms of spinal dysfunction, new therapeutic approaches will undoubtedly emerge, and it will be necessary to keep abreast of these changing concepts to be able to apply effectively the new therapeutic approaches. Therefore an understanding of the microscopic anatomy of the Z joints and the IVDs is extremely important to the clinician and the researcher alike.

The purpose of this chapter is to provide the reader with comprehensive information on the microscopic anatomy of the Z joints and IVDs. A discussion of the normal composition of connective tissue in general and, more specifically, of hyaline cartilage and fibrocartilage in association with the Z joints and IVDs is also included.

MICROSCOPIC ANATOMY OF THE ZYGAPOPHYSEAL JOINTS

Bones in contact with one another are held together by connective tissue. This union forms a joint that, in some instances, is freely movable and is lined by a synovial membrane. This type of joint is known as a synovial (diarthrodial) joint. The Z joints of the spine are of this type. The joints between contiguous vertebral bodies are classified as amphiarthroses and are formed by the IVDs. The IVDs are tough, cushionlike pads consisting mainly of connective tissue, more specifically, specialized fibrocartilage. The IVDs are discussed later in this chapter.

The articular surfaces that form the Z joints, as with all diarthrodial joints, are covered with shiny hyaline cartilage. This cartilage is lubricated by synovial fluid that allows the bones to glide smoothly over each other with minimal friction (Swann et al., 1974). The articular cartilages and joint cavity of the Z joints are enveloped posteriorly by a tough sleeve of dense connective tissue. This connective tissue sleeve is known as the fibrous capsule. Anteriorly, the ligamentum flavum takes the place of the articular capsule of the Z joint (Xu et al., 1991). Lining the joint capsule is a thin inner layer of highly vascularized connective tissue called the synovial membrane. Cells within the synovial membrane manufacture the synovial fluid.

This section discusses the microscopic anatomy of the articular cartilage, the capsule, and the synovial membrane of the Z joints. Because most tissues involved in the formation of the Z joints (and the IVDs) is connective tissue, and because pain arising from the Z joints is a significant cause of back pain (Kirkaldy-Willis, 1988; Mooney & Robertson, 1976), a working knowledge of connective tissue is important in treating pain of spinal origin. Therefore a section on connective tissue, including hyaline cartilage, immediately follows this section on the Z joints.

Zygapophyseal Joint Articular Cartilage

General Considerations. The articular cartilages lining the superior and inferior articular processes of each Z joint are similar in many respects to the articular cartilage associated with most synovial joints of the body. This means that the articular cartilage lining one of the articular processes of a Z joint is made up of a special variety of hyaline cartilage that is very durable, is lubricated by synovial fluid, is compressible, and is also able to withstand large compressive forces (Williams et al., 1989).

Recall that hyaline cartilage is not unique to the Z joints but is widely distributed in the body. Not only does it line the articular facets of Z joints, but it is also found in a portion of the vertebral end plates of the IVDs, the nose, most of the laryngeal cartilages, C rings of the trachea, primary and secondary bronchi, costal cartilages of ribs, most articular cartilages of joints throughout the body, and the xiphoid process. It is also the type of cartilage present in the epiphyseal cartilage plates of growing long bones. Therefore, hyaline cartilage is essential for the growth and development of long bones before and after birth.

The purposes of Z joint articular cartilage is to protect the articular surfaces of the superior and inferior articular processes by acting as a shock absorber and to allow the articular surfaces to move across one another with very little friction. Both functions are carried out efficiently. In fact, the coefficient of friction for typical articular surfaces is less than 0.002, which means that the two surfaces of a typical Z joint glide across each other

with much greater ease than they would if they were both made of ice (coefficient of friction for ice sliding on ice is less than 0.03) (Triano, 1992).

The articular cartilage of a single Z joint surface is rather small, and in fact, the lumbar articular surfaces measure approximately 8 by 10 mm (Giles, 1992a, 1992b). The Z joint articular cartilage is also approximately 1 to 2 mm thick (Figs. 13-1, 13-2, and 13-3). The concavity of the cartilage on lumbar superior articular facets is thicker than the periphery of the same surfaces. This is the opposite from that typically found in other joints of the body where the concavity of a joint surface is usually lined by thinner cartilage than that surrounding the concavity.

Z joint articular cartilage is made up of 75% water and 25% solids (Giles, 1992a, 1992b) and consists of cells embedded in an abundant and firm matrix (Fig. 13-4). The cells that produce the cartilage matrix are chondroblasts, and in mature cartilage they are known as chondrocytes (Table 13-1). The matrix is made up of an intricate network of collagen fibers surrounded by proteoglycans and glycoproteins. The concentration of these constituents of articular cartilage differs from one part of the joint surface to another and also at different depths from the joint surface (Giles, 1992a, 1992b).

Fresh hyaline cartilage is bluish white and translucent. In stained, fixed preparations, the matrix appears glassy, homogeneous, and smooth. Distributed throughout the matrix are spaces called lacunae, and within the lacunae are the chondrocytes. As with all cartilage, Z joint articular cartilage has no nerve supply and no direct blood supply. Chondrocytes must receive nutrients by diffusion across the cartilage matrix from several sources. These sources include the blood vessels within the synovial membrane that is located along the peripheral margin of the nonarticular portion of the cartilage, the synovial fluid, and the blood vessels in the adjacent bone (Williams et al., 1989).

Chondrocytes are found either singly in the lacunae or in clusters of two or more chondrocytes. These clusters are called cell nests or isogenous cell groups (Fig. 13-5). The cells within the nests have arisen from the mitotic activity of a single chondrocyte. Therefore the presence of isogenous cell groups signifies cartilage growth (interstitial cartilage growth). This is supported by electron microscopy findings revealing that the chondrocytes within a cell nest exhibit a well-developed rough endoplasmic reticulum, a Golgi complex, and a large amount of glycogen and lipid.

Articular cartilage differs from typical hyaline cartilage in that the articular surface does not possess a covering of perichondrium (Giles, 1992b; Williams et al., 1989). Instead, the cells of the articular surface appear flat and are closer together than they are farther within the cartilage matrix. In addition, the matrix of the articular

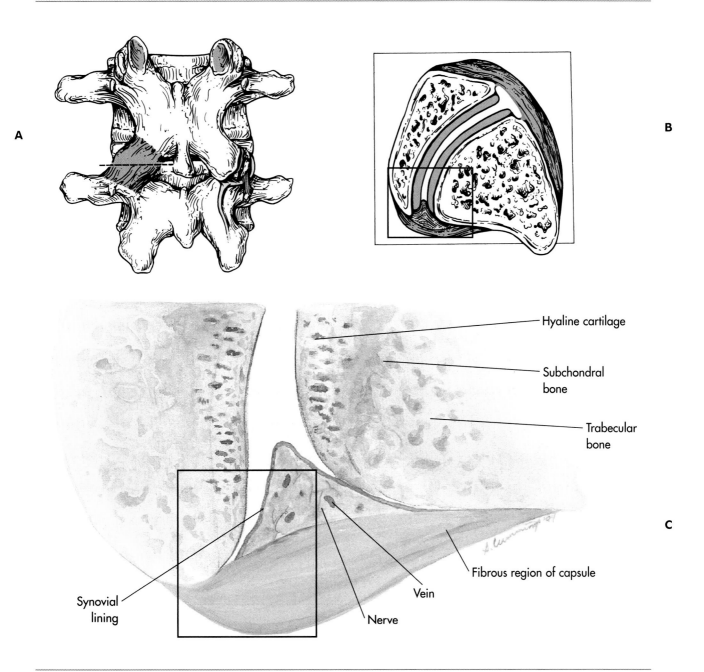

FIG. 13-1 The zygapophyseal joint (Z joint). **A** and **B,** Z joint from a posterior view and a horizontal section, respectively. **C,** Z joint after magnification by approximately a factor of 10. The articular cartilage, subchondral bone, and articular capsule are prominently displayed. In addition, a Z joint synovial fold is prominent. Notice that the articular capsule has an outer, tough fibrous region. The center of the synovial fold is more vascular and contains adipose tissue. A nerve can be seen passing through this latter region. A synovial lining can be seen on the deep surface of the articular capsule and the synovial fold. The box enclosing the synovial fold and a portion of the superior articular process is the region shown at higher magnification in Fig. 13-7.

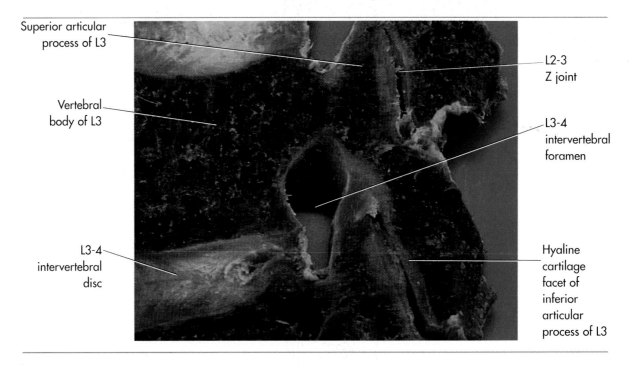

Superior articular process of L3

Vertebral body of L3

L3-4 intervertebral disc

L2-3 Z joint

L3-4 intervertebral foramen

Hyaline cartilage facet of inferior articular process of L3

FIG. 13-2   Parasagittal section through the L3 and L4 region of a cadaveric spine.

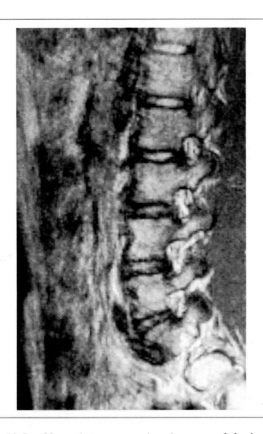

FIG. 13-3   Magnetic resonance imaging scan of the lumbar region performed in a parasagittal plane. The plane of section roughly corresponds to that of Fig. 13-2. Notice the intervertebral discs, the intervertebral foramina, and their contents.

surface becomes dense and fibrous. The collagen fibers, which course perpendicular to the articulating surface from deep within the cartilage matrix, curve as they reach the joint surface and become oriented parallel to the free edge of the articular cartilage.

Cartilage Matrix. The cartilage matrix immediately surrounds the lacunae containing the chondrocytes. The matrix of hyaline cartilage consists of collagen (type II) fibers, a small number of elastic fibers, and an amorphous ground substance. The ground substance consists primarily of proteoglycans and glycoproteins. Each of these components of the cartilage matrix contributes to the strength, longevity, and resilience of this tissue.

Collagen. The collagen component of hyaline cartilage consists of type II collagen fibers. These fibers are relatively thin and course in all directions within the cartilage. They are usually not visible with the light microscope because they are masked by another component of the cartilage matrix, the ground substance. The collagen fibers can be seen easily with an electron microscope.

Collagen functions to bind the cartilage together, protect the chondrocytes, allow for attachment of the articular cartilage to the subchondral bone, and help resist compressive loads (Giles, 1992a). Because collagen is an extremely important constituent of all the connective tissue components of the Z joints and the IVDs, it is discussed in detail in Supporting Cells and Extracellular Matrix of Connective Tissue: Functional Components.

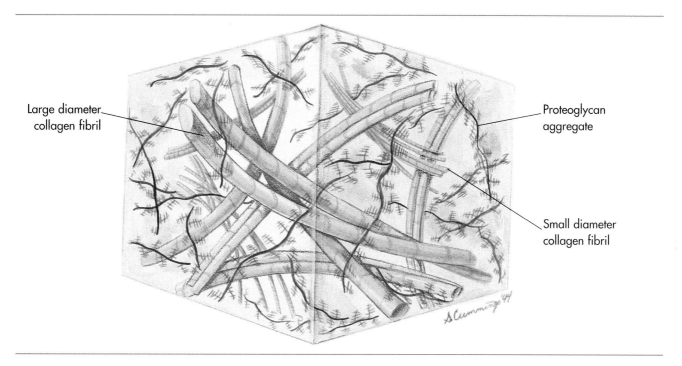

FIG. 13-4   Extracellular matrix of hyaline cartilage. Notice the abundance of collagen fibrils and proteoglycan aggregates.

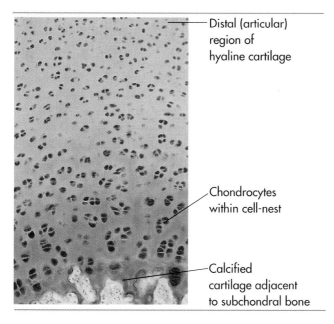

FIG. 13-5   Light micrograph of hyaline (articular) cartilage. The cartilage is from the distal tip of a fetal phalanx (100×). Developing articular cartilage of the zygapophyseal joints is quite similar.

Ground substance. Chemical analysis of the ground substance of the extracellular matrix of hyaline cartilage reveals that it contains a small amount of glycoproteins and a high concentration of three types of glycosaminoglycans: hyaluronic acid, chondroitin sulfate, and keratan sulfate. The chondroitin and keratan sulfates are joined to a core protein to form a proteoglycan mono-

mer. These macromolecules interact with the collagen and elastic fibers of the hyaline cartilage matrix (Fig. 13-6).

The single core protein of the proteoglycan molecule has a molecular weight of 200,000 to 350,000 daltons. The core proteins represent approximately 7% to 12% of the dry weight of cartilage. Bound to each core protein are 80 to 100 chondroitin 4-sulfate and chondroitin 6-sulfate chains, each with a molecular weight of 20,000 daltons. These two glycosaminoglycans make up 80% to 85% of the dry weight of hyaline cartilage. In addition, approximately 50 chains of keratan sulfate, each with a molecular weight of 5000 daltons, are also attached to the core protein. Keratan sulfate contributes approximately 7% of the total dry weight of hyaline cartilage.

At one end of each core protein is a hyaluronic acid–binding region (Fig. 13-6). At this site the proteoglycan units are joined to hyaluronic acid molecules to form long proteoglycan–hyaluronic acid (PG-HA) aggregates. The interaction of the proteoglycan monomer with hyaluronic acid is strengthened by the presence of a link protein (Fig. 13-6). Proteoglycans and glycosaminoglycans are discussed in further detail later in this chapter with regard to the IVD.

Chondronectin is a glycoprotein found in cartilage. Glycoproteins differ from proteoglycans by their low carbohydrate content, different repeating disaccharide units, and the absence of sulfate esters. Chondronectin participates in the adhesion of chondrocytes to type II collagen. Common glycoproteins found in other body tissues include laminin and fibronectin. Laminin is found

Table 13-1 The Cells of Connective Tissue

Cell type	Function	Distribution	Characteristics	Miscellaneous
Fibroblasts	Synthesize and secrete collagen, elastic fibers, reticular fibers, and proteoglycans (among other molecules) Support ligaments, tendons, bone, skin, blood vessels, and basement membranes	Throughout all loose and dense connective tissue	Flat, stellate cells with dark, ovoid, staining nuclei and one or two nucleoli Microscopically, may appear to be of different shapes because of the plane of sectioning	Most abundant cell type found in connective tissue proper
Chondroblasts	Synthesize and secrete extracellular matrix of cartilage Synthesize and secrete collagen, elastic fibers, and glycosaminoglycans Support articular cartilage	Present in hyaline cartilage of articulations (Z joints) and fibrocartilage of intervertebral discs; also found in elastic cartilage	Metabolically active with large vesicular nuclei and prominent nucleoli Cytoplasm pale and vacuolated because of high content of lipid and glycogen	Occupy artificial spaces, called lacunae, which are located in the matrix of cartilage Chondrocytes (mature chondroblasts) similar to chondroblasts except smaller with lower metabolic activity
Osteoblasts	Synthesize and secrete extracellular matrix of bone	In bone	Basophilic cytoplasm resulting from the presence of a large amount of rough endoplasmic reticulum that produces glycosaminoglycans and glycoproteins	Osteocytes (mature osteoblasts) similar to osteoblasts but less active in matrix secretion; occupy spaces in the matrix of bone known as lacunae
Myofibroblasts	Synthesize and secrete components of the extracellular matrix Capable of contractility	In blood vessels and skin throughout the body	Resemble fibroblasts with light microscopy, but ultrastructurally contain actin filaments for contraction	Develop during repair after tissue damage; produce collagen; contractile properties associated with retraction and shrinkage of fibrous (scar) tissue
Adipocytes	Synthesize and store lipids Provide a cushioning and padding function	Throughout body	Small nuclei with abundant lipid in cytoplasm	
Macrophages	Involved in phagocytosis	Throughout body	Derived from monocytes and assume several different forms	Highly motile cells that can move actively from one compartment of the body to another when stimulated by immunoglobulins and antigens
Mast cells	Functionally similar to basophils; granules of basophils and mast cells contain heparin (an anticoagulant), chondroitin sulfate, histamine, and leukotriene 3	In the lamina propria, especially of the digestive and respiratory systems; around blood vessels; and lining serous cavities	Cytoplasm stains basophilic and metrachromatic	

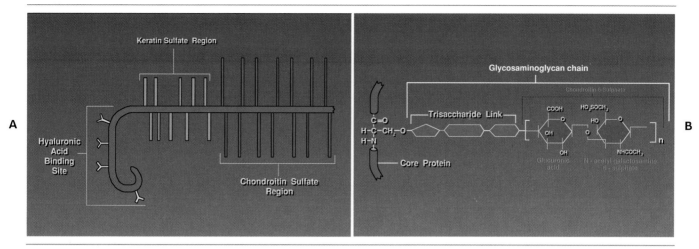

FIG. 13-6   A, Structure of a proteoglycan monomer. Notice several glycosaminoglycan chains (chondroitin sulfate and keratan sulfate) attached to a core protein. The protein molecule can attach to a long hyaluronic acid molecule to help to form a proteoglycan aggregate. **B,** An example of an individual glycosaminoglycan chain, in this case chondroitin 6-sulfate, and its attachment to the core protein. (Courtesy Dino Juarez, The National College of Chiropractic.)

in basal laminae and is partially responsible for the adhesion of epithelial cells. Fibronectin is found in blood, plasma, fibroblasts, and some epithelial cells and helps to mediate normal cell adhesion and migration (Table 13-2).

Clinical and biomechanical considerations. Normally, fluid moves out of articular cartilage when it is compressed and back into the cartilage when the Z joint is distracted. Such movement may help nutrients diffuse through the matrix to the chondrocytes. Articular cartilage can deform considerably when heavy compressive loads are applied to a joint. However, it returns to its previous state when the load is removed. If injured, articular cartilage heals rather slowly (a 1 mm defect heals in about 4 weeks). Passive movement of the joint may stimulate cartilage regeneration, whereas immobility results in the development of adhesions. Intermittent light weight-bearing activity does not stimulate cartilage regeneration but does stop the development of adhesions (Triano, 1992).

Articular cartilage becomes yellow, thinner, and more brittle with age, and undulations that may develop into ragged projections appear as a result of "wear and tear" of the joint surface (Williams et al., 1992). Also with age, fissures or "cracks" may develop in the articular cartilage. The development of such fissures is known as fibrillation of articular cartilage. The fissures may extend from the joint surface to the subchondral bone.

Zygapophyseal Joint Articular Capsule

The Z joint capsules throughout the vertebral column are thin and loose. They are attached to the margins of the opposed superior and inferior articular facets of the adjacent vertebrae (Williams et al., 1989). The capsules are longer and looser in the cervical region than in the lumbar and thoracic regions. The articular capsule of a typical Z joint covers the joint's posterolateral surface. It consists of an outer layer of dense fibroelastic connective tissue, a vascular central layer made up of areolar tissue and loose connective tissue, and an inner layer consisting of a synovial membrane (Giles & Taylor, 1987). The outer, connective tissue layer of the capsule is tough and is essentially made up of parallel bundles of collagen fibers that are primarily oriented in the horizontal plane. A few fibroblasts and fibrocytes and a small amount of ground substance are also found in this layer (see Supporting Cells and Extracellular Matrix of Connective Tissue: Functional Components). The collagen fibers of the capsule attach to the adjacent surfaces of the superior and inferior articular processes, just peripheral to the articular cartilage. In fact, a gradual transition occurs from the joint capsule to fibrocartilage and finally to the articular cartilage of the Z joint. The capsules have a rich sensory innervation (Giles & Taylor, 1987). However, they have a rather poor blood supply, which slows the healing of these structures once they are damaged (Giles, 1992b). The multifidus lumborum muscle attaches to the articular capsule, which lies just medial to the primary attachment of this muscle to the mamillary process. The multifidus lumborum muscle may help to keep the capsule out of the joint space (Taylor & Twomey, 1986).

The articular capsules are thinner superiorly and inferiorly, where they form capsular recesses that cover fat-filled synovial pads. Defects exist within the superior and inferior aspects of the joint capsule and allow for the

Table 13-2 Fibers Found in Connective Tissue

Fiber type	Function	Distribution	Miscellaneous
Collagen	Provides rigid support and tensile strength to tendons, ligaments, cartilage, bone, and intervertebral discs	Throughout body	Most abundant and most important of the extracellular fibrillar proteins in the human body
Fibrillin	Main component of extracellular microfibrils, which are one constituent of elastic fibers. Microfibrils promote adhesion between different components of the extracellular matrix.	Throughout body	Fibrillin is a glycoprotein that forms fibrils
Elastic fibers	Provide elasticity to tissues and allow them to recoil after stretching	Blood vessels, skin, and ligaments. Large elastic fibers found in the ligamenta flava. Also present in elastic cartilage of the ear, epiglottis, lungs, vocal cords, and pleura	Composed of glycoprotein microfilaments (fibrillin) surrounding a core region of elastin
Reticular fibers	Provide a fine scaffolding that supports the extracellular matrix in basal laminae (basement membranes)	Throughout body	Thin fibrils, identical to small collagen fibrils (about 20 nm in diameter); exhibit a 67 nm periodicity of type III collagen (see Table 13-3)
Fibronectin	Serves as an intermediate protein in the extracellular matrix, where it connects cells to other extracellular matrix components, especially collagen and certain glycosaminoglycans (e.g., heparin)	Throughout body	Dimer glycoprotein, synthesized by fibroblasts and some epithelial cells (molecular weight, 230 to 250 kilodaltons)

passage of small nerves and vessels. The synovial joint recesses and the development of synovial joint cysts are discussed in further detail with the lumbar region, where they have been studied the most extensively (see Chapter 7). Also, the specific innervation of the Z joint capsule by the medial branch of the posterior primary division (dorsal ramus) is discussed in Chapter 2.

Ligamentum Flavum. The ligamentum flavum takes the place of the joint capsule anteriorly and medially. As discussed previously, this ligament passes from the anterior and inferior aspect of the lamina of the vertebra above to the posterior and superior aspect of the lamina of the vertebra below. However, the lateral fibers of this ligament course anterior to the Z joint, attach to its margins, and form its anterior capsule. Synovial extensions, or cysts, protrude out of the Z joint and along the attachment sites of the ligamentum flavum to the adjacent superior and inferior articular processes.

The ligamentum flavum is 80% elastic fibers and 20% collagen fibers. The elastic fibers within the ligamentum flavum prevent it from buckling into the intervertebral foramen (IVF) and vertebral canal, thus sparing the contents of these regions.

Synovial Membrane

The synovial membrane (synovium), or joint lining, is a condensation of connective tissue that covers the inner surface of the fibrous capsule, thus forming a sac that encloses the joint cavity (Fig. 13-7). Therefore the region of a diarthrodal joint surrounded by a synovium is known as the synovial cavity. The synovium covers the nonarticular bone that is enclosed within the joint capsule and courses to the margin of the articular cartilage, where a transition zone exists between the synovium and the articular cartilage. The synovium does not cover the load-bearing surface of the cartilage. The joint cavity normally contains a small amount of a highly viscous fluid, rich in hyaluronic acid that lubricates the joint surfaces. This fluid is known as synovial fluid and is produced by the cells within the synovial membrane (see Synoviocytes). The major function of the synovial membrane is to produce synovial fluid. Another function is to absorb waste

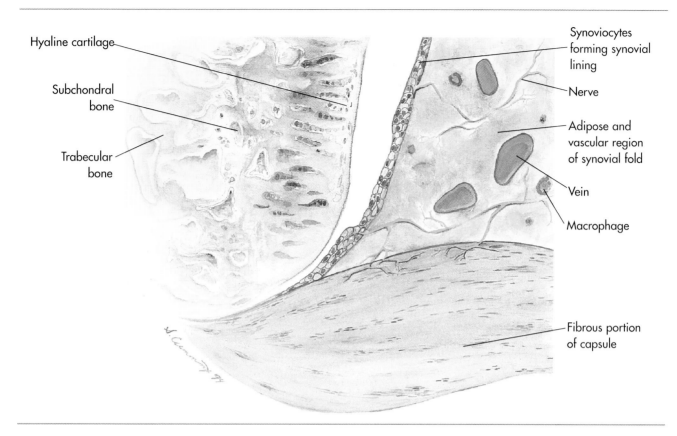

FIG. 13-7 Portion of the Z joint at a magnification of approximately 40 times actual size. The region here is shown by the box in Fig. 13-1. Portions of the articular cartilage, subchondral bone of the superior articular process and mamillary process, the articular capsule, and the Z joint synovial fold can be seen.

products of metabolism and cellular debris before they can accumulate in the Z joint cavity.

The innermost portion of the synovium is composed of one to three layers of specialized cells, known as synoviocytes or synovial lining cells. These cells form the intimal layer. Beneath this layer is a loose network of vascular areolar connective tissue that contains a rich blood supply. This layer is known as the synovial subintimal layer. It possesses many elastic fibers that probably serve to pull the synovium out of the joint cavity. The synovium is innervated by sensory nerve endings.

Typically, projections of the synovial layer extend into the synovial cavity as Z joint synovial folds (Giles, 1992a). Their purpose is to fill in the small gaps along the periphery of the joint, where the articular cartilages of the opposing surfaces do not normally come in contact with one another. These folds also produce synovial fluid and provide an efficient mechanism for the distribution of this fluid directly into the joint cavity.

Z joint synovial folds contain a relatively large amount of adipose tissue at the region of their attachment to the fibrous layer of the articular capsule. They possess a sen-

sory nerve supply, and at times they may extend a considerable distance into the joint, in which case their central tips are usually fibrous. Entrapment of these folds within the Z joint has been implicated as a possible cause of back pain. Giles (1992a) also states that traumatic synovitis of these folds may cause the release of pain-mediating agents and subsequent back pain.

Synoviocytes

Transmission electron microscopy studies reveal that the free surface of the synovial membrane (synovium) is lined by a discontinuous layer of cells, known as synoviocytes. Although synoviocytes resemble other connective tissue cells, they differ from ordinary fibroblasts (see Table 13-1) in their ultrastructural features and metabolic activities.

Synoviocytes have been classified into two types based on their cellular morphologic structure: fibroblast-like cells, or type A synoviocytes, and type B synoviocytes. Type A synoviocytes are somewhat numerous and are characterized by the presence of abundant cytoplasmic organelles such as endoplasmic reticulum. These cells are involved in secretion and are believed to synthesize hyaluronic acid and glycoproteins (see following discussion). Type B synoviocytes are similar to macrophages and are involved in phagocytosis. Types A and B synoviocytes are not connected by junctional complexes and do not rest on a basement membrane, and therefore they do not constitute an epithelial lining of the joint cavity. However, they do create a smooth secreting surface for the synovium. Small folds of synovium, or synovial villi, can be found periodically along the surface of the synovial membrane.

The synovial fluid produced by the type A synoviocytes is rich in hyaluronic acid and also contains protein, although its protein content is less than that of blood plasma (Triano, 1992; Williams et al., 1989). The hyaluronic acid imparts synovial fluid with great viscosity. Coiling of the hyaluronic acid molecules and interlocking between different molecules allow the synovial fluid to act as a shock absorber during compressive loads. During shear forces, however, the coiled hyaluronic acid molecules straighten and the interlocking between molecules decreases, resulting in very smooth, low-friction movement between the adjacent Z joint surfaces.

Supporting Cells and Extracellular Matrix of Connective Tissue: Functional Components

Since the Z joints are composed of connective tissue, a brief discussion of the normal characteristics of this type of tissue is essential for a complete understanding of the structure and function of the Z joints. Therefore, this section discusses the cellular and extracellular components of connective tissue.

Early Connective Tissue (Mesenchyme). The connective tissue appearing in embryonic and early fetal development is called mesenchyme. When examined under the light microscope, this type of tissue is seen to be composed of large stellate or spindle-shaped cells that are separated by an abundant amount of intercellular substance. Early embryonic mesenchymal tissue does not contain fiber bundles. Instead, it is composed of fine reticular fibrils (type III collagen) embedded in a gelatinous, amorphous ground substance that is rich in glycosaminoglycans. Embryonic mesenchymal tissue is described as a multipotent and pluripotent tissue. This suggests that mesenchymal cells undergo extensive mitosis and develop into many different types of connective tissue and related cells during fetal and adult life.

Mature Connective Tissue. Connective tissue is responsible for maintaining structural interrelationships between tissues and cells, including the tissues and cells

of the spine. All connective tissue is composed of cells, extracellular fibers, an amorphous ground substance, and tissue fluid. The extracellular fibers and ground substance form the extracellular matrix. In contrast to other body tissues (e.g., epithelium, muscle), connective tissue contains fewer cells in proportion to the amount of extracellular matrix. Based on the composition of the extracellular matrix, adult connective tissue is classified into three main types: connective tissue proper, cartilage, and bone. The composition of the extracellular matrix varies among these three types. In connective tissue proper the extracellular matrix is soft; in cartilage it is much firmer, is partially calcified, but is flexible in nature; and in bone the matrix is rigid because of the presence of calcium salts, which are in the form of hydroxyapatite crystals.

Cartilage and bone are specialized types of connective tissue. Based on characteristics of the ground substance matrix, three histologic types of cartilage are encountered:

- ◆ Hyaline cartilage
- ◆ Elastic cartilage
- ◆ Fibrocartilage

Hyaline cartilage is discussed in the previous section along with the Z joints, and fibrocartilage is discussed with the IVD. Elastic cartilage is not related to the spine and therefore is not discussed in this chapter.

Cells of connective tissue. As mentioned previously, connective tissue consists of cells, fibers, and ground substance. The type of supportive resident cells found in connective tissue varies considerably and may include fibroblasts, chondroblasts and chondrocytes, and osteoblasts and osteocytes. These cells are important when considering the connective tissue of spinal structures. Adipocytes, mast cells, macrophages, and myofibroblasts are also found in connective tissue in various parts of the body. The functions and primary characteristics of these cells are listed in Table 13-1.

In addition to the resident cells of connective tissue described in Table 13-1, connective tissue also contains immigrant cells. These include all the formed cellular elements found in blood with the exception of erythrocytes. The immigrant cells include the neutrophils, eosinophils, basophils, monocytes, and plasma cells. When inflammation occurs, these immigrant cells leave the circulation and join fibroblasts and other connective tissue resident cells, such as macrophages. Once in the connective tissue, they fight microorganisms that cause inflammation and clean up (phagocytize) the debris that results from this process.

Fibers of connective tissue. Another of the three elements of connective tissue is the fiber component. The types of fibers found in connective tissue are collagen, fibrillin, elastin, reticulum, and fibronectin. The functions of each of these are listed in Table 13-2.

Collagen Synthesis. The most important fiber type of connective tissue is collagen. Collagen is a major component of connective tissue proper, cartilage, and bone. Collagen fibers are found in abundance throughout the articular capsule and hyaline cartilage of the Z joints and also throughout the IVDs. Collagen fibers are composed of collagen macromolecules, which are the most abundant protein in the human body. Collagen fibers are flexible and strong, and they are made up of a bundle of fine, threadlike subunits called collagen fibrils. Collagen is a stable protein under the physiologic conditions that exist in connective tissue; however, collagen is constantly being degraded and replenished by collagen-secreting cells.

For many years, it was believed that collagen synthesis occurred primarily in fibroblasts, chondroblasts, osteoblasts, and odontoblasts, but recent investigations in collagen biology indicate that many other cell types produce this unique protein. Collagen synthesis has been studied quite extensively in fibroblasts (Williams et al., 1989). Fibroblasts have the extensive endoplasmic reticulum and well-developed Golgi apparatus required of cells actively involved in protein synthesis. Labeled amino acids endocytosed by fibroblasts can be followed autoradiographically to the rough endoplasmic reticulum (rER), later to the Golgi complex, then to the outside of the fibroblast, and eventually to the newly formed collagen fibers. This evidence indicates that the collagen synthesis pathway is similar to that of other proteins. Fibroblasts synthesize collagen de novo and secrete it into the extracellular matrix. Fibroblasts also have the ability to break down collagen with specific degradative enzymes called collagenases.

Collagen is a ubiquitous substance that is extremely important in the integrity of both the Z joints and the IVDs. Current research, and possibly future treatments (nutritional and pharmacologic) related to these two regions of the spine, may involve the individual steps of collagen synthesis. Because of the clinical importance of collagen synthesis, this pathway is briefly discussed here.

Collagen synthesis begins inside cells. However, the final processing and assembly into fibers takes place after collagen building blocks have been secreted outside the manufacturing cells. The intracellular events include synthesis of proalpha chains in the rER, hydroxylation and glycosylation of proalpha chains into triple helices in the Golgi apparatus, and formation of secretory granules (vesicles). The extracellular events include cleavage of extension peptides, fibrillogenesis and cross-linking, and assembly of fibrils into mature fibers (Fig. 13-8). The box to the right shows the events (steps) involved in colla-

gen synthesis within the fibroblast (steps 1 through 9) and outside the fibroblast in the extracellular matrix (steps 10 through 12).

COLLAGEN SYNTHESIS

1. Uptake of amino acids via endocytosis
   ↓
2. Formation of messenger ribonucleic acid (mRNA)
   ↓
3. Synthesis, by ribosome, of alpha chains with peptides
   ↓
4. Hydroxylation of amino acids
   ↓
5. Glycosylation of specific hydroxyl-1 residues in rough endoplasmic reticulum (rER)
   ↓
6. Formation of procollagen in rER and movement into transfer vesicles
   ↓
7. Packaging of the procollagen by the Golgi complex into secretory vesicles
   ↓
8. Movement of vesicles to plasma membrane assisted by microfilaments and microtubules
   ↓
9. Exocytosis of procollagen
   ↓
10. Cleavage of procollagen to form tropocollagen
    ↓
11. Polymerization of tropocollagen into collagen microfibril
    ↓
12. Polymerization of collagen microfibrils into a complex, 1 to 12 μm collagen fiber

---

The amino acid composition of collagen is one of the features that makes collagen such a unique protein. Four amino acids compose most of the polypeptides in the collagen macromolecules. The principal amino acids that make up collagen are glycine (35%), proline (12%), hydroxyproline (10%), and alanine (11%). In the cytoplasm of the fibroblast, approximately 250 to 300 amino acids are combined by polyribosomes associated with rER to form a polypeptide with a molecular weight of 30,000 daltons. This step of "translation" is performed under the control of messenger ribosomal ribonucleic acid (mRNA). Three polypeptide chains are combined

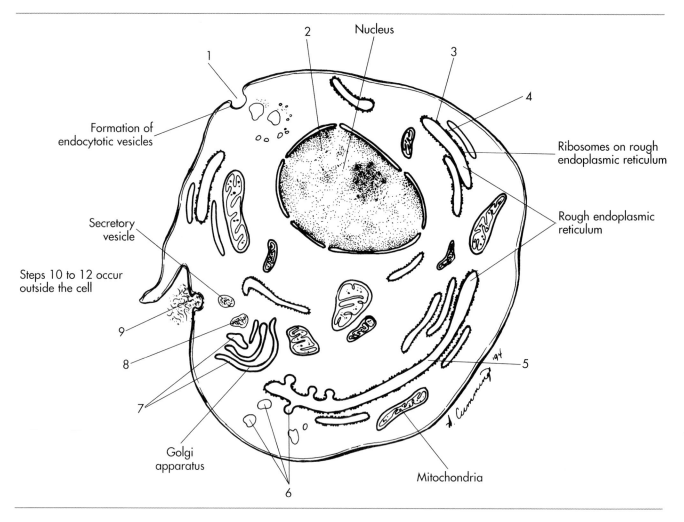

FIG. 13-8 Intracellular steps involved in collagen synthesis. The numbers refer to the box on p. 403.

into polypeptide alpha triple helices with a molecular weight of approximately 100,000 daltons. These triple helices are released into the cisternae of rER (see the box on p. 403, steps 1 through 3). The third amino acid in each alpha chain of the newly formed triple helix is glycine. The amino acid following glycine is frequently proline, and the amino acid preceding the glycine is frequently hydroxyproline. Differences in the chemical structure of the alpha chains are responsible for at least 11 different types of collagen that have been identified to date (Table 13-3).

Several modifications of the polypeptide chains occur within the cisternae of rER and the Golgi apparatus (see the box, steps 4 to 6 and Fig. 13-8). Disulfide bonds are formed within each polypeptide chain and between adjacent chains. Vitamin C is required for the formation of the disulfide bonds, and its absence results in certain collagen-related diseases such as scurvy. This bonding gives shape and stability to the triple-helix collagen mac-

romolecule. The structure formed now constitutes a procollagen molecule. The procollagen molecule moves to the exterior of the cell via secretory granules (see the box, steps 7 to 9 and Fig. 13-8). Further modifications are made outside the cell. For example, enzymes cleave most of the uncoiled amino acids, thereby converting procollagen to tropocollagen molecules. These eventually aggregate to produce collagen fibrils (see the box, steps 10 to 12). Cross-links between lysine and hydroxylysine are then formed, giving the molecule its tensile strength.

The tropocollagen molecules are 300 nm long and 1.5 nm in diameter. They consist of three polypeptide chains that are twisted around one another to form a right-handed superhelix with a head and a tail end. Numerous tropocollagen molecules lie end to end and also in parallel chains or rows. All the molecules face the same direction, and between the parallel rows, approximately one quarter of the length of the tropocollagen

Table 13-3   Characteristics of Collagen Types I to XI

Collagen type	Distribution	Light microscopy	Ultrastructure	Produced by	Function
I	Outer anulus fibrosus, loose fibrous tissue, skin dermis, tendons, bones, ligaments, fascia, sclera, dentin, organ capsules, fibrocartilage	Large-banded collagen fiber, closely packed, thick, nonargyrophilic	Densely packed, thick fibrils with marked variation in diameter	Fibroblast, chondroblast, osteoblast, odontoblast	Resistance to tension
II	Z joint articular cartilage, intervertebral disc (anulus fibrosus, nucleus pulposus), cartilage end plate, hyaline and elastic cartilage, vitreous of eye	Loose collagenous network visible only with picro-Sirius stain and polarized microscope	Very thin fibrils, embedded in abundant ground substance	Chondroblast	Resistant to intermittent pressure
III	Blood vessels, smooth muscle, endoneurium, bone marrow, uterus, lymphoid tissue, kidney, lung	Small-banded collagen fiber, forms reticular networks, weakly birefringent greenish fibers	Loosely packed, thin fibrils with more uniform diameter	Smooth muscle cells, fibroblast, reticulocyte, hepatocyte	Structural maintenance
IV	Epithelial and endothelial basement membranes, lens capsule	Sheetlike layers	Neither fibers nor fibrils	Endothelial and epithelial cells, muscle cells	Support and filtration
V	Basement membranes of placenta, smooth and skeletal muscle	Thin fibrils	*	Fibroblast	*
VI	Fine filaments of elastic tissue	Thin fibrils	*	Endothelial cells	*
VII	Anchoring fibrils in basement membrane of skin and amnion	Short, striated fibrils	*	Endothelial cells	*
VIII	Placental membranes, endothelium	*	*	Endothelial cells	*
IX	Cartilage	*	*	Chondrocytes	*
X	Mineralized cartilage	*	*	Hypertrophic chondrocytes	*
XI	Cartilage	*	*	Chondrocytes	*

*Insufficient data.

molecule overlaps. Therefore a tropocollagen molecule of one row ends approximately one quarter of the distance along the length of another tropocollagen molecule of an adjacent row. This configuration results in a regular 64 to 67 nm periodicity that is clearly visible on an electron micrograph. Fig. 13-10 shows collagen fibers within the IVD.

The finest strand of collagen that can possibly be seen with the light microscope is the fibril, which is about 0.2 to 0.3 μm in diameter. A fibril is made up of still smaller units that have a diameter of 45 to 100 nm. These are referred to as microfibrils. Newly formed microfibrils are only about 20 nm in diameter, and evidence shows that they increase in size with age. Most microfibrils are visible only with the electron microscope and demonstrate

the characteristic cross-banding with a periodicity of 64 to 67 nm. The parallel assembly of microfibrils forms fibrils. The fibrils, in turn, aggregate in bundles to form the thicker collagen fibers. These fibers have a diameter ranging from 1 to 12 μm or more.

Types of Collagen. At present, 11 different types of collagen have been positively identified. They are designated as types I through XI (Table 13-3). Types I to V are the most abundant types of collagen. Types VI to XI are considered to be less important because they occur in small quantities.

Types I, II, and III are arranged as ropelike fibrils and are the main forms of fibrillar collagen. Type I collagen consists of two alpha-1 chains and one alpha-2 chain and represents 90% of all collagen fibers distributed in connective tissue. Because type I fibers resist tensile stresses, their orientation and cross-linking vary according to the local environment. Type I collagen is found in bone, tendon, and the anulus fibrosus of the IVD. It is also found in the skin and cornea (Table 13-3).

Type II collagen fibers are small, banded fibrils averaging 20 nm in diameter. They help to form the extracellular matrix of hyaline cartilage, including that of the Z joints and end plates of the IVDs. Type II collagen is found in the nucleus pulposus of the IVD. It is also found in elastic cartilage and the cornea and vitreous body of the eye. These fibers demonstrate a high electrostatic attraction for the chondroitin sulfate glycosaminoglycans. Type II collagen contains a higher degree of lysine hydroxylation than type I collagen.

Type III and type IV collagen are well distributed throughout the body but are not found to any great extent in Z joints, the IVDs, or other spinal structures. The key features of these fibers and collagen types V through XI are listed in Table 13-3.

Ground Substance. The cells and fibers of connective tissue are surrounded by a translucent, fluidic, homogeneous, gel-like matrix called amorphous ground substance (Bloom & Fawcett, 1986). The ground substance exhibits no structural organization that is visible with light microscopy. Extracellular amorphous ground substance plays a vital role in the regulation of tissue nutrition, support, and maintenance of proper water content. Based on chemical analysis, the extracellular ground substance of connective tissue has the physical properties of a viscous solution or thin gel and consists of proteoglycans and glycosaminoglycans of various types. Proteoglycans and glycosaminoglycans are an important part of the hyaline cartilage of the Z joints and the vertebral end plates of the IVDs. They are also being studied with regard to the anulus fibrosus and nucleus pulposus of the IVD. Therefore, glycosaminoglycans and proteoglycans are discussed in further detail with the articular cartilage of the Z joint (see previous discussion) and with the IVD (see following discussion).

MICROSCOPIC AND MOLECULAR STRUCTURE OF THE INTERVERTEBRAL DISCS

The vertebral bodies are united by symphyseal joints, and these joints are made up of the IVDs. The IVDs permit a limited amount of movement between the vertebral bodies while maintaining a union of great strength. The intrinsic stability of the motion segment (two adjacent vertebrae and the ligaments, including the disc, between them), and therefore of the whole spine, results mainly from the IVDs and the ligaments associated with them (Bogduk & Twomey, 1991). The spine's extrinsic stability is provided by the paraspinal and trunk muscles.

IVDs (Fig. 13-9) are important parts of the spinal column and play an active and important role in the spine's physiologic function. The physical properties, elasticity, and resiliency of the IVDs allow them to give support to the spine and act as soft cushions and shock absorbers. The IVDs also allow the spine to return back to its original shape after being compressed or stretched (Chai Ben-Fu & Tang Xue-Ming, 1987).

The IVD consists of three main parts: the outer anulus fibrosus, which consists of a series of fibrocartilaginous rings; the inner gelatinous nucleus pulposus; and the cartilaginous end plates of hyaline-like cartilage. The end plates are located between the bony vertebrae and the other parts of the IVD (Ghosh, 1990).

Each IVD is reinforced peripherally by circumferential ligaments (Fig. 13-9, *A*). A thick anterior longitudinal ligament extends down the anterior aspect of the spinal column and is attached to the vertebral end plates. It provides additional anterior support to the anulus fibrosus. A thinner posterior longitudinal ligament spans across the posterior aspect of each disc and is firmly attached to the IVD's posterior aspect.

The IVD is specialized connective tissue designed to provide strength, mobility, and resistance to strain. All three parts of the IVD listed previously (Figs. 13-9, *B*, and 13-10). consist of water, cells, proteoglycans (PGs), and collagen. These components are found in varied concentrations in the different regions of the disc. In fact, the varied concentrations of these basic components within the IVD make it a specialized type of connective tissue.

Collagen fibers within the IVD become taut during movements of the spine and tend to restrain the PGs. The PGs, in turn, allow the IVD to deform. Because of its ability to absorb fluid (swell) and then to maintain its hydration, the PG gel of the nucleus pulposus is able to resist compression under large external loads (Weiss, 1988). Therefore the IVD is able to act as a lubricating cushion that prevents adjacent vertebrae from being eroded by abrasive forces during movement of the spinal column. The hydrated gelatinous nucleus pulposus serves as a shock absorber to reduce the impact between adjoining vertebrae (Junquera et al., 1992).

The histologic changes that take place in the IVD with advancing age have been described in postmortem studies by several investigators (Brown, 1971; Pritzker, 1977; Roberts et al., 1989). These changes include loss of distinction between the nucleus pulposus and the anulus fibrosus, desiccation and fibrosis of the nucleus pulposus with fibrillation of the matrix, brown discoloration of the nucleus, fissuring of the nucleus and anulus fibrosus, fractures of the vertebral end plate, and osteophyte formation. Fig. 13-11 demonstrates a series of events asso-

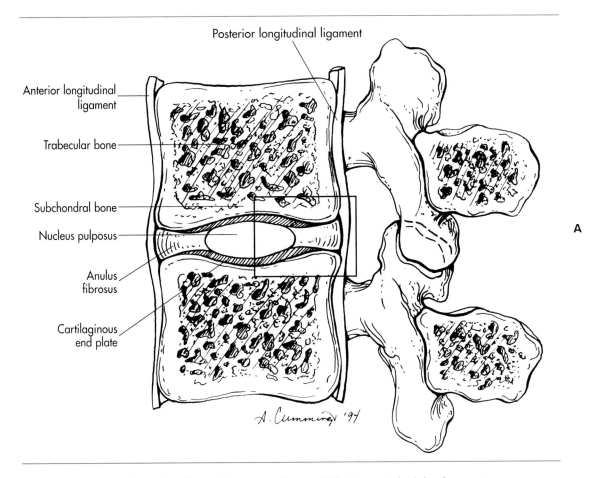

Posterior longitudinal ligament

Anterior longitudinal ligament

Trabecular bone

Subchondral bone

Nucleus pulposus

Anulus fibrosus

Cartilaginous end plate

A

FIG. 13-9   A, Sagittal section of two adjacent vertebrae and the intervertebral disc between them.   *Continued.*

ciated with degeneration of the IVD. Based on plain x-ray films, the fundamental features of disc degeneration are reported to be disc space narrowing and osteophytosis. Chapter 7 describes the consequences of these changes and the development of internal disc disruption. Chapter 2 describes the gross anatomic features of the IVD and the clinical relevance of these features.

The remainder of this chapter focuses on the typical microscopic anatomy and the composition of the anulus fibrosus, the nucleus pulposus, and the cartilaginous vertebral end plate. The chapter concludes with sections covering PGs and fibrocartilage. These last two sections have been included for readers interested in acquiring a deeper understanding of the biology of the IVD.

Anulus Fibrosus

The anulus fibrosus (AF) is the rigid, outer series of rings (lamellae) that forms the peripheral portion of the IVD (Figs. 13-12 and 13-13). It functions to absorb pressure from the central jellylike shock absorber, the nucleus

pulposus. The tightly packed collagen fibers of the AF normally do not allow the large PG molecules of the nucleus pulposus to pass between them, even when the IVD is subjected to large compressive forces. The adult AF is not distinctly separated from the nucleus pulposus or from the cartilage of the vertebral end plates (Inerot & Axelsson, 1991).

The histologic features of the AF do not change much from childhood to maturity. The outer ring of the AF consists of an external tough layer of dense collagenous connective tissue, while the remainder of the AF is primarily composed of overlapping concentric layers of fibrocartilage. The outer part of the AF attaches to the margins of adjacent cartilage end plates in infancy and childhood and to the outer rims of adjacent vertebral bodies in adolescence.

Light and electron microscopy indicate that the AF is composed of fibrocartilage and has a lamellar structure. Anteriorly, the AF consists of more than 20 moderately thick lamellae. The outer lamellae are entirely fibrous and contain thick, tightly packed bundles of type

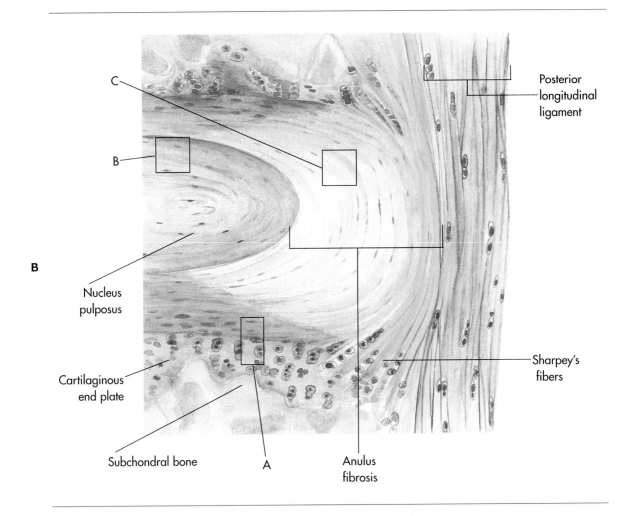

B

Posterior longitudinal ligament

C

B

Nucleus pulposus

Cartilaginous end plate

Subchondral bone

A

Anulus fibrosis

Sharpey's fibers

FIG. 13-9, cont'd.   B, Shows the boxed region in **A** at higher magnification (approximately 15×). In addition to showing the anulus fibrosus, nucleus pulposus, and cartilaginous end plate, the vertebral body and posterior longitudinal ligament are shown. Notice that the outer fibers of the anulus fibrosus attach to the cortical and subchondral bone of the vertebral body. These attachment sites are known as Sharpey's fibers. The collagen fibers of the inner layers of the anulus fibrosus enter the end plate and curve to run parallel to the discal surface of the vertebral body. (The boxes labeled *A, B,* and *C* refer to the regions shown in Fig. 13-10.)

I collagen fibers (Ghosh, 1990). Although the outer AF is composed of type I collagen (Table 13-3), the fibers of the inner AF are composed of type II collagen (Bishop, 1992). The lamellae of the inner part of the AF also have a richer PG ground substance associated with them, which increases the capacity to resist compression (McDevitt, 1988). The collagen fibers in each lamella are orientated parallel to one another and form an angle of inclination (of approximately 25° to 30°) with the horizontal axis of the bony vertebral rims. The fibers of each consecutive layer form approximately a 120° to 130° angle with the fibers of adjacent lamellae. The lamellar

structure and the angle of inclination of the collagen fibers enable the AF to sustain the normal forces of compression, torsion, and flexion that occur during movements of the IVD (Chai Ben-Fu & Tang Xue-Ming, 1987).

As mentioned previously, the anterior and lateral parts of the AF are composed of more than 20 moderately thick lamellae. The outer lamellae are loosely attached to the strong anterior longitudinal ligament (Ghosh, 1990). The posterior and posterolateral parts of the AF are much thinner. They consist of 12 to 15 more closely arranged, thinner lamellae that follow the contour of the

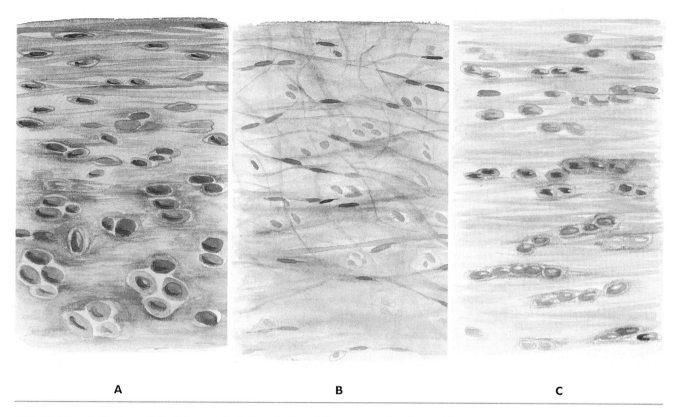

FIG. 13-10 **A,** Regions of the intervertebral disc. **A, B,** and **C** correspond to lettered boxes of Fig. 13-9, *B*. **A,** Cartilaginous end plate. **B,** Nucleus pulposus. **C,** Anulus fibrosus. **A, B,** and **C** represent a magnification of approximately 100 times actual size.

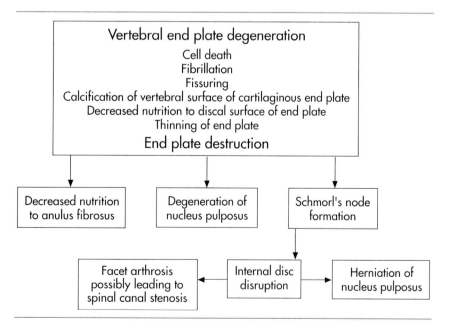

FIG. 13-11 Flowchart demonstrating a series of events leading to degeneration of the intervertebral disc.

A

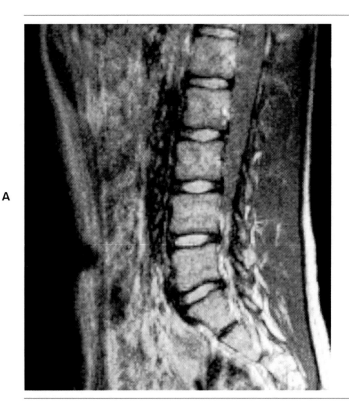

B

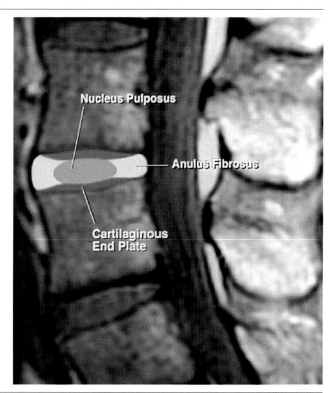

FIG. 13-12 **A,** Midsagittal magnetic resonance imaging scan of the lumbar region showing the intervertebral disc with adjacent vertebral bodies. **B,** Similar view with the parts of the intervertebral disc labeled. (Photograph courtesy Ron Mensching and illustration courtesy Dino Juarez, The National College of Chiropractic.)

posterior parts of the adjacent vertebral bodies. The outer collagen fibers of the AF are fused with the thin posterior longitudinal ligament (Ghosh, 1990) and also attach to the posterior vertebral rims. The inner fibers of the AF are continuous with the cartilaginous end plates (see following discussion) (Fig. 13-9, *B*).

PG extraction from ground human lumbar AFs suggests that the PGs contain three regions: a chondroitin sulfate–rich region, a keratan sulfate–rich region, and a region that binds to hyaluronic acid (Table 13-4 and Fig. 13-6). By binding to hyaluronic acid, the PGs are permitted to aggregate into PG macromolecules. Because of the immense clinical importance of PGs as they relate to the IVDs, a section devoted to this topic is found later in this chapter. However, characteristics of PG content specific to the AF are covered here.

Previous investigations of glycosaminoglycans and PGs of the IVDs have found that the PG subunits from the AF contain approximately 75% chondroitin sulfate and 25% keratan sulfate and hyaluronic acid (Antonopoulos et al., 1974; Stevens, Dondi, & Muir, 1979). These percentages are determined by analyzing the glucosamine/galactosamine ratios (Table 13-4) (Inerot & Axelsson, 1991). Both the hyaluronic acid and

the keratan sulfate concentrations are higher in the AF than in hyaline cartilage (Antonopoulos, Gardell, & Szirmai, 1964; Hardingham & Adams, 1976). Also, the keratan sulfate region appears to be larger in AF PGs than in hyaline cartilage PGs. Fibrocartilage of human knee joint menisci has been shown to also contain dermatan sulfate. This molecule has not been detected in the human AF. Biochemically, the absence of dermatan sulfate and the presence of type I and type II collagen fibers suggest that the AF may be classified as an intermediate between hyaline cartilage and fibrocartilage (Inerot & Axelsson, 1991).

A study of the aging of IVD PG composition of canines and humans has shown that the keratan sulfate–rich region of the PG core protein is more resistant to proteolysis than the chondroitin sulfate–rich region. In addition, the number of keratan sulfate–rich fragments in human disc tissue increases with aging (Cole, Ghosh, & Taylor, 1986).

CLINICAL CONSIDERATIONS

During the day, fluid moves in and out of the nucleus pulposus, providing nutrients to the disc. During sleep-

Table 13-4 Glycosaminoglycans*

Name	Molecular weight (daltons)	Sulfation	Protein linked	Disaccharide composition	Distribution
Hyaluronic acid	10^6	No	No	D-Glucuronic acid + N-acetylglucosamine	Intervertebral disc, cartilage (including Z joint articular cartilage), synovial fluid, skin, vitreous body of eye, loose connective tissue, umbilical cord support fluid (Wharton's jelly)
Chondroitin sulfate	20,000	Yes	Yes	D-Glucuronic acid + N-acetylgalactosamine	Intervertebral disc, cartilage (including Z joint articular cartilage), bone, skin, cornea, aorta, notochord
Dermatan sulfate	55,000	Yes	Yes	L-Iduronic acid or D-glucouronic acid + D-galactosamine	Skin, tendons, ligaments, fibrocartilage, blood vessels, heart
Heparan sulfate	15,000	Yes	Yes	D-Glucuronic acid or L-iduronic acid + D-galactosamine	Basement membranes, lung, liver, aorta
Keratan sulfate (I)	7000	Yes	Yes	D-Galactose + D-galactosamine	Cornea
Keratan sulfate (II)	7000	Yes	Yes	D-Galactose + D-galactosamine	Intervertebral disc (nucleus pulposus and anulus fibrosus), cartilage (including Z joint articular cartilage)

*Five main groups of glycosaminoglycans with different tissue distributions exist. Chondroitin sulfate exists as chondroitin sulfate-4 and chondroitin sulfate-6; both possess high levels of interaction with collagen type II. Dermatan sulfate demonstrates low levels of interaction, mainly with collagen type I. Heparan sulfate demonstrates intermediate levels of interaction with collagen types III and IV. **Sulfation causes the molecules to be highly ($-$) charged and contributes to their ability to attract and bind Na^+ and water.**

ing hours, the nucleus pulposus fills with fluid and presses against the AF. Therefore, when an individual arises in the morning, the AF is tense and less flexible. This increase in AF tension after approximately 5 hours of rest may render it more vulnerable to injury after a period of rest.

Sudden movements of the lumbar spine, especially torsion coupled with flexion, can produce small tears. These tears usually occur in the posterior part of the AF, where the distribution of collagen fibers is less concentrated. Sometimes, tears in the AF may allow some of the soft jellylike nucleus pulposus to squeeze out into the vertebral canal. This latter condition is known as a prolapsed or herniated intervertebral disc. IVD herniation is not as common a cause of back pain as once thought (see Chapter 7). However, the discs can be a source of pain without rupture or herniation (Bogduk, 1990). Contrary to previous reports (Malinsky, 1959; Wyke, 1987) that the IVD could not produce pain because it lacks nerve supply, several investigators (Bogduk et al., 1981; Yoshzawa, O'Brien, & Thomas-Smith, 1980) have confirmed that the lumbar discs do have a nerve supply and that nerve fibers and nerve endings have been demonstrated to exist in at least the outer third and possibly as far as the outer half of the AF. Most of these authors conclude that the lumbar disc is supplied with the necessary apparatus for the transmission of nociception and subsequent perception of pain. Chapters 2 and 7 discuss the gross anatomy, including the innervation, of the IVD in further detail.

Nucleus Pulposus

Both fetal and infant discs have large notochordal nuclei pulposi with abundant fluid mucoid matrices. The nucleus of a young disc is encapsulated along the periphery by the AF and on the superior and inferior surfaces by the cartilaginous end plates (see following discussion). Perinatally, the AF and the cartilaginous end plates are vascular, but their blood supply declines dramatically with childhood growth (Taylor, 1990); by 4 years of age, none of the blood vessels that earlier supplied the IVD can be found. In fact, the adult nucleus pulposus (NP) is the largest avascular structure of the body. It receives nutrition primarily by means of diffusion from blood vessels within the subchondral bone of the adjacent vertebral bodies. This diffusion process by which the IVD receives its nutrients is known as imbibition.

The human NP is a highly hydrated tissue at birth, with a water content of 88% of its dry weight. This falls to 69% at 77 years of age. By comparison, the water content of the AF declines from 78% at birth to approximately 70% at 30 years, and thereafter it stays relatively constant (Gower & Pedrini, 1969). In adults, as the hydration declines with age, the tissues become firmer and lose their translucency, and the boundaries between the NP and the AF become less distinguishable. Table 2-2 shows the relative concentrations of water, collagen, and PG (nonaggregated/aggregated ratio) of the NP and AF.

The higher water content of the NP, compared with that of the AF, is accompanied by a lower concentration of collagen in the NP. In addition, the collagen found in the NP is type II rather than type I, which is found in the AF. The individual fibrils of type II collagen are much smaller than those of type I (see Table 13-3). The fibers are also loosely arranged and are surrounded by a more abundant ground substance. In the NP, this ground substance contains a high percentage (65%) of very hydrophilic, nonaggregated PGs.

Therefore the NP is a thick, jellylike region with a high concentration of fluid. It draws this fluid from the surrounding vertebral bodies. The fluid, a distillate of plasma, passes through the cartilaginous end plates on its way to the NP. The NP also has relatively few cells. The cells are primarily notochordal cells (in the young; see following discussion), fibroblasts, and chondrocytes. The adult NP makes up 35% to 50% of the IVD (Bishop, 1992). It normally lies slightly posterior to the IVD's center. Normal nuclear material moves backward and forward with flexion and extension movements of the spine, respectively.

The region of the adult NP that is adjacent to the vertebral end plates contains a relative abundance of chondrocytes. The matrix surrounding the chondrocytes stain deeply with safranin and alcian blue because of the presence of abundant PG macromolecules. Also in this region, vertically oriented collagen fibers extend from the end plate to the NP (Oda, Tamaka, & Tsukuki, 1988). These collagen fibers seem to be independent of the anchoring fibers of the AF. The attachment of these fibers to the end plate and the NP of the IVD may give stability to the IVD at times when the cartilaginous end plate is calcified or replaced by bone.

Controversial Role of the Notochord in the Formation of the Nucleus Pulposus. As previously mentioned, the NP is located in the center of the AF and occupies 35% to 50% of the IVD volume. In children the NP is large and is derived from the notochord (see Fig. 12-12). Gradually, the transparent embryonic notochordal cells are replaced by a sparse population of chondrocytes and fibroblasts. In time these cells are partially replaced by fibrocartilage, which makes the NP more opaque and no longer transparent (Junqueira et al., 1992).

Several investigators have proposed that embryonic notochordal cells undergo degeneration and disappear soon after birth and that these cells have no further participation in the formation of the NP. Virchow (1857) wrote that the NP was formed from connective tissue. Luschka (1856, 1857) maintained that both the notochordal cells and the liquefaction of the inner layers of the surrounding connective tissue contributed to the formation of the NP. Peacock (1951) concluded that the NP was produced by mucoid degeneration of notochordal cells, which caused the disappearance of these cells and increased the mucoid matrix. However, Woelf and colleagues (1975) studied enzymes present in the NP and described the presence of enzymes that were associated with PG synthesis and oxidative activity. This indication of PG synthesis led them to conclude that human notochordal cells **do** contribute to the matrix of the NP in fetal and postnatal life. Recent investigators have demonstrated that some notochordal cells persist up to the third decade of life and that they play a significant role in producing and maintaining the NP. Trout and colleagues (1982) were successful in identifying notochordal cells in the NPs of individuals from 8 weeks of fetal life to 32 years of age. However, they could not definitely identify notochordal cells in the specimens from individuals older than 32 years.

The notochordal cells found by Trout and colleagues (1982) in individuals up to 32 years of age were large, with a single, generally round to oval nucleus. The Golgi complex was small, two to four cisternae per stack, with many vesicles near the mature face. Centrioles were found near the nucleus in some cells, and autophagic vacuoles and lysosomes were also present. One unusual feature of these cells was the consistent presence of rER. The rER surrounded poorly developed mitochondria that contained tubular cisternae.

Oda and colleagues (1988) found that the NP was composed of tissue derived from the notochord in specimens collected from individuals ranging in age from 1 month to midteens. They also found a fine fibrous tissue derived from the AF. No notochordal cells were demonstrated in the NP in the specimens that came from individuals 16 to 19 years of age. However, in specimens from individuals older than 20 years, notochordal originating cells were found. Also, the NP of the specimens had been replaced by fibrocartilage and dense collagenous fibrous tissue. Pritzker (1977) and Bishop (1992) suggested that the cells of the vertebral cartilaginous end plates may be responsible for synthesizing the gelatinous matrix of the NP in mature IVDs. Therefore, notochordal cells probably contribute to the formation, development, and maintenance of the NP. However, this role declines as individuals reach age 30. After age 30, the vertebral end plate may continue to help the few cells left within the NP maintain the PG and collagen makeup of the NP.

Cartilaginous End Plate

As mentioned previously, the IVD is composed of a tougher, peripheral fibrocartilaginous AF and a central gelatinous NP, both of which are located between the superjacent and subjacent cartilaginous end plates (EPs) (Chai Ben-Fu & Tang Xue-Ming, 1987) (Figs. 13-12 and 13-13). The adult cartilaginous EP is a thin strip (about 3 mm thick) of hyaline-like cartilage that contains many fine collagenous fibrils (similar to fibrocartilage) (Bishop, 1992). The EPs separate the NP and medial aspect of the AF from the subchondral bone of the adjacent vertebral bodies (Figs. 13-9, 13-12, and 13-13).

The subchondral bone of the vertebral bodies consist of a thin peripheral ring of compact bone that surrounds the EP and a large central region that is cribriform in appearance, containing many small holes that pass to the cancellous bone of the vertebral body.

Developmentally, each EP is a part of the cartilage model of the vertebral body. However, the EP does not have a firm attachment to the vertebral body. In fact, no fibrillar connections have been found between the EP and the adjacent vertebral body (Bishop, 1992), but the collagen fibers of the AF and NP enter the EP and become enclosed in the EP's ground substance (Fig. 13-9, B). In addition, the EP plays a vital role in the nutritional support of the IVD and may be the source of PG synthesis for the NP and AF (Bishop, 1992). Because the EP is more closely related to the AF and NP than to the subchondral bone of the adjacent vertebral body, it is usually considered to be an integral part of the IVD.

Each cartilaginous EP is composed of parallel lamellae of cells (primarily chondrocytes) and collagen fibers, arranged horizontally (Ghosh, 1990). As mentioned previously, the collagen fibers from the AF appear to continue into the EP at the IVD-EP junction (Roberts et al., 1989). The EP's ground substance consists of water within an amorphous matrix of PGs.

The EPs have important mechanical functions. They contribute to the resilience of the motion segment. In addition, the EPs participate in the hydrostatic distribution of the pressure absorbed by IVDs during loading (Broberg, 1983).

The cartilaginous EPs are also thought to play an important role in the IVD's nutrition. Nutrients must diffuse from the blood vessels within the vertebral bodies, which contact the periphery of each EP, through the cartilage matrix, eventually to reach the cells deep within the cartilaginous EP. Only 10% of the bony EP of the vertebral body is perforated by small vascular buds that make contact with the cartilaginous end plate (Maroudas, 1975). The vascular contacts are more plentiful in the central part of the EP than in the peripheral regions (Roberts et al., 1989). The cartilaginous EP and the NP have both a close anatomic and a close physiologic relationship with each other. The latter relationship is demonstrated by the fact that degeneration of a cartilaginous EP may initiate the "degeneration" of the NP (see Chapter 7).

The ability to transport nutrients through cartilaginous tissues is known to depend on the makeup of the cartilage matrix, particularly the PG content of the matrix (Nachemson et al., 1970). The PG content (i.e., types of PGs present) and PG concentration control the diffusion and distribution of charged solutes and macromolecules within the cartilage matrix. The EP near the NP has a higher PG and water concentration than does the EP adjacent to the AF. The EP close to the AF also has a higher concentration of PGs, as well as a lower concentration of collagen, than the neighboring AF (Roberts et al., 1989). Therefore, permeability is enhanced close to the NP and probably tapers off near the periphery of the EP.

The permeability of the EP declines with age. If this permeability decreases to the point that the path for nutrients to the IVD and waste products from the IVD is blocked, metabolic waste products increase within the IVD. This may initiate the processes of internal disc disruption and "disc degeneration" (Chai Ben-Fu & Tang Xue-Ming, 1987; Crock, 1986).

Formation of bone inside the cartilaginous EP, which occurs in some EPs of certain individuals, initiates a reduction of the nutritional route to the IVD as a whole. Bone formation may first cause the destruction of the discal surface of the EP, which eventually contributes to the degeneration of the NP. Oda and colleagues (1988) found that when bone formation remained outside the cartilaginous EP, no adverse degenerative changes were observed in the NP. This important finding might indicate the particular significance of the EP in the maintenance of the NP.

Detailed histologic changes of the human cervical IVD from the neonate to the ninth decade, with special emphasis on the age changes of the NP and the cartilaginous EP, were investigated by Oda and colleagues (1988). They found that the cartilaginous EP can be divided into two regions: the growth cartilage layer, which corresponds to the growth plate of a growing long bone, and the articular cartilage layer, which faces the NP (Fig. 13-14). They also noted a fine fibrous tissue between the material derived from the notochordal cells in the NP and the articular cartilage layer of the EP of the cervical discs of 1-month-old infants. The cartilaginous EP of specimens collected from individuals 1 year old to the teenage years also contained the same two layers. The cartilaginous EP of specimens from individuals over 20 years of age had lost the growth layer and were

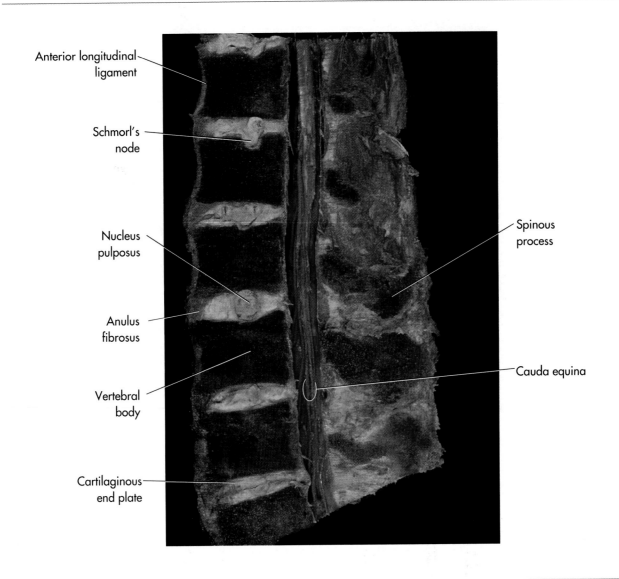

Anterior longitudinal ligament

Schmorl's node

Nucleus pulposus

Anulus fibrosus

Vertebral body

Cartilaginous end plate

Spinous process

Cauda equina

FIG. 13-13 Midsagittal section through a cadaveric lumbar spine. Notice that the cartilaginous end plates, the anuli fibrosi, and nuclei pulposi can be seen at several levels. Also notice the Schmorl's node, which has been labeled (compare with Figs. 13-15 and 13-16).

composed only of the articular layer. In the age group from 20 to 30 years, the cartilaginous EP began to calcify, and the calcified areas were invaded by blood vessels from the adjacent vertebral bodies. Calcification of the vertebral EP has been related to degenerative change within the IVD as a whole (Bishop, 1992) (see Fig. 13-11).

End Plate Fracture (Schmorl's Nodes). Hydrostatic loading of the NP of the IVD causes bulges of the nu-

cleus into the EP. If the compressive force is great enough, fracture of the EP can occur. EP fractures, also known as traumatic Schmorl's nodes, have at times been noted in postmortem studies as features of disc degeneration (Sachs et al., 1987; Vernon-Roberts & Pirie, 1977) (Fig. 13-13).

Schmorl's nodes are defined as herniations of the IVD through the EP (Figs. 13-13, 13-15, and 13-16). They were first described in 1927 by a German pathologist, Christian G. Schmorl. These lesions are believed to be as

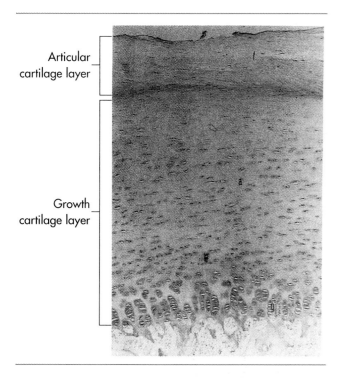

Articular cartilage layer

Growth cartilage layer

FIG. 13-14 Cartilaginous end plate of a newborn. Notice that it can be divided into two regions: the growth cartilage layer, which corresponds to the growth plate of a growing long bone, and the articular cartilage layer, which faces the nucleus pulposus. (From Oda, J., et al. *Spine*, 1988, *13*, 1205-1211.)

sociated with trauma and occur most frequently in the lumbar and thoracic regions. Even though trauma is the most likely cause of Schmorl's node formation, a possible congenital origin of EP defects has also been suggested (Pate, 1991). Such congenital defects could predispose one to a later EP fracture.

Schmorl's nodes probably predispose the IVD to early degenerative change, especially when observed in younger age groups. These nodes are as common in adolescents as in adults. They are found most frequently in the lower thoracic or upper lumbar vertebrae.

A dorsolumbar kyphosis, seen in adolescents, may be associated with Schmorl's nodes. Therefore, EP fractures should be considered a possible etiologic cause of back pain when an active adolescent patient has back pain of the thoracolumbar region.

Compression injury frequently results in an EP fracture. This may completely resolve in some patients, or in others, inflammatory repair processes may extend into the NP and result in disc degradation (see Chapter 7). Such inflammatory disc degradation initiates internal disc disruption, which may become symptomatic. If the AF remains intact, isolated IVD resorption may follow,

but if fissures and tears develop in the AF, the degraded nuclear material may herniate (Bogduk, 1990).

Glycosaminoglycans and Proteoglycans

The topic of glycosaminoglycans (GAGs) and proteoglycans (PGs) was introduced with connective tissue earlier in this chapter. GAGs and PGs are covered in further detail here because of their extreme importance in the IVD's proper functioning. Much of the relevant current research related to the IVD involves GAGs and PGs. In fact, "proteoglycans are now thought to be the chief cellular indicators of disc functional capacity and appear to be the key to understanding the pathogenesis of disc degeneration" (Bishop, 1992).

The main function of GAGs and therefore PGs is structural; they interact with collagen fibers to provide support. In addition to providing support, GAGs, because of their ionic charge, are able to form electrostatic interactions with cationic molecules. This serves to transport electrolytes, water, and metabolites. The gel-like or viscous nature of the GAGs allows them to have a lubricating function in connective tissue and joints and also allows them to act as shock absorbers in the IVD.

Proteoglycan Monomers and Proteoglycan Aggregates. PG monomers are complex macromolecules composed of many GAGs covalently bonded to a core protein of varying length. Three dimensionally, the side chains attached to the core protein form the shape of a "bottle brush" (see Fig. 13-6). The short branches of the bottle brush represent keratan sulfate, and the long ones represent chondroitin sulfate. PG monomers group together to form PG aggregates. The backbone of a PG aggregate is hyaluronic acid. Hyaluronic acid is a long coil-like chain composed of alternating molecules of glucuronic acid and glucosamine. The PG monomers are attached to hyaluronic acid by a link protein.

Glycosaminoglycans. GAGs refer to long-chain, unbranched carbohydrate polymers composed of repeating disaccharide units of glucosamine (or galactosamine) and glucuronic acid attached to a protein core. The hexosamine (glucosamine and galactosamine) is usually sulfated (see Table 13-4). However, an exception among the GAGs to this general pattern is hyaluronic acid, which is the longest GAG and has no sulfated hexosamines. Most of the sugar molecules of GAG chains are negatively charged and repel each other. This negative charge attracts numerous Na^+ ions, which are osmotically active. This causes a large amount of water to rush into the matrix and creates a swelling hydrostatic pressure. This hydrostatic pressure enables the matrix of cartilage and the IVD to withstand compressive forces.

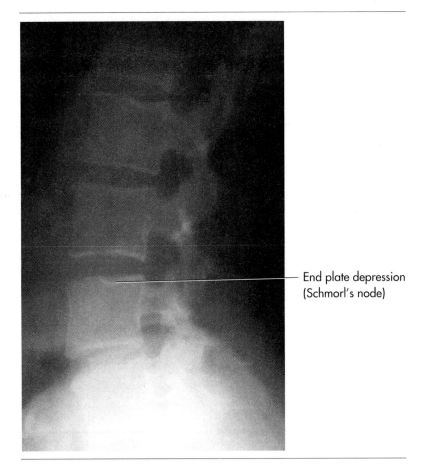

End plate depression
(Schmorl's node)

FIG. 13-15 X-ray film demonstrating a Schmorl's node (compare with Figs. 13-13 and 13-16).

GAGs are synthesized within the cells of the connective tissue in which they are found. For instance, the fibroblast is the primary cell type of connective tissue proper, and it produces and maintains the ground substance (which consists of GAGs) of this tissue. Chondroblasts are cells that produce the ground substance of cartilage, and osteoblasts produce the ground substance of bone. The GAGs for the entire IVD are probably primarily produced by the cells within the cartilaginous EP. The time it takes to replace the PGs in the human IVD is considerable (approximately 3 years) and is longer than the replacement time of other species (Table 13-5). Therefore, much time is needed before complete repair of pathologic conditions or damage to the IVD can take place, and in some cases (especially if the EP is damaged) repair may not be possible.

The principal GAGs of the extracellular matrix include the following:

- Hyaluronic acid
- Chondroitin sulfate
- Dermatan sulfate
- Heparan sulfate
- Keratan sulfate

Table 13-5 Comparison of Turnover Time (Days) for Proteoglycan Molecules from Various Regions of the Intervertebral Discs of Dogs, Pigs, and Humans

Region of disc	Dog (3 years of age)	Pig (3 years of age)	Human* (30 years of age)
Nucleus pulposus	750	900	1350
Outer anulus (anterior)	350	500	900
Inner anulus (anterior)	420	700	1050
Outer anulus (posterior)	510	630	990
Inner anulus (posterior)	630	800	1170

*Note that for a 30-year-old human, it takes more than 3 years to replace proteoglycan molecules.

These five types of GAGs differ in the following important ways: molecular weight, length of the chain, and type of disaccharide units. Table 13-4 summarizes the major characteristics of the principal GAGs. GAGs tend to exist in various configurations, which results in a variety of electrostatic charges among GAGs and allows them to participate in various degrees of interactions

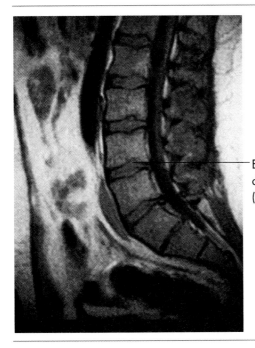

End plate
depression
(Schmorl's
node)

FIG. 13-16 Midsagittal magnetic resonance imaging scan demonstrating a Schmorl's node (compare with Figs. 13-13 and 13-15).

with adjoining chains. This variety of configurations and interactions of GAGs contributes to the formation of additional physical and chemical characteristics of the extracellular matrix.

Hyaluronic acid is by far the largest GAG, consisting of an estimated 2500 disaccharide units. Its molecular weight is approximately 10^6 daltons. Hyaluronic acid is the major GAG of synovial fluid and many other tissues (see Table 13-4). It is partially responsible for swelling within the extracellular matrix and also for attracting cells to the site of an injury. PG monomers also bind to hyaluronic acid to form PG aggregates.

Chondroitin 4-sulfate and chondroitin 6-sulfate consist of glucuronic acid and N-acetylgalactosamine. These two GAGs are similar in structure and function (Table 13-4). Chondroitin 4-sulfate is the most abundant GAG found in the body and is present in immature cartilage.

Chondroitin 6-sulfate is distributed in mature cartilage and other tissues.

Dermatan sulfate is the major GAG of skin, from which it derives its name. It is also distributed in tendons, ligaments, fibrocartilage, and other tissues. However, it is not found in the IVD or Z joints. Dermatan sulfate has a high affinity to associate closely with collagen type I fibers (see Tables 13-3 and 13-4).

Keratan sulfate is the shortest of the GAGs (see Table 13-4). It is found in skeletal tissue, as well as the cornea (type I). Along with hyaluronic acid and chondroitin sulfate, karatan sulfate is a main contributor of cartilage PGs. It is also found in abundance in the NP of the IVD.

Heparan sulfate is associated with collagen type III reticular fibers, which are found in large amounts in basal laminae. Heparan sulfate is also distributed in the lungs, liver, and aorta. However, it is not found to any great extent in the Z joints or IVDs.

Fibrocartilage

Because the AF and NP of the IVDs are considered to be specialized fibrocartilage, a brief discussion of the general characteristics of this type of cartilage is included here.

Light microscopy reveals that fibrocartilage appears similar to dense connective tissue and hyaline cartilage (Fig. 13-17). Its matrix contains obvious thick bundles of type I collagen fibers (Table 13-3). The collagen bundles are distributed in parallel beams among rows of chondrocytes. The chondrocytes are smaller than those of hyaline or elastic cartilage and are easily distinguished from the fibroblasts, also present in fibrocartilage, because chondrocytes lie within round or oval lacunae. Because of the presence of the collagen fibers and a lesser amount of GAGs, the matrix of fibrocartilage stains more eosinophilic than hyaline or elastic cartilage. Also, fibrocartilage, unlike hyaline and elastic cartilage, is not enveloped by a perichondrium. Fibrocartilage is distributed in the IVD (see the previous discussion) and articular cartilages. It is also found in the pubic symphysis, ligamentum teres femoris capitis, glenoid ligament, and the interarticular cartilages of some joints.

Cartilaginous end plate

A

B

Subchondral bone

C

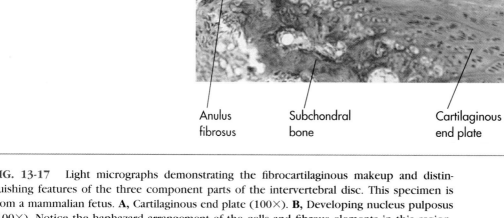

Anulus fibrosus

Subchondral bone

Cartilaginous end plate

FIG. 13-17 Light micrographs demonstrating the fibrocartilaginous makeup and distinguishing features of the three component parts of the intervertebral disc. This specimen is from a mammalian fetus. **A,** Cartilaginous end plate (100×). **B,** Developing nucleus pulposus (100×). Notice the haphazard arrangement of the cells and fibrous elements in this region. **C,** Portion of the anulus fibrosus.

REFERENCES

Antonopoulos, C.A. et al. (1964). Determination of glycosaminoglycans from tissue on the microgram scale. *Biochem Biophys Acta, 83,* 1-19.

Antonopoulos, C.A. et al. (1974). Extraction and purification of proteoglycans from various types of connective tissue. *Biochem Biophys Acta, 338,* 108-119.

Bishop, P. (1992). Pathophysiology of the intervertebral disc. In S. Haldeman (Ed.), *Principles and practice of chiropractic* (2nd ed). East Norwalk, Conn: Appleton & Lange.

Bloom, W. & Fawcett, D. (1986). *Textbook of histology* (3rd ed). Philadelphia: WB Saunders.

Bogduk, N. (1990). Pathology of lumbar disc pain. *Manual Med, 5,* 72-79.

Bogduk, N. & Twomey, L.T. (1991). *Clinical anatomy of the lumbar spine.* London: Churchill Livingstone.

Bogduk, N. et al. (1981). The nerve supply to the human lumbar intervertebral discs. *J Anat, 132,* 39-56.

Broberg, K.B. (1983). On the mechanical behavior of intervertebral disc. *Spine, 8,* 151-161.

Brown, M.D. (1971). The pathophysiology of disc disease. *Orthop Clin North Am, 2,* 359-370.

Buckwalter, J. et al. (1989). Articular cartilage and intervertebral disc proteoglycans differ in structure: An electron microscopic study. *J Orthop Res, 7,* 146-151.

Chai Ben-Fu & Tang Xue-Ming (1987). Electron microscopic observation of normal, protruding and ruptured lumbar intervertebral discs, *Chinese Med J, 100*(9), 723-730.

Cole, T.C., Ghosh, P., & Taylor, T.K. (1986). Variations of the proteoglycans of the canine intervertebral disk with aging. *Biochem Biophys Acta, 19,* 209-219.

Crock, H.V. (1986). Internal disc disruption: A challenge to disc prolapse fifty years on. *Spine, 1,* 650-653.

Ghosh, P. (1990). Basic biochemistry of the intervertebral disc and its variation with ageing and degeneration. *J Man Med, 5,* 48-51.

Giles, L.G. (1992a). The pathophysiology of the zygapophyseal joints. In S. Haldeman (Ed.), *Principles and practice of chiropractic* (2nd ed). East Norwalk, Conn: Appleton & Lange.

Giles, L.G. (1992b). The surface lamina of the articular cartilage of human zygapophyseal joints. *Anat Rec, 233,* 350-356.

Giles, L.G. & Taylor, J.R. (1987). Human zygapophyseal joint capsule and synovial fold innervation. *Br J Rheumatol, 26,* 93-98.

Gower, W.E. & Pedrini, V. (1969). Age related variations in protein-polysaccharides from human nucleus pulposus, anulus fibrosus, and costal cartilage. *A J Bone Joint Surg, 51,* 1154-1162.

Hardingham, T.E. & Adams, P.A. (1976). A method for the determination of hyaluronate in the presence of glycosaminoglycans and its application to human intervertebral disc. *Biochem J, 159,* 143-147.

Inerot, S. & Axelsson, I. (1991). Structure and composition of proteoglycans from human anulus fibrosus. *Connect Tissue Res, 26,* 47-63.

Junqueira, C.L. et al. (1992). *Basic histology* (7th ed). East Norwalk, Conn: Appleton & Lange.

Kirkaldy-Willis, W.H. (1988). The pathology and pathogenesis of low back pain. In W. Kirkaldy-Willis (Ed.), *Managing low back pain* (2nd ed). New York: Churchill Livingstone.

Luschka, H. (1856). Die altersveranderungen der zwischenwirbelnorpel. *Virchows Arch, 11,* 8.

Luschka, H. (1857). Uber gallertartige auswuchse am clivus blumenbachii. *Virchows Arch, 11,* 8.

Malinsky, J. (1959). The ontogenetic development of nerve terminations in the intervertebral discs of man. *Acta Anat, 38,* 96-113.

Maroudas, A. et al. (1975). Factors involved in the nutrition of the human intervertebral disc. *J Anat, 120,* 13-130.

McDevitt, C.A. (1988). Proteoglycans of the intervertebral disc. In P. Ghosh (Ed.), *Biology of the intervertebral disc.* Boca Raton, Fla: CRC Press.

Mooney, V. & Robertson, J. (1976). The facet syndrome. *Clin Orthop Res, 115,* 149-156.

Nachemson, A. et al. (1971). In vitro diffusion of dye through the end plates and the annulus fibrosus of human lumbar intervertebral disks. *Acta Orthop Scand, 41,* 589-607.

Oda, J., Tamaka, H., & Tsukuki, N. (1988). Intervertebral disk changes with aging of human cervical vertebra: From the neonate to the eighties. *Spine, 13,* 1205-1211.

Pate, D. (1991). Roentgen report: Schmorl's nodes, *MPI's Dynam Chiro, Sept. 13.*

Peacock, A. (1951). Observation on the prenatal development of the intervertebral disc in man. *J Anat, 185,* 260-274.

Pritzker, P.H. (1977). Aging and degeneration in the lumbar intervertebral disc. *Orthop Clin, 8,* 65-77.

Roberts, S. et al. (1989). Biochemical and structural properties of the vertebral end plate and its relation to the intervertebral disc. *Spine, 14,* 166-174.

Sachs, B.L. et al. (1987). Dallas discogram description: A new classification of CT/discography in low-back disorders. *Spine, 12,* 287-294.

Stevens, R.L., Dondi, P.G., & Muir, H. (1979). Proteoglycans of the intervertebral disk: Absence of degradation during the isolation of proteoglycans from the intervertebral disk. *Biochem J, 179,* 573-578.

Swann, D.A. et al. (1974) Role of hyaluronic acid in joint lubrication. *Annu Rev Dis, 33,* 318-326.

Taylor, J.R. (1990). The development and adult structure of lumbar intervertebral discs. *J Man Med, 5,* 43-47.

Taylor, J.R. & Twomey, L.T. (1986). Age changes in lumbar zygapophyseal joints: Observations on structure and function. *Spine, 11,* 739-745.

Triano, J. (1992). Interaction of spinal biomechanics and physiology. In S. Haldeman (Ed.), *Principles and practice of chiropractic* (2nd ed). East Norwalk, Conn: Appleton & Lange.

Trout, J.J. et al. (1982). Ultrastructure of the human intervertebral disc. I. Changes in notochordal cells with age. *Tissue Cell, 14*(2), 359-369.

Vernon-Roberts, B. & Pirie, C.J. (1977). Degenerative changes in the intervertebral disks of the lumbar spine and their sequelae. *Rheumatol Rehabil, 16,* 13-21.

Virchow, R.L. (1857). *Untersuchung uber die entwickelung des schadel grindes in gesunden und krankhaften zustande und uber den eintfuss derselben auf schadelform, gesichsbildun und gehirnbau.* Berlin: G. Reimer.

Weiss, L. (1988). *Histology* (6th ed). New York: McGraw-Hill.

Williams, P.L. et al. (Eds.) (1989). *Gray's anatomy* (37th ed). Edinburgh: Churchill Livingstone.

Woelf, H.J. et al. (1975). Role of the notochord in human intervertebral disc. I. Fetus and infant. *Clin Orthop Rel Res, 39,* 205-212.

Wyke, B. (1987). The neurology of back pain. In M.I.V. Jayson (Ed.), *The lumbar spine and back pain* (3rd ed). New York: Churchill Livingstone.

Xu, G.L. et al. (1991). Normal variations of the lumbar facet joint capsules. *Clin Anat, 4,* 117-122.

Yoshizawa, H., O'Brien, J., & Thomas-Smith, W. (1980). The neuropathology of the intervertebral discs removed for low back pain. *J Pathol, 132,* 95-104.

Index

---

t indicates table; *f* indicates footnote; *(box)* indicates box.